AF703522

20
IDEOS

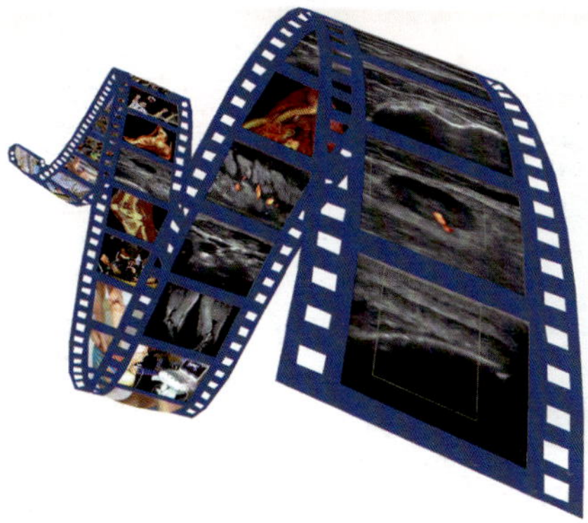

SONOGRAPHIC ATLAS
for Common Musculoskeletal Pathologies

FOUR STEPS TO ACCESS DIGITAL CONTENT

1	**CONNECT**	Go to the website indicated on the label that includes the access code
2	**REGISTER**	Register at the Publisher Portal (first time only) for a username and password
3	**ACCESS**	Enter your username and password to access the restricted contents
4	**TYPE THE CODE**	In the web page dedicated to the work or on the homepage of the publishing house, type the personal access code placed under the protection of the label applied to this page

The **online access** provides for the acceptance of the **personal license** limited to a **single user** for each code. The **access is allowed to the individual user** and does not allow library or institutional access licenses.

The **sharing of passwords and/or code is not allowed** and any attempt to misuse the personal code will invalidate and lock it. The access cannot be shared and will expire according to the time frames set out in the license agreement that you subscribe to at first access. Further details may be provided upon acceptance of the license agreement. The use of the codes is subject to acceptance of the conditions. Any violation or attempted violation of code protection will not be accepted.

The protection can be removed by scraping with slight pressure from a coin

EE5763001425
www.learningoncloud.eu/en

LEARNING ON CLOUD
LOC
www.learningoncloud.eu

Hardware and software requirements:
PC with Windows, Macintosh or Linux,
latest generation of internet browser such as Internet Explorer (version 8.0 onwards, 9 is recommended), Firefox, Chrome etc., with Adobe Flash Player plug-ins installed; Internet connection.

Technical Help Desk: Available by email at support@ediermes.com

LEVENT ÖZÇAKAR
Editor

SONOGRAPHIC ATLAS

for Common Musculoskeletal Pathologies

MURAT KARA EDA GÜRÇAY
ŞULE ŞAHİN ONAT MARTINE DE MUYNCK
Associate Editors

FRANCO FRANCHIGNONI
Project Manager

Under the auspices of

edi·ermes

SONOGRAPHIC ATLAS
for Common Musculoskeletal Pathologies
by Levent Özçakar (Editor)
Murat Kara, Eda Gürçay, Şule Şahin Onat, Martine De Muynck (Associate Editors)
Franco Franchignoni (Project Manager)

ISBN 978-88-7051-576-3 - Paper edition

ISBN 978-88-7051-577-0 - Digital edition

Notices

Knowledge and best practice in this field are constantly changing. As new research and experience broaden our understanding, changes in research methods, professional practices, or medical treatment may become necessary.

Practitioners and researchers must always rely on their own experience and knowledge in evaluating and using any information, methods, compounds, or experiments described herein. In using such information or methods they should be mindful of their own safety and the safety of others, including parties for whom they have a professional responsibility.

With respect to any drug or pharmaceutical products identified, readers are advised to check the most current information provided (i) on procedures featured or (ii) by the manufacturer of each product to be administered, to verify the recommended dose or formula, the method and duration of administration, and contraindications.

It lies within the responsibility of practitioners, relying on their own experience and knowledge of their patients, to make diagnoses, to determine dosages and the best treatment for each individual patient and to take all appropriate safety precautions. To the fullest extent of the law, neither the Publisher nor the authors, contributors, or editors, assume any liability for any injury and/or damage to persons or property as a matter of products liability, or arising from negligence or otherwise, or from any use or operation of any methods, products, instructions, or ideas contained in the material herein.

A book is the final product of a very complex series of operations that requires numerous tests on texts and images. It is almost impossible to publish a book with no errors. We will be grateful to those who find them and notify us. For enquiries or suggestions about this volume, please use the following address:

External relations - Edi.Ermes srl - Viale Enrico Forlanini, 65 - 20134 Milan (Italy)
Voice +39.02.70.21.121 - Fax +39.02.70.21.12.83

Paper edition printed in October 2017 by Faenza Printing Industries Spa
for Edi.Ermes - viale Enrico Forlanini, 65 - 20134 Milan, Italy
http://www.ediermes.it - Tel. +39 02 7021121 - Fax +39 02 70211283

Forewords

International Society of Physical and Rehabilitation Medicine

The International Society of Physical and Rehabilitation Medicine (ISPRM) is pleased to support the publication of the book *Sonographic Atlas for Common Musculoskeletal Pathologies* edited by Professor Levent Özçakar. This is the second book on this topic published by the author, together with Professor Franco Franchignoni as project manager.

The PRM specialist treats and rehabilitates persons with conditions of the musculoskeletal (MSK) system on a daily basis. Sonographic imaging has become an important diagnostic and therapeutic tool for many physiatrists. This technique has become a unique complement to the more traditional clinical history and physical examination, enhancing the quality of the clinical services provided to the patient. MSK ultrasonography is an accurate and cost effective option for the appropriate diagnosis of soft tissues and articular injuries and for the application of pharmacologic agents with local injections.

To become an expert in sonographic exploration of the MSK system continuous learning and constant mentoring are needed. The PRM specialist must understand the theory of ultrasonography and how to apply it to the MSK system. A few years ago, the authors published a first and very successful book on *Musculoskeletal Ultrasound in Physical and Rehabilitation Medicine*. This second publication, an Atlas, is in fact a "hands on course" with a large number of images, relevant figure explanations, as well as "expert notes". The reader will have the impression that he/she is discussing the images with an expert on MSK ultrasonography.

ISPRM wishes to continue to support this project and the development of MSK ultrasound. Because of our commitment to the training and education of PRM residents and specialists in the various areas of our specialty we believe that the *Sonographic Atlas for Common Musculoskeletal Pathologies* represents an important contribution to the specialty of PRM.

Jorge Lains
President

Walter Frontera
President-elect

Leonard Li
Vice President

Physical and Rehabilitation Medicine Board of the European Union of Medical Specialists

Physical and Rehabilitation Medicine Section of the European Union of Medical Specialists

A bit longer than one year ago, the American Journal of Physical Medicine and Rehabilitation published "Nineteen reasons why physiatrists should do musculoskeletal ultrasound" by the European Musculoskeletal Ultrasound Study Group (EURO-MUSCULUS) and the Ultrasound Study Group in Physical and Rehabilitation Medicine (USPRM). Beyond all general aspects supporting the use of ultrasound imaging (US) as a not-invasive, portable, cost-effective diagnostic tool, able to describe multiple alterations in neuro-musculoskeletal structures as well as in peripheral arteriovenous vessels, one statement sounded especially intriguing: "*in the hands of clinicians, US becomes a great tool immediately after physical examination*". It is certainly true that the diagnostic phase starting with clinical and functional assessment of motor behavior finds its natural completion in the discrimination of the anatomical backgrounds of signs and symptoms. Through mastering US imaging, PRM physicians can better accomplish their leading role as clinicians, gathering all the relevant information needed to provide a differential diagnosis of musculoskeletal conditions suitable to be approached with a conservative treatment. Similarly, some neuromuscular conditions can also be quickly diagnosed through the combination of expert eye and cost-effective not-invasive ultrasound imaging.

The Physical & Rehabilitation Medicine physicians should therefore claim for the acquisition of advanced skills in the use of US. On behalf of the UEMS PRM Board and the UEMS PRM Section, we are proud to endorse the diffusion of this Atlas, that represents like the natural consequence of the previous book "Musculoskeletal ultrasound in Physical and Rehabilitation Medicine", edited by Levent Özçakar and Martine De Muynck.

With the present Atlas, the Editor achieves the difficult goal of bringing the US laboratory to the reader: the book is a collection of high-quality US pictures and videos taken during routine diagnostic practice and exemplifying several scenarios of normal and abnormal findings in the assessment of musculoskeletal body structures.

This is the recommended educational resource not only for those who already have some expertise in the field and wish to challenge their diagnostic ability, but also for those who move their first steps in the US laboratory. The detailed legends and the expert notes accompanying the iconographic material will allow even the less expert reader to decipher the US findings.

Again, we wish to congratulate the Editor (Levent Özçakar) and the Project Manager (Franco Franchignoni) for this excellent work, and finally thank them for giving us the honor and privilege of writing this foreword.

Maria Gabriella Ceravolo
President UEMS PRM Board

Nicolas Christodoulou
President UEMS PRM Section

Preface

After our first book *Musculoskeletal Ultrasound in Physical and Rehabilitation Medicine*, we are very much pleased and honored to announce that a 'new product' of the same project has now been launched. We strongly believe that this second book *Sonographic Atlas for Common Musculoskeletal Pathologies* will help to move one step forward in the lengthy training process of musculoskeletal US in our PRM discipline.

As you might well be aware, the first book (which has been distributed worldwide, in both English and Spanish versions) comprised basic technical and clinical skills and some pathological examples as regards several joints and groups of diseases. Herewith, being a strongly 'mentor-necessitating' training, one of the most important challenges that physiatrists are facing with during their musculoskeletal US experience is actually 'maintenance' once they start. Accordingly, the main purpose of this second book is to provide plenty of examples concerning the most commonly scanned pathologies in physiatry, and thus to fill the gap of long-term supervised education in our specialty.

The sections of the book are organized as regions in an anatomy atlas, i.e. starting from head and neck down to ankle and foot. In each section, the subsections are arranged in accordance with the anatomical structures. The text is based mainly on the long figure legends, which also include clinical/physical examination findings.

In total, we will take you through 500 images and 20 related videos. Additionally, in some of the figures, you will find 3D reconstruction of the local anatomy along with schematic drawings of probe positionings. Importantly, while reading the book, you will see parts referred as "Expert Note", at the bottom of many pages. These comments are, for sure, the most distinguishing part of the book, because they provide valuable, practical explanations, making the readers feel as if they are revising and discussing that particular US image with an expert sitting next to them.

In closing, I convey my gratitudes to the international bodies of our specialty which once again supported (ISPRM and UEMS PRM Section & Board) or endorsed (ESPRM and European Academy of Rehabilitation Medicine) our book, making it indisputably more valuable. Last but not least, I need to highlight the great efforts of my associate editors and project manager, without whom this book would have never been actualized.

With my best wishes for a pleasant and fruitful reading!

September 2017

Levent Özçakar
Ankara, Turkey

List of Contributors
(in alphabetic order)

Giuseppe ANASTASI, MD, Professor
University of Messina, Medical School
Department of Biomedical Sciences
and Dental Sciences
and Morphological Imaging
Messina, Italy

Martine DE MUYNCK, Professor
Ghent University Medical School
Department of Physical
and Rehabilitation Medicine,
Ghent, Belgium

Eda GÜRÇAY, MD, Associate Professor
Gaziler Physical and Rehabilitation Medicine
Education and Research Hospital,
Ankara, Turkey

Murat KARA, MD, Associate Professor
Hacettepe University Medical School
Department of Physical
and Rehabilitation Medicine,
Ankara, Turkey

Şule Şahin ONAT, MD, Associate Professor
Ankara Physical and Rehabilitation
Medicine Education
and Research Hospital,
Ankara, Turkey

Levent ÖZÇAKAR, MD, Professor
Hacettepe University Medical School
Department of Physical
and Rehabilitation Medicine,
Ankara, Turkey

To my parents

&

to my wife and daughters

Contents

SECTION 3 Lower limb

VIDEO INDEX

Video 1	Supraspinatus tendon tear in a 53-year-old woman with shoulder pain and anterolateral tenderness
Video 2	Calcifying supraspinatus tendon in a 35-year-old woman with severe shoulder pain after a slip and fall injury
Video 3	Bilateral calcifying supraspinatus tendons in a diabetic woman
Video 4	Shoulder osteoarthritis in an elderly man with pain during activities and worsening at night
Video 5	Synovitis in a 40-year-old woman with active rheumatoid arthritis
Video 6	Repaired flexor pollicis longus tendon in a 34-year-old woman after a glass injury
Video 7	An elderly woman with trigger finger
Video 8	A small foreign object following a penetrating trauma
Video 9	Intra-articular effusion in a 50-year-old woman with groin pain especially during passive hip internal rotation
Video 10	Lateral collateral ligament injury in a 34-year-old man with knee pain and mild focal tenderness
Video 11	Chronic tenosynovitis of the tibialis posterior tendon in a patient with rheumatoid arthritis
Video 12	Partial tear of the Achilles tendon in a 38-year-old man
Video 13	Repaired Achilles tendon in a 43-year-old man who had recurrent ruptures due to long-distance running
Video 14	Anterior talofibular ligament tear in a patient with ankle pain and swelling after repetitive inversion injuries
Video 15	Metatarsophalangeal joint arthritis in a 17-year-old girl diagnosed with juvenile idiopathic arthritis
Video 16	Radial nerve injury after humeral shaft fracture in a 28-year-old man
Video 17	Posterior interosseous neuropathy in a 40-year-old woman who had burning pain and tenderness over the lateral elbow
Video 18	Surgical transposition of the ulnar nerve in a 38-year-old man with medial elbow pain
Video 19	Plexiform neurofibromas in the sciatic nerve of a 45-year-old woman who is otherwise asymptomatic
Video 20	Morton's neuroma in a patient who defines sharp pain at the base of the web space radiating to the toes

Section 1
HEAD AND NECK - TRUNK

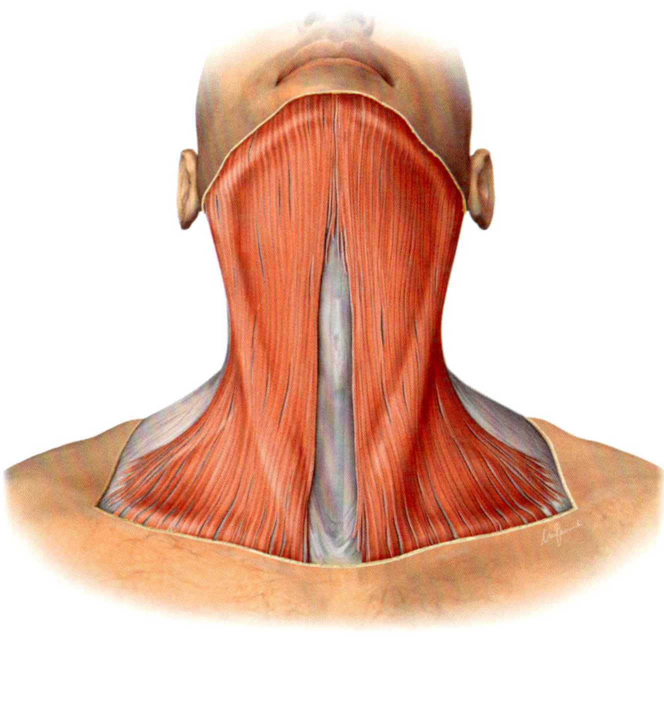

1 Head and Neck Trunk

- **Sternocleidomastoid**
- **Lymph node**
- **Subcutaneous tissue** - Lateral neck
- **Cervical rib**
- **Nerve** - Axilla
- **Sternoclavicular joint**
- **Sternum**
- **Nerve** - Thoracodorsal
- **Subcutaneous tissue** - Thoracodorsal
- **Subcutaneous tissue** - Low back
- **Infraspinatus**
- **Latissimus dorsi**

STERNOCLEIDOMASTOID

1.1 Torticollis in a 3-year-old boy with a firm palpable mass resembling an olive on the lateral neck region

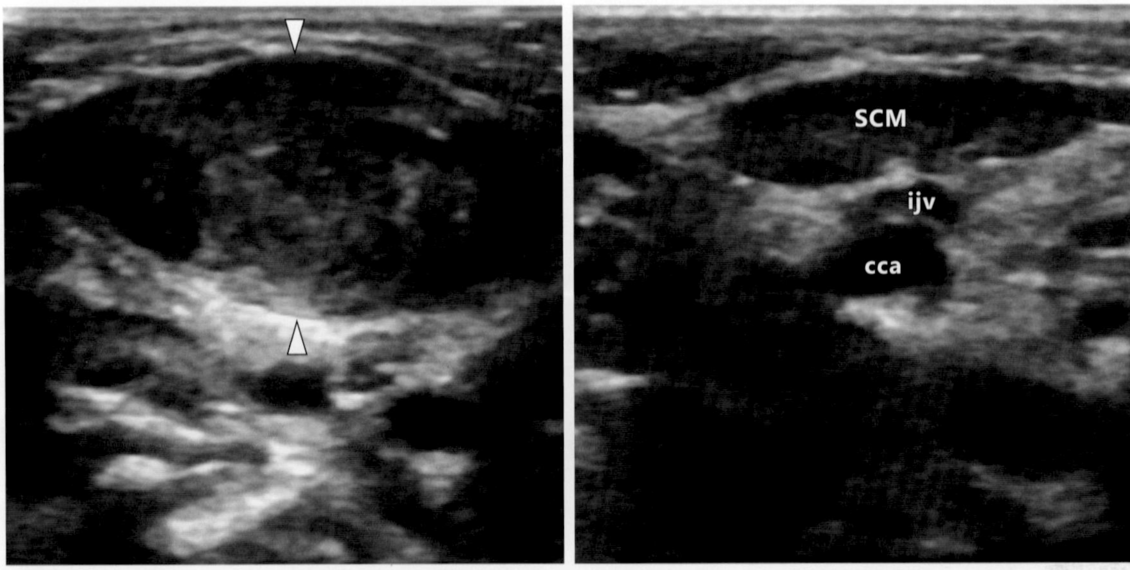

a b

Axial US imaging reveals fusiform thickening (*arrowheads*) of the sternocleidomastoid muscle (**a**). Normal side (**b**).

cca common carotid artery
ijv internal jugular vein
SCM sternocleidomastoid

Expert note

Intramuscular (organized) hematoma within the muscle can be seen as a small mass or diffuse enlargement of the sternocleidomastoid muscle.

Apart from individual cases, US imaging is of extra importance for children in general [1]. Yet, it does not contain radiation and it is patient friendly. At any time/position, the baby/child can be scanned without any need for strict immobilization or sedation. One concrete example would be the imaging for torticollis in the newborns whereby "a simple/short touch" with the probe on the baby would be conclusive at once.

One practical suggestion would be to let the mother sit on the examination table and hold the baby lying or sitting on her lap. The baby will be much more quiet than when you let it lie on the table.

Torticollis in a 7-year-old girl with limited neck rotation **1.2**

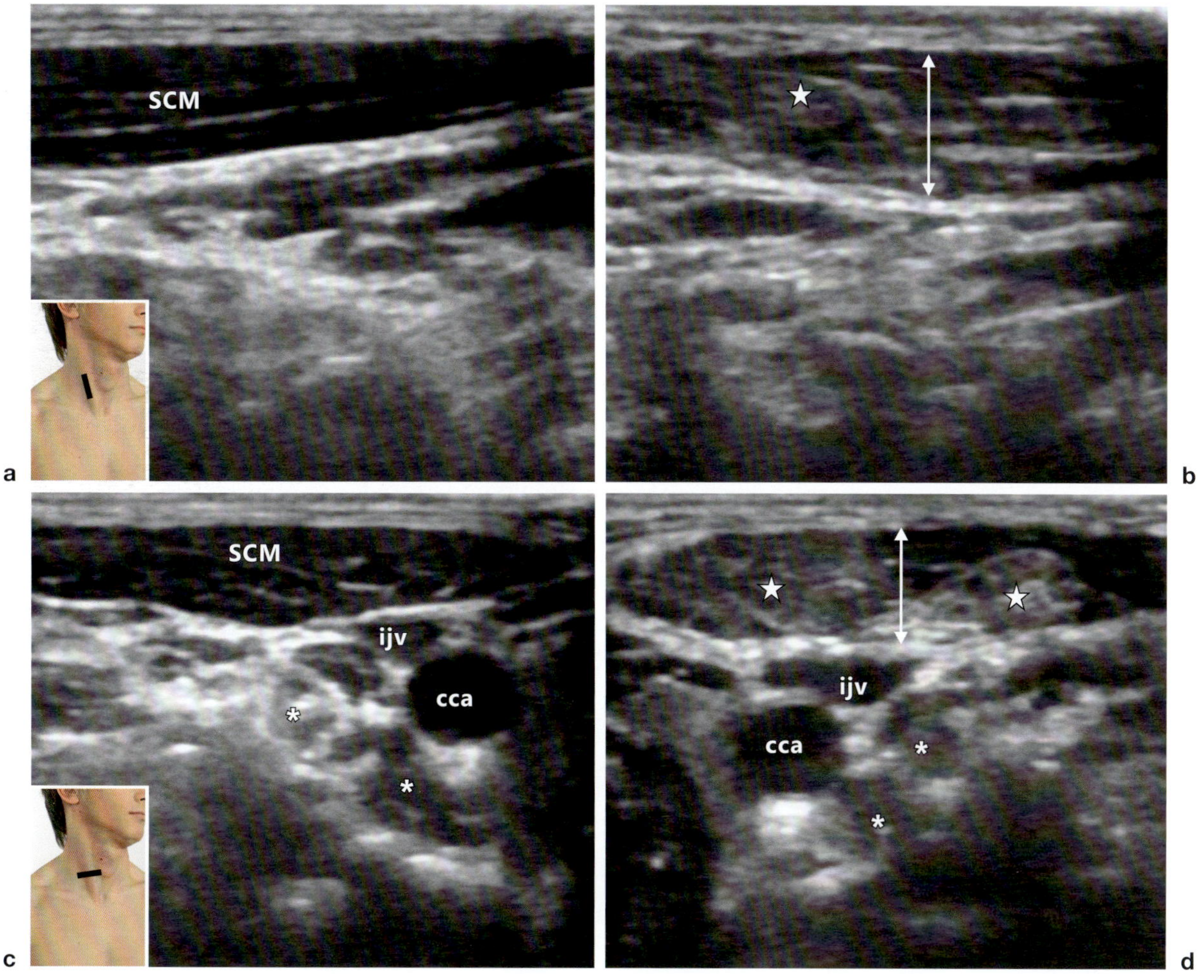

Images **a** and **b** show longitudinal scans, while **c** and **d** axial scans. When compared with the normal side (**a**, **c**), longitudinal (**b**) and axial (**d**) US images reveal fusiform thickening (*double arrow*) of the sternocleidomastoid muscle (**SCM**) with hyperechoic intramuscular foci (*stars*). Please also note the close relation of the SCM and the deeper neurovascular structures i.e. brachial plexus (*asterisks*), internal jugular vein (**ijv**) and common carotid artery (**cca**).

Expert note

Fibromatosis colli is the most common cause of neonatal torticollis which usually appears sonographically as a hyperechoic mass or diffuse sternocleidomastoid enlargement of mixed echogenicity [2].

1.3 Lymphadenopathy in a 30-year-old man with a palpable mass on the anterolateral part of the neck

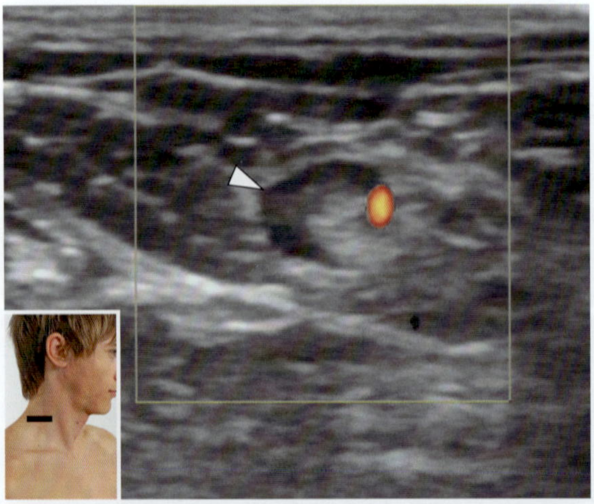

Power Doppler image reveals a reactive enlarged lymph node (*arrowhead*) with a hypoechoic peripheral zone, hyperechoic centre, and slow-flowing blood.

Expert note

This is the typical appearance of a lymph node in echogenicity and vascularity. For sure, clarifying that the palpable mass is a lymph node or understanding its nature of involvement (benign vs malignant) is possible and highly important in US imaging. The number of lymph nodes, their size, shape (oval vs rounded), the proportion center/halo and vascularization (centrifugal/centripetal) should be assessed.
Please note that one exam might not always enable to differentiate between reactive/benign/malignant nodes and follow-up exams might be helpful.

1.4 Lymphadenopathy in a 35-year-old woman with a painful palpable lump on the lateral side of the neck

a 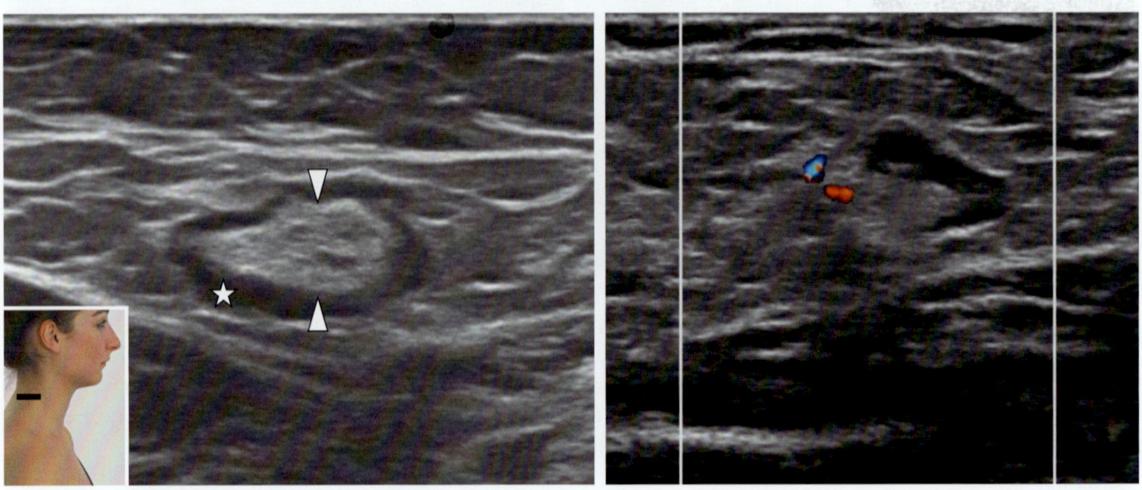 b

Axial US images illustrates an enlarged reactive lymph node with hypoechoic peripheral zone (*star*) and hyperechoic centre (*arrowheads*) on B-mode (**a**) and low flow signal on power Doppler imaging (**b**).

Expert note

Ultrasound image of a reactive lymph node comprises hypoechoic cortex with a thickened, hyperechoic hilum and frequently increased flow signals [3].

Epidermal inclusion (sebaceous) cyst in a 48-year-old man who had a swelling on the posterolateral side of the neck for the last 2-month

1.5

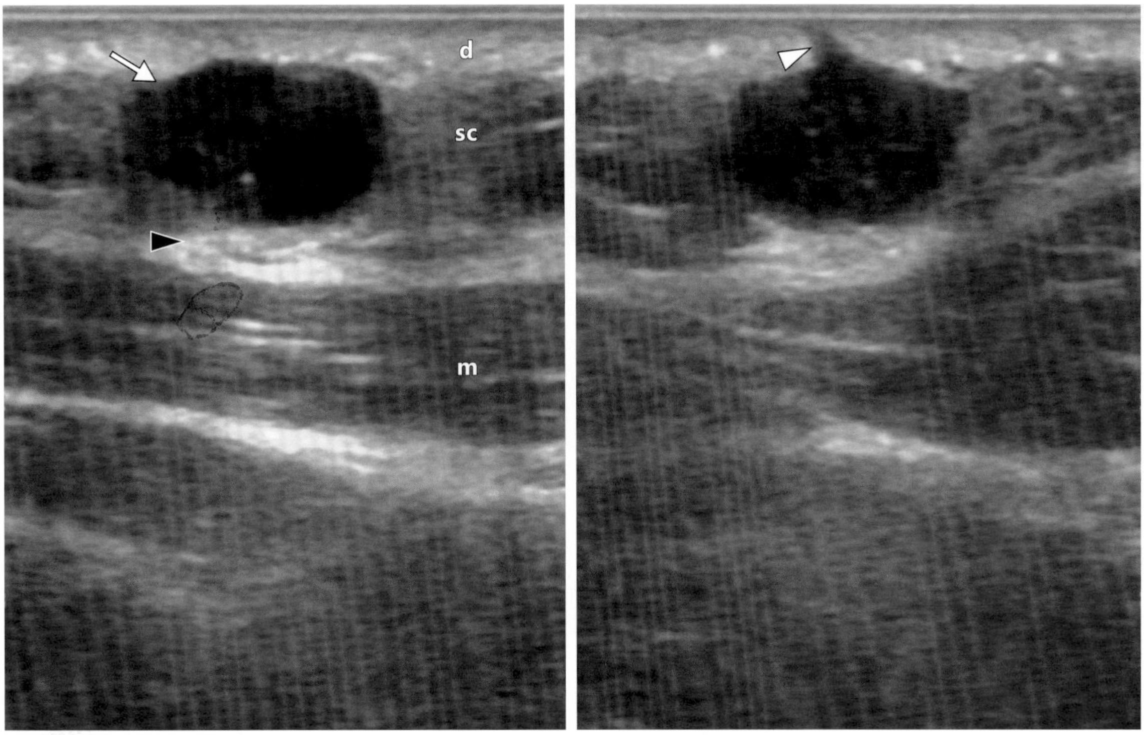

a b

Longitudinal US image demonstrates a rounded well-defined hypoechoic mass (*arrow*) within the subcutaneous tissue (**sc**) presenting posterior acoustic enhancement (*arrowhead*) (**a**). Please note the tract of drainage (*arrowhead*) to the skin in the axial view (**b**).

d dermis
m muscle

Expert note

Using high frequencies (12-20 MHz), imaging of the superficial tissues like epidermis, dermis and subcutaneous fat can be performed in details. Sensitivity and specificity for the diagnosis of epidermal cysts with US are 91.8 and 92.2%, respectively [4].

1.6 Thoracic outlet syndrome in a young woman with "pins and needles" feeling and numbness in the whole upper extremity

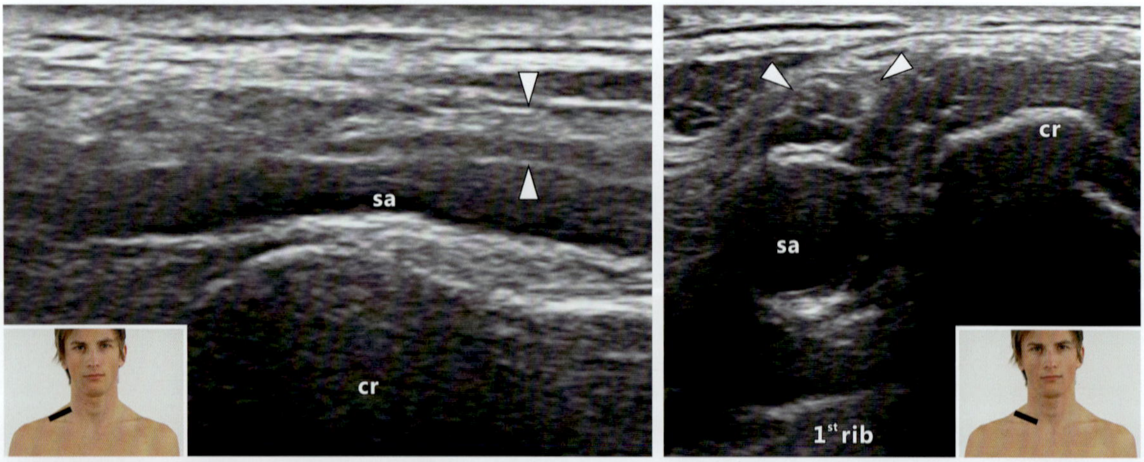

a b

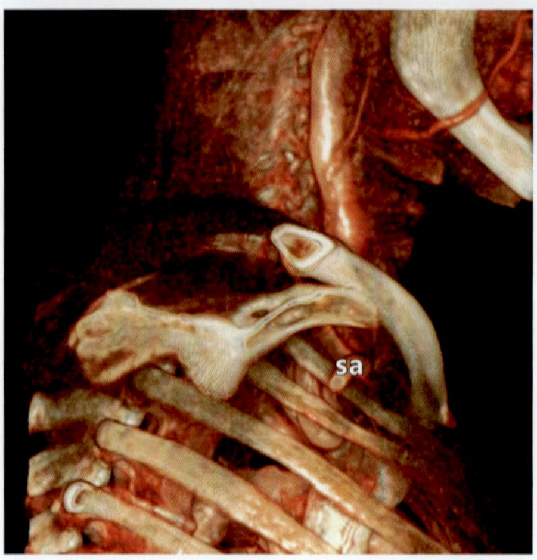

Longitudinal (**a**) and axial (**b**) US images obtained in the supraclavicular region illustrates the close proximity of the cervical rib (**cr**; extra rib which arises from the 7th cervical vertebra) with the subclavian artery (**sa**) and the brachial plexus (*arrowheads*).

Expert note

While radiographs would definitely provide a better snapshot on the bony architecture, the relationship between the (compressive) aberrant structures and the neurovascular bundle can be promptly/readily be demonstrated with the use of B-mode and Doppler US imaging. Dynamic examination during the provocative maneuvers for thoracic outlet syndrome definitely gives additional information as regards the type (of the syndrome) as well.

Schwannoma of the median nerve in the axilla of a 41-year-old woman with a painless lump

1.7

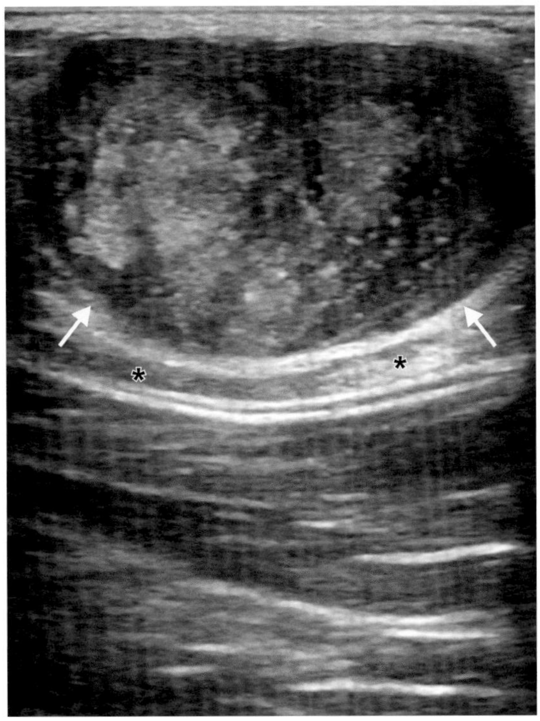

Longitudinal US image demonstrates a huge, well-defined, globoid and hyperechoic mass (*arrows*) adjacent to another nerve trunk (*asterisks*).

Expert note

Owing to the crowdedness of the axillary region, proximal-distal scanning would be necessary to better understand the origin of the schwannoma.

1.8 Sternoclavicular joint arthritis in an old man with a diagnosis of lymphoma

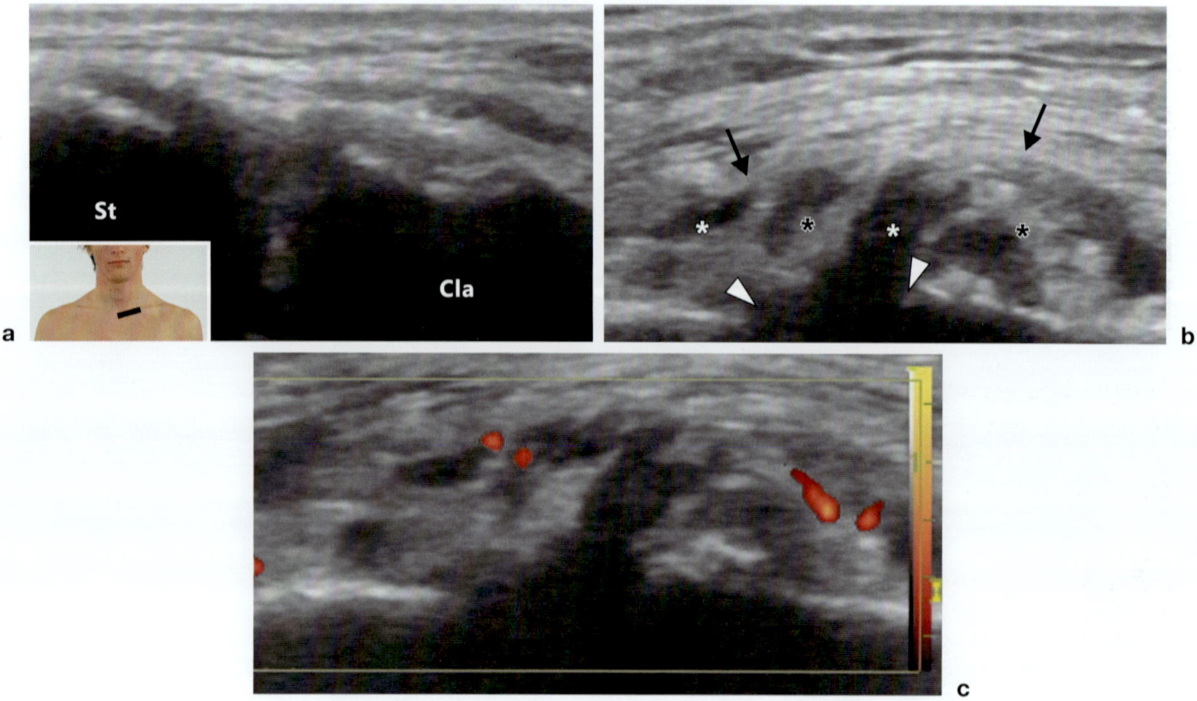

This lymphoma patient was admitted with complaints of pain on the anterior part of the chest.

When compared with the normal side (**a**) longitudinal US imaging over the sternoclavicular joint shows mild joint space widening (*arrowheads*), enlargement of the articular capsule (*black arrows*), synovial effusion (*white asterisks*) and hypertrophy (*black asterisks*) (**b**). Hyperemia is also detected on power Doppler imaging (**c**).

Cla clavicle
St sternum

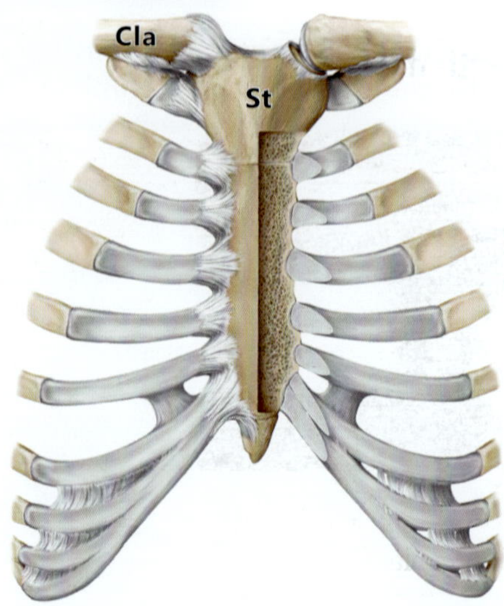

Expert note

Like in the periphery, joints of the axial skeleton can readily be scanned with US imaging. This availability is of great importance for various rheumatic diseases or any other uncommon condition that might involve these joints, indisputably not only for diagnostic but also for interventional purposes.

Degenerative osteoarthritis of the sternoclavicular joints in an old woman with pain in the upper anterior chest wall **1.9**

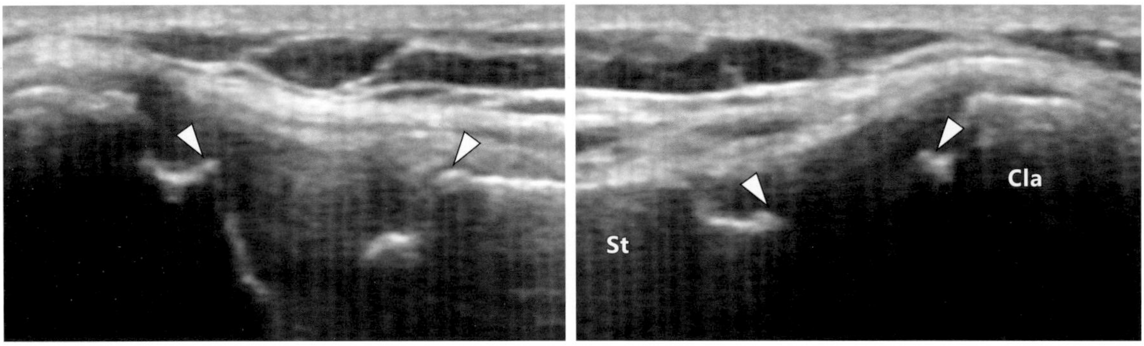

a b

Longitudinal US images over the stenoclavicular joints show small irregularities and marginal osteophytes (*arrowheads*) at the articular surfaces of the clavicle and sternum bilaterally.

Cla clavicle **St** sternum

Expert note
In thin patients, a lot of gel would be necessary to visualize these joints.

Sternoclavicular joint arthritis in a 45-year-old woman with mass-like lump and recalcitrant pain limiting her recreational activities **1.10**

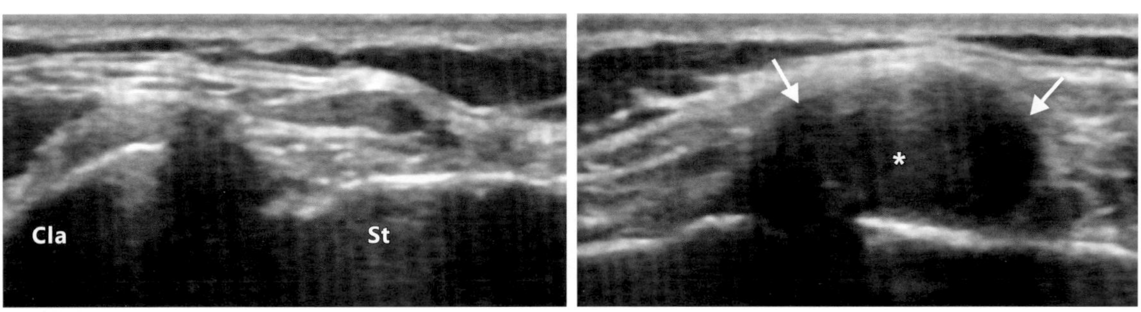

a b

When compared with the normal side (**a**), longitudinal US imaging demonstrates chronic synovial hyperplasia (*asterisk*) distending the joint capsule (*arrows*) (**b**).

Expert note
During daily clinical practice, the possible role of an immediate US examination in providing an initial understanding on the nature of a mass-like lesion is invaluable.

1.11 A 32-year-old woman who had chest pain and tenderness after an antecedent blunt trauma to the sternum three weeks ago

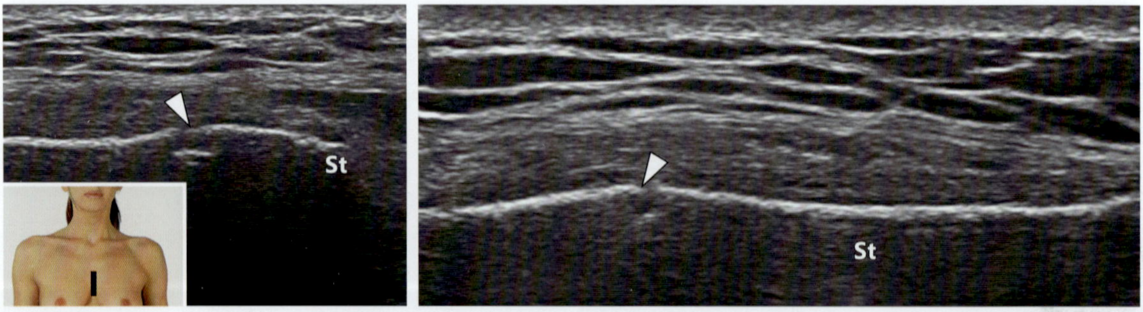

a b

Axial (**a**) and longitudinal (**b**) US images show a small cortical defect at the sternal bone (*arrowheads*).

St sternum

Expert note

Sono-palpation was positive in this patient and it actually/clearly guided the localization of this very small cortical lesion. The diagnosis might have otherwise turned out to be an impasse with conventional radiographs.

Diffuse neurofibromas in a 7-year-old child with a painless lump underlying one of the café-au-lait spots **1.12**

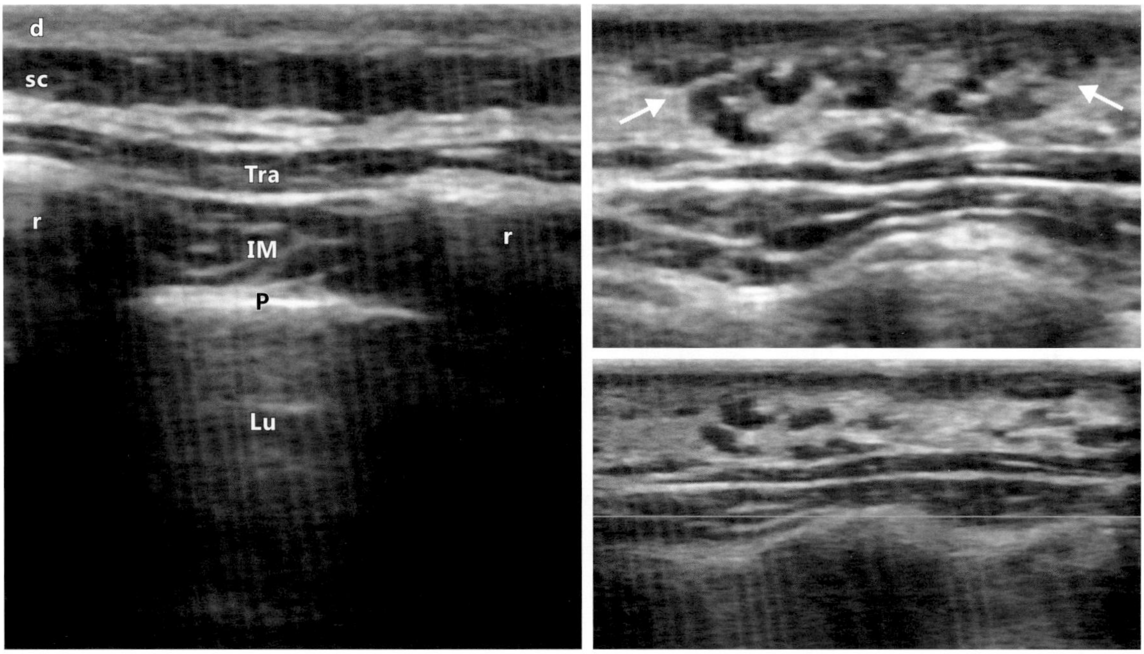

a b c

When compared with the normal side (**a**), axial US image over the trapezius muscle (**Tra**) on the dorsal region shows diffuse neurofibromas (*arrows*) expanding inside the subcutaneous tissue (**b**). No flow signal is observed with power Doppler imaging (**c**).

d	dermis	**P**	pleura
IM	internal intercostal muscle	**r**	rib
Lu	lung	**sc**	subcutaneous tissue

Expert note

Power Doppler imaging is typically negative in neurofibroma(tosi)s; however plexiform types might sometimes be quite vascular [5]. This feature is again very important to be diagnosed promptly; for the surgeon as well.

1.13 A 41-year-old woman with diffuse neurofibromas in the lower trunk and back

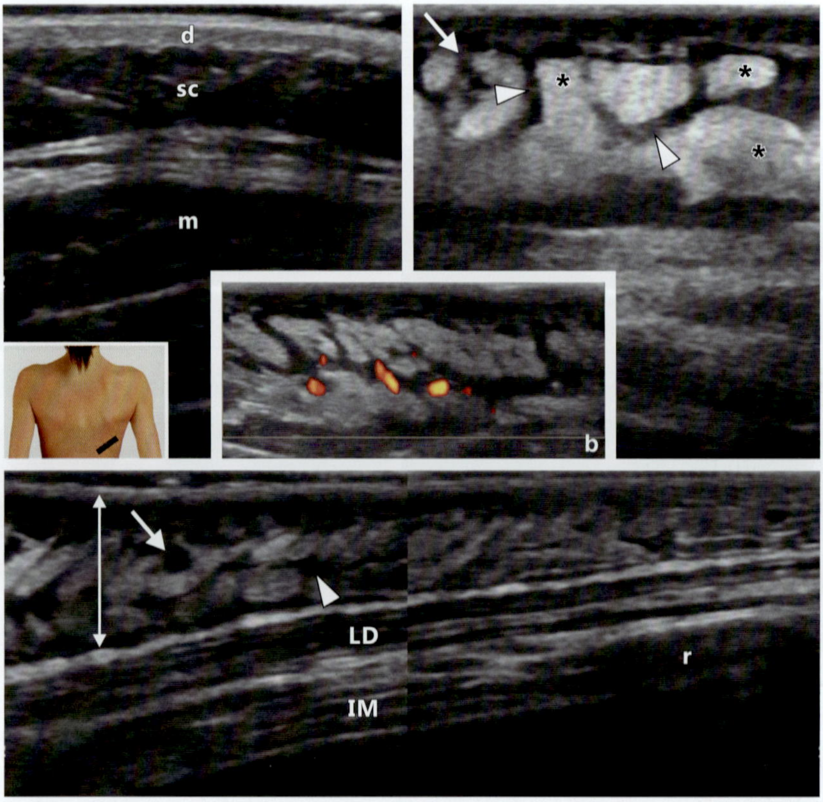

When compared with the normal side (**a**), longitudinal US image obtained over the lateral trunk region demonstrates hypoechoic tubular (*arrowheads*) and nodular (*arrows*) structures within the hyperechoic subcutaneous lesion (*asterisks*) (**b**-**d**). A few vascular signals were present in power Doppler imaging (**b**). Split-screen image shows the diffuse thickening of the subcutaneous tissue (**sc**, *double arrow*) (**d**).

d	dermis	**LD**	latissimus dorsi	**r**	rib
IM	internal intercostal muscle	**m**	muscle		

Expert note

Neurofibromas are categorized in three forms: localized (90%), diffuse or plexiform. A localized neurofibroma is typically seen as the "onion skin image" or the "target sign" with a centrally hyperechoic and peripherally hypoechoic mass apperance. The diffuse type involves the subcutaneous tissue, particularly of the head and neck. The plexiform neurofibroma is defined as "bag-of-worms" formed by diffuse tortuous nerve thickenings and is pathognomonic sign for neurofibromatosis syndromes by which two thirds have malignant potential [5]. Depending on the type of neurofibroma(tosi)s, US imaging may reveal various findings. Sensitivity and specificity for the diagnosis of nerve sheath tumors have been reported as 42.9% and 100%, respectively [4].

Subcutaneous lipoma in an elderly man with diffuse and painless lump over the scapula **1.14**

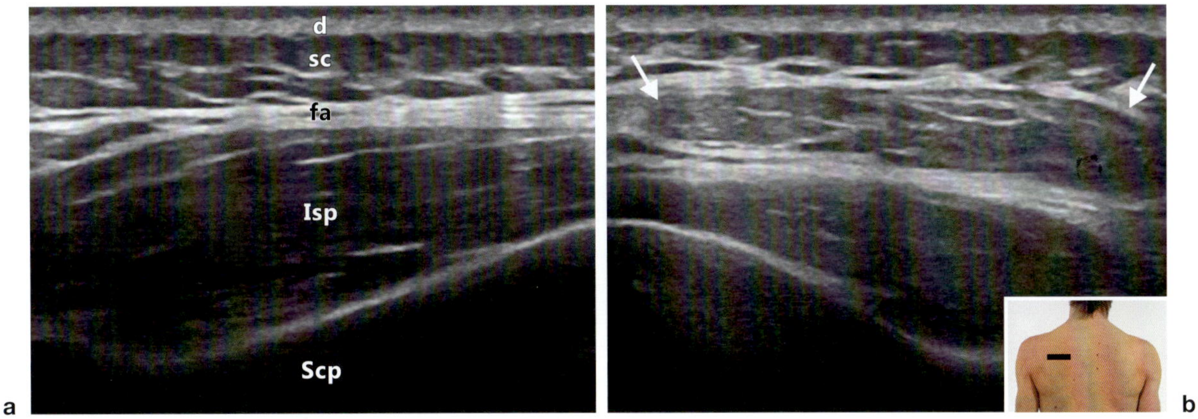

When compared with the normal side (**a**), longitudinal US image shows an elongated, well-defined subcutaneous mass (*arrows*) with intrinsic heterogenous echoes (**b**).

d	dermis	**sc**	subcutaneous tissue
fa	fascia	**Scp**	scapula
Isp	infraspinatus		

Lipoma in a 47-year-old woman with painless swelling over the dorsal region **1.15**

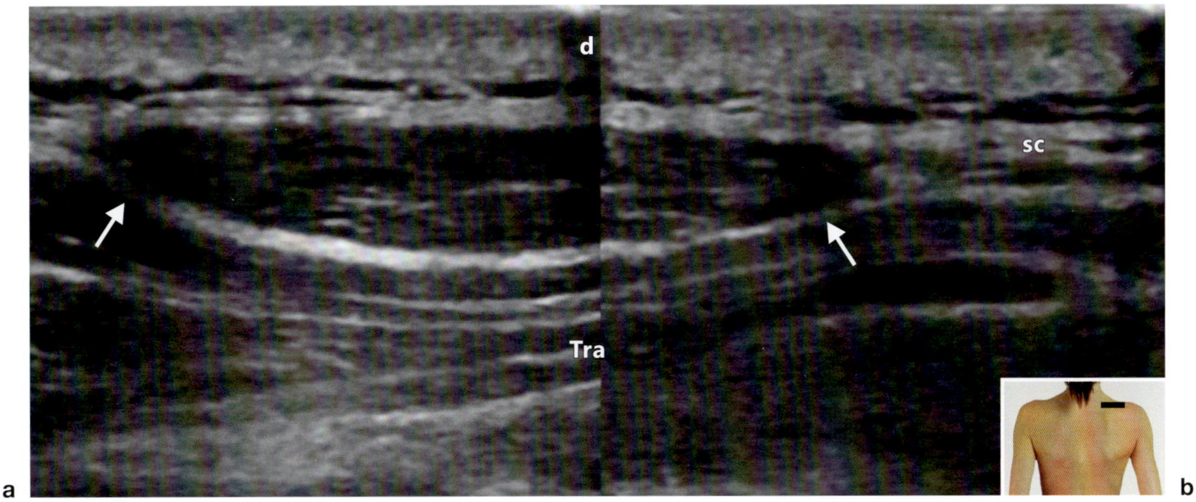

Split-screen longitudinal US image illustrates an oval, hypoechoic soft-tissue mass (*arrows*) located above the trapezius muscle (**Tra**). Note that the lipoma shows enlargement towards the underlying muscle compartment.

1.16 Episacroiliac lipoma (Copeman's nodule) in a 44-year-old obese woman who had pain on the lumbosacral region

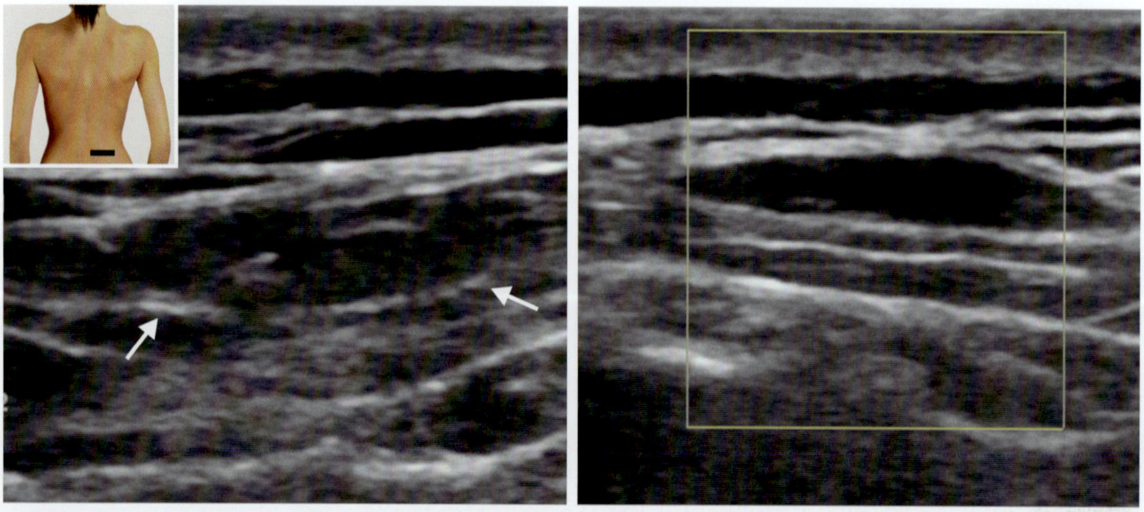

a b

Axial US image shows fusiform, hypoechoic subcutaneous nodule formation (*arrows*) (**a**) without any flow signal by power Doppler imaging (**b**).

Expert note

Mobile nodules that are commonly located at the sacroiliac, posterior superior iliac, and the lumbar paraspinal regions may display fatty tissue that has herniated through fascial layers [6].

Infraspinatus muscle strain in a 34-year-old man with a gradual-onset pain, worsening while he tried to reach his back pocket **1.17**

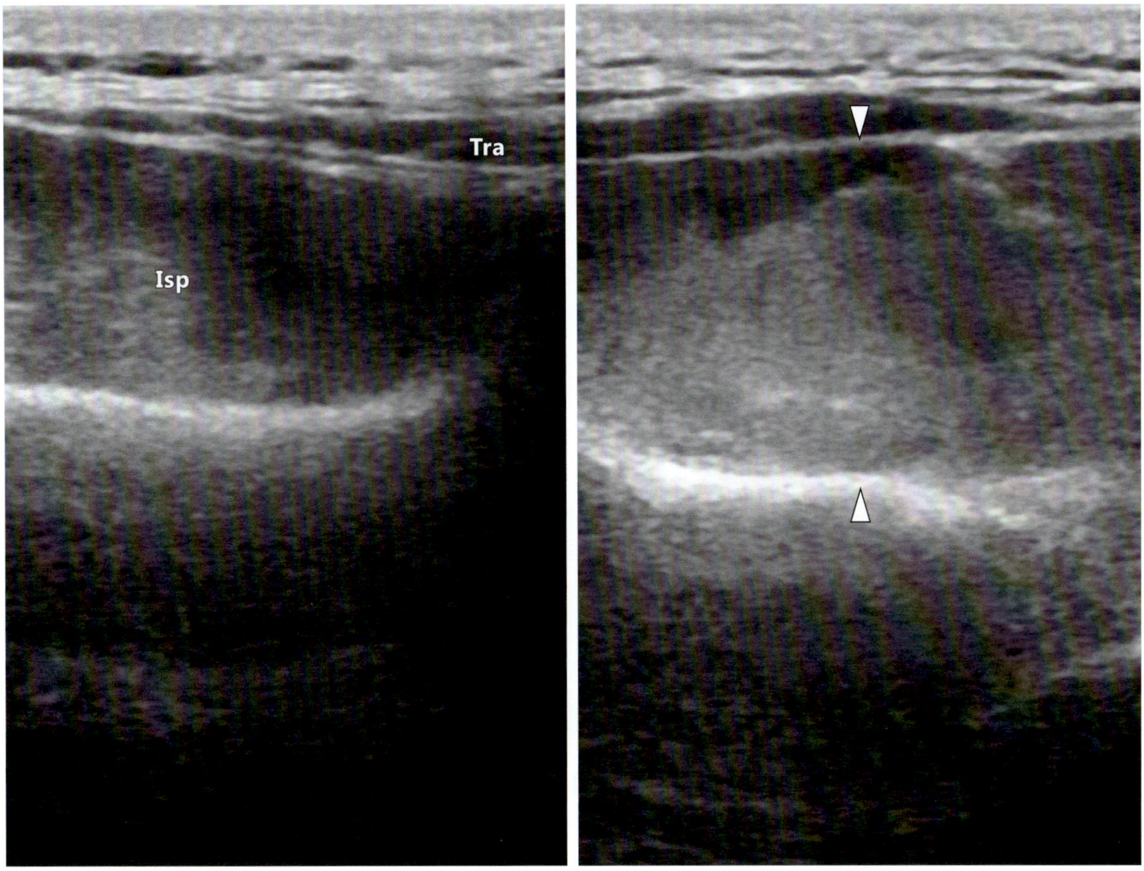

When compared with the normal side (**a**), axial US imaging shows diffuse hyperechoic enlargement of the infraspinatus muscle (*arrowheads*) consistent with healing process of the strain (**b**).

Isp infraspinatus
Tra trapezius

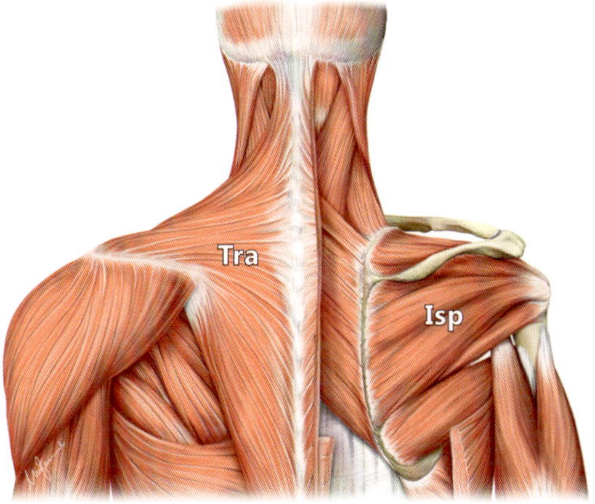

1.18 Latissimus dorsi strain in an elderly woman after lifting a heavy object

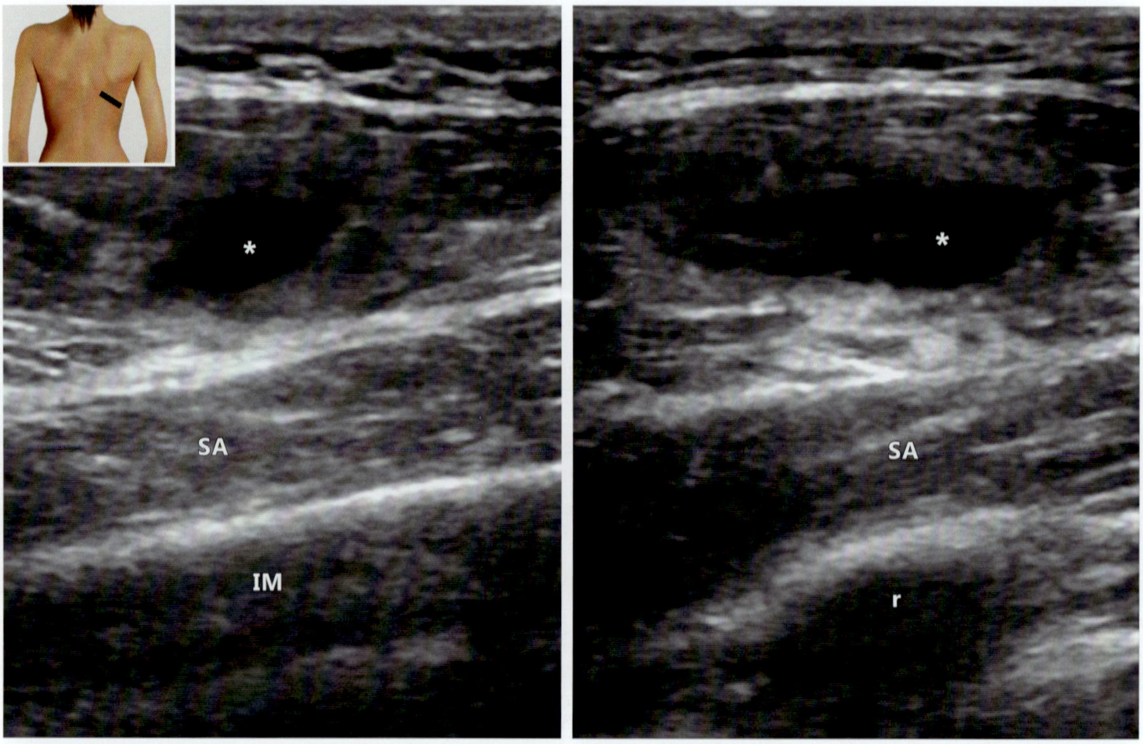

a b

Longitudinal (**a**) and axial (**b**) US images reveal hemorrhagic disruption of the latissimus dorsi muscle fascicles with hypo-/an-echoich appearance (*asterisks*).

IM internal intercostal muscle
r rib
SA serratus anterior

Expert note

Muscle injuries comprise one of the most important groups of musculoskeletal pathologies that can readily/thoroughly be scanned by US imaging. Yet, they are invariably located over the bones and dynamic imaging is of great significance in their prompt evaluation. Especially for sports injuries, the problem can even be examined on-site in the sports arena. Further, repeated evaluations can easily be performed as frequently as requested. Herewith, its use in the decision for return to the play/field should be balanced between the clinical and sonographical findings, i.e. not solely be based on either one of them.

A muscle tear has two components: the disruption of the fibers and the hematoma (usually larger than the former). In US imaging, what we often evaluate is the hematoma and this takes some time to develop. So if the initial examination is negative, repeated imaging after 12-24 hours would be reasonable.

REFERENCES

1. Chang KV, Şahin Onat Ş, Lee CW, Kara M, Hung CY, Özçakar L. EURO-MUSCULUS/USPRM basic scanning protocols revisited in children. Eur J Phys Rehabil Med. 2016; 52: 887-901.
2. Bedi DG, John SD, Swischuk LE. Fibromatosis colli of infancy: variability of sonographic appearance. J Clin Ultrasound. 1998; 26: 345-8.
3. Bianchi S, Martinoli C. Elbow. In: Bianchi S, Martinoli C, editors. Ultrasound of the musculoskeletal system. Berlin: Springer; 2007. p. 349-405.
4. Hwang EJ, Yoon HS, Cho S, Park HS. The diagnostic value of ultrasonography with 5-15-MHz probes in benign subcutaneous lesions. Int J Dermatol. 2015; 54: e469-75.
5. Kara M. Ultrasound imaging for peripheral nerve problems. In: Özçakar L, De Muynck M, editors. Musculoskeletal ultrasound in physical and rehabilitation medicine. Milan: Edi.Ermes; 2014. p. 141-60.
6. Bicket MC, Simmons C, Zheng Y. The best-laid plans of "back mice" and men: a case report and literature review of episacroiliac lipoma. Pain Physician. 2016; 19: 181-8.

Section 2
UPPER LIMB

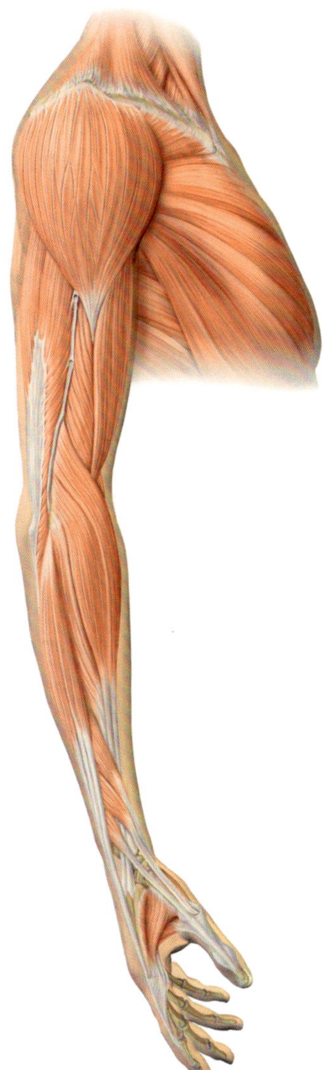

Shoulder 2

- **Biceps tendon**
- **Subdeltoid bursa**
- **Subscapularis tendon**
- **Supraspinatus tendon**
- **Glenohumeral joint** - Posterior
- **Infraspinatus tendon**
- **Acromioclavicular joint**

2.1 Bicipital tenosynovitis in a 42-year-old woman with a 2-month history of shoulder pain

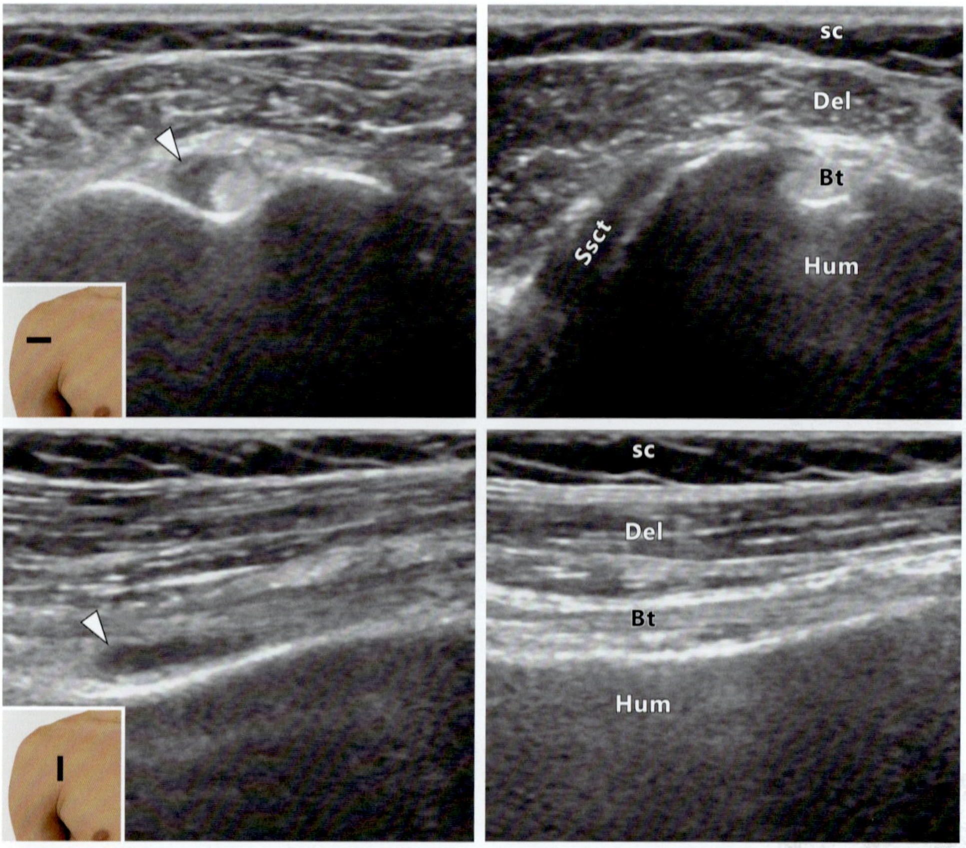

a b c d

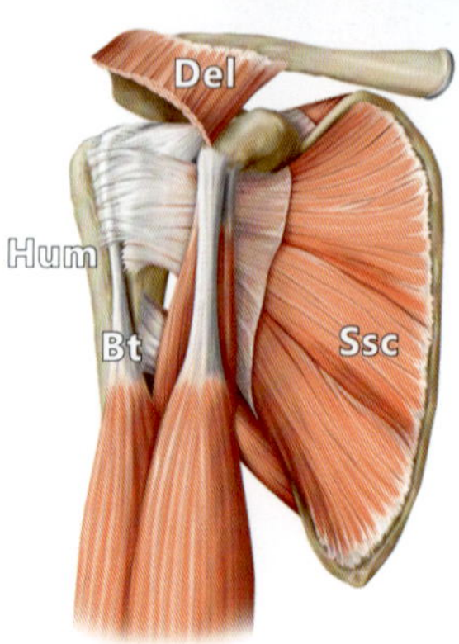

Pain was associated with any movement of the shoulder and she had a positive Speed's test.

Axial (**a**) and longitudinal (**c**) US images reveal effusion (*arrowheads*) within the biceps tendon (**Bt**) sheath. The tendon itself also seems to be a little edematous especially in the long-axis view. Normal side (**b**, **d**).

Del deltoid muscle
Hum humerus
sc subcutaneous tissue
Ssct subscapularis tendon

Expert note

Unless marked changes in the bicipital tendon are present, it is more likely that the fluid in its sheath will be attributed to joint effusion [1, 2]. Again, this can be confirmed better after a substantial shoulder imaging.

Shoulder joint effusion in a 43-year-old woman with anterior shoulder pain

2.2

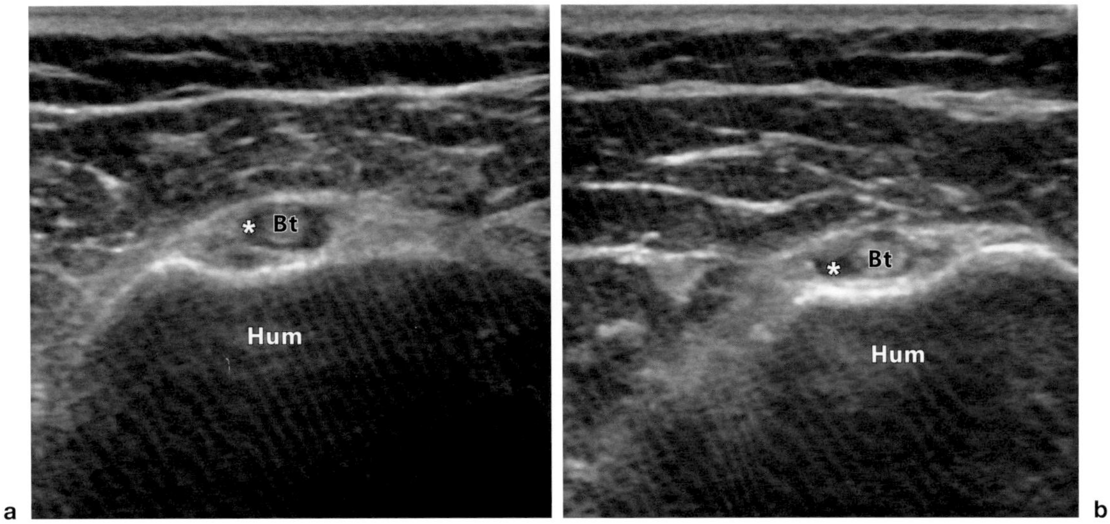

Anterior axial US images show bilateral fluid (*asterisks*) around the biceps tendon (**Bt**).

Chronic joint effusion in a middle-aged man who had shoulder pain radiating down to the anterior arm

2.3

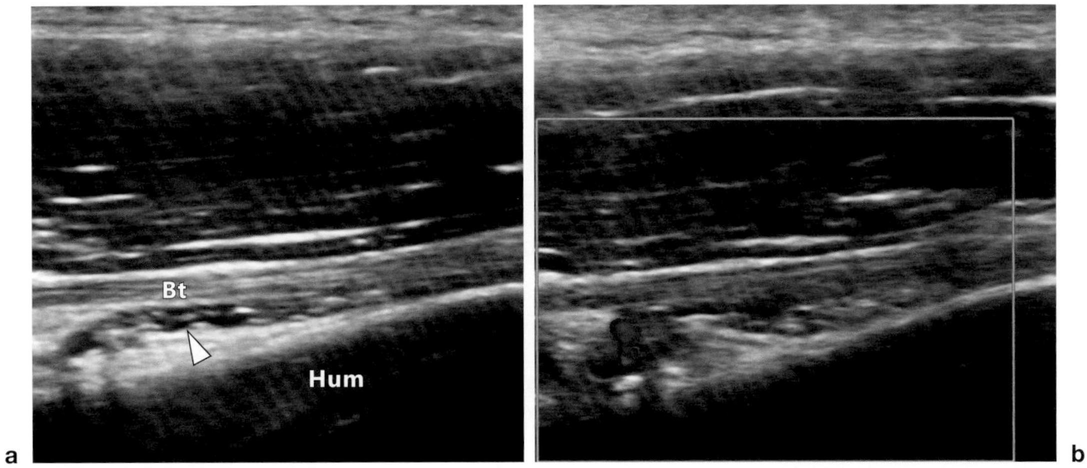

Longitudinal US image shows mild effusion (*arrowhead*) inside the biceps tendon (**Bt**) sheath (**a**). Power Doppler imaging is positive only for the anterior humeral circumflex artery (**b**).

Hum humerus

2.4 Mild bicipital tendinitis in a 50-year-old man with pain on the anterior side of the shoulder especially during movements

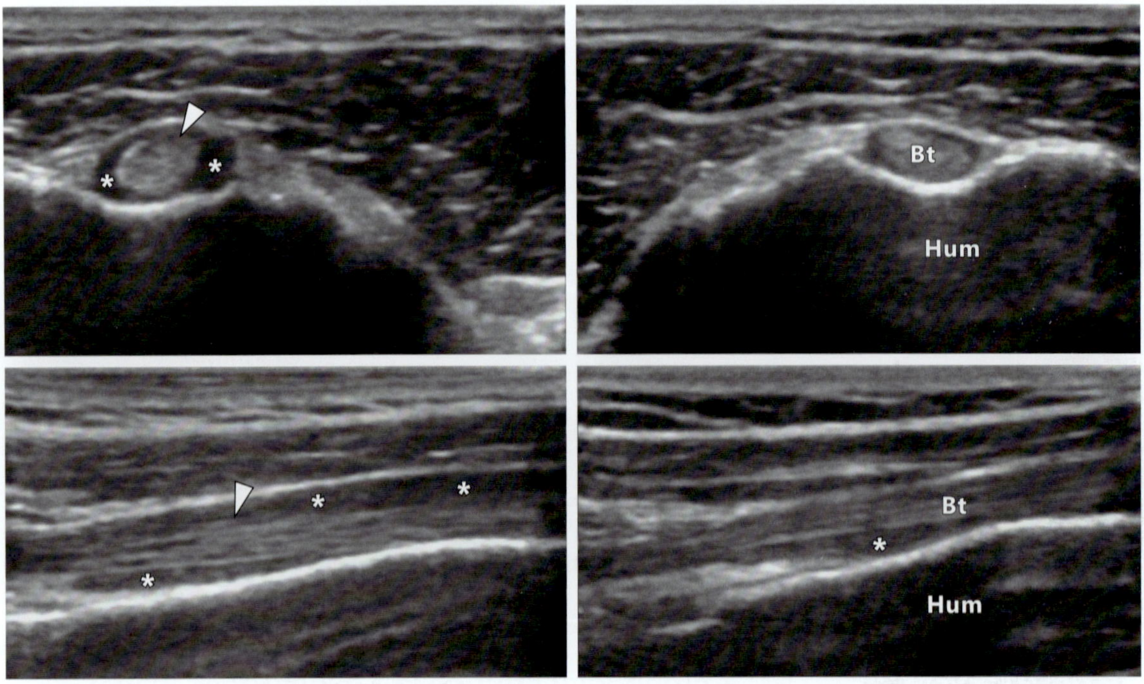

Axial (**a**) and longitudinal (**c**) US images demonstrate mildly swollen biceps tendon (*arrowheads*) containing effusion (*asterisks*) around it. Normal biceps tendon (**Bt**) with a small amount of physiologic fluid within its sheath (**b**, **d**).

Hum humerus

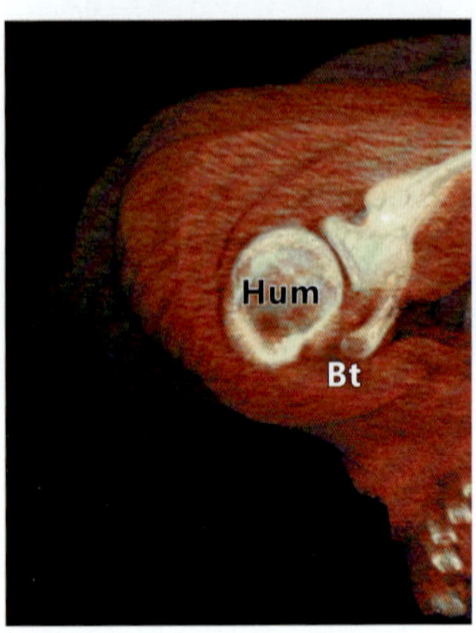

Expert note

Polymyalgia rheumatica is one of the inflammatory diseases whereby US findings (synovitis in the shoulder/hip) have been included in the recent diagnostic criteria [3]. In addition to relevant hip findings (effusion and/or trochanteric bursitis); the presence of subdeltoid bursitis, biceps tenosynovitis, glenohumeral synovitis have been accepted to improve the specificity of the diagnosis in polymyalgia rheumatica.

Shoulder joint effusion in a 73-year-old woman with polymyalgia rheumatica **2.5**

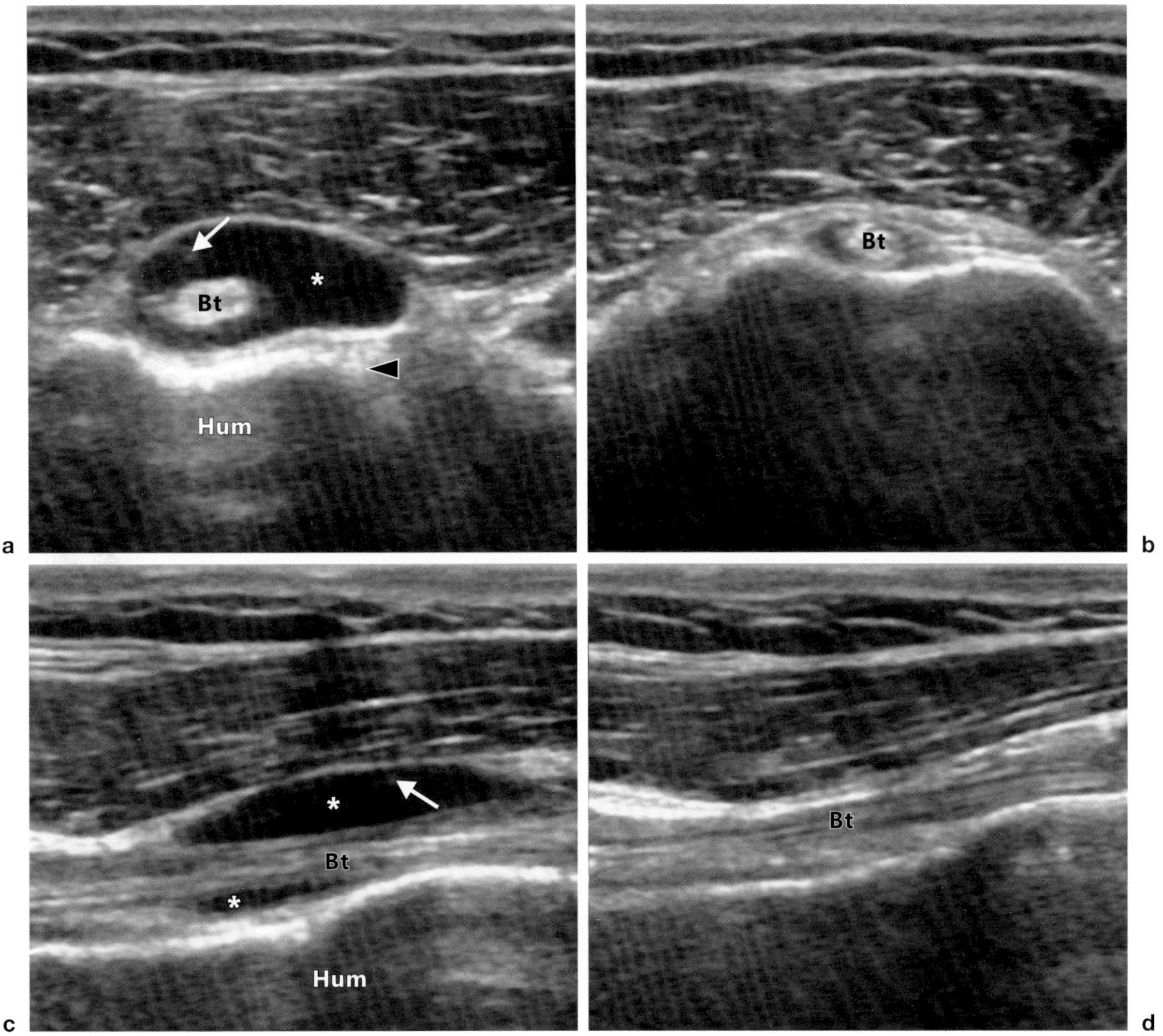

Anterior axial (**a**) and longitudinal (**c**) US images reveal fluid (*asterisks*) and a few synovial folds (*arrows*) around the biceps tendon (**Bt**). The tendon itself appears quite normal and there is also enhanced-through transmission artifact (*arrowhead*) due to anechoic fluid accumulation (**a**). Contralateral side (**b**, **d**).

Hum humerus

2.6 Bicipital tenosynovitis in a 66-year-old woman with anterior shoulder pain after lifting an object

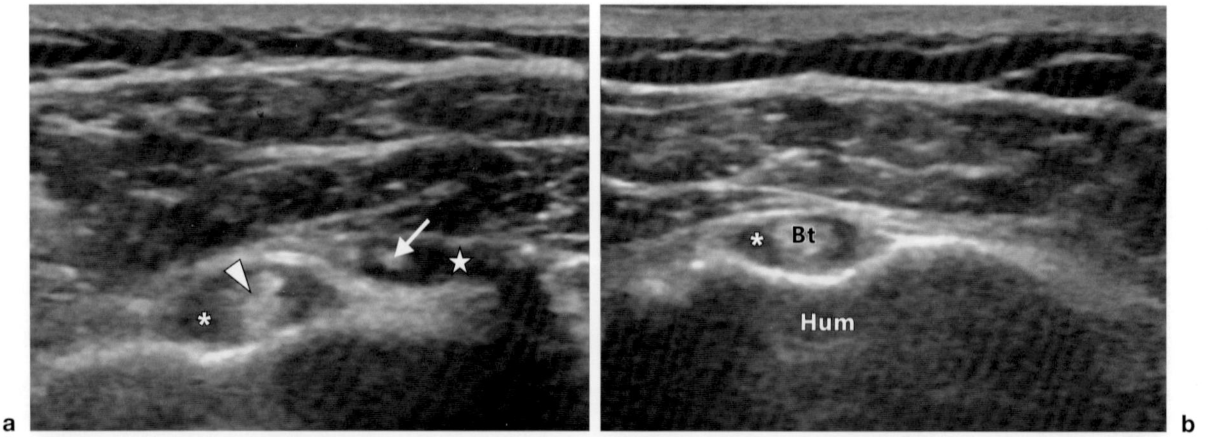

Axial US imaging shows fluid (*asterisk*) around the thickened (*arrowhead*) biceps tendon (**Bt**). Chronic subacromial bursitis containing the fluid (*star*) and synovial thickening (*arrow*) is also seen medially (**a**). Contralateral asymptomatic side with mild effusion (*asterisk*) (**b**).

Hum humerus

Expert note

Some fluid can be physiological; certainly above the age of 60, one often finds fluid in asymptomatic joints.

Biceps tenosynovitis in a 40-year-old man with anterior shoulder pain during arm movements for the last two months **2.7**

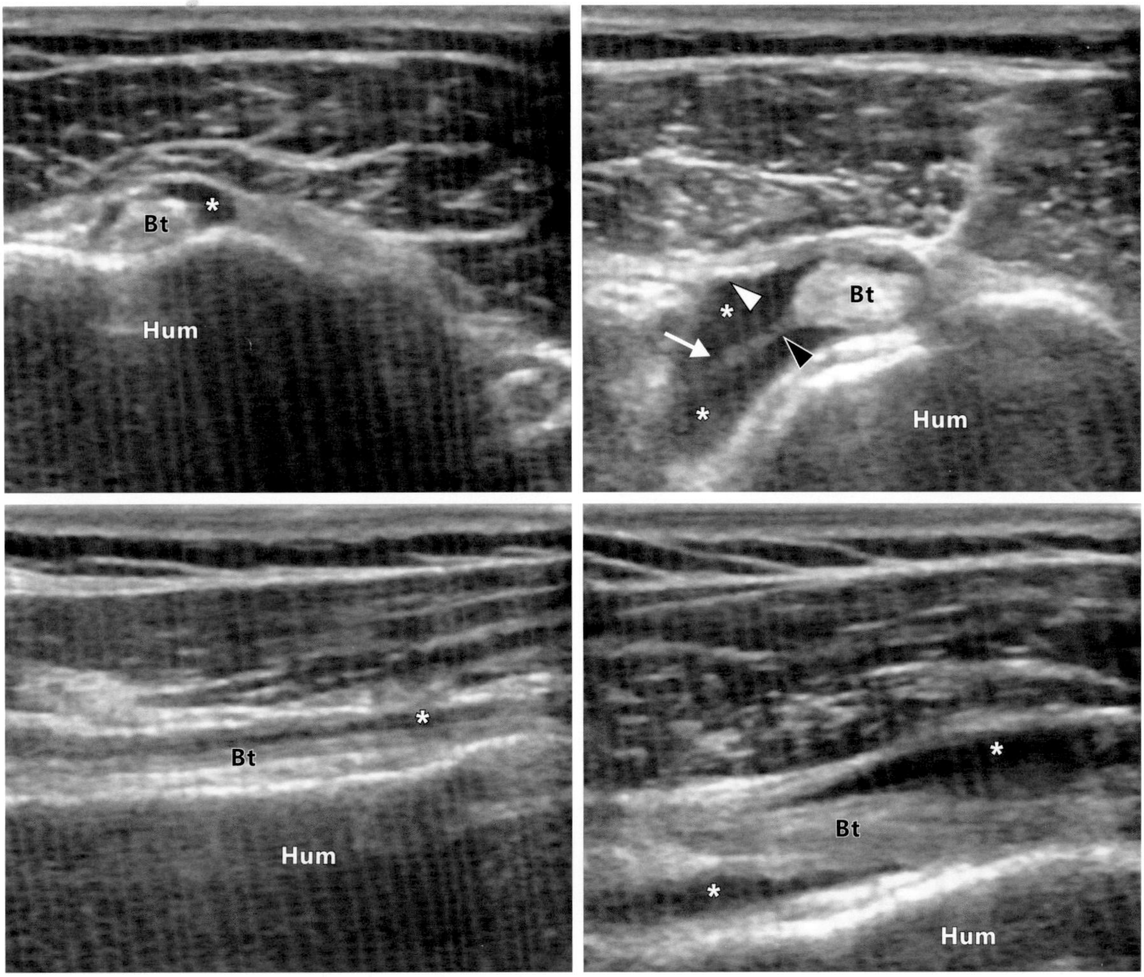

When compared with the normal biceps tendon (**Bt**) which displays a small amount of effusion (*asterisk*) (**a**, **c**), axial (**b**) and longitudinal (**d**) US images show enlarged biceps tendon with marked fluid (*asterisks*) around it. Please note that the presence of synovial effusion allows clear detection of the mesotenon (*arrow*) which connects the visceral (*black arrowhead*) and parietal (*white arrowhead*) layers of the synovial sheath and also serves as a passage for the feeding vessels.

Hum humerus

Expert note

The axial diameter of the long head of the biceps tendon is around 5.0 mm (less than 7.1 mm) [4].

2.8 Biceps tenosynovitis in a 56-year-old man with anterior shoulder pain 2 weeks after strenuous painting activity

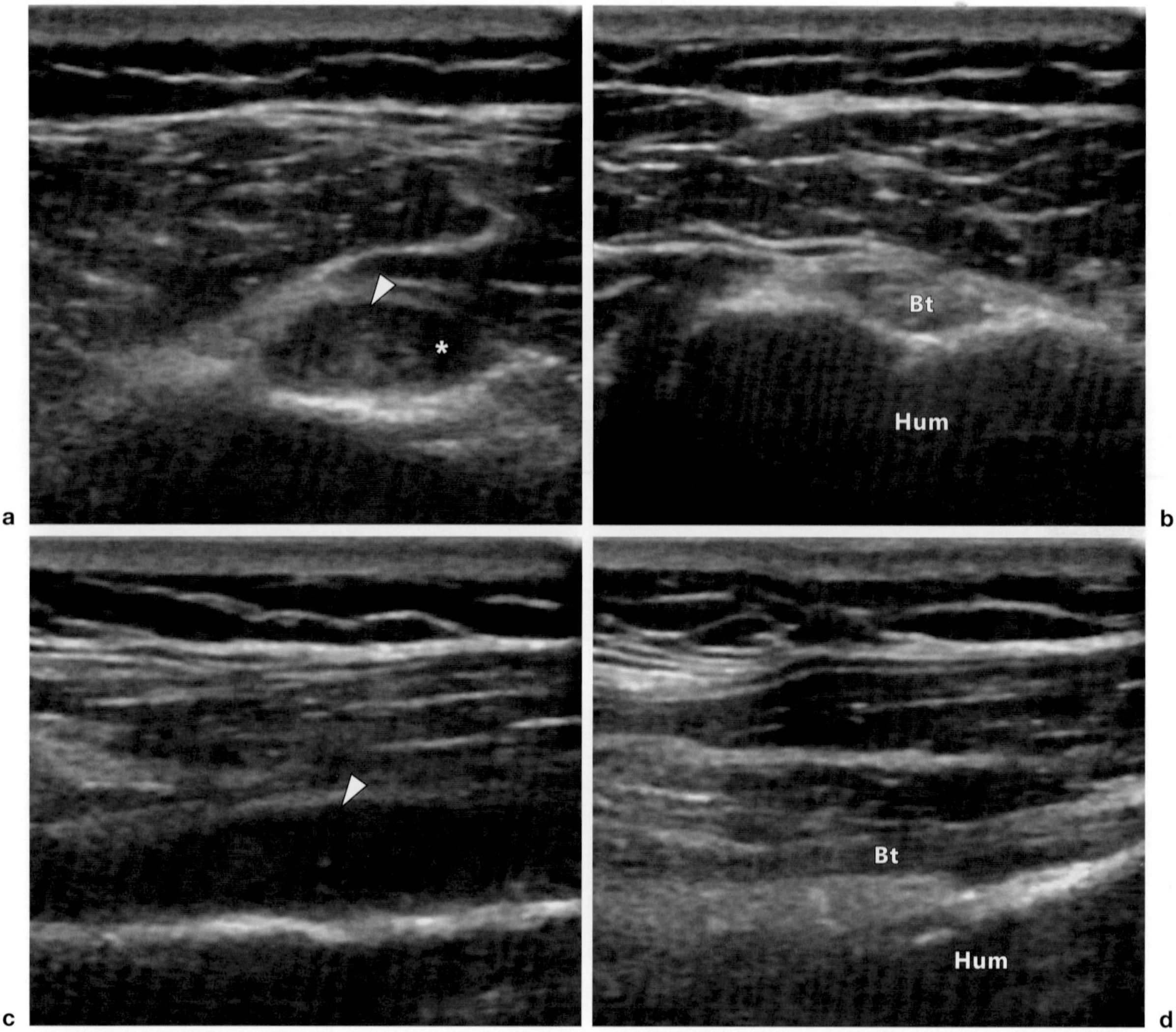

Axial (**a**) and longitudinal (**c**) US images demonstrate edematous and hypoechoic (*arrowheads*) biceps tendon (**Bt**) with some fluid (*asterisk*) around it. Normal side (**b**, **d**).

Hum humerus

Expert note

As elsewhere, imaging of the tendons also needs to be carried out in the following fashion: i. is the tendon present (as expected); ii. how is the shape (e.g. swollen, global or focal thinning); iii. how is the echogenicity and mobility?

Bicipital tenosynovitis in a 60-year-old man with chronic shoulder pain and vague weakness 2.9

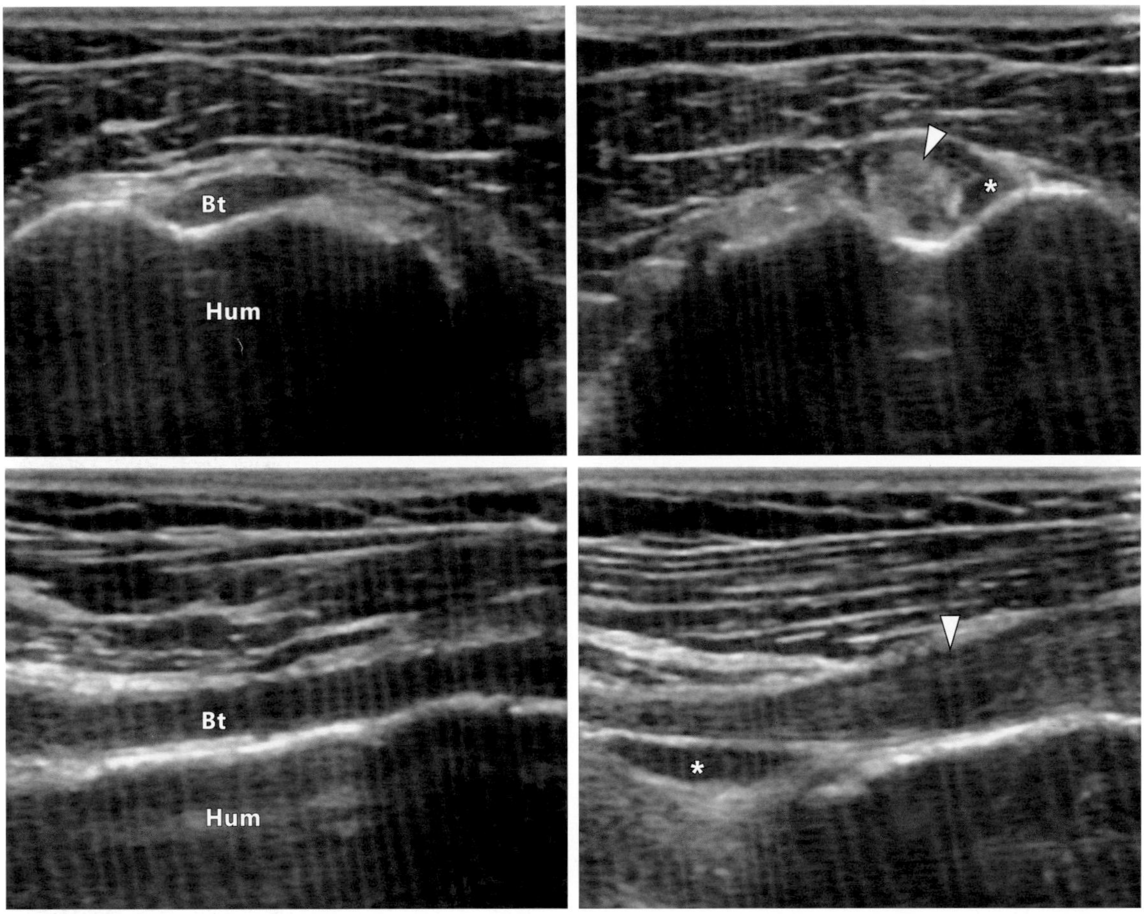

a b c d

When compared with the normal side (**a**, **c**), axial (**b**) and longitudinal (**d**) US images demonstrate heterogeneous and thickened appearance (*arrowheads*) of the biceps tendon (**Bt**) containing some fluid (*asterisks*) in the tendon sheath.

Hum humerus

Expert note

Depending on the probe angle (being parallel to the biceps tendon or not), anisotropy artifact can be seen and should not be misinterpreted as fluid.

2.10 Biceps tenosynovitis in a 45-year-old man suffering from chronic pain and tenderness in his shoulder

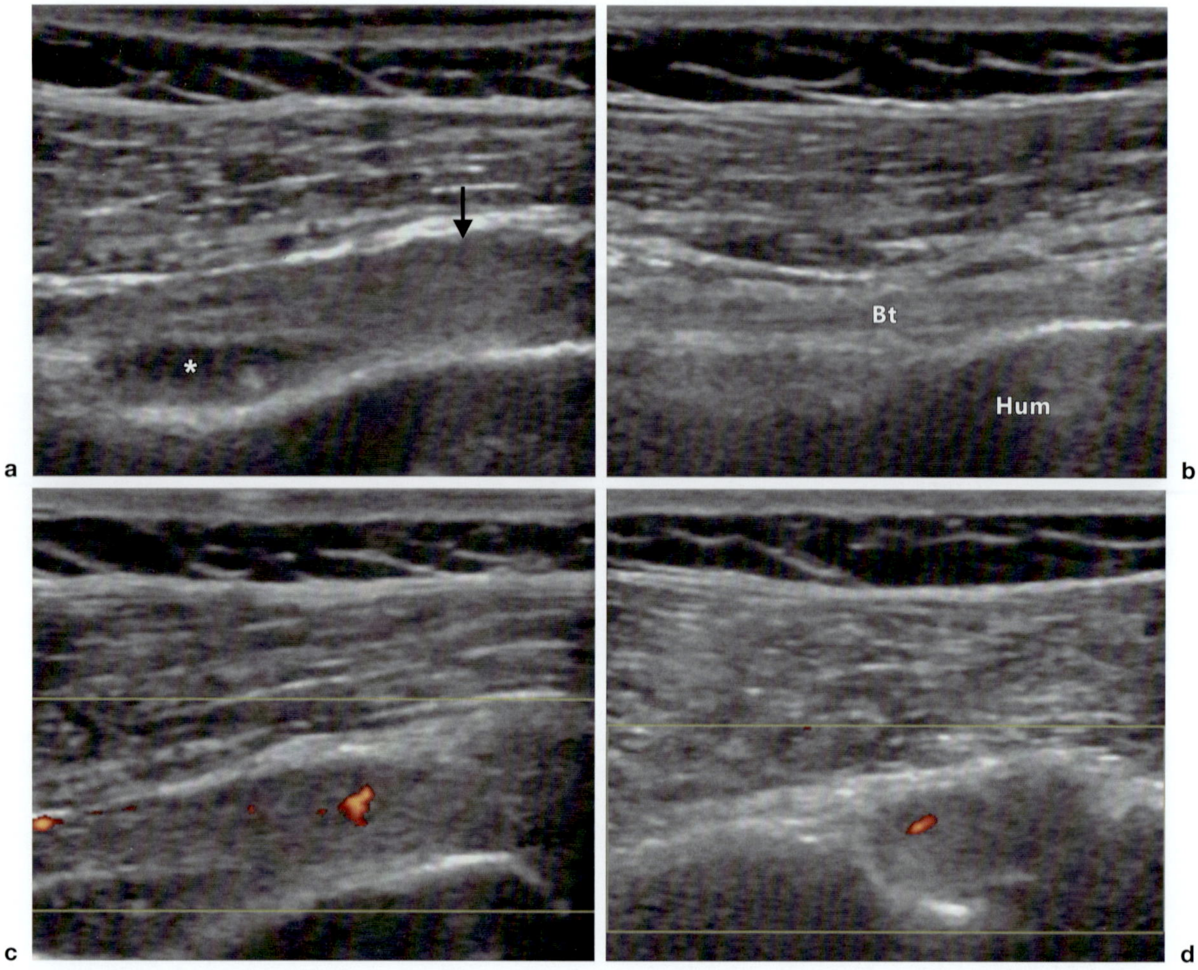

Longitudinal US image shows fluid (*asterisk*) around the biceps tendon (**Bt**) which appears as hypoechoic and swollen (*arrow*) (**a**). Normal contralateral side (**b**).
Power Doppler images show mild hyperemia as a sign of acute local inflammation inside the swollen tendon in both longitudinal (**c**) and axial (**d**) views.

Hum humerus

Biceps tenosynovitis in a 38-year-old woman suffering from tenderness over the proximal biceps groove after shoulder injury

2.11

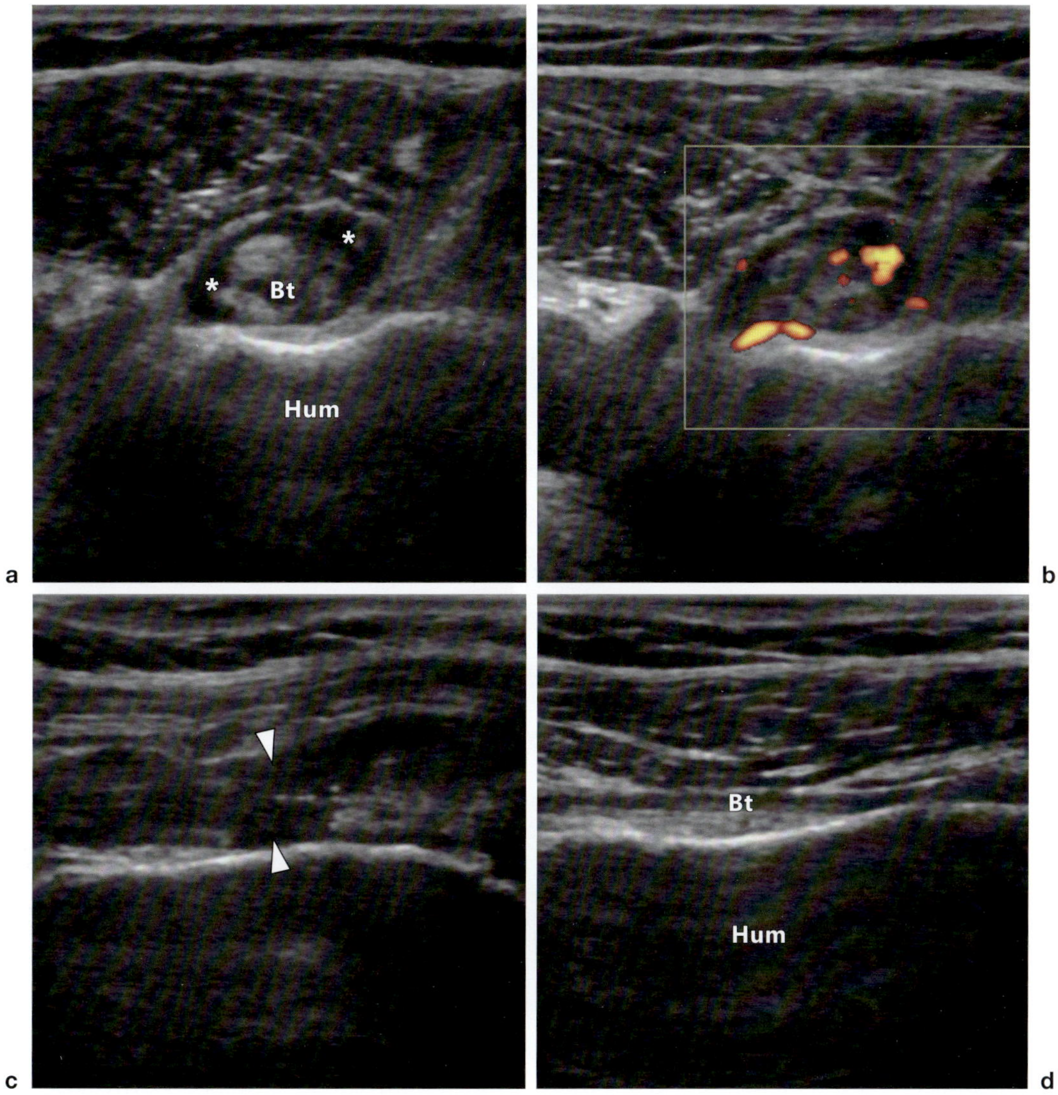

Speed's test was positive in physical examination.

Axial US images reveal swollen biceps tendon (**Bt**) with surrounding effusion (*asterisks*) (**a**), and moderate blood flow signals at power Doppler imaging (**b**). Comparative US images demonstrate the irregular/swollen (**c**) (*arrowheads*) and normal (**d**) tendons in the longitudinal view.

Hum humerus

2.12 Bilateral chronic biceps tendinopathy in a 47-year-old woman who had deep pain and discomfort in the anterior shoulder

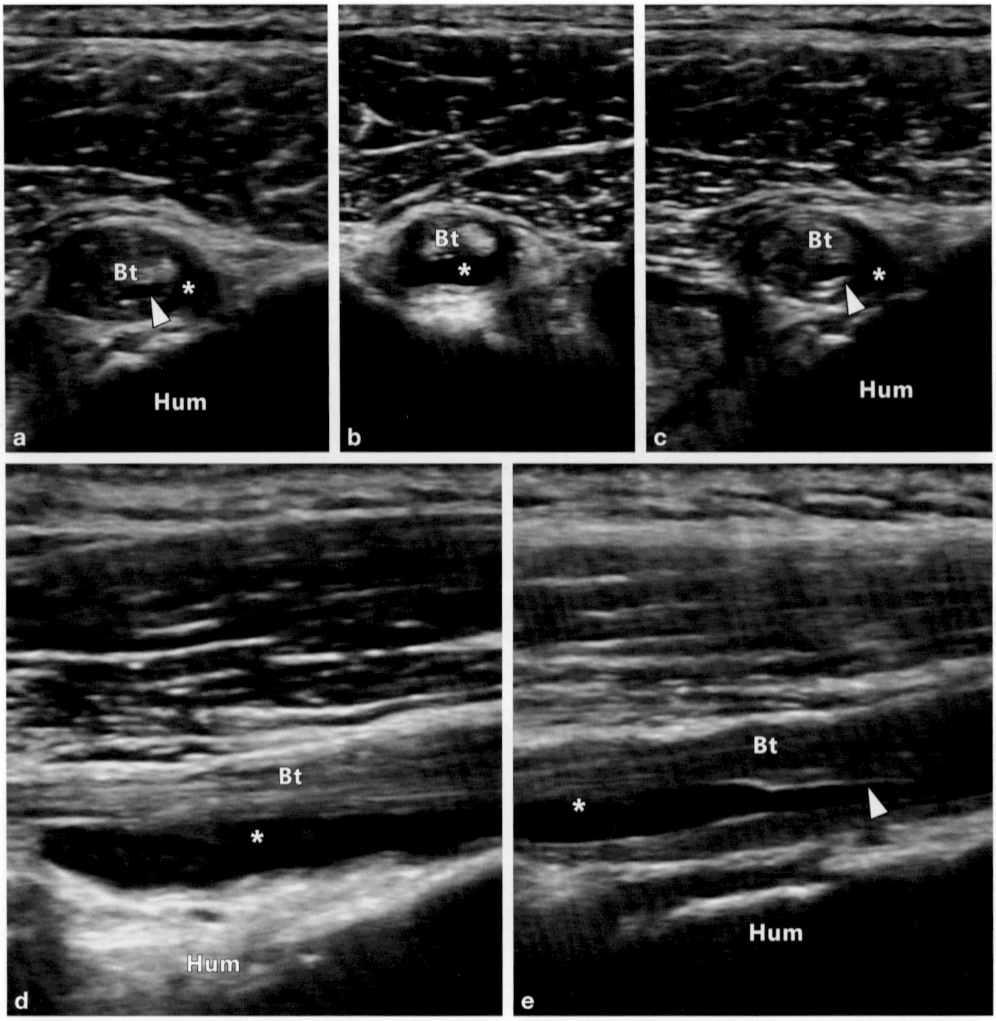

Axial US images of the biceps tendons (**Bt**) show mild (**a**) and moderate (**b**, **c**) amounts of fluid at different levels (*asterisks*) bilaterally (**b**). Corresponding longitudinal US images confirm the tendinopathies on both sides (**d**, **e**). Please note that the longitudinal views clarify that the small anechoic areas (*arrowheads*) are the extensions of fluid accumulation not intratendinous tears.

Hum humerus

Expert note

Once again, it is very important to perform imaging at least in two-axes and dynamically (from proximal to distal) to better understand the pathology from three-dimensional perspective.

Calcifying biceps tendinitis in an adult patient with adhesive capsulitis for about three months 2.13

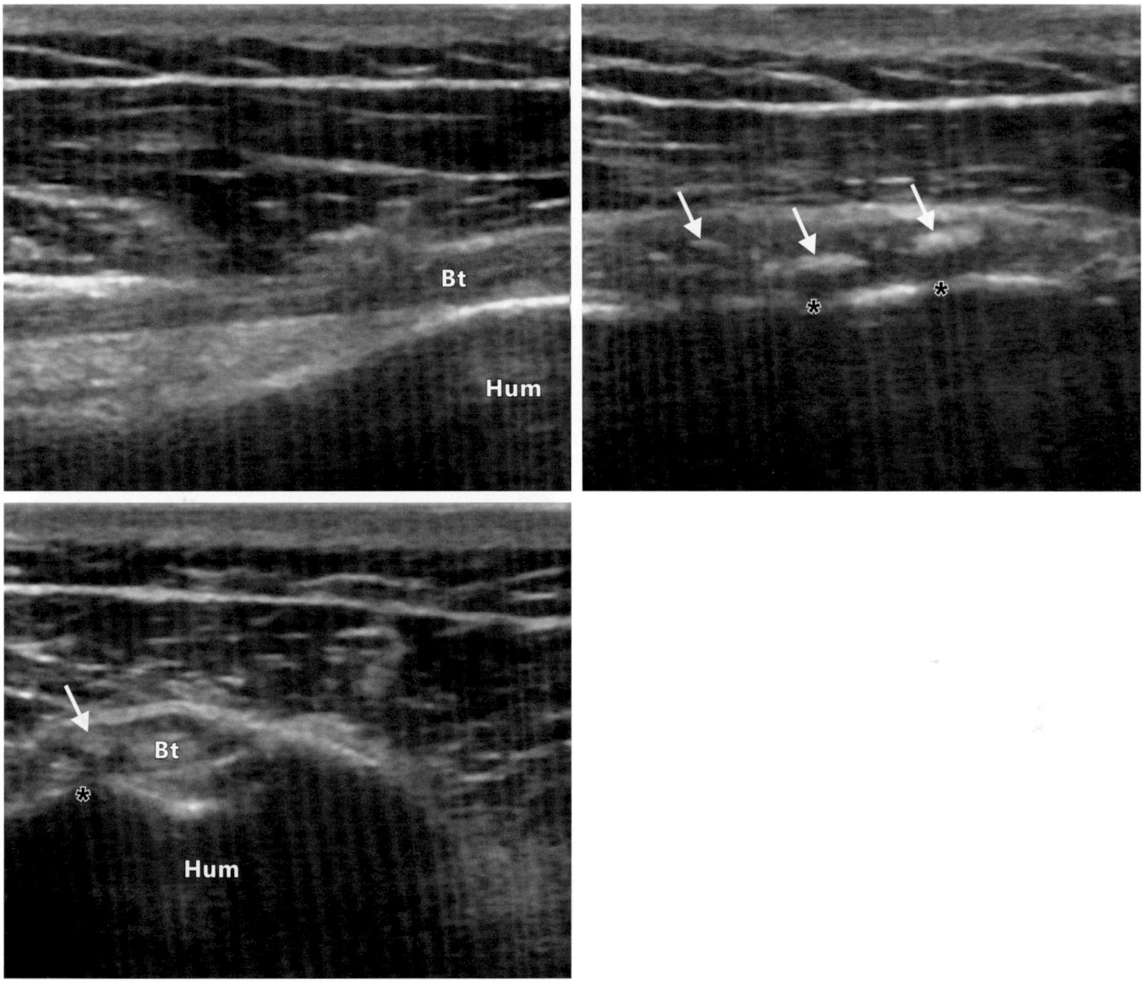

a b c

When compared with the normal biceps tendon (**Bt**) (**a**), longitudinal (**b**) and axial (**c**) US images illustrate hypoechoic and thickened tendon with Grade II hyperechoic calcifications (*arrows*) giving incomplete posterior acoustic shadowing artifacts (*asterisks*).

Hum humerus

2.14 Biceps tendon partial rupture in a 46-year-old man who reported pain and weakness around the shoulder

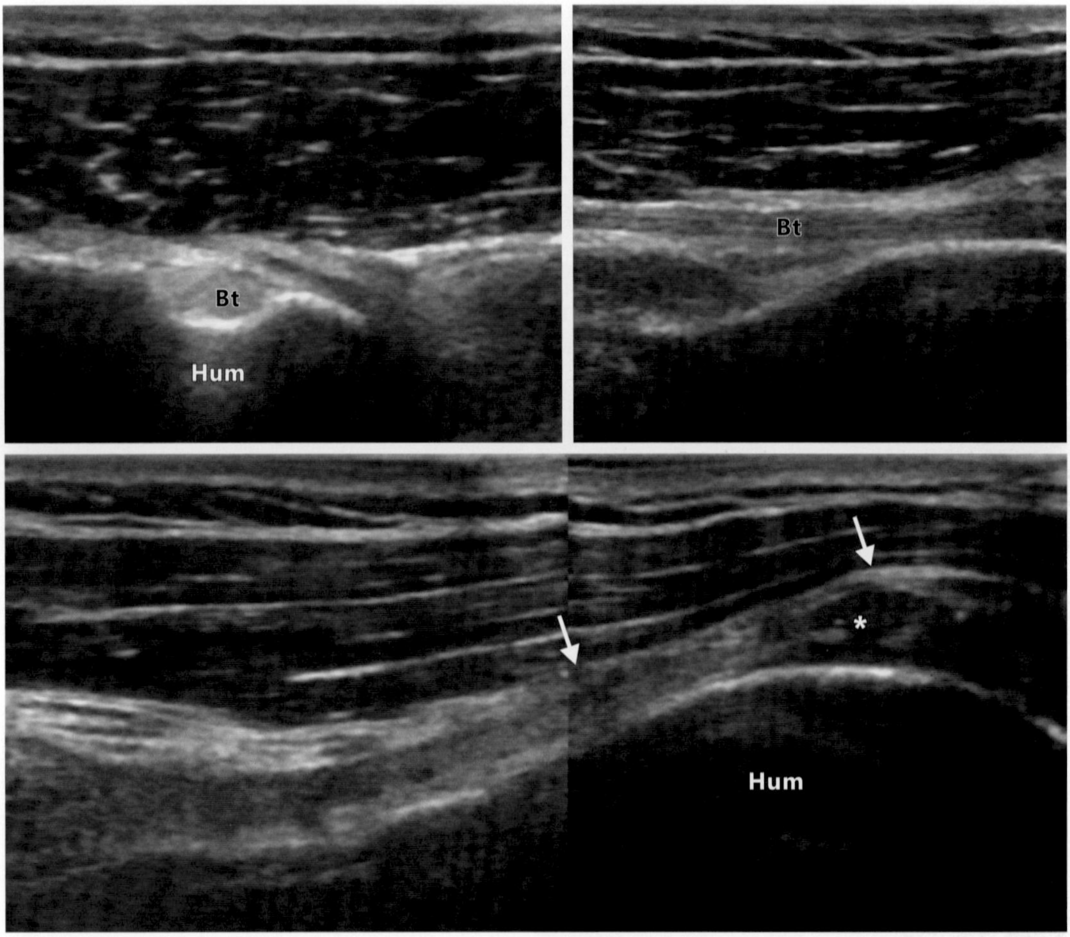

a b c

When compared with the normal axial (**a**) and longitudinal (**b**) US views of the biceps tendon (**Bt**); split-screen longitudinal image (**c**) illustrates irregular thickening of the proximal portion of the tendon (*arrows*) including hypoechoic defects (*asterisk*), consistent with chronic tear.

Expert note

Dynamic imaging (active/passive) would definitely yield additional findings as regards the ends of the rupture zone.

Acute biceps tendon tear in a 46-year-old woman who injured the arm while lifting weights **2.15**

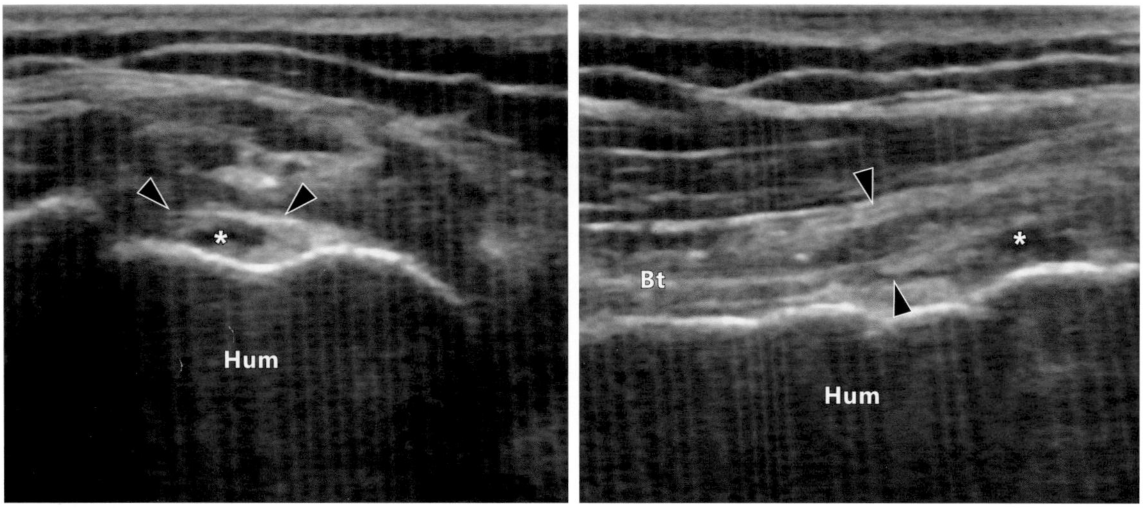

a b

She had tenderness and pain with no clear weakness.

Anterior axial (**a**) and longitudinal (**b**) US images illustrate small anechoic zone (*asterisks*) within the biceps tendon (**Bt**) which is heterogeneous and irregular (*arrowheads*).

Hum humerus

Proximal humeral epiphyseal growth plates in an otherwise healthy 9-year-old boy **2.16**

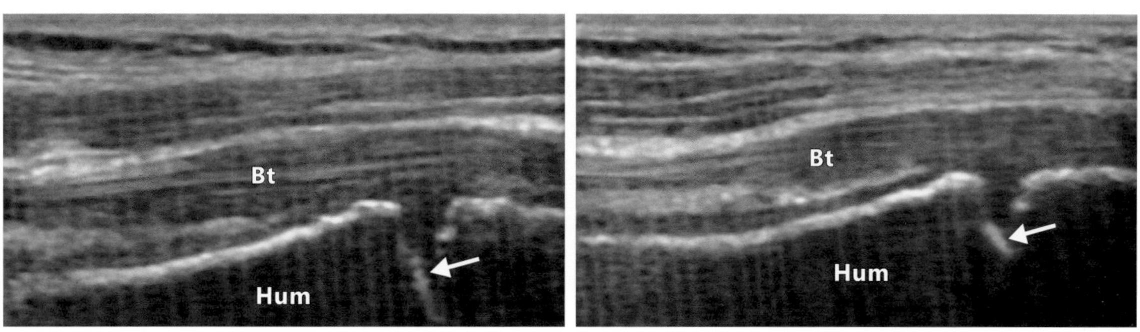

a b

Anterior longitudinal US images show normal epiphyses (*arrows*) of the humerus (**Hum**) and the overlying biceps tendons (**Bt**) (**a**, **b**).

Expert note

When two interrupted white lines are observed in US imaging, the possibility is one of the three: fracture, joint and epiphyseal plate.

2.17 Biceps tendon subluxation in a 49-year-old woman with painful clicking sensation while rotating her arm

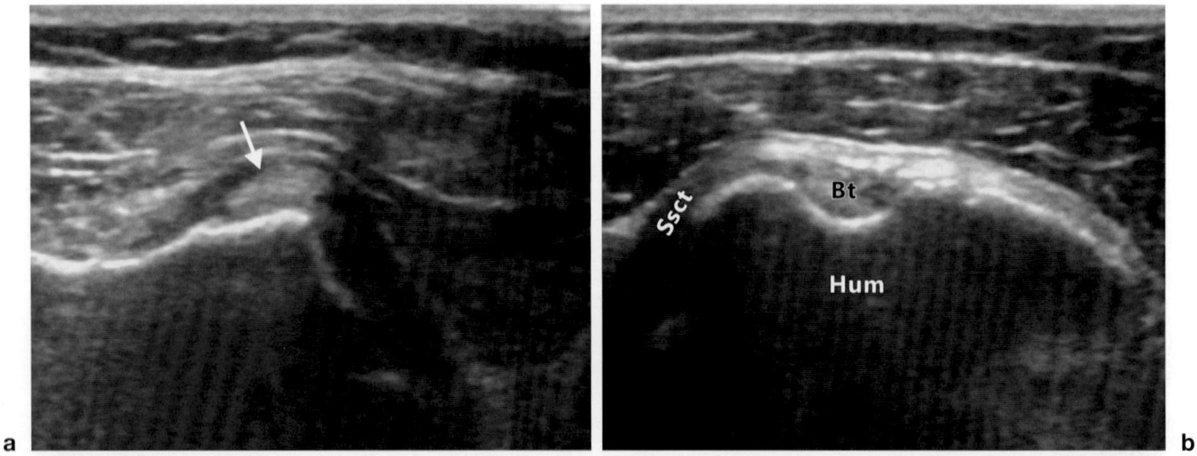

Anterior axial US image reveals subluxation of the biceps tendon (**Bt**) (*arrow*) medially (**a**). Normal contralateral side (**b**).

Hum humerus
Ssct subscapularis tendon

Subluxation of the biceps tendon in a 57-year-old man with bilateral shoulder pain during overhead activities 2.18

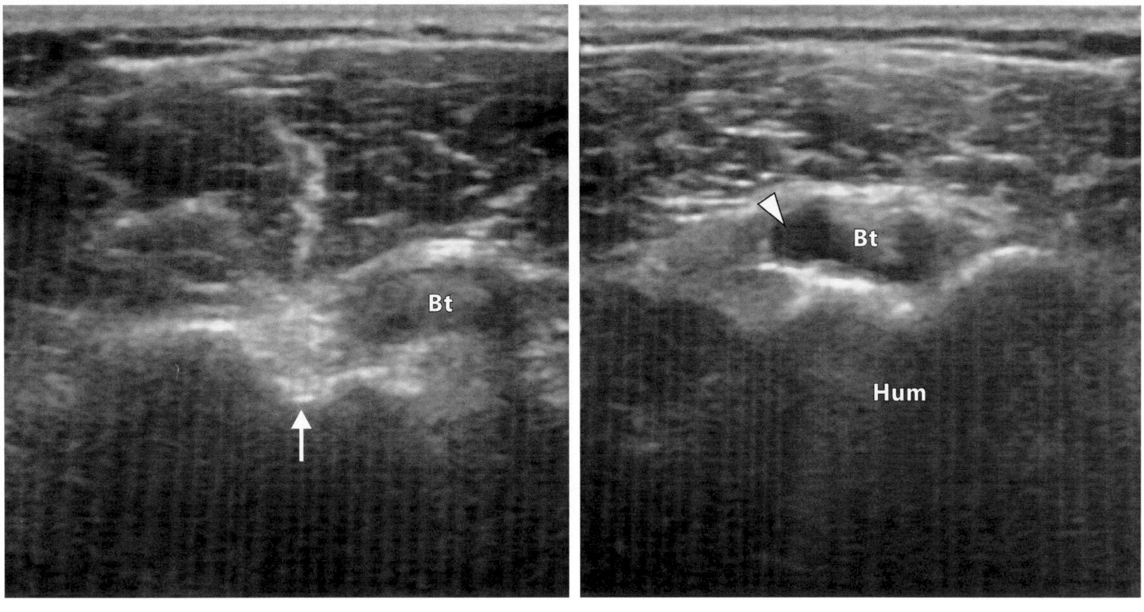

a b

Anterior axial US images demonstrate medial subluxation of the biceps tendon (**Bt**) from the bicipital groove (*arrow*) on one side (**a**), and a small amount of fluid (*arrowhead*) around the tendon on the other side (**b**).

Hum humerus

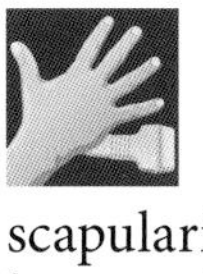

Expert note

Biceps tendon subluxation is usually towards the medial side; i.e. if the tendon is not present in its normal anatomical localization, it should initially be searched nearby the subscapularis tendon [5]. In case of biceps (sub)luxation, one should carefully examine the subscapularis tendon and look for a subscapularis rupture as well.

2.19 Bilateral biceps tendon subluxation in a 52-year-old man with painful snapping sensations

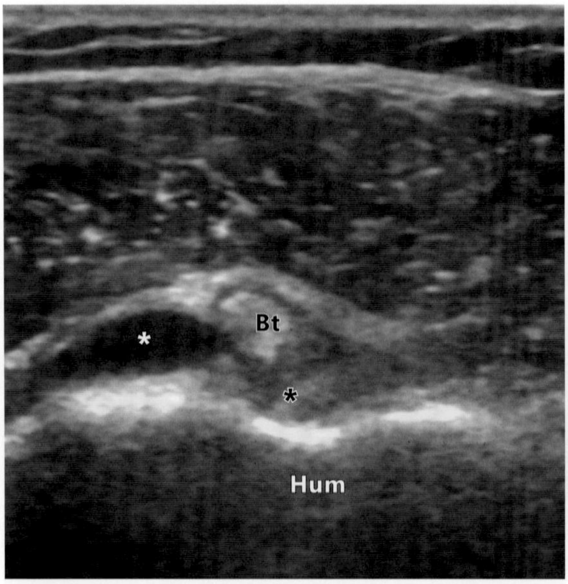

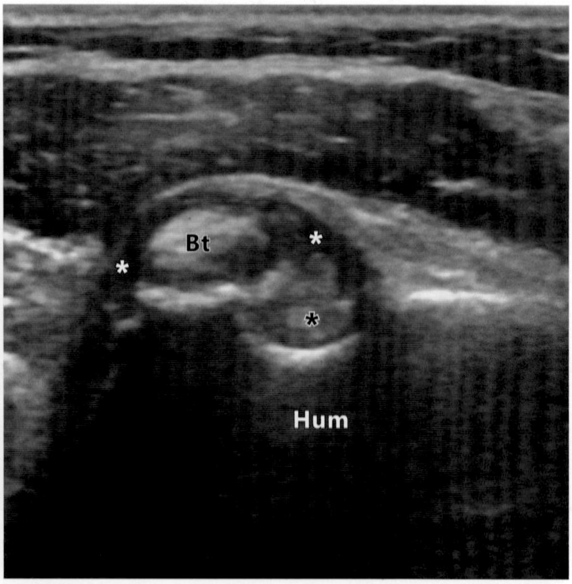

Anterior axial US images (**a**, **b**) illustrate abnormal fluid (*white asterisks*) around the subluxated biceps tendons (**Bt**). The hyperechoic fibrous scar tissue (*black asterisks*) within the groove -referred as "pseudobiceps" tendon- can be viewed on both sides.

Hum humerus

Biceps tendon rupture in a 75-year-old man after a sudden heavy lifting **2.20**

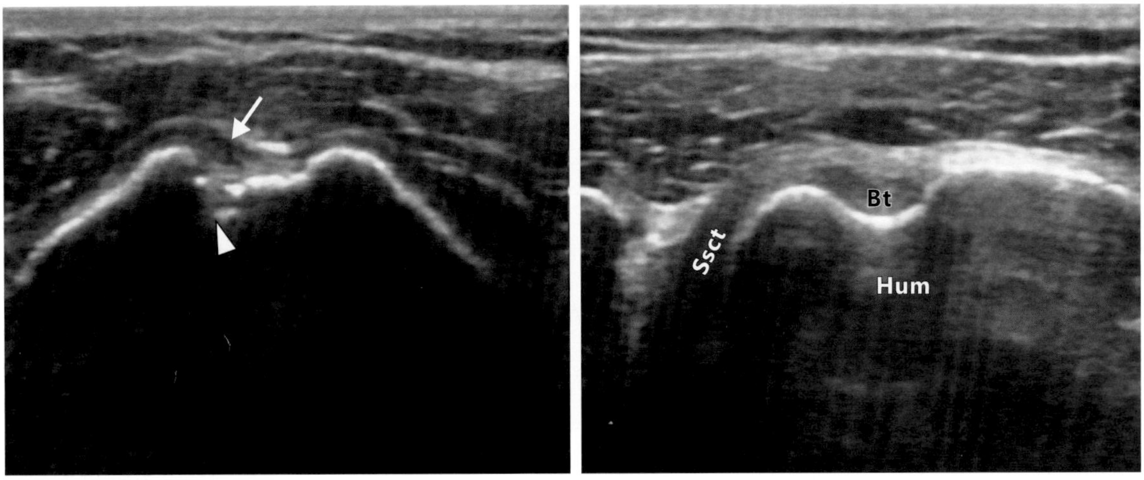

Anterior axial US imaging (**a**) demonstrates absence of the biceps tendon (**Bt**) (*arrow*) at the irregular groove (*arrowhead*). Normal side (**b**).

Hum humerus
Ssct subscapularis tendon

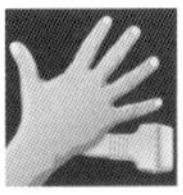

Expert note

Like in other rotator cuff ruptures, finding such irregularities on the bony cortex might raise suspicion as regards the cause of the overlying tendon tear. The vice versa might also be the case i.e. after a rupture, as not being protected by the overlying tendon anymore, the underlying cortex can become irregular after some time.

2.21 Subdeltoid bursitis in a 55-year-old man who had deep throbbing pain in the anterior shoulder

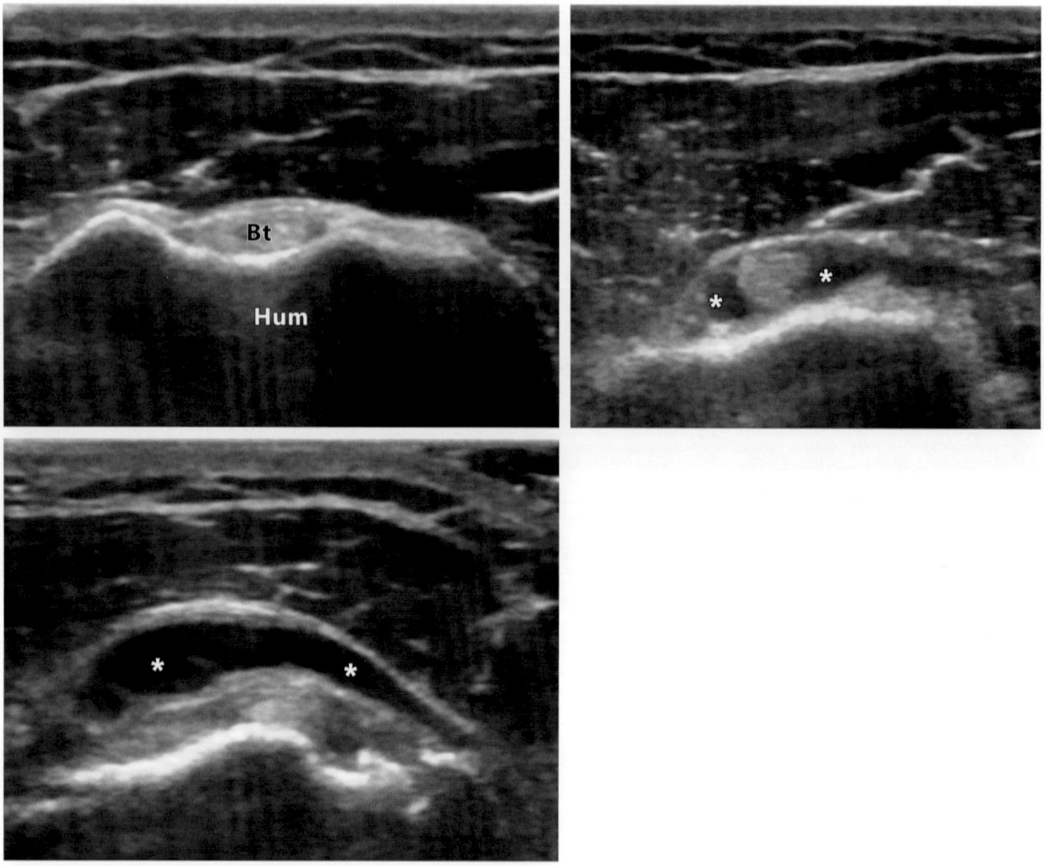

a b c

Speed's and Neer's tests were positive in physical examination.

When compared with the normal side (**a**), axial US images at different levels in the same patient revealed effusion (*asterisks*) around the biceps tendon (**Bt**) (**b**) and within the subdeltoid bursa (*asterisks*) (**c**).

Hum humerus

Expert note

Findings of both joint and bursal effusions have low sensitivity (22%) and high specificity (99%) in the diagnosis of rotator cuff tears [6]. As such, in case of fluid in two compartments (articular and bursal), one should do a very careful examination of the rotator cuff tendons to look for a full-thickness rupture.

Subdeltoid bursitis in a 50-year-old man who had night pain when he slept lying on the affected shoulder 2.22

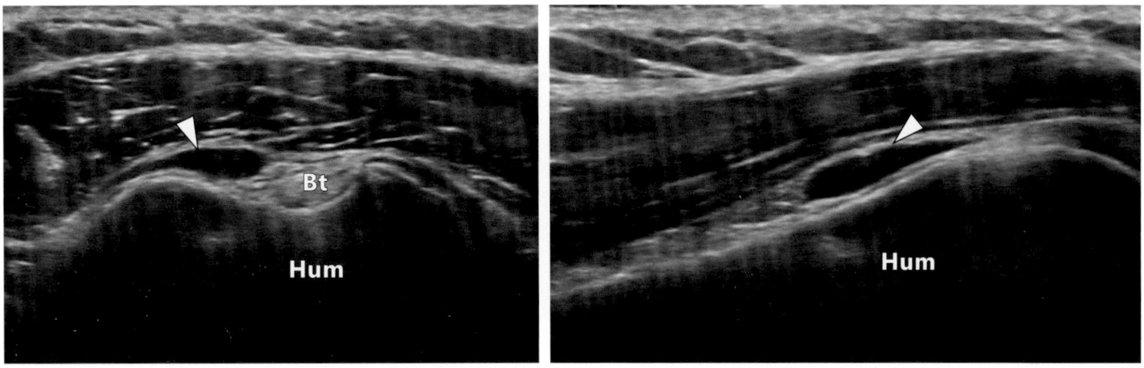

a b

Axial (**a**) and longitudinal (**b**) US images demonstrate moderate amount of fluid (*arrowheads*) inside the subdeltoid bursa extending distally.

Bt biceps tendon
Hum humerus

Expert note

Owing to its appearance, the extension of the subdeltoid bursa over the lateral side of the humerus in the longitudinal view is referred as "teardrop" sign.

2.23 Chronic subdeltoid bursitis in a 40-year-old woman with dull shoulder pain disturbing her sleep at night

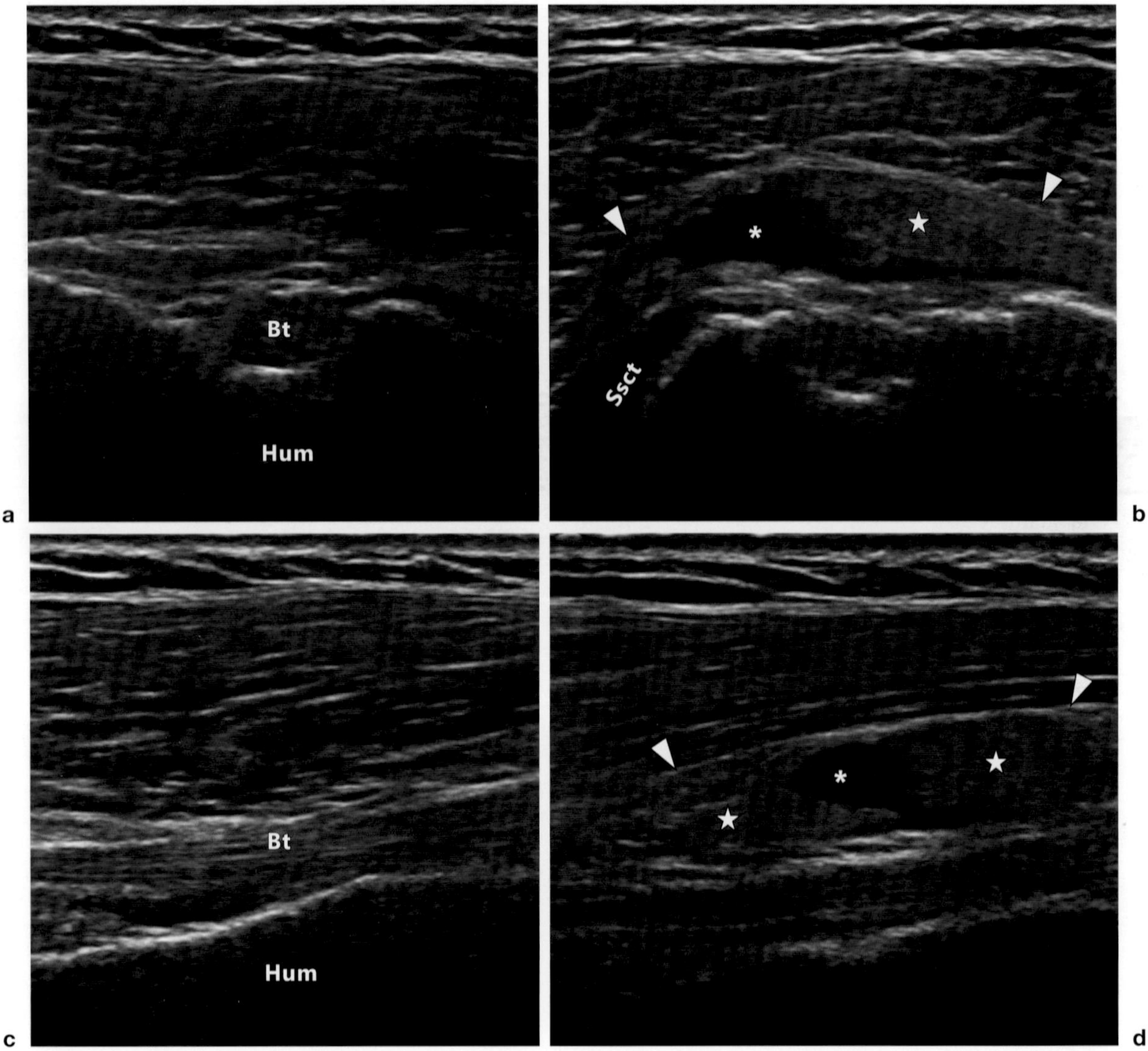

When compared with the normal side (**a**, **c**), axial (**b**) and longitudinal (**d**) images reveal fluid (*asterisks*) and marked synovial hypertrophy (*stars*) within the subdeltoid bursa (*arrowheads*).

Bt biceps tendon
Hum humerus
Ssct subscapularis tendon

Chronic subdeltoid bursitis in a 45-year-old woman with severe night pain **2.24**

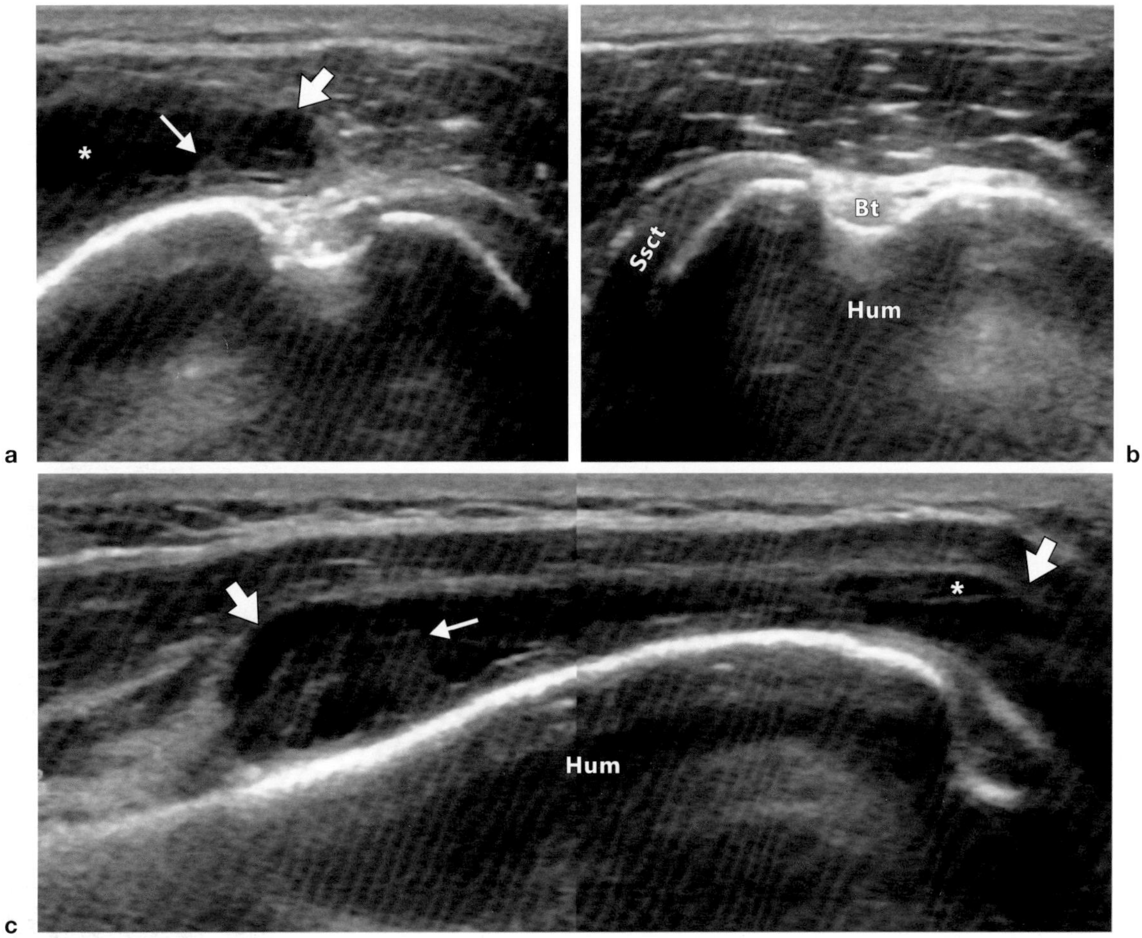

Anterior axial (**a**) and longitudinal split-screen (**c**) US images show chronic subdeltoid bursitis (*thick arrows*). Normal contralateral side in the axial view (**b**). Please note the presence of synovial hypertrophy (*thin arrows*) in addition to fluid (*asterisks*), suggesting chronicity.

Bt biceps tendon
Hum humerus
Ssct subscapularis tendon

Expert note

Detection of synovial hypertrophy is important during the examination for two reasons: first, it implies that the effusion is more likely to be chronic; second, if an intervention is planned, US-guidance will definitely help for prompt/complete drainage.

2.25 Chronic subacromial bursitis in a 66-year-old woman with a 6-month history of shoulder pain without any trauma

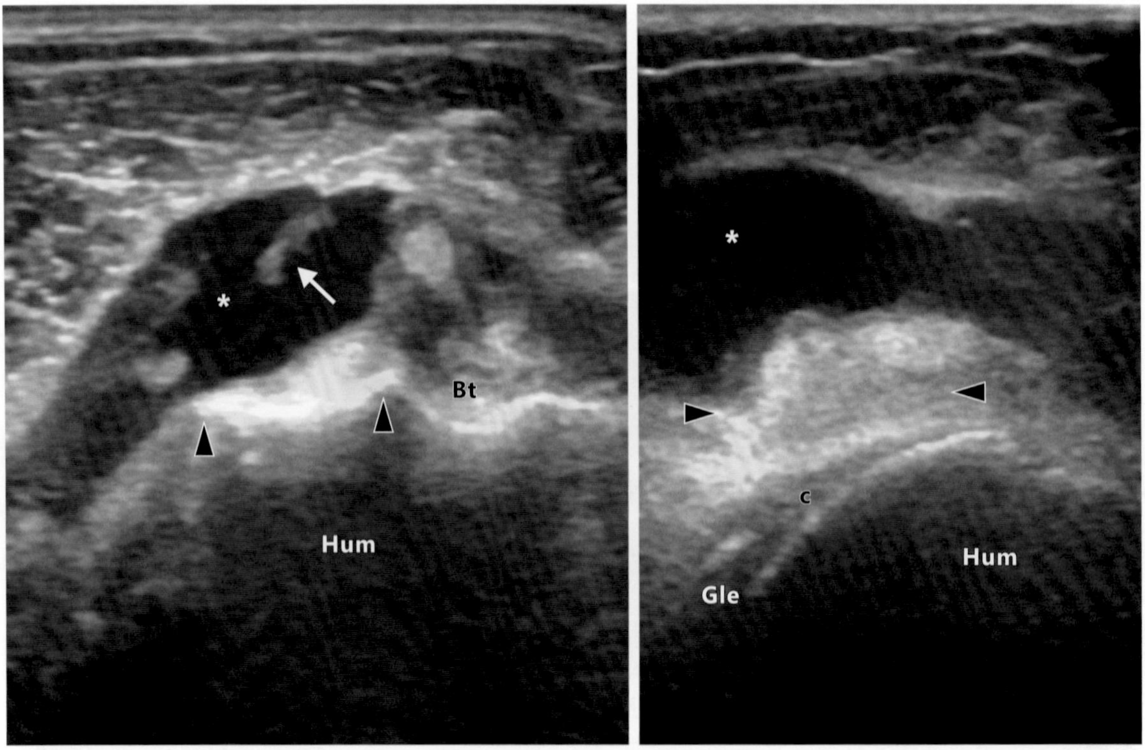

a b

Anterior (**a**) and posterior (**b**) axial US images clearly depict significant anechoic fluid collection (*asterisks*) and synovial hypertrophy (*arrow*) in the subdeltoid bursa. Also note the underlying enhanced through-transmission artifacts (*arrowheads*).

Bt	biceps tendon	**Gle**	glenoid
c	cartilage	**Hum**	humerus

Expert note

Since the subdeltoid bursa is an irregularly shaped 3-dimensional potential space, especially in acute fluid collections (like elsewhere), probe compressions might easily displace the fluid within the bursa. While this could cause a misdiagnosis initially, it might erroneously guide (i.e. easily refrain from) a necessary intervention as well. Yet, aside from "seeing is believing", another general rule for US-guided interventions would be "if/where you see, you can have access to it". In case of chronic bursitis, one should also/carefully examine the different cuff tendons; yet, there is very often an underlying tendon problem.

Chronic subdeltoid bursitis in a 52-year-old man with severe shoulder pain and tenderness on the anterior shoulder

2.26

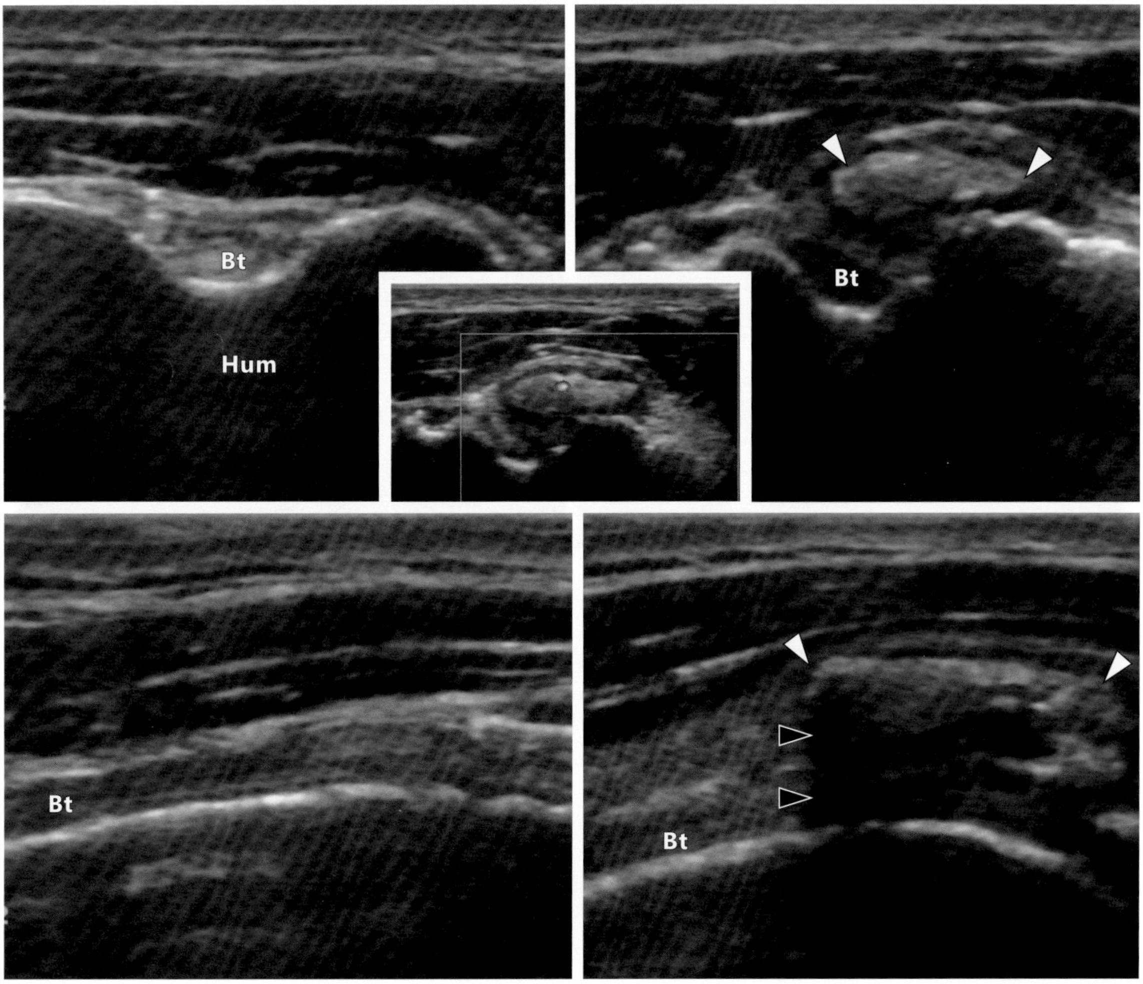

a b c d

When compared with the normal side (**a**, **c**), axial (**b**) and longitudinal (**d**) US images obtained over the anterior shoulder show Grade II calcification (*white arrowheads*) inside the subdeltoid bursa with incomplete posterior acoustic shadowing artifact (*black arrowheads*). Power Doppler imaging depicts a single blood flow signal (*small figure*).

Bt biceps tendon
Hum humerus

Expert note

Although this calcification might be an immature one, it should be kept in mind that the other possibility would be a disintegrating one.

2.27 Chronic subacromial bursitis in a 50-year-old woman with rheumatoid arthritis

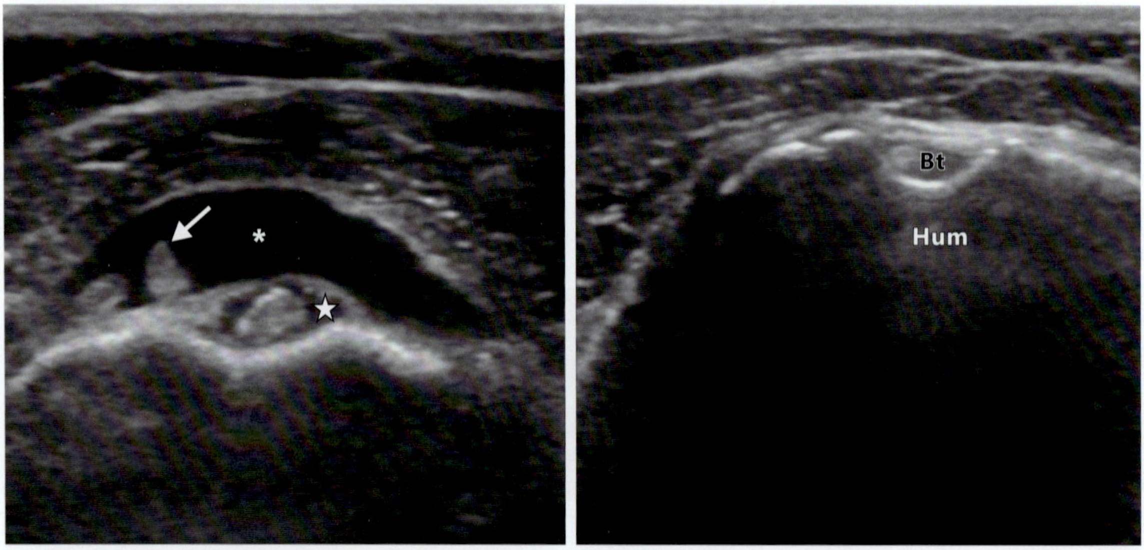

a b

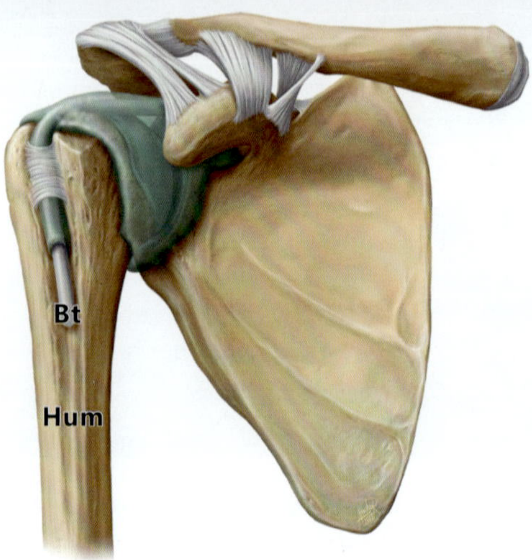

She described anterolateral shoulder pain particularly with abduction and flexion.

Anterior axial US imaging shows fluid accumulation (*asterisk*) with synovial folds (*arrow*) in the subdeltoid bursa and a small amount of fluid within the biceps tendon (**Bt**) sheath (*star*) (**a**). Normal contralateral side (**b**).

Hum humerus

Expert note

When the rotator cuff is intact, these two areas (subdeltoid bursa and bicipital tendon sheath) do not have any communication. Accordingly, there needs to be separate punctures if one plans to have access to both spaces. On the other hand, in case of a full-thickness rupture, injection/aspiration to either compartment would suffice.

Chronic subdeltoid bursitis in a 51-year-old man with anterior shoulder pain and rheumatoid arthritis **2.28**

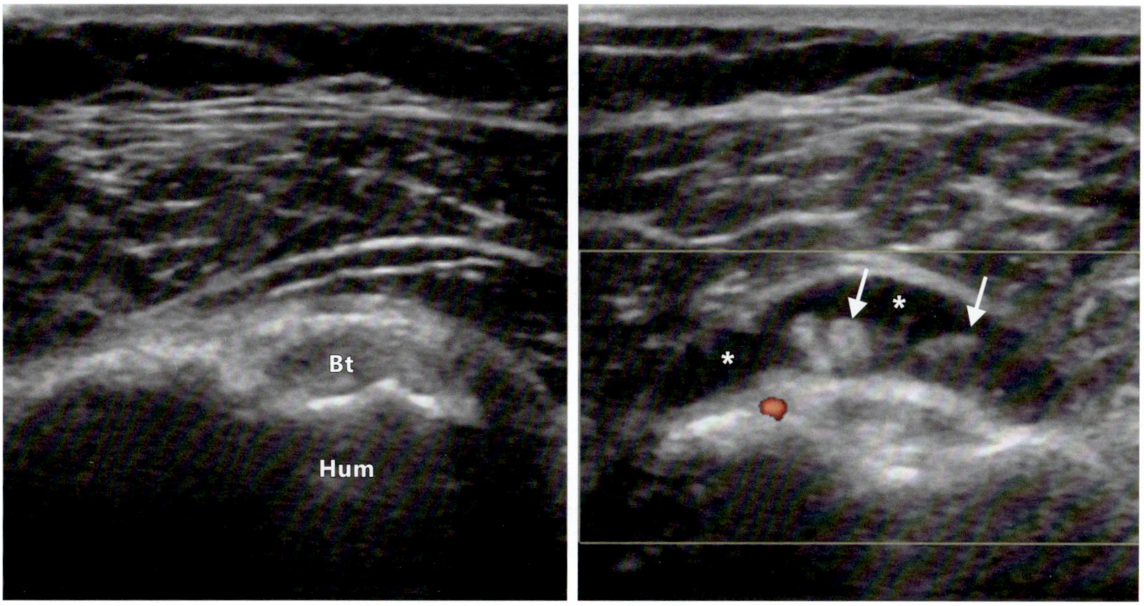

a b

When compared with the normal side (**a**), axial US image shows extensive effusion (*asterisks*) and synovial folds (*arrows*) within the subdeltoid bursa (**b**). Power Doppler image shows no signal for active inflammation but only the ascending branch of the anterior circumflex humeral artery (**b**).

Bt biceps tendon
Hum humerus

2.29 Subdeltoid bursitis and bicipital tenosynovitis in an elderly patient with Parkinson disease

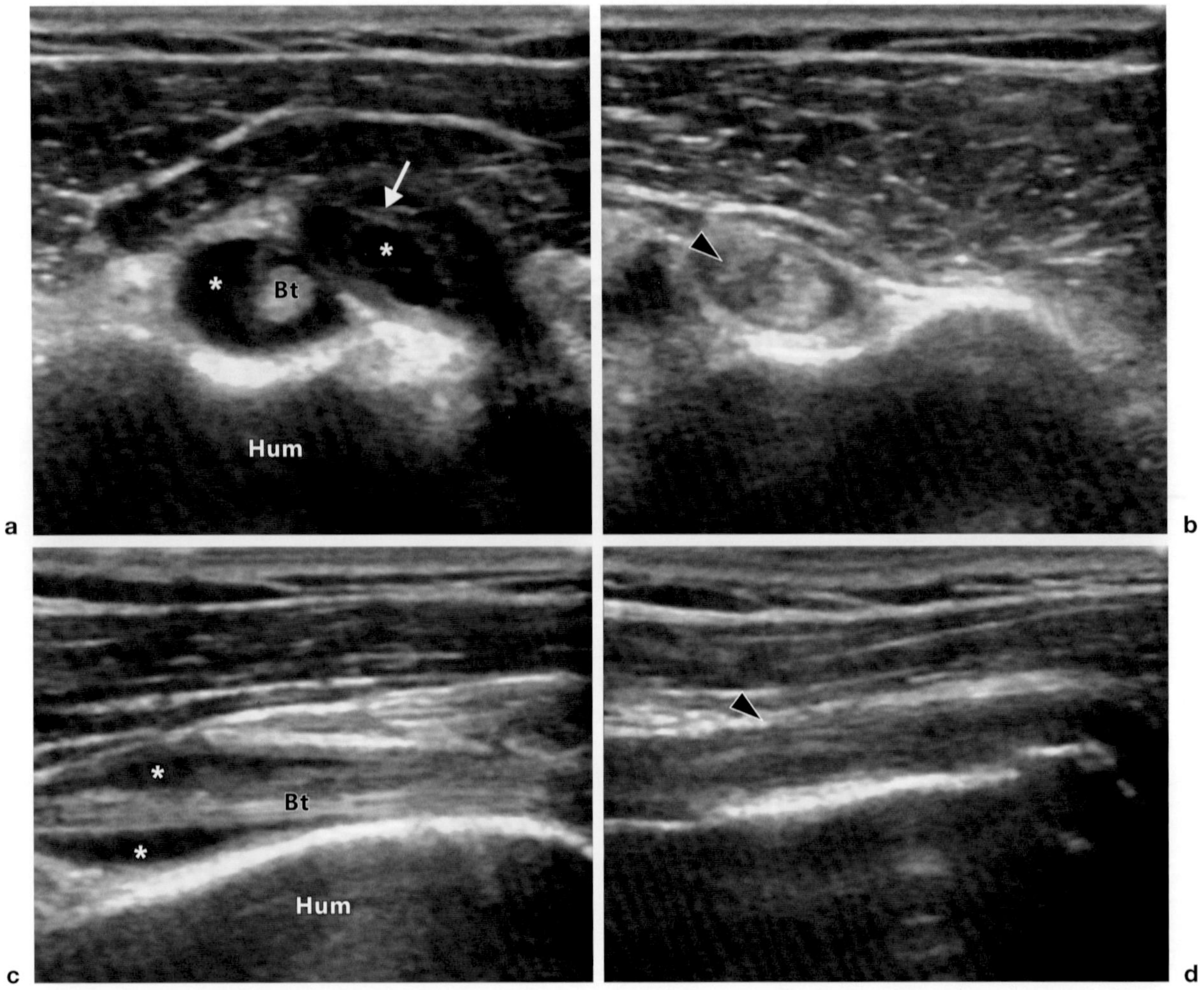

Axial US image demonstrates effusion (*asterisks*) around the biceps tendon (**Bt**) and inside the subdeltoid bursa which also contains synovial thickenings (*arrow*) (**a**). Bicipital tendinopathy (*arrowhead*) is more due to tendon edema than effusion on the contralateral side (**b**). Corresponding longitudinal images are confirmatory (**c**, **d**).

Hum humerus

Subacromial bursitis and bicipital tenosynovitis in a 55-year-old woman with severe shoulder pain 2.30

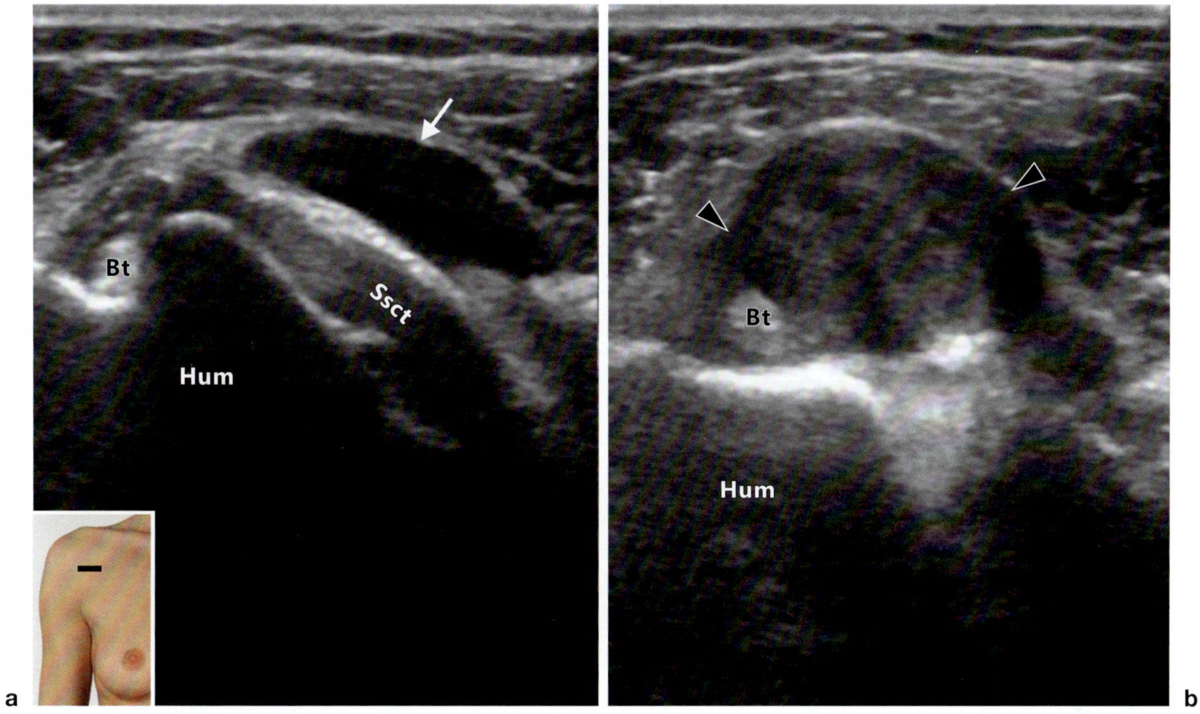

Axial US imaging obtained over the anterior shoulder demonstrates extensive fluid (*arrow*) distending the subdeltoid bursa (**a**). Contralateral side demonstrates significant enlargement of the biceps tendon (**Bt**) sheath which is almost completely filled with hypertrophied synovium (*arrowheads*) (**b**).

Hum humerus
Ssct subscapularis tendon

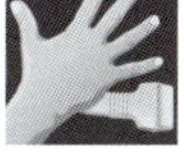

Expert note

The role of US imaging is paramount for clinical decision making; i.e. in this patient where and how to enter [2]. Yet, while "blind injectors" would prefer to use the lateral approach, appropriate way of injection would be more anterior and perhaps also easily with a smaller needle. Likewise, for the contralateral side, this image would prompt only a corticosteroid injection and avoid unnecessary attempts of aspiration.

2.31 Chronic bursitis in a 51-year-old man with pain and discomfort (particularly at night)

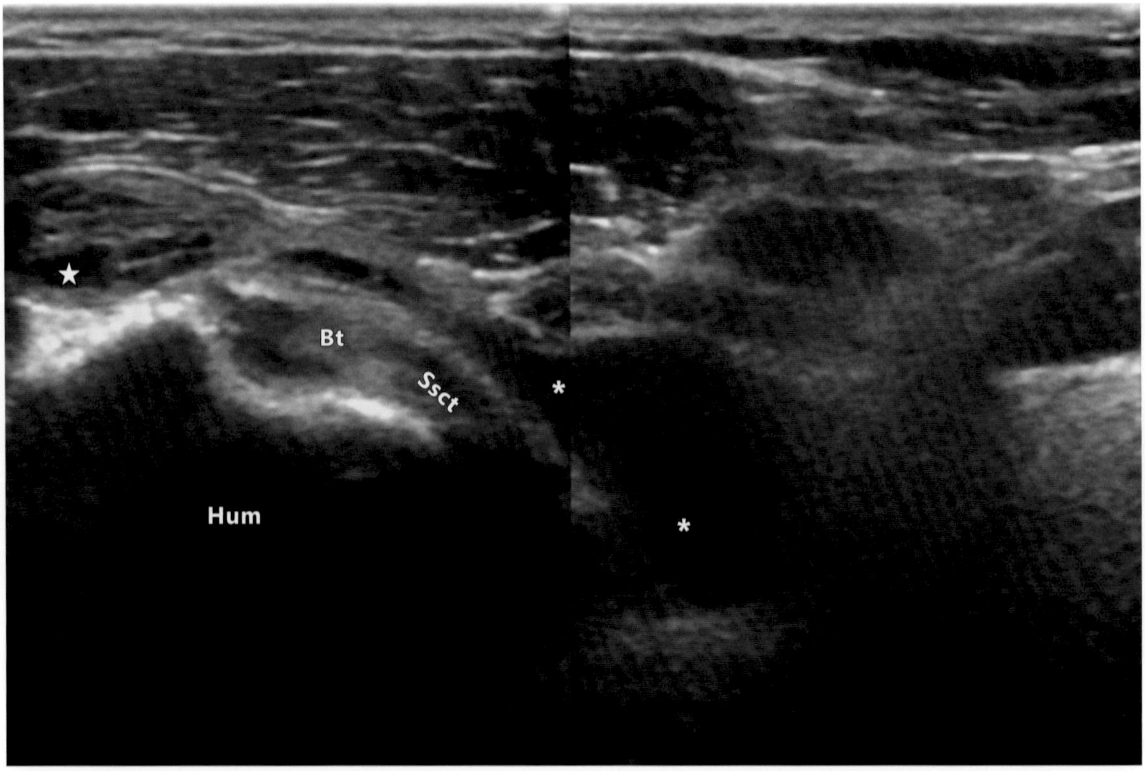

Split-screen axial US imaging demonstrates effusion and synovial thickenings (*star*) in the subdeltoid bursa whereby the collection is seen to extend and accumulate more medially (*asterisks*) over the subscapularis tendon (**Ssct**).

Bt biceps tendon
Hum humerus

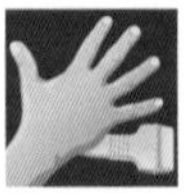

Expert note

Once again, this atypical localization of the fluid exemplifies how challenging the drainage of such a bursa would be unless performed with the guidance of US imaging.

Shoulder

Subacromial bursitis in a 73-year-old diabetic woman with severe shoulder pain (worse at night) 2.32

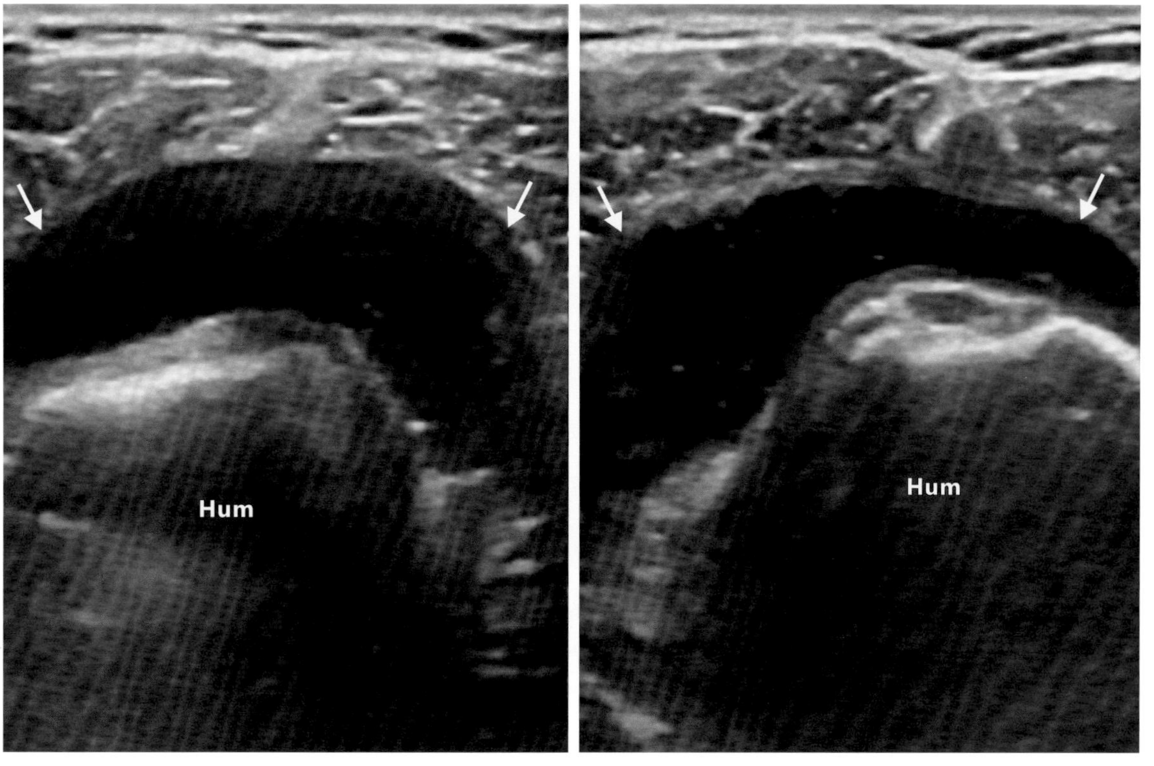

Axial US images over the anterior aspect of the shoulder reveal bilateral subdeltoid bursitis with abundant fluid (*arrows*) (**a**, **b**).

Hum humerus

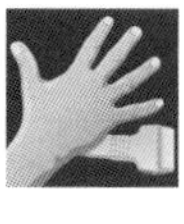

Expert note

Especially in patients with night pain, simple detection/drainage of the bursal fluid would have a tremendous effect on the patient's quality of life.

2.33 Chronic subacromial bursitis in a 45-year-old rheumatoid arthritis patient with shoulder pain and discomfort

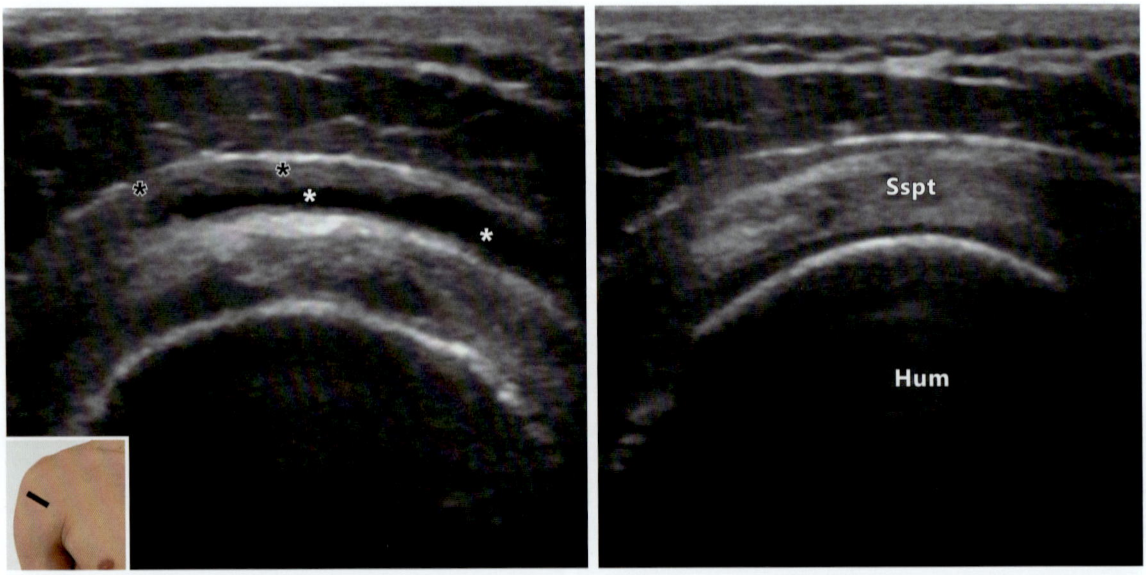

a b

Axial US imaging in Crass position shows some fluid (*white asterisks*) and chronic synovial changes (*black asterisks*) in the subdeltoid bursa (**a**). Normal side (**b**).

Hum humerus
Sspt supraspinatus tendon

Expert note

Like elsewhere, the nature of bursitis might give an idea as regards the duration/nature of the process which would definitely be prompting the relevant intervention as well.

Subacromial bursitis in a 21-year-old woman with shoulder pain and tenderness for about two months **2.34**

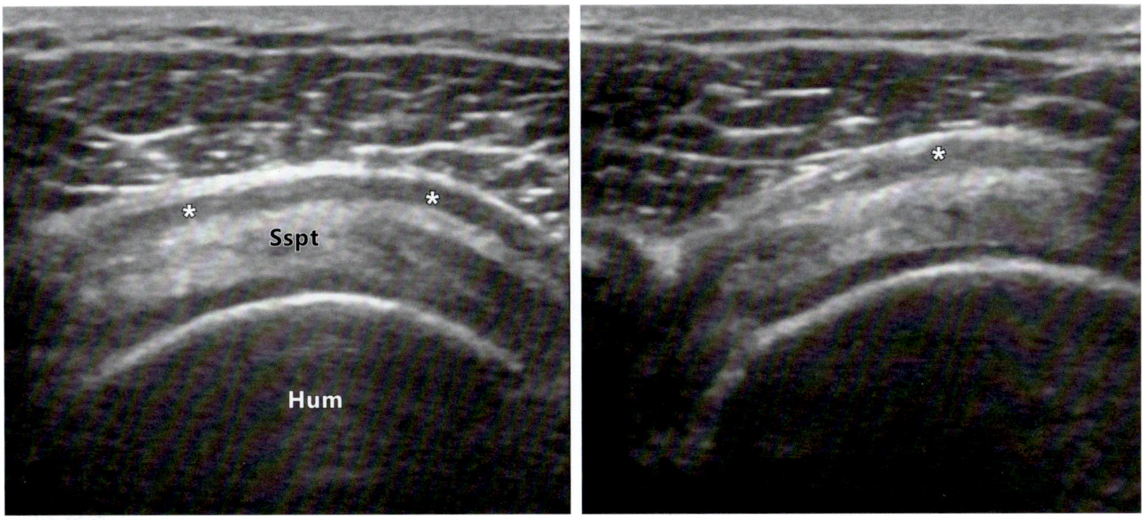

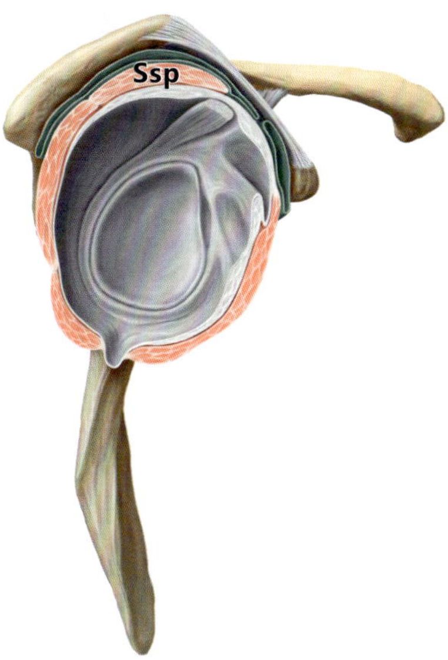

Axial US images in Crass position show bilateral mild enlargement of the subdeltoid bursae (*asterisks*) with hypoechoic effusion. Supraspinatus tendons (**Sspt**) seem to retain normal appearance.

Hum humerus

Expert note

Normal subdeltoid-subacromial bursa can be seen as a very thin an/hypoechoic line (less than 2 mm) between the deltoid muscle and the supraspinatus tendon. This space might be a little increased (the layers separated) in Crass position though. As such, before diagnosing as bursitis, sonographers should think twice (also in accordance with the clinical findings) and perform side-to-side comparison as well [2].

2.35 Bilateral subdeltoid bursitis in a 59-year-old woman with a 3-week history of shoulder pain that is worse by movement and at night

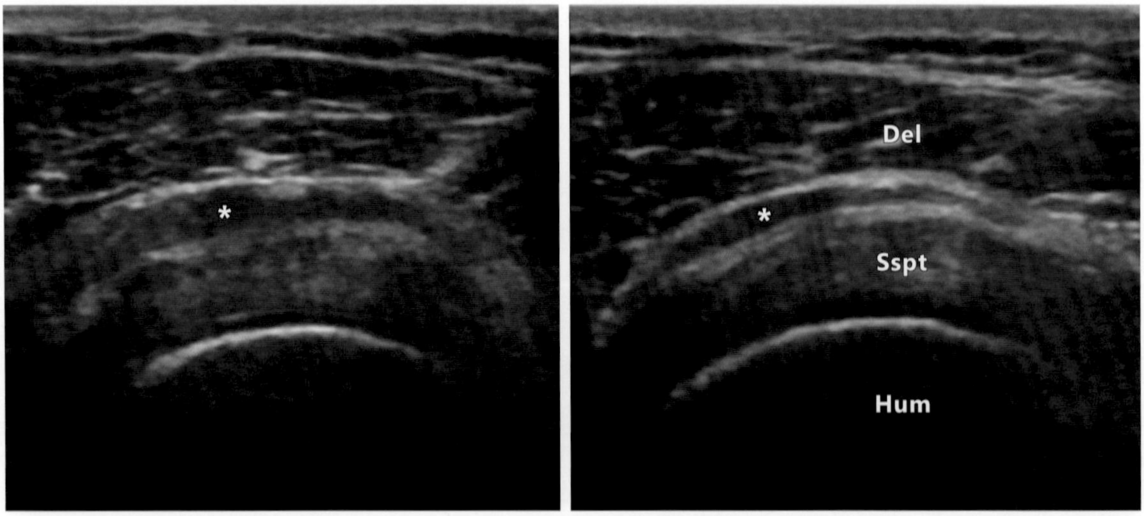

a b

Axial US images over the rotator cuff reveal bilateral fluid within the bursal lumen (*white asterisks*) (**a**, **b**). The amount of fluid is more on the left image and echogenicity of the supraspinatus tendon (**Sspt**) seems to be more heterogenous (**a**).

Del deltoid
Hum humerus

Chronic subacromial bursitis in a 31-year-old man with bilateral shoulder pain for the last one year

2.36

a

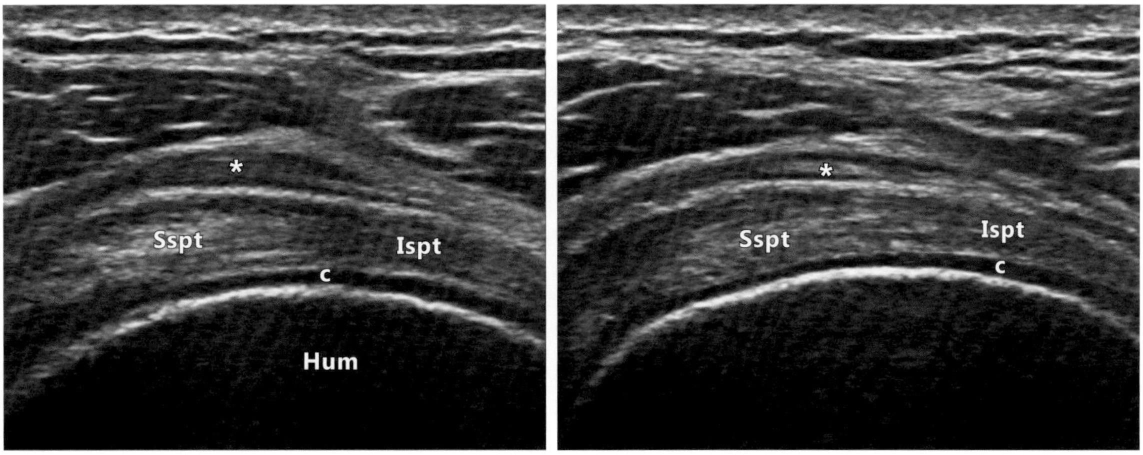

b

Axial US images obtained over the rotator cuff (during Crass position) show bilateral hypoechoic synovial thickenings (*asterisks*) in the subdeltoid bursa (**a**, **b**).

c cartilage
Hum humerus
Ispt infraspinatus tendon
Sspt supraspinatus tendon

Expert note

Occasionally, the appearance of (chronic) bursitis could be confined to only synovial thickening rather than any fluid accumulation. Of note, in these images, the transition zone (intermingling fibers) between the supraspinatus and infraspinatus tendons is perfectly visualized with the gradual decrease in the thickness of the rotator cuff.

2.37 Chronic subacromial bursitis in a 42-year-old woman with shoulder pain (> 3 months)

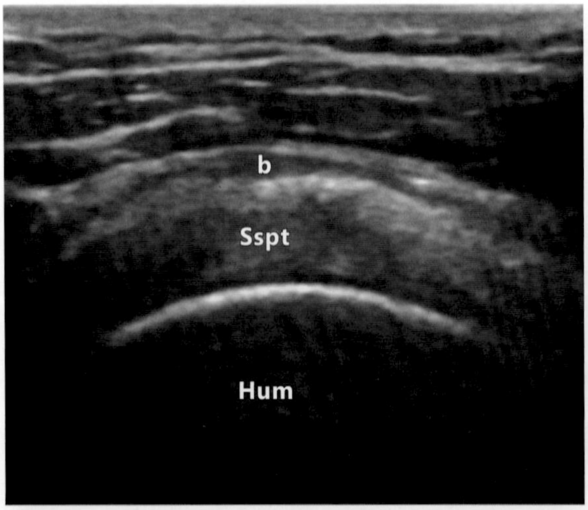

a

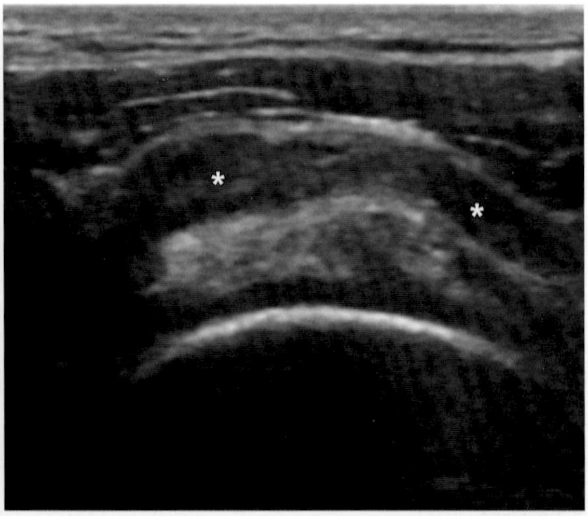

b

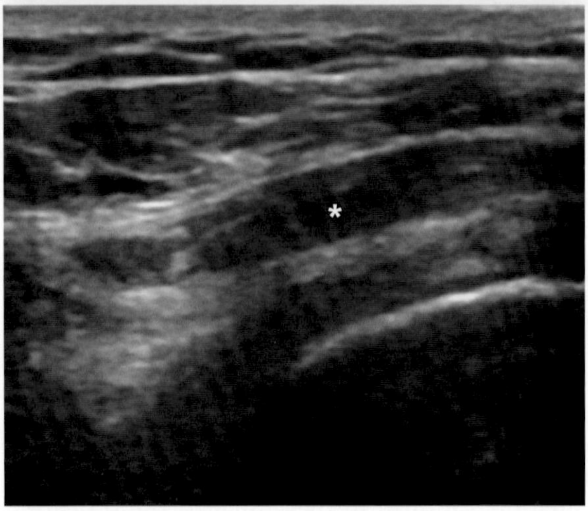

c

The pain is worse at night, interrupting sleep and also limiting her movements.

When compared with the normal side (**a**), axial (**b**) and longitudinal (**c**) US images over the supraspinatus tendon (**Sspt**) illustrate that the subdeltoid bursa is markedly distended by hypoechoic synovial hypertrophy (*asterisks*).

b	subdeltoid bursa
Hum	humerus

Expert note

Recognizing the epiphyseal plates in children is noteworthy [8]; otherwise an interrupted bony surface might indicate a fracture (or a joint elsewhere).
The other unossified area in these images (acromion) may also let the sound waves be transmitted through itself. This way, proximal cuff can easily be scanned in children which otherwise requires extra techniques and can only/partially be imaged in adults.
Especially in children (and certainly if one is not used to examine children), it is important to compare both sides. The same applies for patients above the age of 65 as well. Very often, one finds bilateral small amounts of fluid, calcifications or degenerative tendon changes in asymptomatic people.

Subacromial bursitis in a 9-year-old girl with anterior shoulder pain after a blunt trauma **2.38**

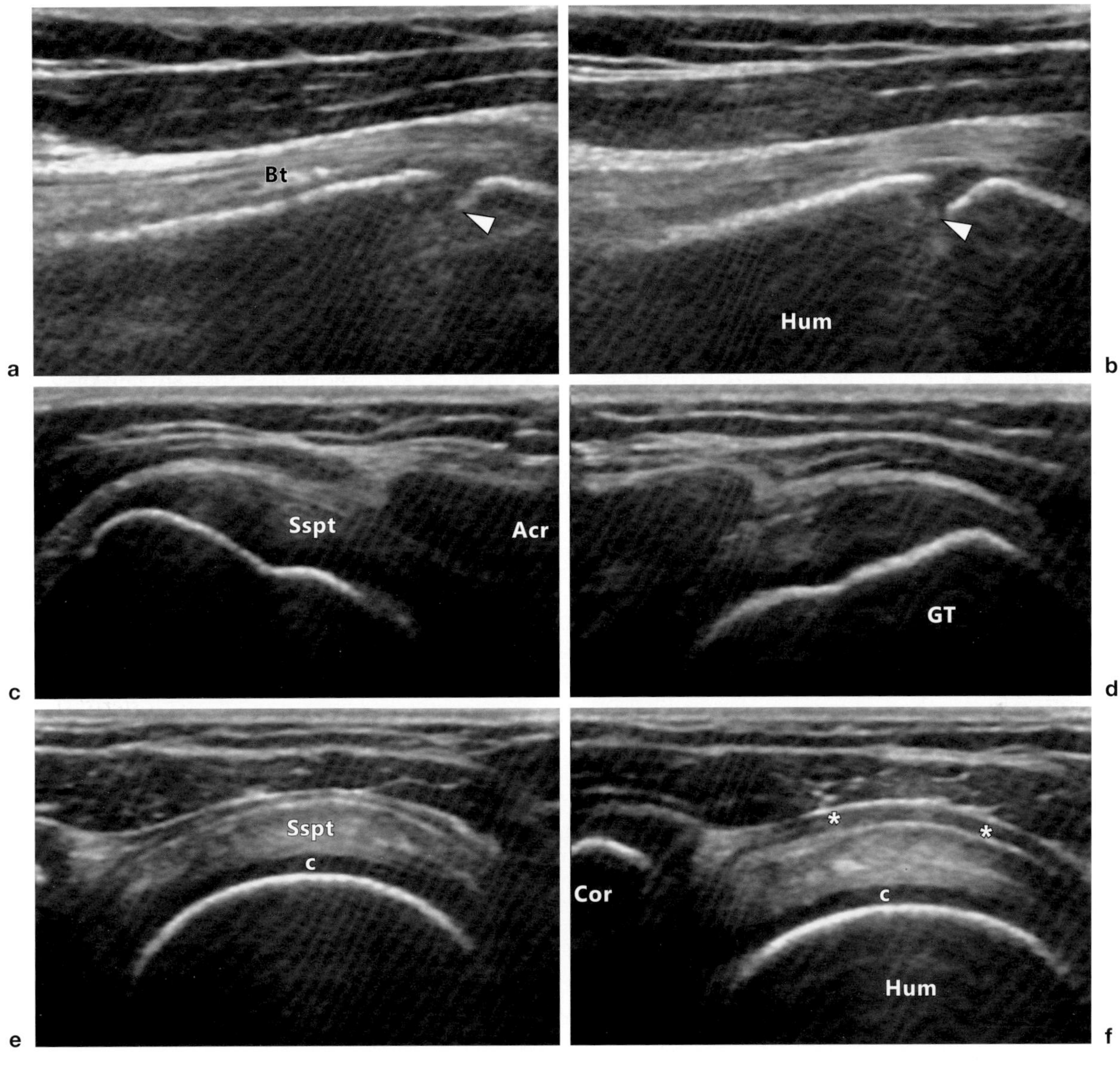

When compared with the asymptomatic side (**a**, **c**, **e**), anterior longitudinal image (**b**) shows the normal appearance of the long head of the biceps tendon (**Bt**) and lateral longitudinal view (**d**) demonstrates the normal view of the supraspinatus tendon (**Sspt**). Axial view during Crass position (**f**) depicts mild effusion in the subdeltoid bursa (*asterisks*). Please note the epiphyseal plates (*arrowheads*) in figures **a** & **b** and the hypoechoic appearance of the unossified acromion (**Acr**) in figures **c** & **d**.

c	cartilage	**GT**	greater tubercle
Cor	coracoid process	**Hum**	humerus

2.39 Subscapularis tendon tear in a 45-year-old man who had pain during internal rotation of the arm

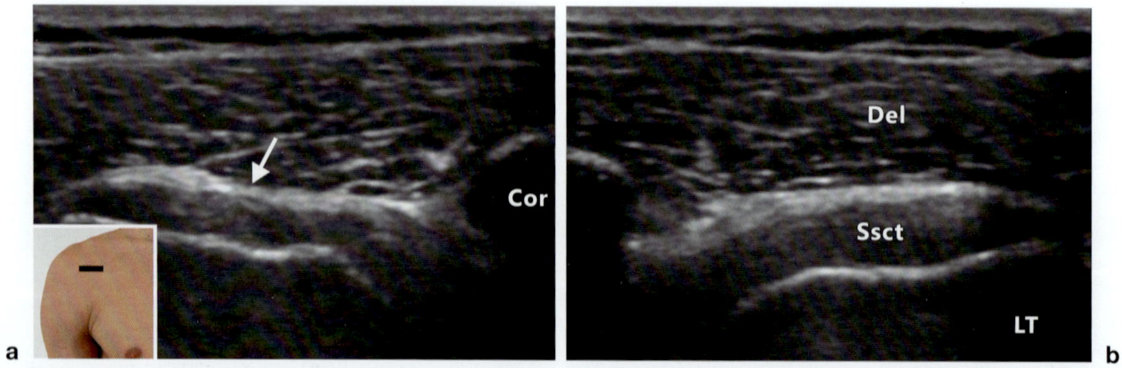

Anterior axial US image reveals flattening or diffuse thinning (*arrow*) in the upper portion of the subscapularis tendon (**Ssct**) (**a**). Normal side (**b**).

Cor coracoid process
Del deltoid
LT lesser tubercle

Expert note

During comparative imaging, correlating the US findings with medical history and clinical examination is paramount. For instance, instead of diffuse thinning on one side, diffuse thickening (e.g. subscapularis tendinitis) on the other side would be another possibility should the rest of the physical examination be likely.

2.40 Subscapularis tendinopathy in a 43-year-old female tennis player with a 3-month history of shoulder pain

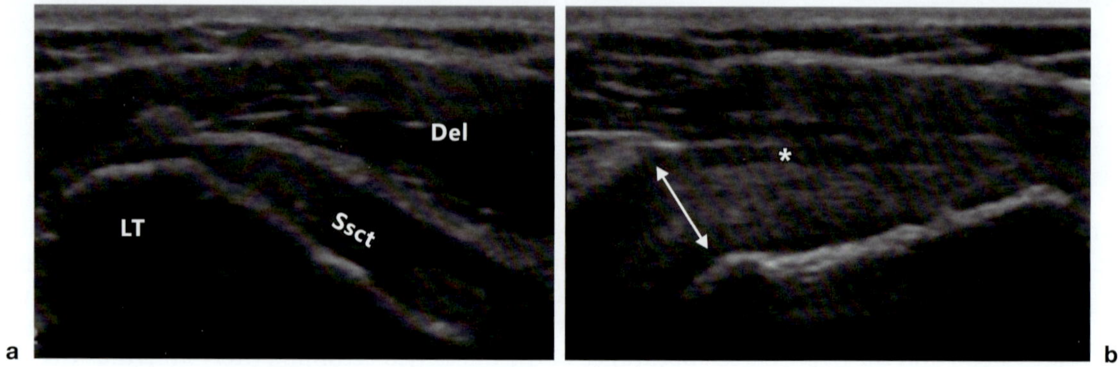

When compared with the normal subscapularis tendon (**Ssct**) (**a**), axial US image over the anteromedial shoulder demonstrates diffuse/regular thickening of the tendon (*double arrow*) and mild fluid in the subscapularis bursa (*asterisk*) (**b**).

Incomplete subscapularis tendon tear in a 53-year-old man tennis player

2.41

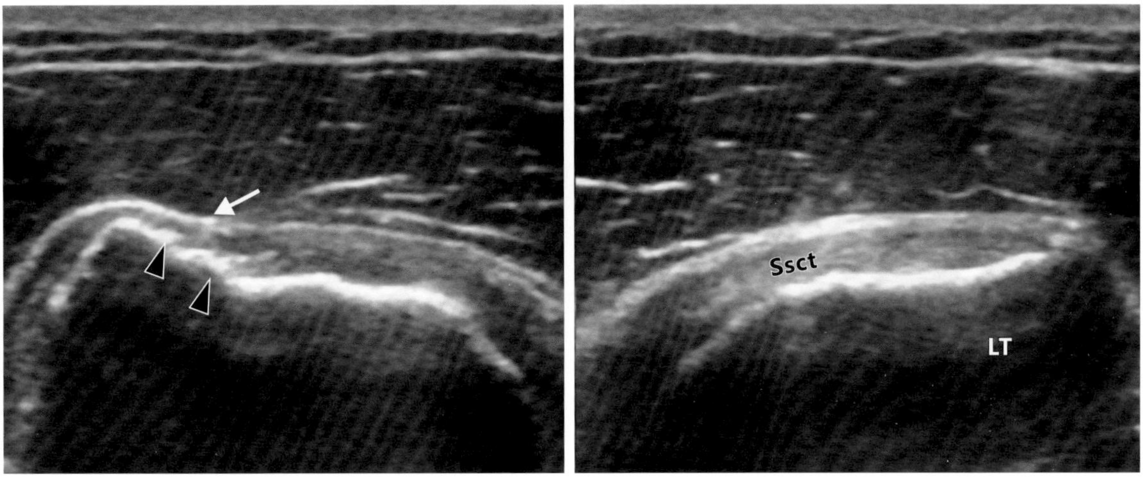

a b

The patient had a 3-month history of 'deep' shoulder pain which was elicited when he was serving overhead.

Axial US imaging shows partial-thickness tear (*arrow*) of the subscapularis tendon (**Ssct**) and cortical irregularities (*arrowheads*) of the lesser tubercle (**LT**). Normal contralateral side (**b**).

Expert note

While change in the convex appearance (focal thinning) of the subscapularis tendon might indicate a direct sign of rupture, underlying cortical irregularities could also be considered as supportive (indirect) findings of a rupture.

2.42 Subscapularis tendon tear in a 35-year-old man after a strenuous ball throw with forceful shoulder external rotation

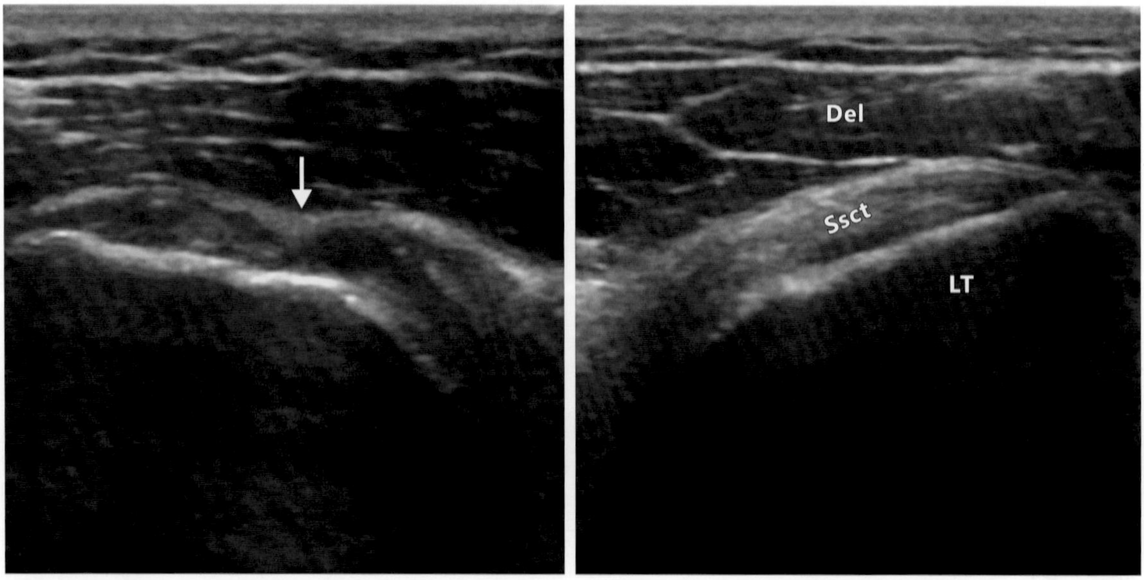

Axial US imaging demonstrates partial-thickness tear (*arrow*) of the subscapularis tendon (**Ssct**) (**a**). Normal side (**b**).

Del deltoid
LT lesser tubercle

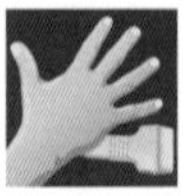

Expert note

Note the change in shape and the focal hypoechoic zone as direct signs of rupture and the enhancement artifact (bright image of the cortex).

It is very important to do a complete examination of the shoulder every time [2]. Most rotator cuff ruptures will be ruptures of the supraspinatus tendon. Although rare, isolated ruptures of the subscapularis and infraspinatus tendons do occur. Extensive (combined) ruptures of subscapularis and supraspinatus or supraspinatus and infraspinatus (and teres minor) tendons can also be seen [1].

Shoulder

A 41-year-old woman with anterior shoulder pain which gradually worsened in the last six months following a shoulder injury

2.43

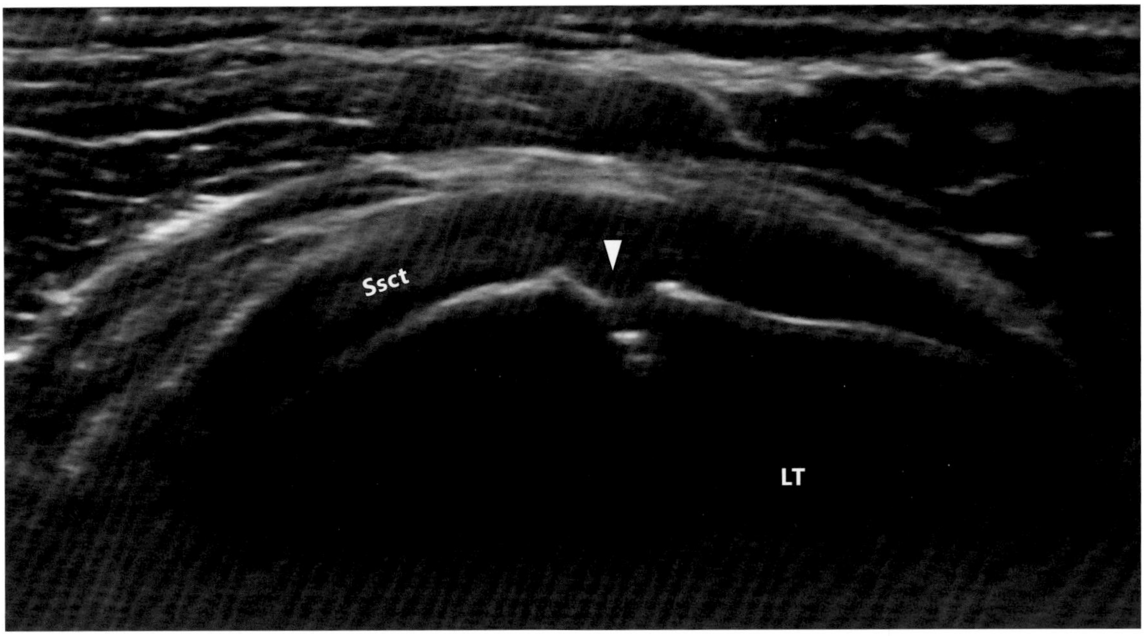

Axial US image over the anteromedial shoulder demonstrates a cortical defect (*arrowhead*) just deep to the subscapularis tendon (**Ssct**).

LT lesser tubercle

2.44 A 56-year-old man with history of shoulder trauma one year ago

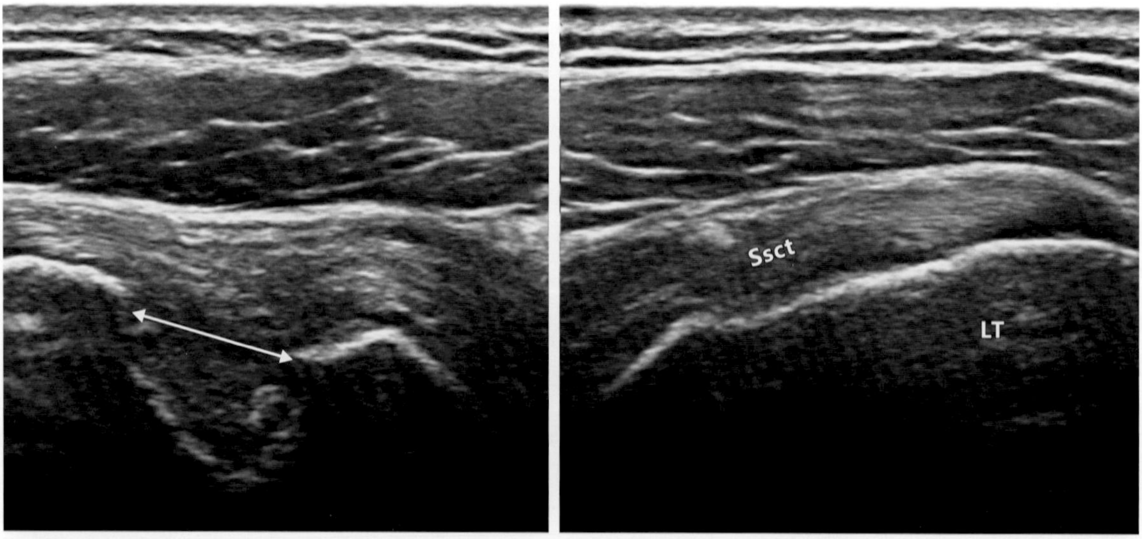

a b

Axial US image obtained over the anteromedial aspect of the humerus demonstrates a large cortical defect (*double arrow*) deep to the subscapularis tendon (**Ssct**) (**a**). Normal view of the structures on the other side (**b**).

LT lesser tubercle

Subscapularis tendon rupture in a 57-year-old man with anterior shoulder pain

2.45

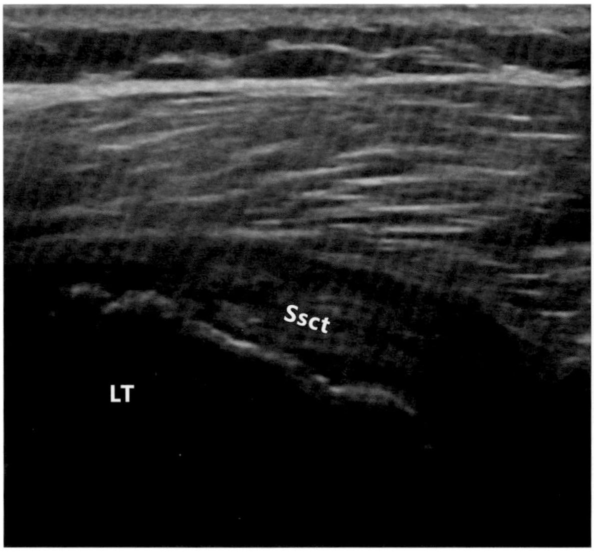

a

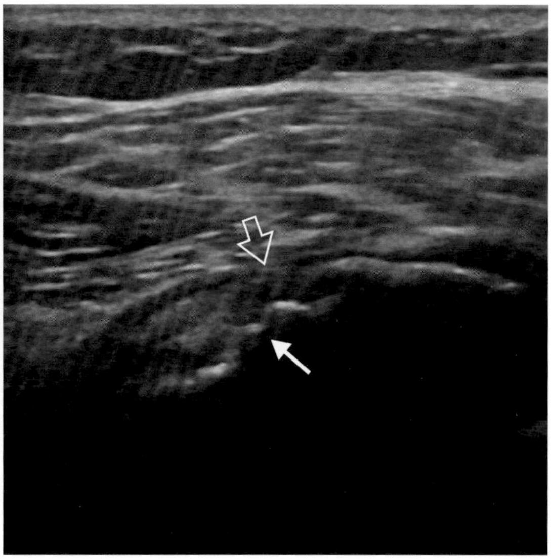

b

When compared with the relatively normal subscapularis tendon (**Ssct**) (**a**), axial US image shows a partial full-thickness tear (*thick arrow*), possibly due to the underlying cortical irregularities (*thin arrow*) of the humerus (**b**).

LT lesser tubercle

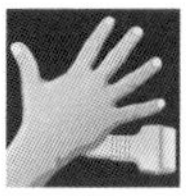

Expert note

As mentioned before: “the egg or the chicken” i.e. whether the tendon rupture or the cortical irregularity is the preceeding component can not always/easily be ascertained.

2.46 Partial tear of the subscapularis tendon in a 48-year-old man with anteromedial shoulder pain for about five months

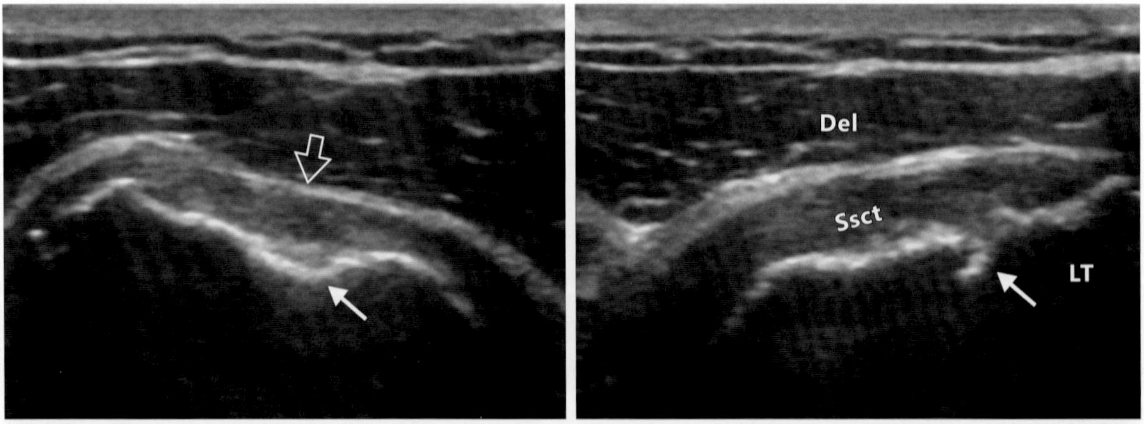

a b

Anterior axial US images show cortical irregularities (*thin arrows*) on both sides (**a**, **b**) with a partial subscapularis tendon (**Ssct**) rupture (*thick arrow*) on the symptomatic side (**a**).

Del deltoid
LT lesser tubercle

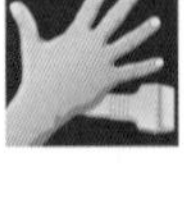

Expert note

Thinning and changed (convex) contour of the tendon are suggestive of a tear which otherwise does not display any anechoic defect. Again, compression of the tendon might be contributory for the diagnosis.

Calcifying subscapularis tendon in a 51-year-old man with anterior shoulder pain and positive lift-off test **2.47**

a 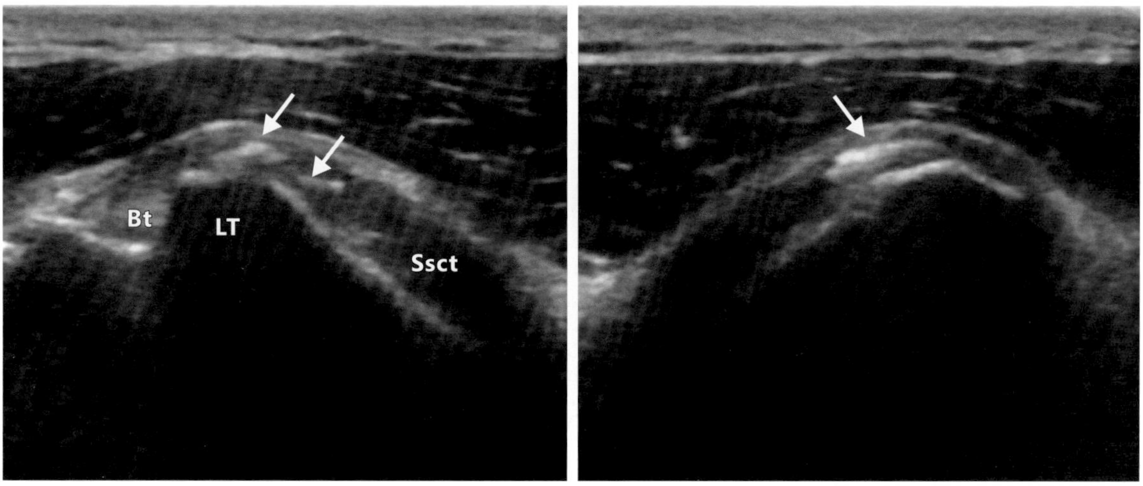 b

Anterior axial US images reveal bilateral intratendinous type II calcifications (*arrows*) in the distal attachment site of the subscapularis tendon (**Ssct**).

Bt biceps tendon
LT lesser tubercle

Expert note

While the posterior acoustic shadowing artifact makes the recognition of calcifications very easy; sonographers should not forget that depending on their stage and/or size, calcifications might not always display acoustic shadowing. One could wonder whether these insertional calcifications are the same type of calcifications as the midsubstance ones (and hence can be treated in the same way or not). Of note, insertional calcifications in the subscapularis are often asymptomatic.

2.48 Calcifying subscapularis tendon in a 67-year-old woman with frozen shoulder

a 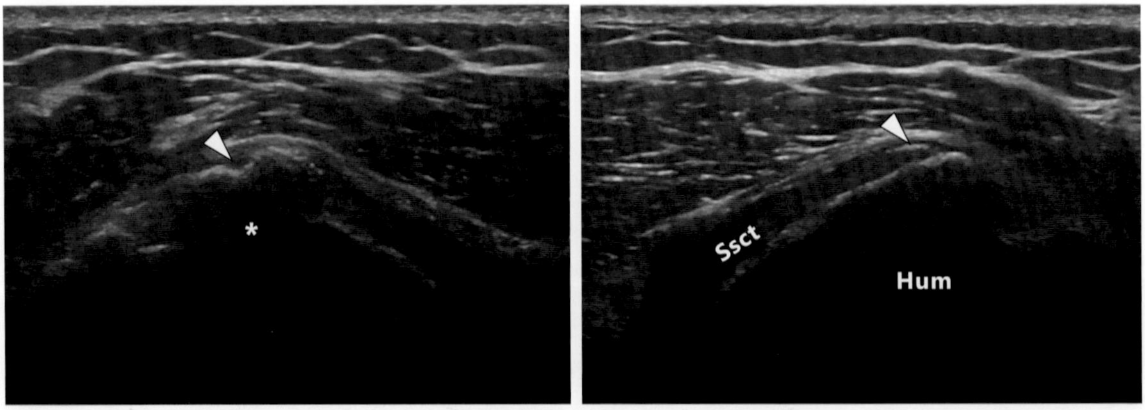 b

Anterior axial US images over the subscapularis tendons (**Ssct**) illustrate a type I calcification (*arrowhead*) with posterior acoustic shadowing artifact (*asterisk*) on the symptomatic side (**a**) and a small type III calcification (*arrowhead*) on the asymptomatic side (**b**).

Hum humerus

Expert note

When compared with other imaging modalities that are usually performed for the symptomatic extremity, especially in subjects with degenerative problems, comparison is an important advantage of US imaging which can provide extra information.

Herewith, in case of frozen shoulder, limitation of passive external rotation can make it difficult to examine the subscapularis tendon. Hence, also considering the fact that adhesive capsulitis does not have any pathognomonic finding on US, imaging might perhaps be used only to unmask the possible accompanying findings in such cases.

Calcifying subscapularis tendon in a 49-year-old farmer with recurrent anterior shoulder pain for the last nine months 2.49

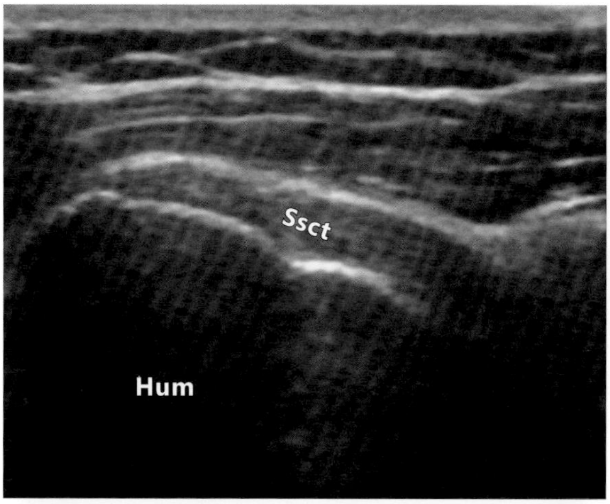

a

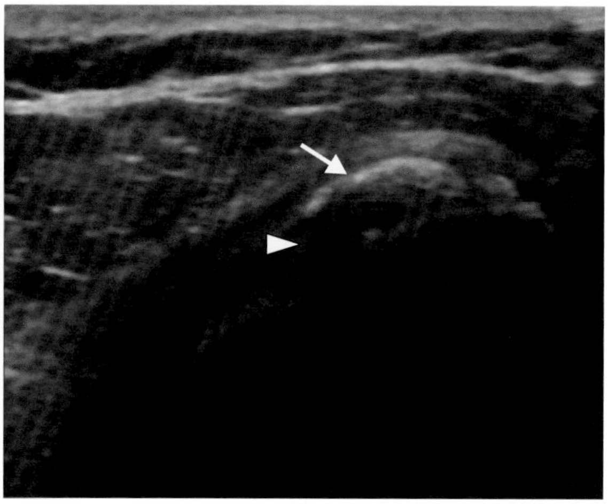

b

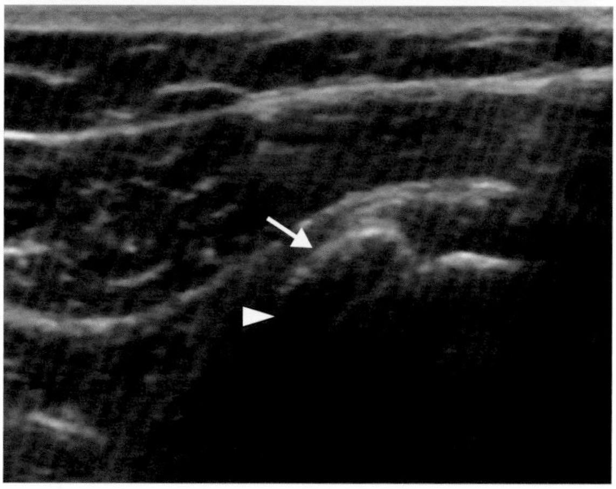

c

When compared with the normal side (**a**), anterior axial US images over the subscapularis tendon (**Ssct**) reveal hyperechoic foci (*arrows*) with incomplete acoustic shadowing (*arrowheads*), reflecting calcific deposits (**b**, **c**). Note that the tendon is mildly thickened as well.

Hum humerus

2.50 Bilateral calcifications in the subscapularis tendon in an older woman with chronic pain and limited movements of the shoulder

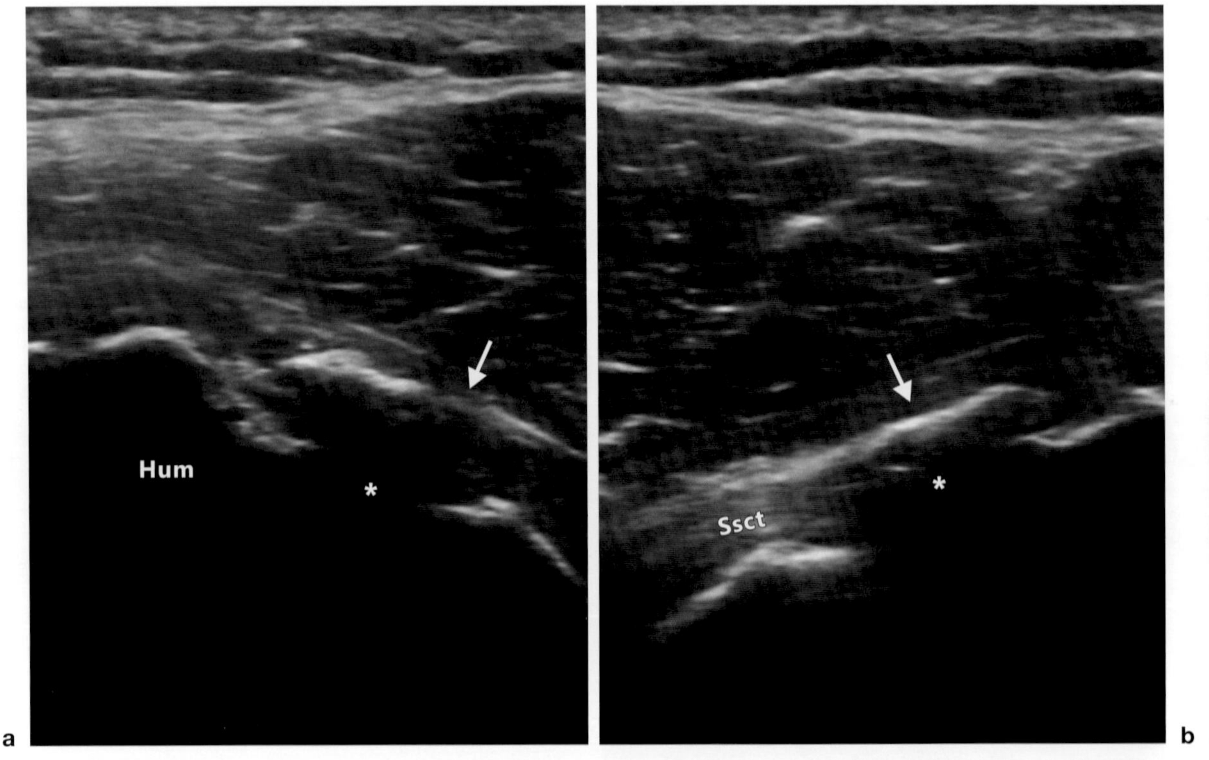

Anterior axial US images over the subscapularis tendon (**Ssct**) illustrate linear type II calcifications (*arrows*) inside the tendon with incomplete posterior acoustic shadowing artifacts (*asterisks*) (**a**, **b**).

Hum humerus

Shoulder

Supraspinatus tendinopathy in a 42-year-old woman with shoulder pain **2.51**

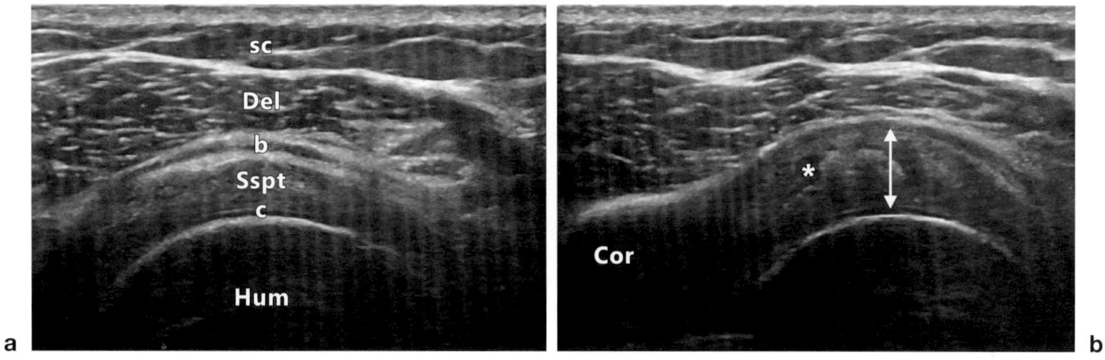

When compared with the normal side (**a**), axial image during Crass position (**b**) shows a swollen (*double arrow*) and irregularly hypoechoic supraspinatus tendon (**Sspt**) with a small intrasubstance tear (*asterisk*).

b	subdeltoid bursa	**Cor**	coracoid process	**Hum**	humerus
c	cartilage	**Del**	deltoid	**sc**	subcutaneous tissue

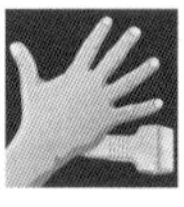

Expert note

The thickness of supraspinatus tendon is about 6 mm and similar to the overlying deltoid muscle thickness. Side to side difference of >2 mm usually suggests tendinopathy [9].

Chronic supraspinatus tendinopathy in a 49-year-old man initiated after a previous minor trauma **2.52**

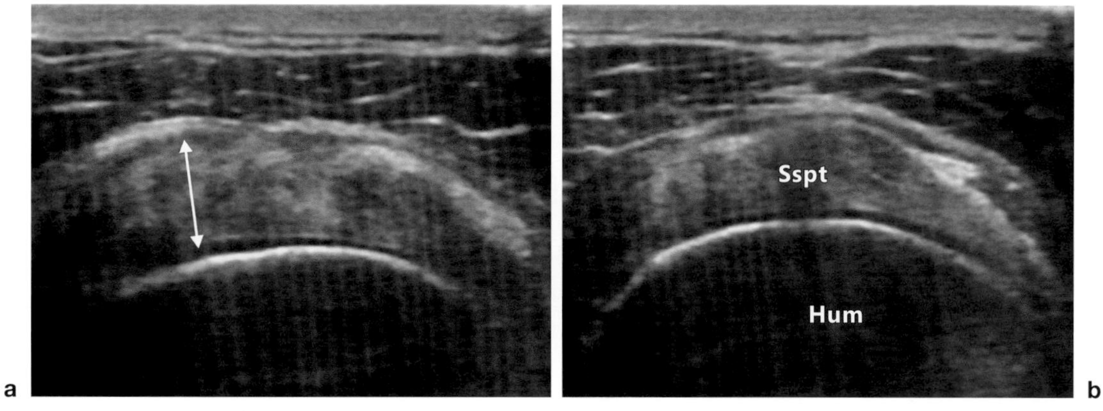

Axial US image illustrates thickening of the affected supraspinatus tendon (**Sspt**) with heterogeneous and hypoechoic echotexture (*double arrow*) (**a**). Contralateral side (**b**).

2.53 Supraspinatus tendinopathy in a young woman with shoulder pain during movements

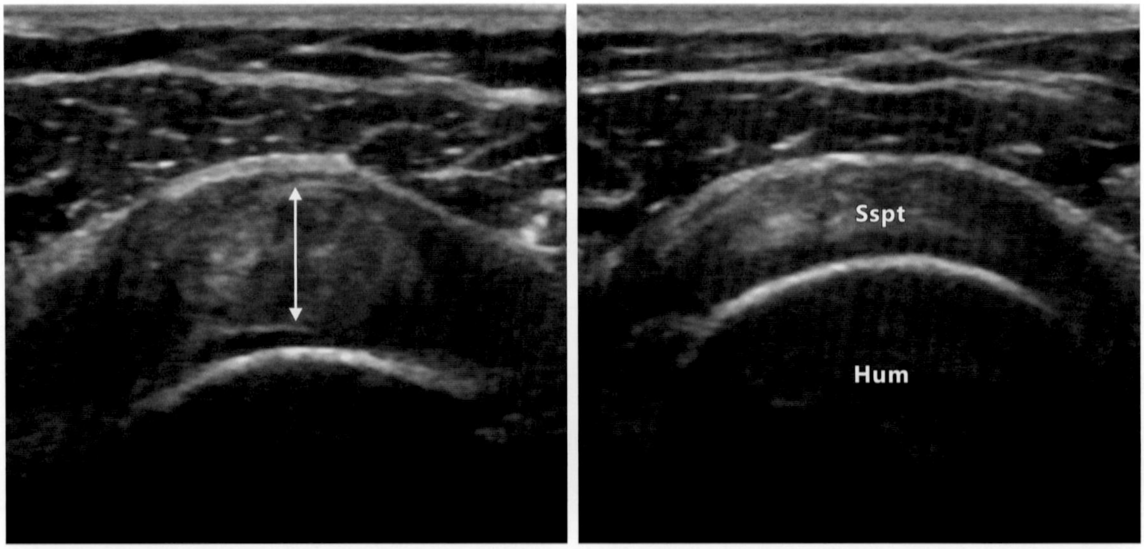

Axial US image obtained over the supraspinatus tendon (**Sspt**) in Crass position shows diffuse thickening with heterogenous echogenicities (*double arrow*) (**a**). Normal contralateral view of the rotator cuff (**b**).

Hum humerus

Axial (**a**) and longitudinal (**c**) US images over the proximal humerus illustrate irregular, hypoechoic thickening (*arrowheads*) of the biceps tendon (**Bt**) and a small amount of fluid (*asterisk*). Axial image in Crass position (**e**) reveals abnormally swollen supraspinatus tendon (**Sspt**) with a heterogenous appearance (*double arrow*). Corresponding images of the normal side (**b**, **d**, **f**).

Hum humerus

Expert note

Although fluid around the biceps tendon might be an initial sign for rotator cuff lesions, concomitant problems can also ensue. Therefore, substantial US imaging is advocated in each and every "shoulder patient".

Biceps tenosynovitis and supraspinatus tendinopathy in a middle-aged woman with continuous shoulder pain

2.54

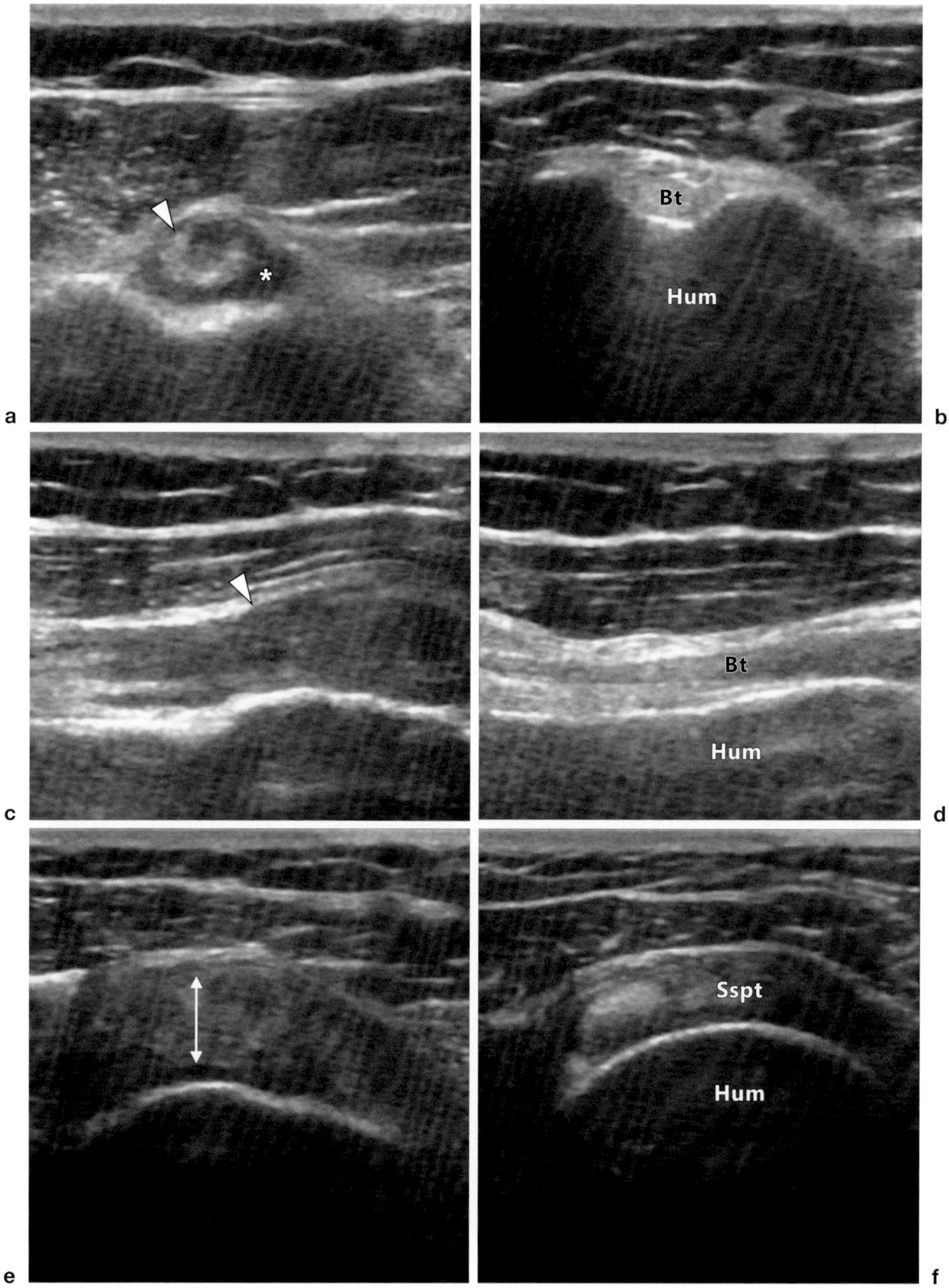

2.55 Supraspinatus tendon tear in a 65-year-old man with intermittent shoulder pain in the last two months

a 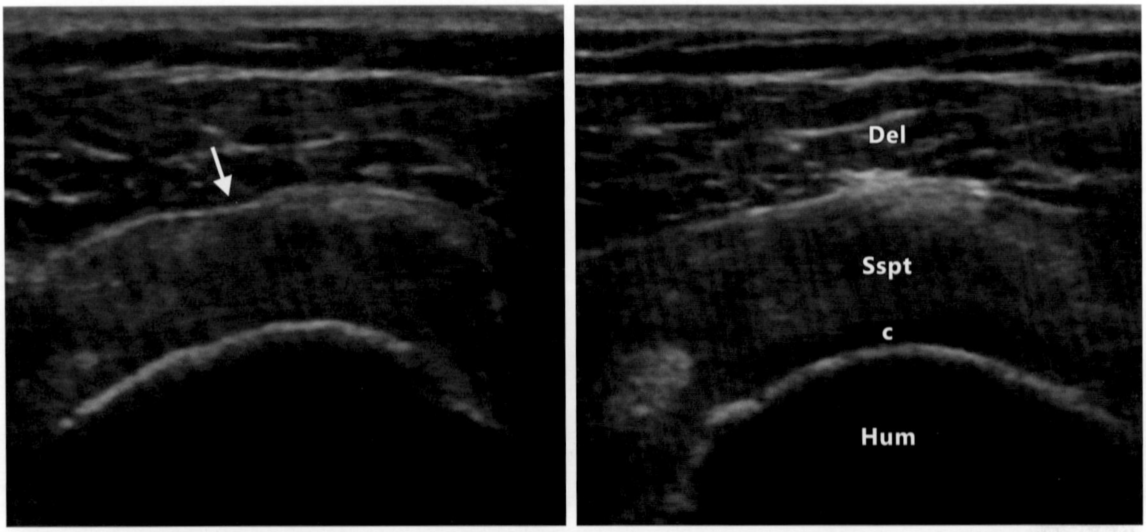 b

Axial US image of the rotator cuff illustrates a slump (*arrow*) in the supraspinatus tendon (**Sspt**), reflecting a small tear (**a**). Normal view of the rotator cuff (**b**).

c cartilage
Del deltoid
Hum humerus

Expert note

Focal thinning seems to appear as a direct sign of partial thickness tear at the bursal side of the supraspinatus tendon.

Supraspinatus tendon tear in a 49-year-old woman with persistent shoulder pain and a positive Jobe's sign

2.56

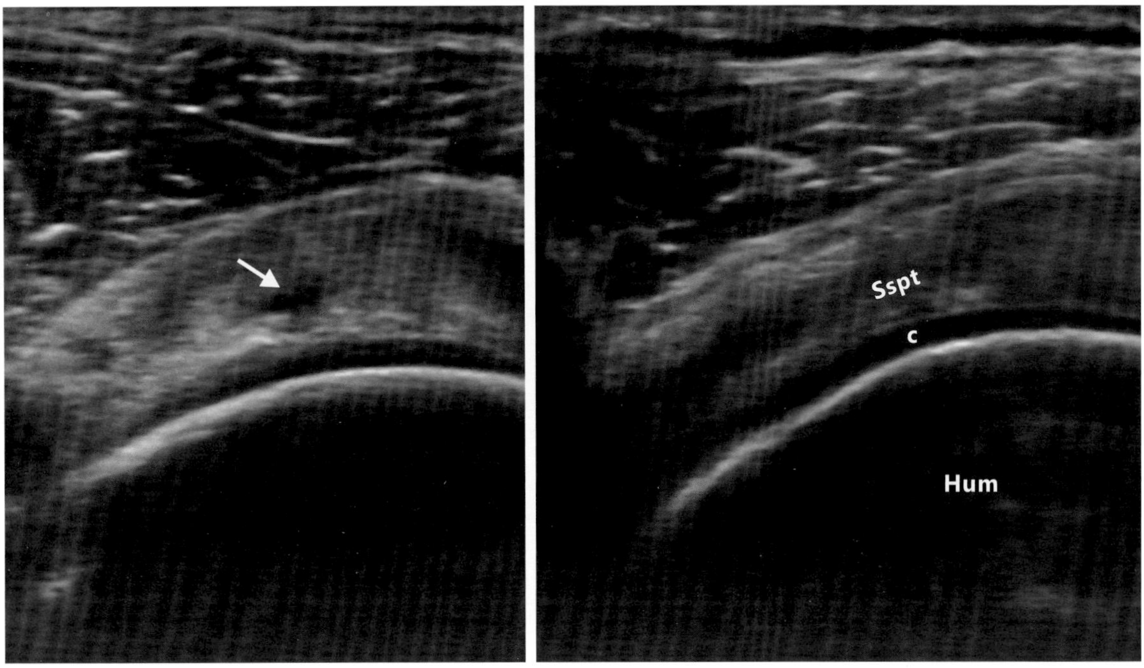

a b

Axial US image over the rotator cuff demonstrates a small intrasubstance tear (*arrow*) (**a**). Normal view of the supraspinatus tendon (**Sspt**) on the asymptomatic side (**b**).

c	cartilage
Hum	head of humerus

Expert note

There is a focal anechoic zone inside the tendon; if this is compressible, it is an absolute direct sign of a rupture.

2.57 Supraspinatus tendon tears in an elderly patient who had chronic intermittent shoulder pain especially during overhead activities

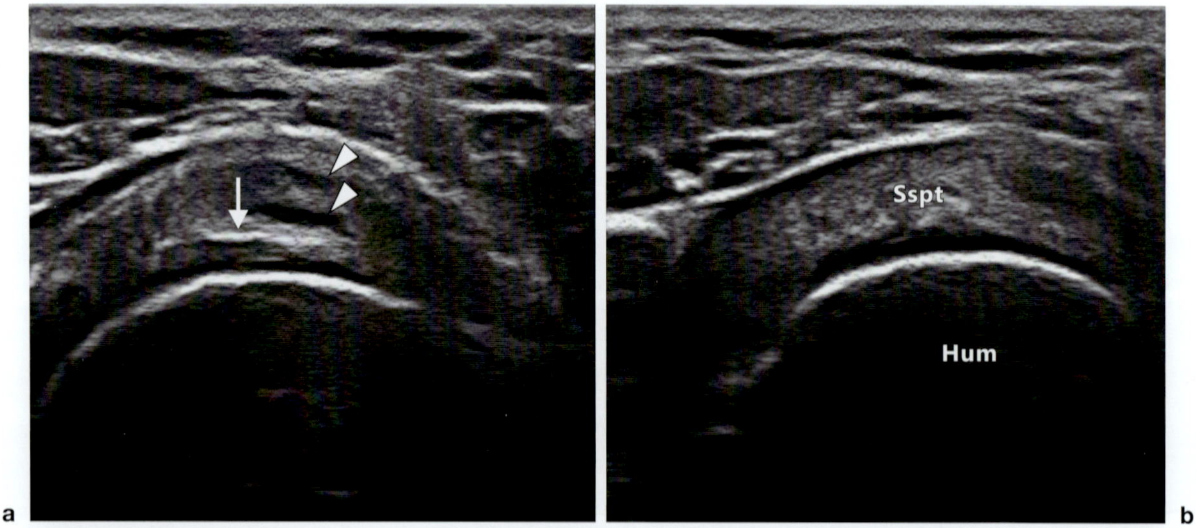

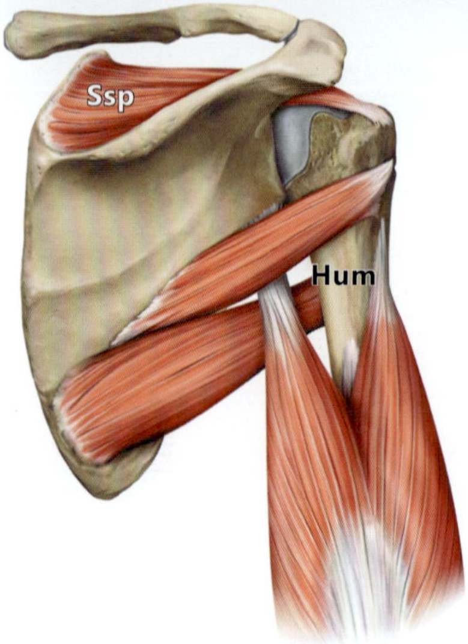

Axial US imaging in Crass position reveals two small intratendinous tears (*arrowheads*) and a hyperechoic fibrous scar tissue (*arrow*) (**a**). Normal side (**b**).

Hum humerus
Ssp supraspinatus
Sspt supraspinatus tendon

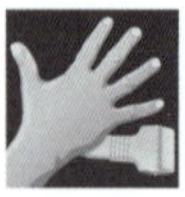

Expert note

In this case, there is no change in shape, but a change in echogenicity -as a direct sign of rupture. Focal hypoechoic zones are definitely suspicious and if they are compressible, they are absolute direct signs of rupture.

Hyperechoic zones within the cuff are quite likely to be indicative for previous tears. Of note, US imaging are quite sensitive for detecting these lesions as well. Unfortunately, this patient had undergone a magnetic resonance imaging before and it was reported to be normal.

Rupture of the supraspinatus tendon in a 50-year-old woman **2.58**

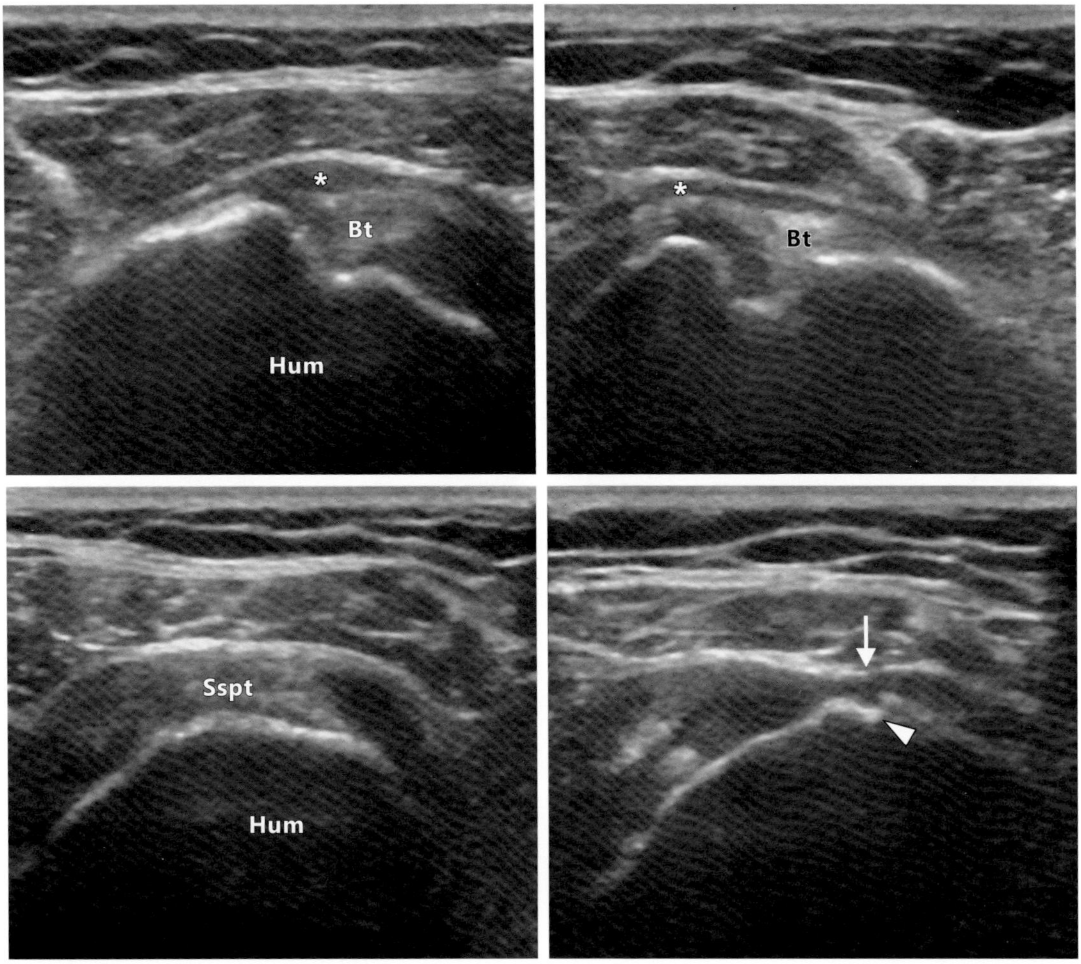

a b c d

She had shoulder pain which was aggravated on abduction and flexion, and relieved by medications and keeping the shoulder adducted.

US imaging of the biceps tendon (**Bt**) in anterior axial view shows bilateral mild fluid in the subdeltoid bursae (*asterisks*) (**a**, **b**). Imaging for the supraspinatus tendon (**Sspt**) in Crass position (**c**, **d**) shows an incomplete full-thickness tear (*arrow*) overlying a cortical irregularity (*arrowhead*) of the humerus (**Hum**).

Expert note

In contrast to focal lesions, a global thinning of the tendon is more likely to be due to degeneration.

2.59 Supraspinatus tendon tear in a 45-year-old painter who spends much of his professional time painting ceilings

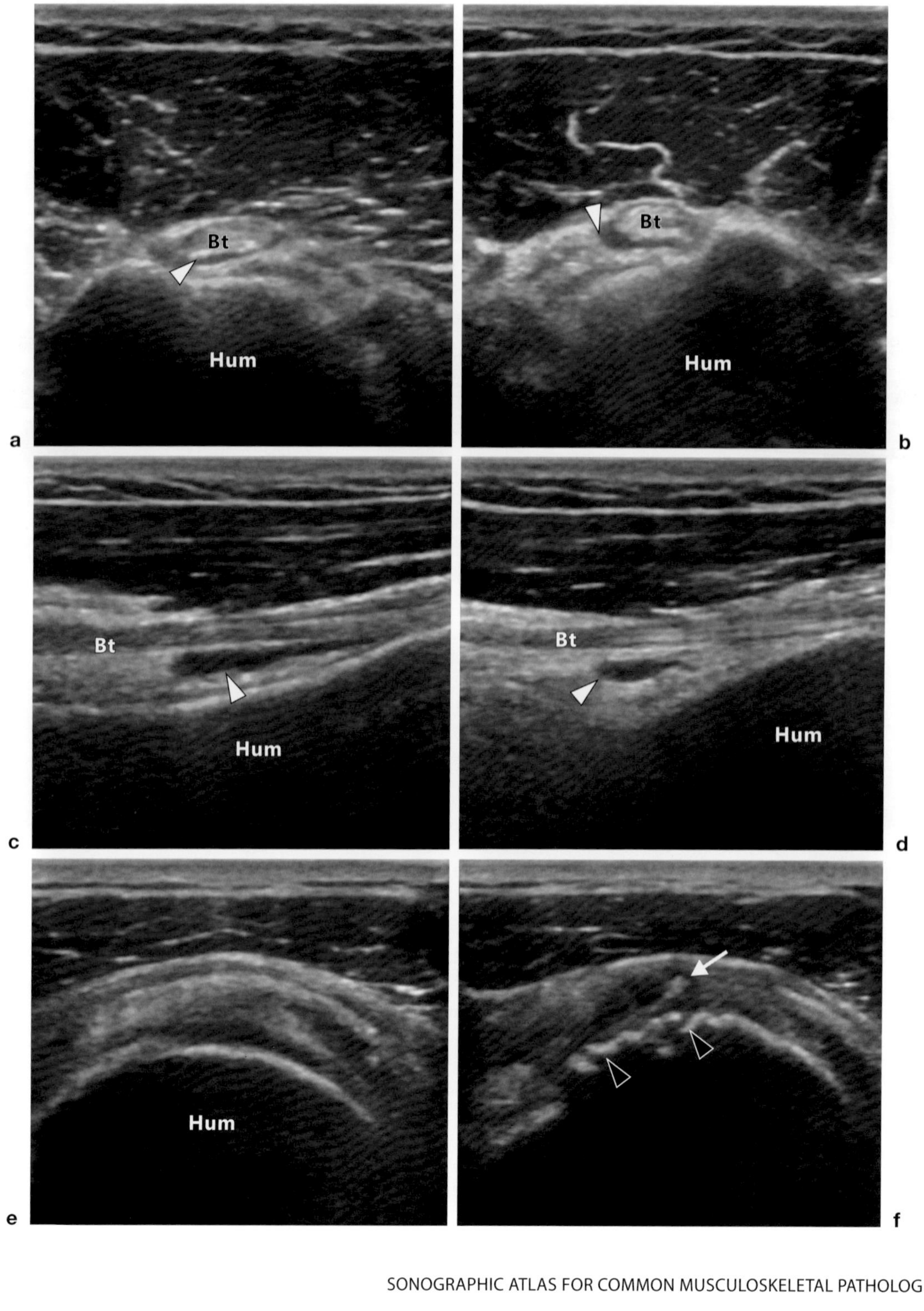

The patient complains of shoulder pain, and inability to raise his arm above the shoulder level in the last 8 months.

Axial (**a**, **b**) and longitudinal (**c**, **d**) US images of the biceps tendon (**Bt**) demonstrate a small amount of joint effusion in the tendon sheath (*white arrowheads*).
When compared with the normal side (**e**), axial US imaging in Crass position reveals an incomplete partial-thickness rupture (*arrow*) of the supraspinatus tendon (**Sspt**) and underlying cortical irregularities (*black arrowheads*) of the humerus (**Hum**) (**f**).

Expert note

One of the reasons why shoulder examination starts with anterior axial view is that the double-layer synovial sheath around the proximal portion of the biceps tendon is often the initial place to search for joint fluid. Likewise, in case fluid is present, the rest of the examination is tailored accordingly i.e. performed more diligently while exploring additional findings (e.g. rotator cuff pathologies).
The presence of cortical irregularities (indirect sign of ruptures) usually necessitates caution as regards overlying cuff injuries. Yet, if not present currently, they might possibly lead to tears due to abnormal friction. On the other hand, they could as well be caused due to the overlying rupture i.e. the tendon not "protecting" the cortex anymore.

2.60 Normal anterior and lateral shoulder views in a healthy man

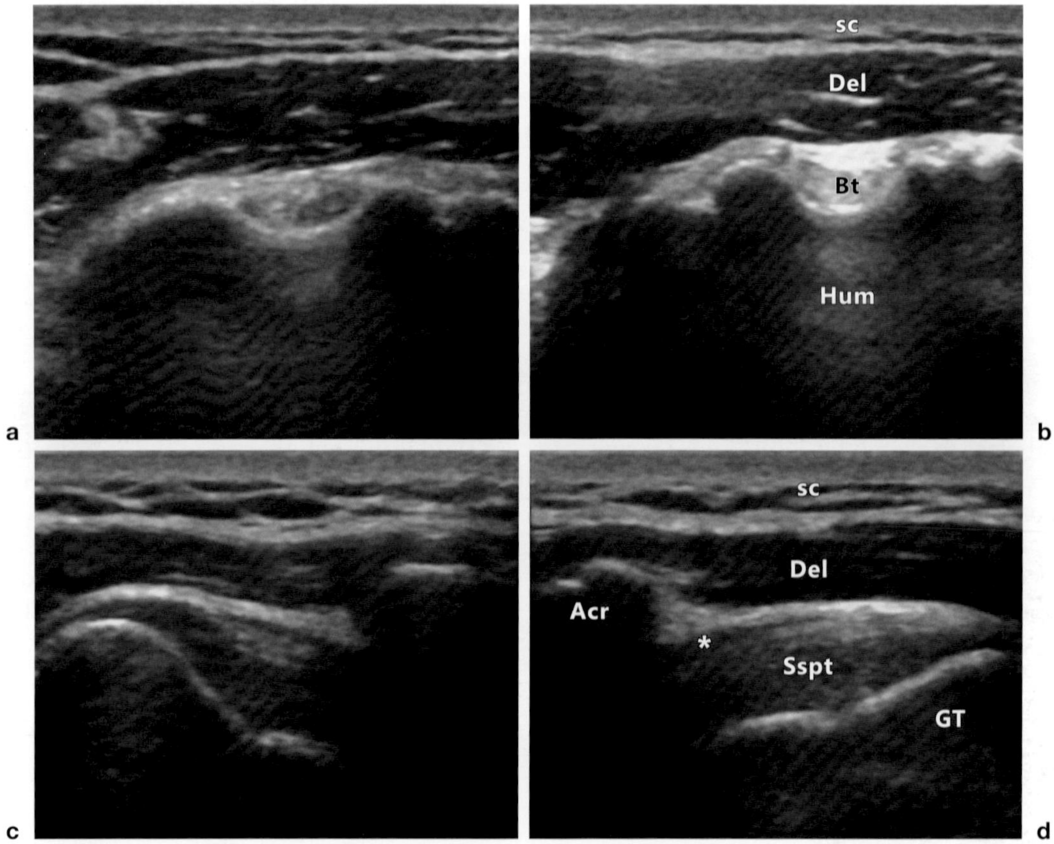

Anterior axial US images (**a**, **b**) show normal appearances of the biceps tendons (**Bt**). Lateral longitudinal scans (**c**, **d**) show normal appearances of the supraspinatus tendons (**Sspt**) and the subacromial-subdeltoid bursa (*asterisk*).

Acr	acromion	**Hum**	humerus
Del	deltoid	**sc**	subcutaneous tissue
GT	greater tubercle		

Expert note

In obese patients, it can be difficult to obtain this coronal view of supraspinatus tendon which is also referred as "bird's beak". Due to the fat tissue between the arm and the trunk, the upper limb will already be in a relatively abducted position -making the tendon glide and disappear beneath the acromion. As such, the elbow should be held firmly against the body in obese subjects for better imaging [1].

Supraspinatus tendon tear in a 55-year-old man with painful shoulder movements **2.61**

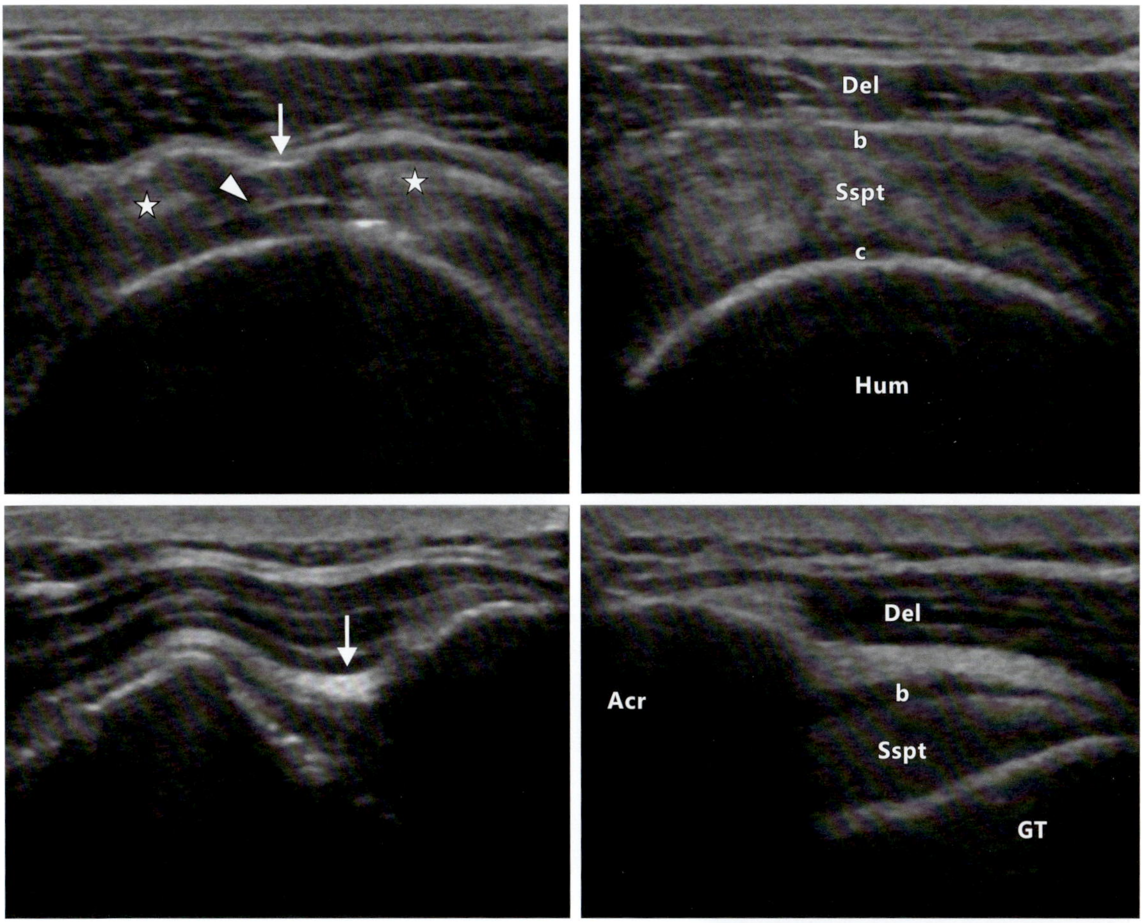

Anterior axial (**a**) and lateral longitudinal (**c**) US images show the retracted fibers (*stars*) on both sides of the incomplete full-thickness rupture, the cartilage interface sign (*arrowhead*) and deltoid muscle (**Del**) herniation (*arrow*). Normal contralateral views (**b**, **d**).

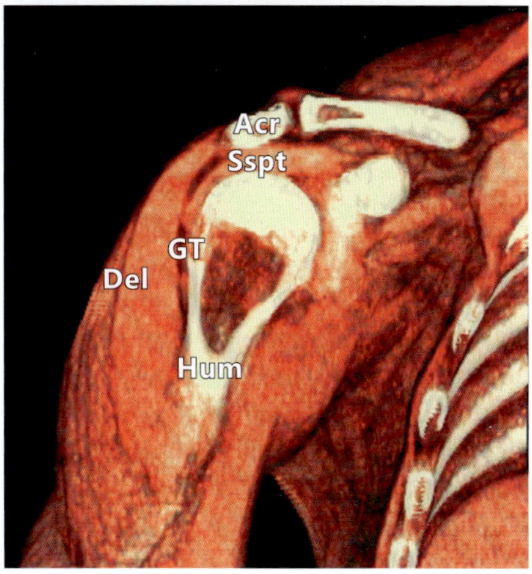

Acr	acromion
b	subdeltoid bursa
Bt	biceps tendon
c	cartilage
GT	greater tubercle
Hum	humerus
Sspt	supraspinatus tendon

2.62 Rupture of the supraspinatus tendon in an elderly man with limited painful shoulder

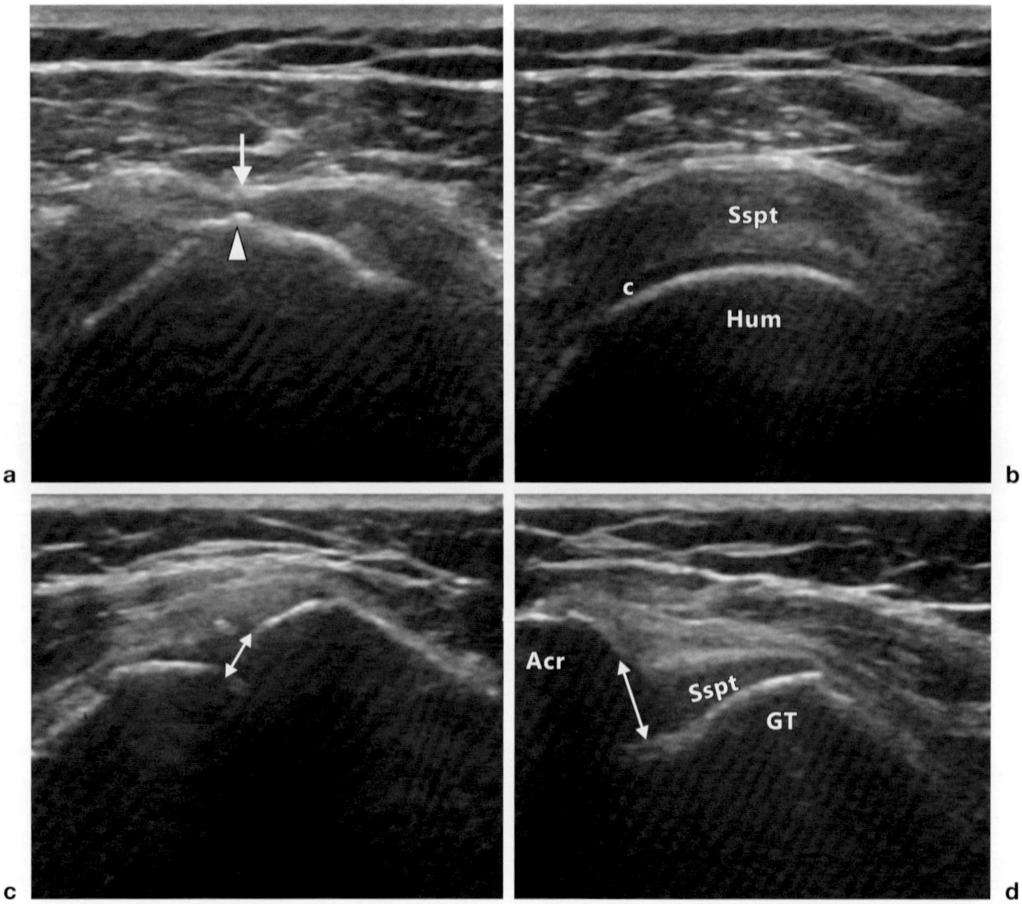

Axial US imaging in Crass position reveals incomplete full-thickness tear (*arrow*) of the supraspinatus tendon (**Sspt**) over the cortical irregularity (*arrowhead*) (**a**). Normal side (**b**). Lateral coronal US imaging illustrates decreased subacromial space (*double arrow*) on the ruptured area (**c**). Normal side (**d**).

Acr	acromion	**GT**	greater tubercle
c	cartilage	**Hum**	head of humerus

Expert note

Superior subluxation of the glenohumeral joint (an indirect sign of tear) resulting in an acromial humeral distance of <6 mm is reported to be specific for a rotator cuff tear [10].

Supraspinatus tendon tear in 40-year-old woman who suffered pain during shoulder movements **2.63**

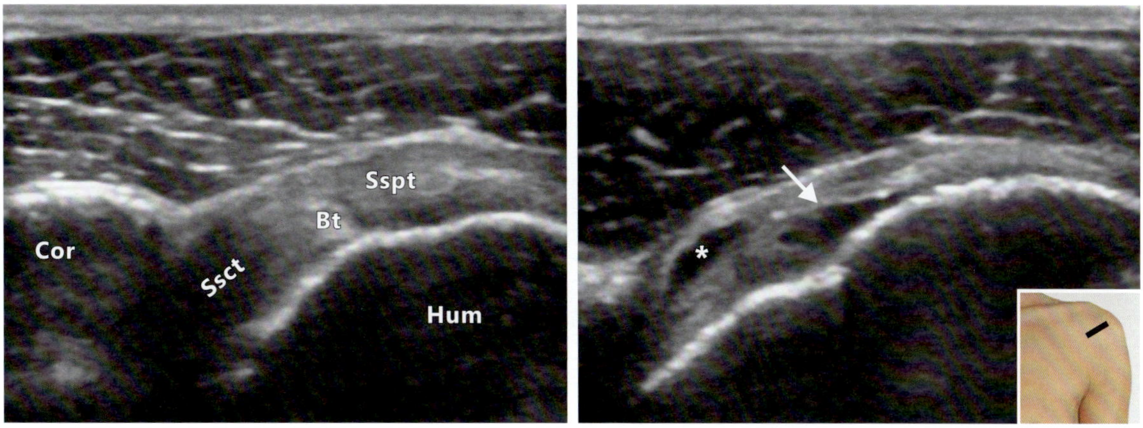

When compared with the normal side (**a**), US imaging (coracoacromial view) reveals a small amount of fluid in the bursa (*asterisk*) and an articular-sided partial tear (*arrow*) of the supraspinatus tendon (**Sspt**) (**b**).

Bt	biceps tendon	**Hum**	humerus
Cor	coracoid process	**Ssct**	subscapularis tendon

Expert note

Majority of the supraspinatus ruptures ensue in the distal ("critical") zone of the tendon and can be scanned in different views. Herewith, proximal lesions -or proximal extensions of the distal tears- need to be scanned in certain conditions and coracoacromial view (over the rotator cuff interval) would be elucidatory in that sense [1].
If there is fluid in two compartments, this is an indirect sign of a full thickness rupture of a rotator cuff tendon (cause of a connection between the two compartments).

2.64 Suprapinatus tendon tear in a 55-year-old woman with anterior shoulder pain especially during dressing and washing herself

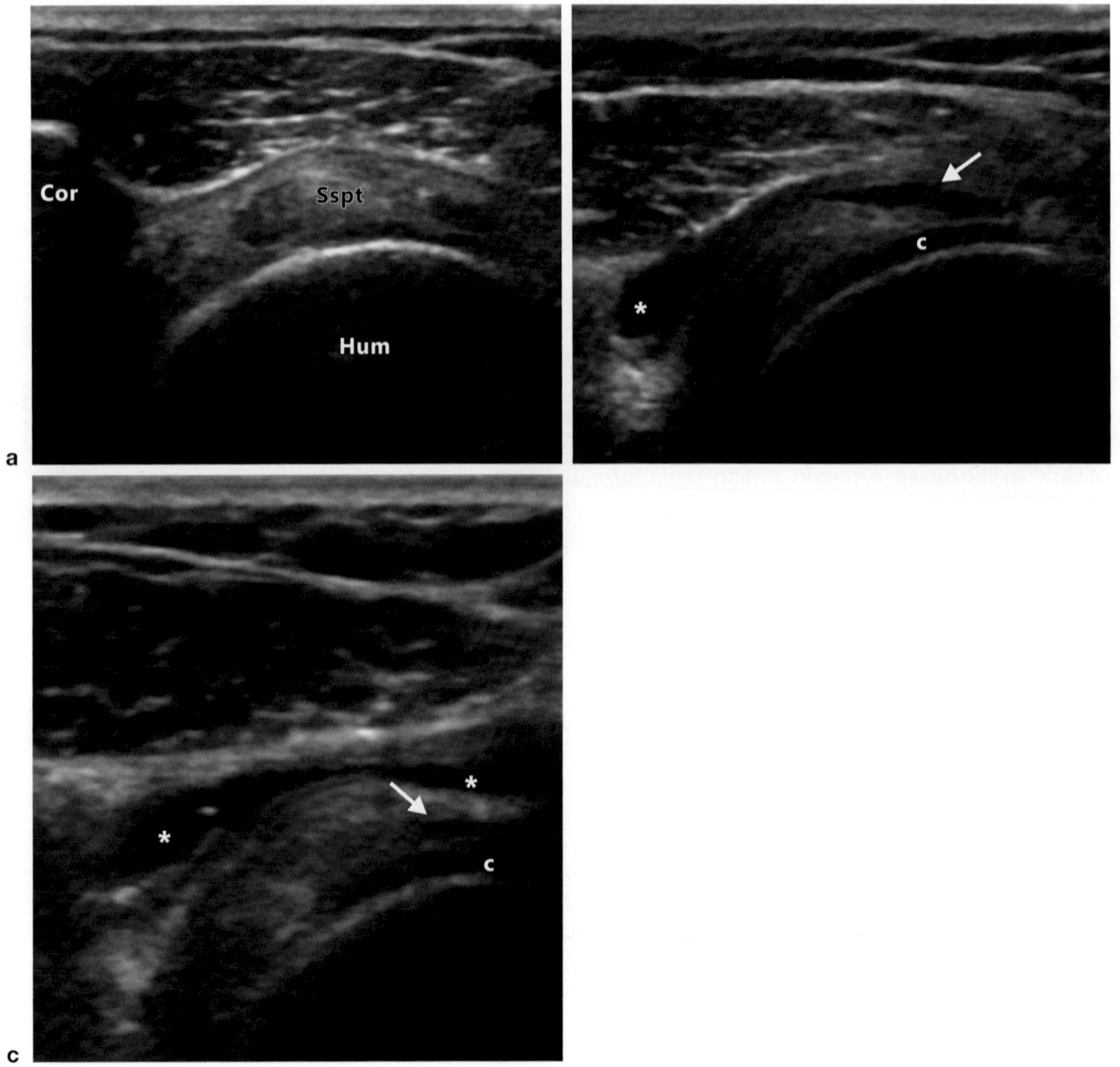

When compared with the normal look of the supraspinatus tendon (**Sspt**) (**a**), axial US images demonstrate incomplete partial-thickness tear of the tendon (*arrows*), and a small amount of fluid (*asterisks*) within the subdeltoid bursa at different zones (**b**, **c**).

c cartilage
Cor coracoid process
Hum humerus

Supraspinatus tear in a young girl who had shoulder pain with limited range of abduction **2.65**

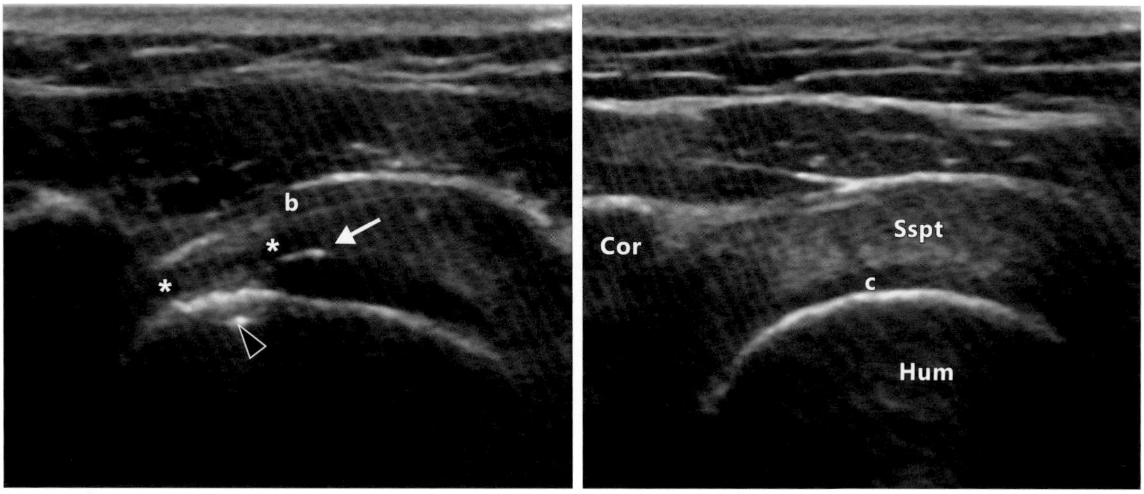

a b

Axial US image in Crass position shows full-thickness tear (*asterisks*) of the supraspinatus tendon (**SSpt**) and a focal cortical irregularity (*arrowhead*) on the head of the humerus (**a**). Please note the interface sign (*arrow*) between the anechoic defect area and the hyaline cartilage (**c**). Normal side (**b**).

b subdeltoid bursa
Cor coracoid process
Hum humerus

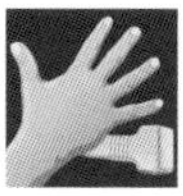

Expert note

Focal absence of the tendon (direct sign) and cartilage interface sign overlying the cortical irregularities (indirect sign) coexist in this patient.

2.66 Partial rupture of the supraspinatus tendon in a 55-year-old woman with severe shoulder pain

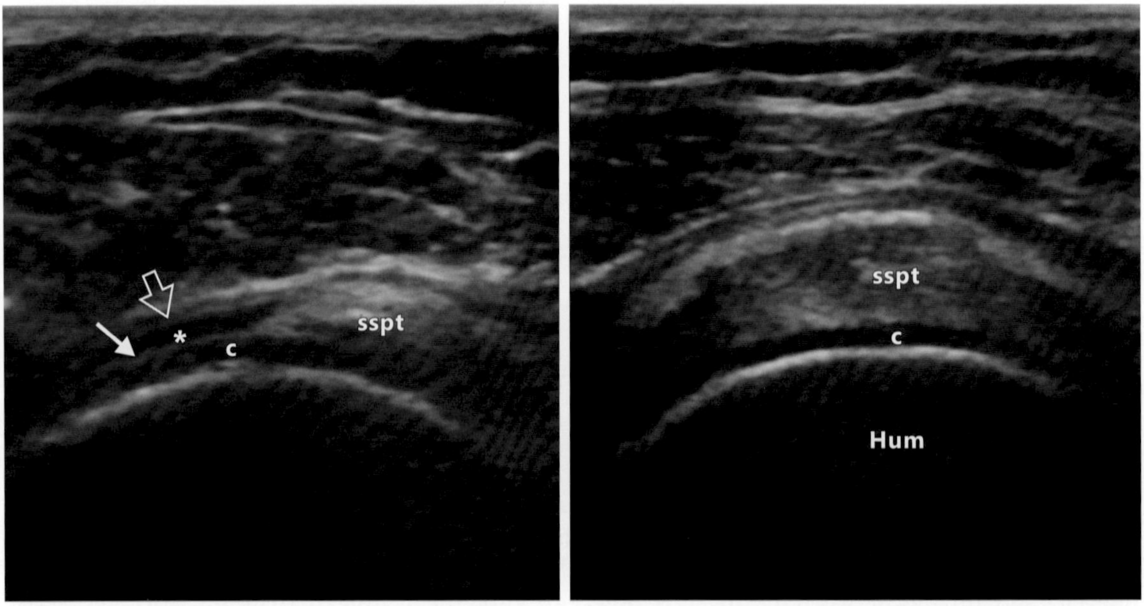

a b

Axial US imaging (**a**) reveals an incomplete full-thickness tear (*thick arrow*) of the supraspinatus tendon (**Sspt**) with a clear interface sign (*thin arrow*) between the fluid-filled defect (*asterisk*) and the hyaline cartilage (**c**). Normal side (**b**).

Hum humerus

Expert note

In this patient, the interface sign can easily be detected between the two anechoic layers which are themselves already apparent. However, in other cases where the rupture might not be so evident, the use of this artifact can help the sonographer localize the overlying tear/fluid. Yet, the underlying anechoic layer (covering the humeral head) is always articular/hyaline cartilage.

Rotator cuff tendinopathy in an elderly man with chronic shoulder pain **2.67**

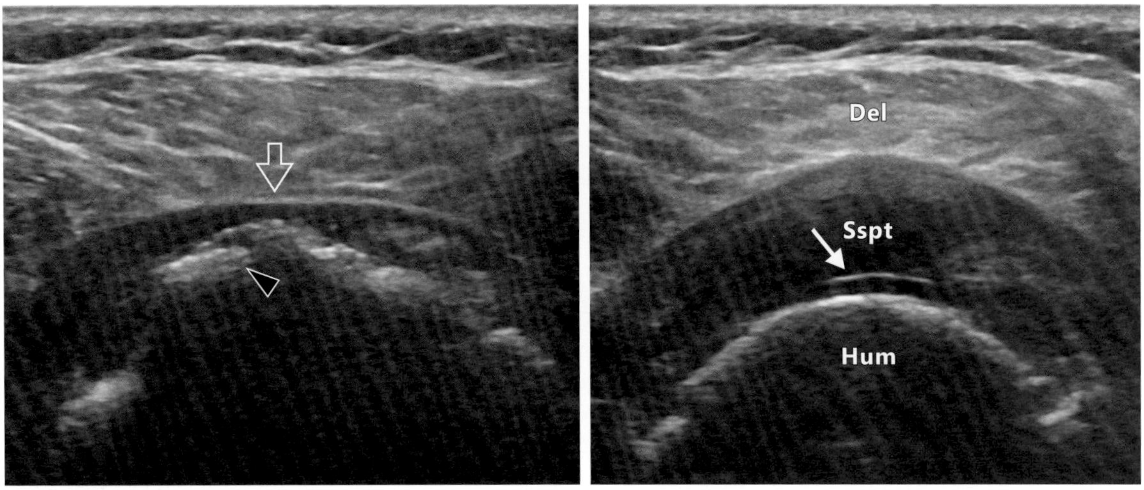

a b

Axial US image in Crass position (**a**) demonstrates an incomplete full-thickness rupture (*thick arrow*) of the supraspinatus tendon (**Sspt**) and widespread cortical irregularities (*arrowhead*) of the humerus (**Hum**). The tendon is edematous/swollen but has a normal contour on the other side (**b**).

Del deltoid

Expert note

It should be kept in mind that the interface sign (*thin arrow*) only indicates two adjacent an/hypoechoic zones, not necessarily a rupture being one of them. Like in this case, an edematous tendon might also be overlying the articular cartilage; therefore, compression or correlation with the clinical findings might again help interprete the US findings promptly.

2.68 Supraspinatus tendon tear in a 53-year-old woman with shoulder pain and anterolateral tenderness

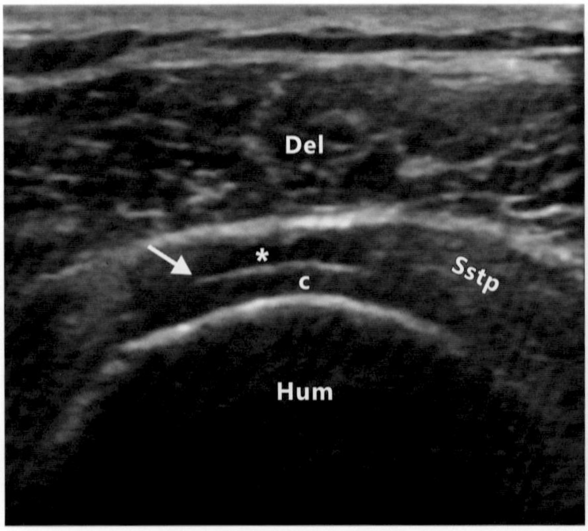

a

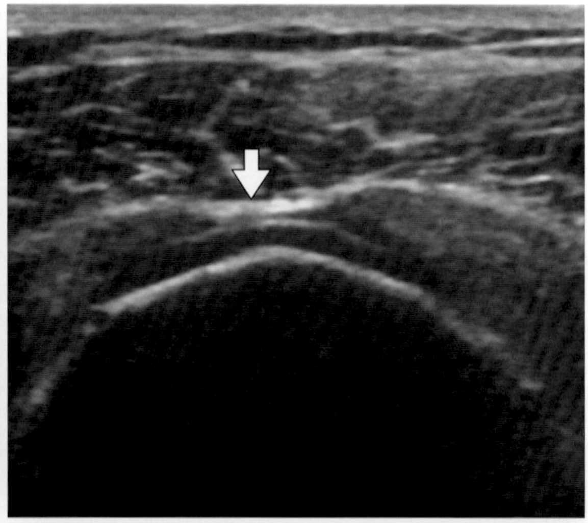

b

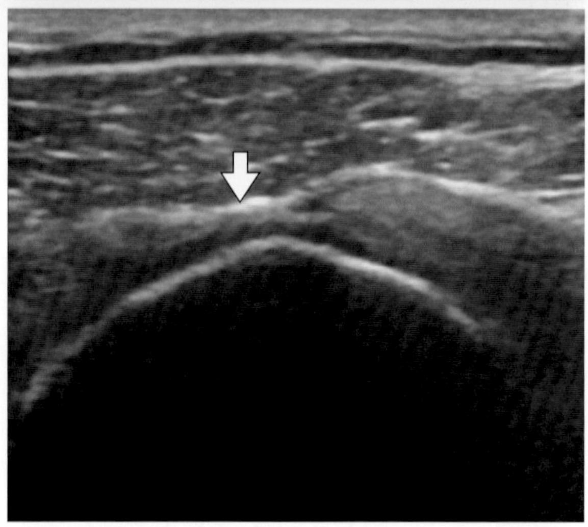

c

Video 1

Axial US imaging reveals fluid-filled (*asterisk*) incomplete full-thickness tear of the supraspinatus tendon (**Sspt**) (**a**). Herniation of the deltoid muscle (**Del**) into the defect (*thick arrows*) is seen with mild (**b**) and moderate compression (**c**) applied with the transducer. Please note the interface sign as a bright linear echo (*thin arrow*) between the bursal fluid and the articular cartilage (**c** in figure **a**).

Hum humerus

Expert note

In this case, the purpose of compression with the probe would be two-fold: first, it unmasks that the rotator cuff can be compressed (due to rupture), second, it also shows that the fluid can be displaced. For sure, the cartilage interface sign can be taken into consideration as an indirect sign of rupture as well.

Supraspinatus tendon tear in an elderly man who suffered pain when he lied on the affected arm 2.69

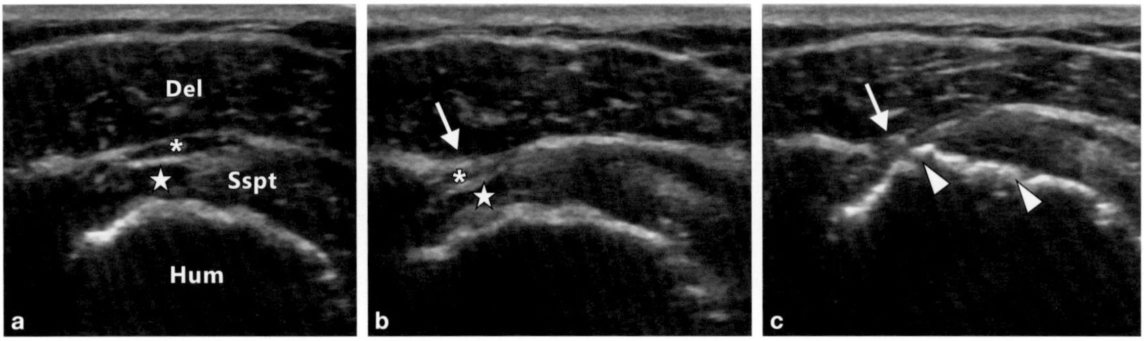

Axial US images in Crass position (**a**-**c**) show anechoic disruption of the supraspinatus tendon (**Sspt**) fibers (*stars*), a small amount of effusion in the subacromial bursa (*asterisks*) and cortical irregularities (*arrowheads*) of the humerus (**Hum**). Depending on the size of the rupture and the underlying irregularities, mild probe compressions yield different appearances (*arrows*) at various/nearby areas (**b**, **c**).

Del deltoid

2.70 Supraspinatus tendon in a 50-year-old man with a 3-month history of anterolateral shoulder pain

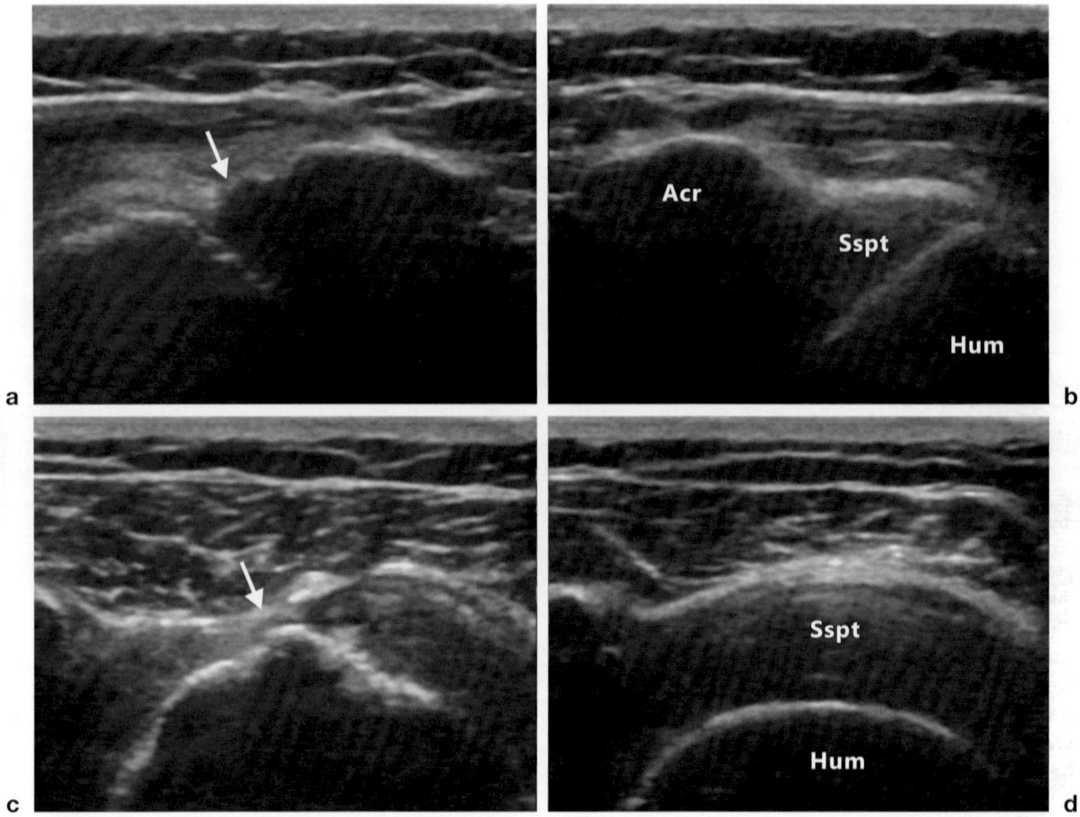

Lateral longitudinal US images (**a**, **b**) show asymmetric "bird's beak" i.e. blunt/absent (*arrow*) on the left image (**a**). Axial US image (**c**) clearly demonstrates an incomplete full-thickness tear (*arrow*) of the supraspinatus tendon (**Sspt**). Normal side (**d**).

Acr acromion
Hum humerus

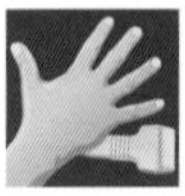

Expert note

In addition to static imaging, dynamic evaluation can also be performed with probe compression [2]. Yet, the two overt criteria for a cuff rupture would be absence of a tendon or its compressibility (healthy tendons are not compressible). Therefore, if the classical ("car tire") appearance is not present and replaced by a "flat tire" on static/dynamic imaging, the diagnosis of a rupture can be established.

While axial views are generally used to have/explain more details concerning the rotator cuff tears, lateral coronal view ("bird's beak" appearance) can provide an initial/overall snapshot as well.

Additionally, the narrowing of the subacromial space can be taken as an indirect sign (change seen in the environment not directly in the tendon) of a rupture.

Supraspinatus tendon rupture in a 50-year-old man who had pain when lifting and lowering his arm or during sudden movements **2.71**

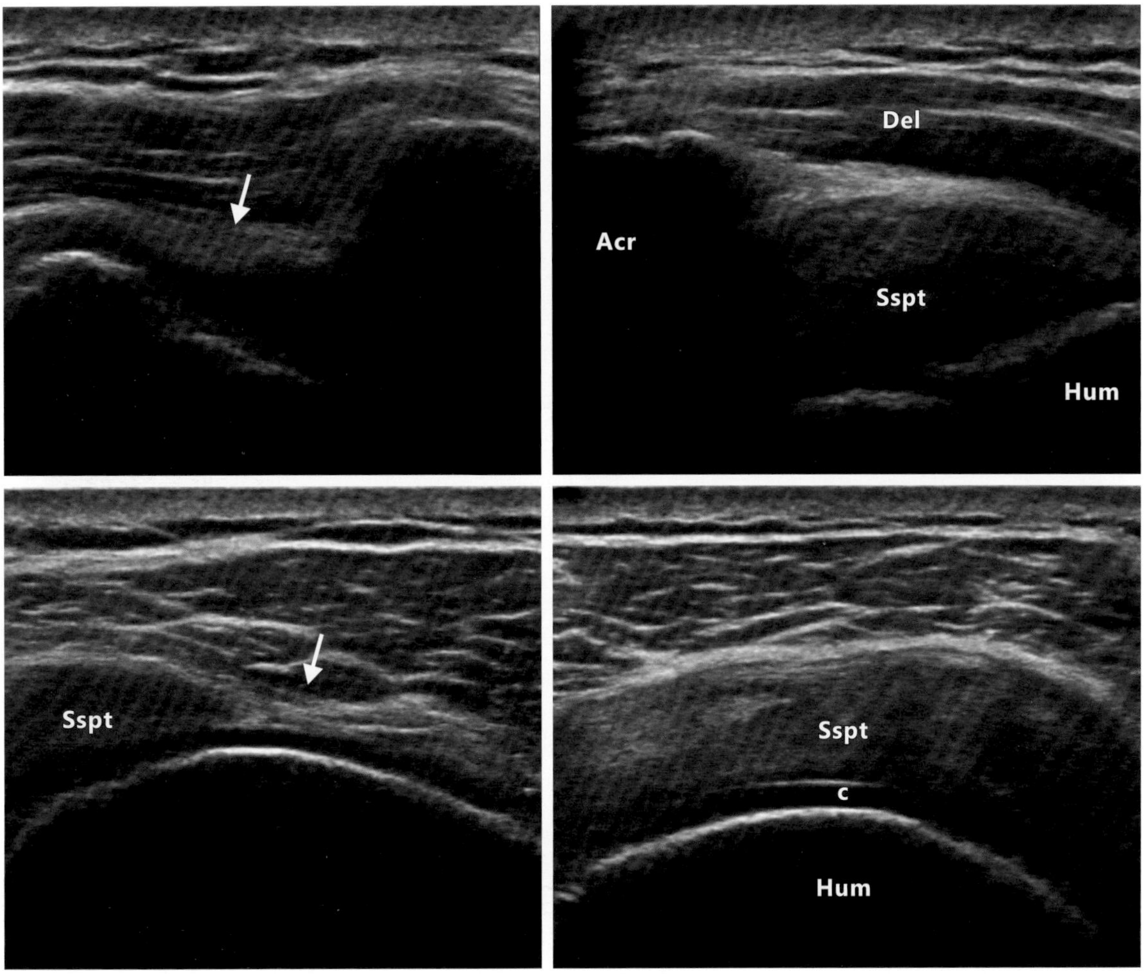

a b c d

Longitudinal (**a**) and axial (**c**) US images over the cranial aspect of the humeral head (**Hum**) shows herniation (*arrows*) of the deltoid muscle (**Del**) secondary to an incomplete full-thickness supraspinatus tendon (**Sspt**) tear. Corresponding contralateral views show normal appearance of the tendon (**b**, **d**).

Acr acromion
c cartilage

Expert note

If the small interface sign on figure **d** is reproducible with different probe angulations, one likely reason would be a focal edema or subtle tear in the tendon.

2.72 Supraspinatus tendon tear and severe enthesopathy in a patient with reactive arthritis

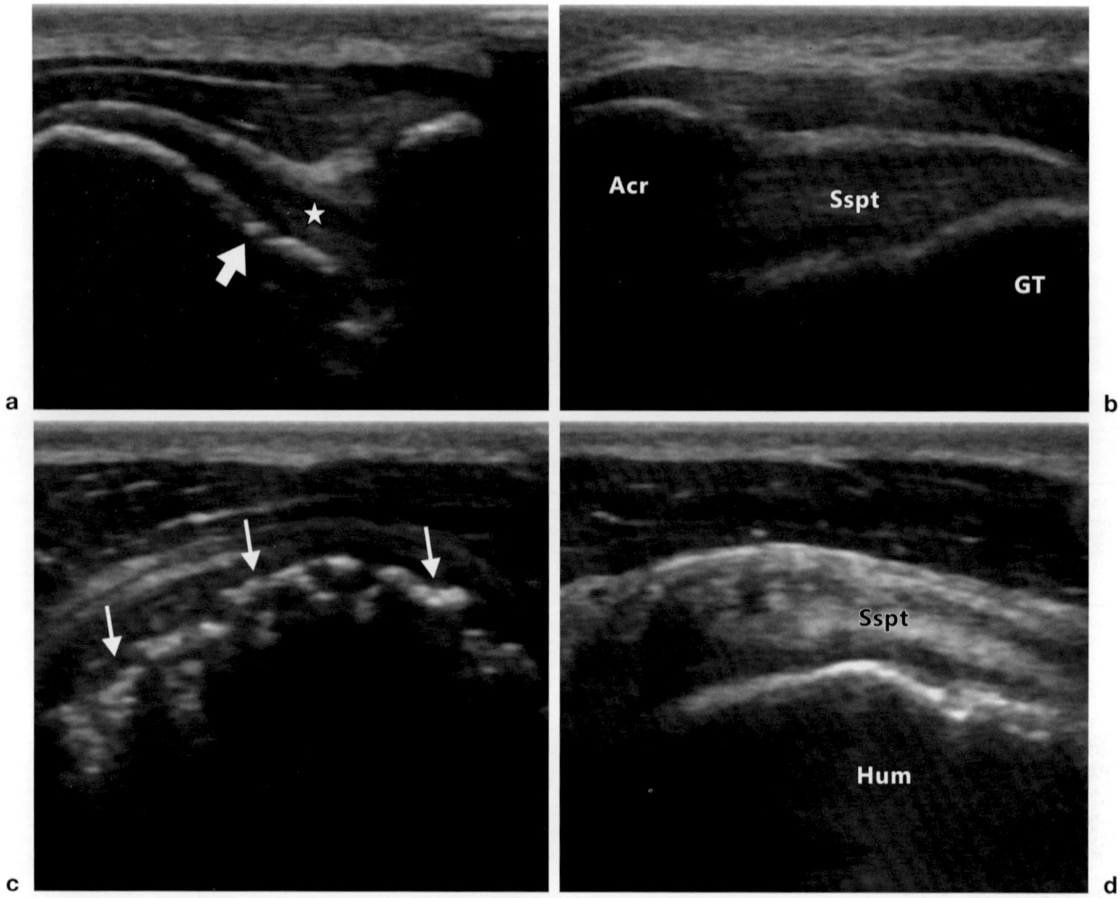

Initial lateral coronal US image shows the absence of "bird's beak" appearance (*star*) of the supraspinatus tendon (**Sspt**) and mild cortical irregularities (*thick arrow*) (**a**). Normal side (**b**). Axial imaging with Crass position clearly reveals a wide full thickness tear with severe enthesopathy (*thin arrows*) on the humeral head (**Hum**) (**c**). Normal side (**d**).

Acr acromion
GT greater tubercle

Expert note

As noted elsewhere, axial imaging is much more demonstrative for enthesopathies. These massive irregularities are seldom seen in "classical" traumatic or degenerative tendon problems.

Supraspinatus tendon tears in a 77-year-old woman who had restricted shoulder motions in all planes 2.73

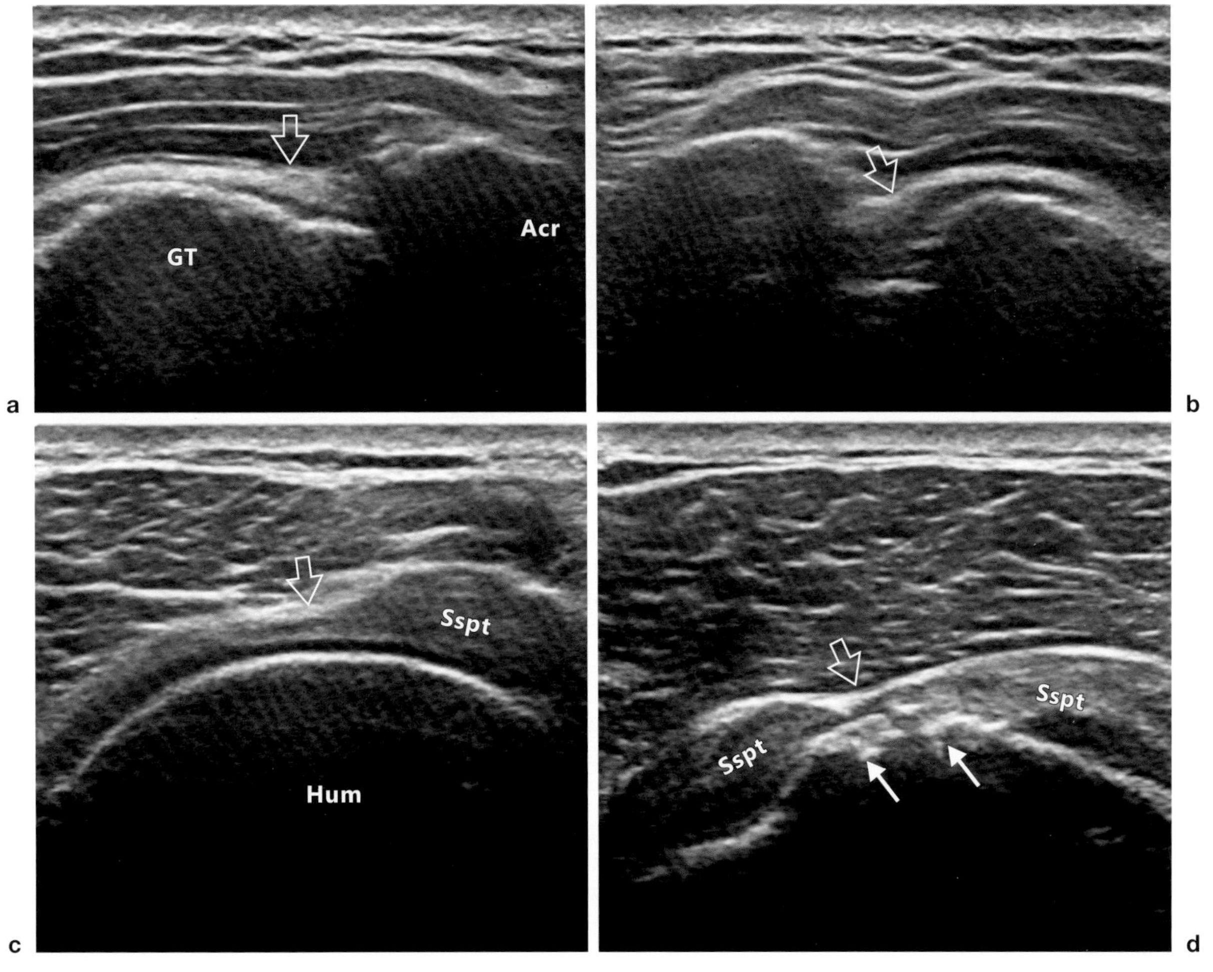

Lateral longitudinal (**a**, **b**) and axial images show bilateral large (**c**) and small (**d**) full-thickness tears (*thick arrows*) of the supraspinatus tendons (**Sspt**) accompanied by unilateral cortical irregularities (*thin arrows*).

Acr acromion
GT greater tubercle
Hum head of humerus

2.74 Bilateral incomplete tears of the supraspinatus tendon in an elderly patient who had dull shoulder pain and weakness in abduction

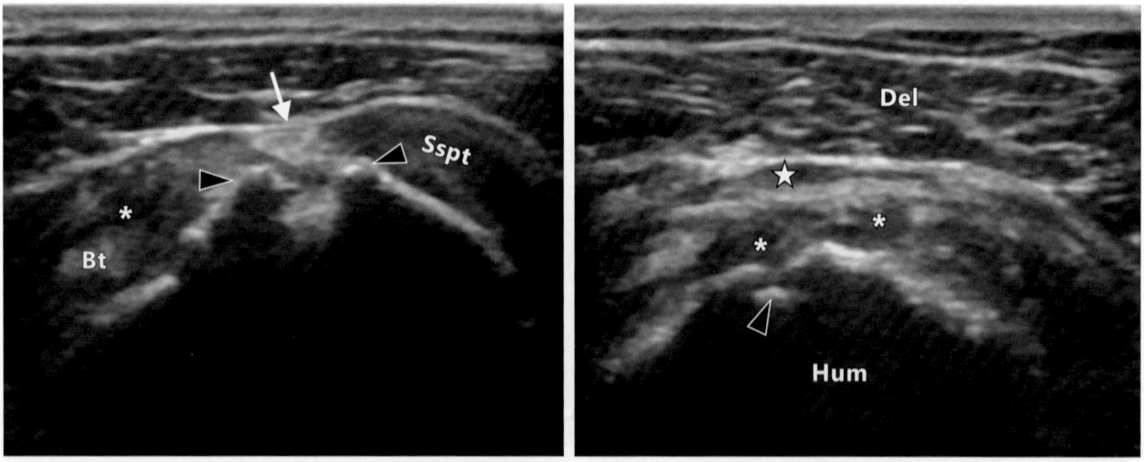

a b

Axial US images demonstrate a full thickness tear (*arrow*) of the supraspinatus tendon (**Sspt**) on the symptomatic side (**a**) and an irregular articular-sided partial-thickness tear on the asymptomatic side (**b**). Please note the hypoechoic appearance of the disrupted tendon fibers (*asterisks*) and the cortical irregularities (*arrowheads*) of the humerus (**Hum**) on both sides. *Star* indicates the mild accompanying subdeltoid bursitis.

Bt biceps tendon

Expert note

One important advantage of US imaging in the elderly is definitely comparison. Yet, several pathologies can also be found on the asymptomatic sides of the patients and they can be reassured as regards their joint problems in advance.

On the symptomatic side, there are changes in shape and echogenicity as direct signs of rupture; the cortical irregularities are indirect signs. On the asymptomatic side, there are changes in echogenicity (focal hypoechoic zones) with enhancement (bright cortex). The cortex is also irregular on that side. Above the age of 65, one very often finds asymptomatic ruptures of the supraspinatus tendon. Herewith, in symptomatic ruptures, one often finds accompanying bursitis or biceps tenosynovitis.

Supraspinatus tears in an elderly woman with shoulder pain and weakness on abduction

2.75

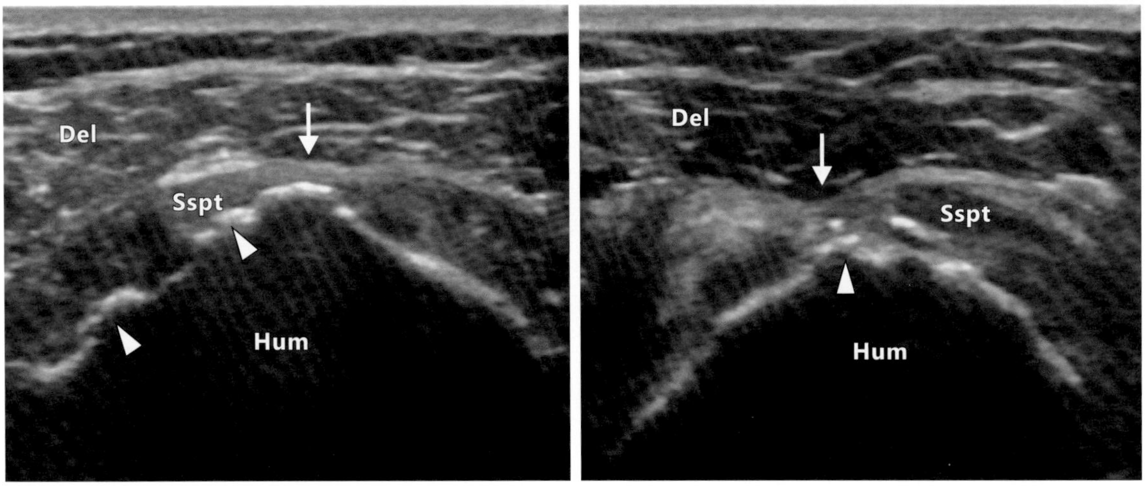

Axial US images in Crass position show incomplete full-thickness tears (*arrows*) of the supraspinatus tendon (**Sspt**) and cortical irregularities (*arrowheads*) on the humerus (**Hum**) (**a**, **b**). During sono-palpation, it is observed that the deltoid (**Del**) fills (bulges into) the area where the Sspt is torn (and thus compressible) (**b**).

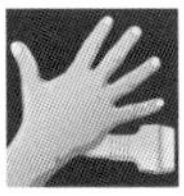

Expert note

Just to remind the criteria for rotator cuff tears [2]:

- *Direct*
  - Changes in shape (focal thinning -"flat tire"- or absence of a tendon) and echogenicity (hypoechoic focus and central echogenic band)
  - Hypoechoic lesion with articular or bursal extension
  - Fluid-filled defect
  - Compressibility
- *Indirect*
  - Narrowing of the subacromial space
  - Fluid in two compartments
  - Cortical irregularity on greater tubercle
  - Interface sign

2.76 Rupture of the supraspinatus tendon in a 58-year-old man after falling from a bicycle

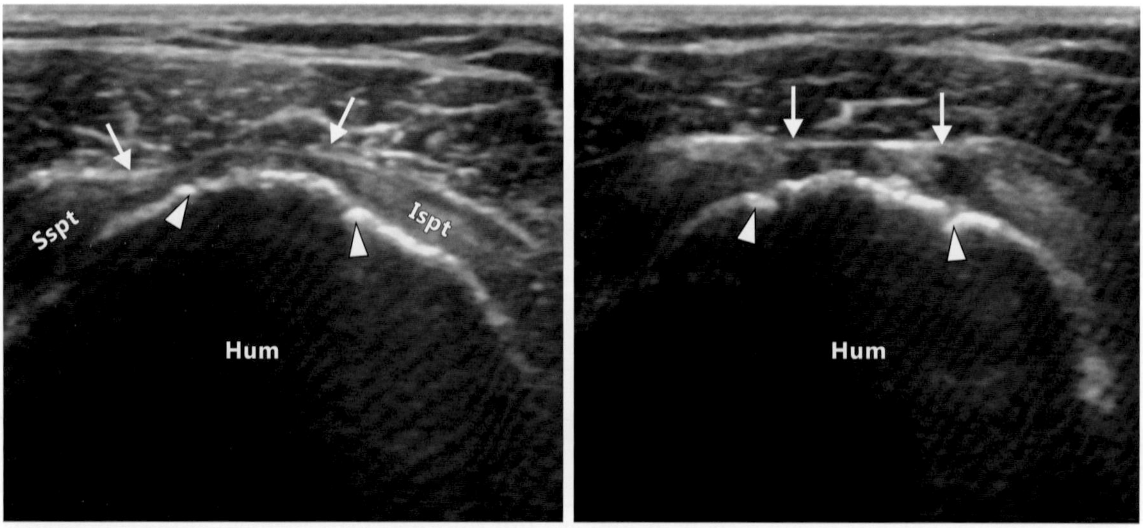

a b

He had a positive drop sign during evaluation of the rotator cuff.

Axial US images in Crass position show incomplete full-thickness rupture (*arrows*) of the supraspinatus tendons (**Sspt**) and mild cortical irregularities (*arrowheads*) on the humeral heads (**Hum**) bilaterally (**a**, **b**).

Ispt infraspinatus tendon

Expert note

The term "full-thickness" refers to the extent of the rupture in a particular area. In case of "partial thickness" ruptures, it would also be important to further note the exact localization i.e. bursal side, articular side or intratendinous. On the other hand, the terms "partial" or "incomplete" *vs* "complete" refer more to the width of the rupture i.e. how wide the tear expands within the tendon.
A rupture has in fact three dimensions [2]: thickness and width, which we are used to evaluating with US, but also "length" (the retraction between the proximal and distal stumps) which we do/can not evaluate.

Supraspinatus tendon tear in a 60-year-old man with shoulder pain especially during overhead activities **2.77**

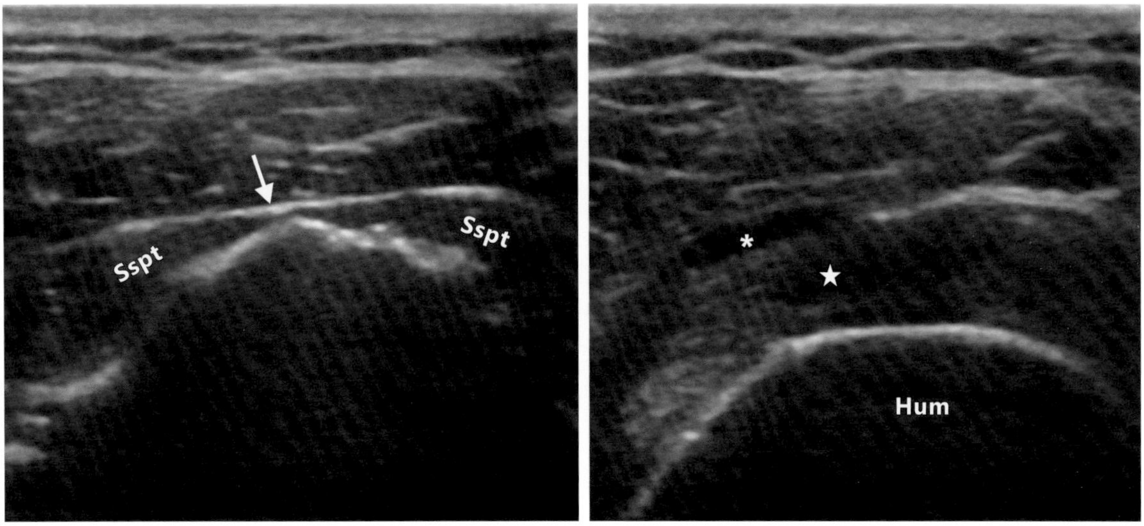

a b

Axial image in Crass position demonstrates full-thickness supraspinatus tendon (**Sspt**) tear (*arrow*) on the asymptomatic side (**a**). Only partial-thickness tear (*star*) and mild effusion in the subdeltoid bursa (*asterisk*) are seen on the symptomatic side (**b**).

Hum head of humerus

Expert note

It is noteworthy that the painful complaints of the patients do not necessarily stem only from the cuff tears but -for instance- that mild bursitis might well turn out to be a more disturbing scenario.

2.78 Bilateral supraspinatus tendon ruptures in a 60-year-old man with complaints of severe pain and restricted shoulder movements

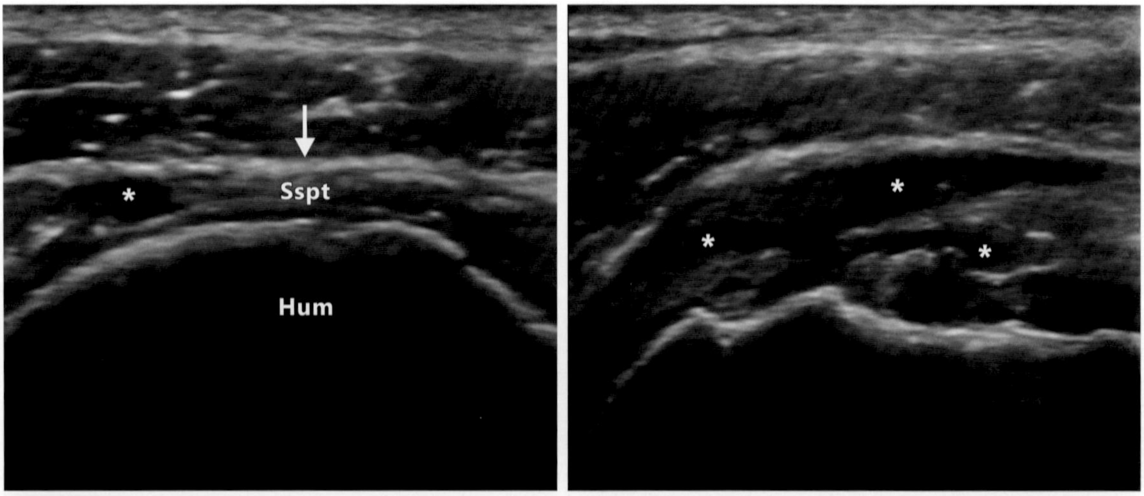

a b

Axial US image in Crass position demonstrates neighboring zones of focal tear (*asterisk*) and thinning of the supraspinatus tendon (**Sspt**) (*arrow*) (**a**). Although the tendon contour seems to be preserved, tears (*asterisks*) involving a large area and extending towards the bursa are seen on the contralateral side (**b**).

Hum head of humerus

Expert note

On both sides, there is a focal anechoic zone in the tendon, in contact with articular and bursal sides (direct sign of a full-thickness rupture). In figure **b**, there is a filled bursa, probably with thickened synovial wall. This is actually a good example/image to demonstrate how (otherwise non-communicating) subdeltoid bursa and the joint space may somehow be connected.

Bilateral supraspinatus rupture in a 75-year-old man with shoulder pain worse at night and during daily activities **2.79**

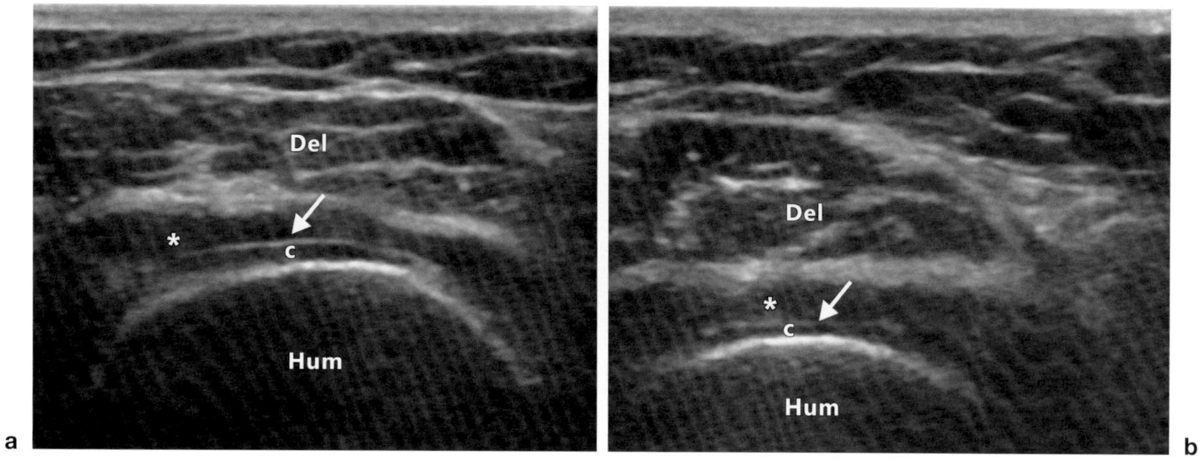

Axial US images in Crass position reveal bilateral full-thickness rupture of the supraspinatus tendon. Interface sign (*arrows*) between the effusion in the subdeltoid bursa (*asterisks*) and the surface of the articular cartilage (**c**) is also observed bilaterally.

Del deltoid

Hum head of humerus

Supraspinatus tendon tear in a 76-year-old man who had gradually increasing shoulder problems over the last five years **2.80**

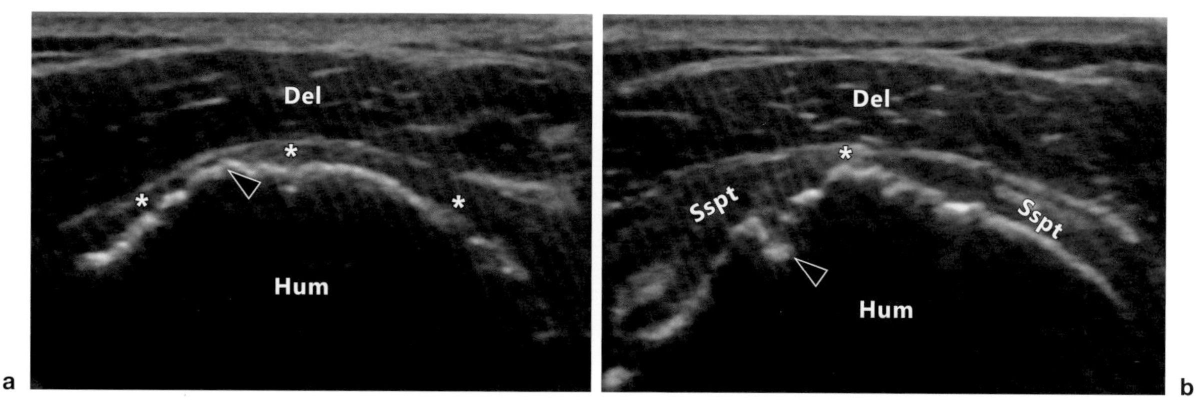

Axial US images over the supraspinatus tendon (**Sspt**) illustrate complete (**a**) and partial (**b**) full-thickness tears (*asterisks*) together with bony irregularities (*arrowheads*).

Expert note

Although the humeral head is totally "naked" in figure **a**, substantial scanning for the supraspinatus tendon should be done before one can say it is a massive complete rupture.

2.81 Bilateral supraspinatus tendon tear in a 77-year-old woman with pain and limited movements in the shoulders

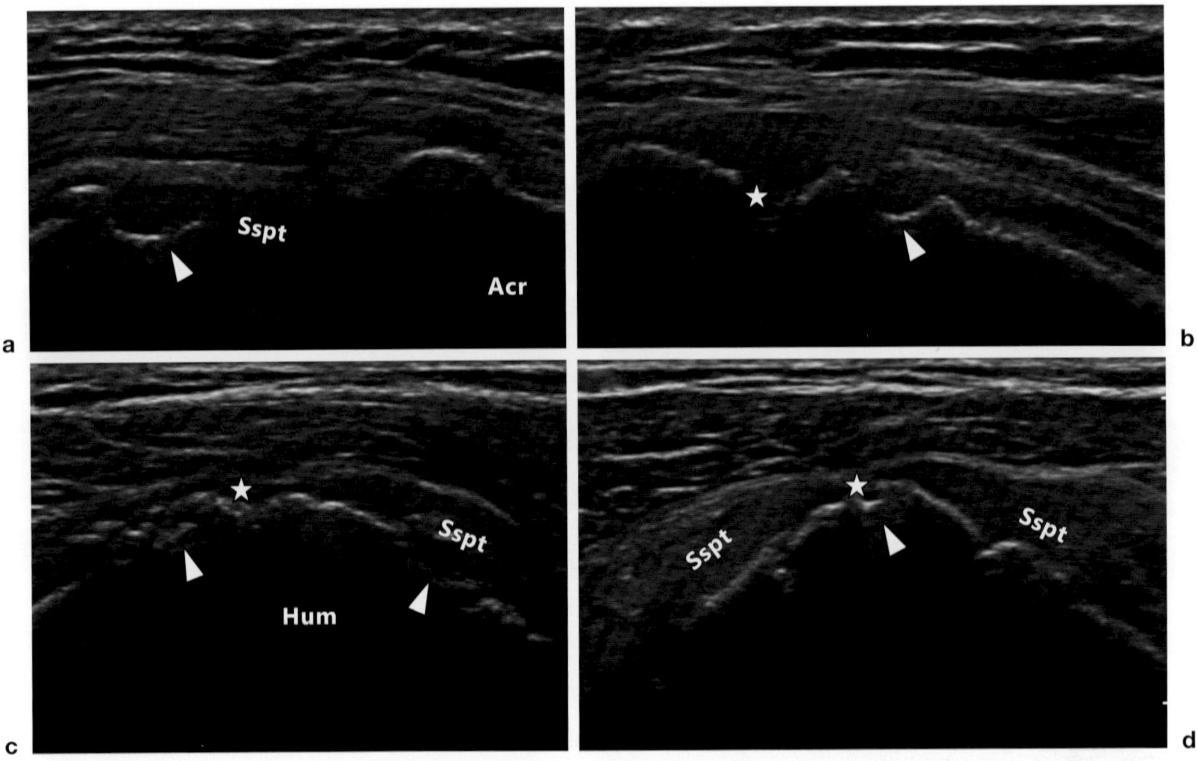

Longitudinal (**a**, **b**) and axial US images reveal large (**c**) and small (**d**) full-thickness supraspinatus tendon (**Sspt**) tears (*stars*) and severe cortical irregularities (*arrowheads*) on the humeral head (**Hum**) on both sides.

Acr acromion

Expert note

In case of full-thickness tears, the humeral head would likely dislocate superiorly. This would either make it very difficult to distinguish the two bones (acromion and humerus) like in figure **b** or distort the classical appearance of "parrot's beak" in coronal view [11]. It is especially true when there are significant changes in the bony contours (e.g. degeneration).
The radiographs will probably show severe ascending arthrosis in this case.

Bilateral complete rupture of the supraspinatus tendon in an elderly woman with inability to abduct her shoulders

2.82

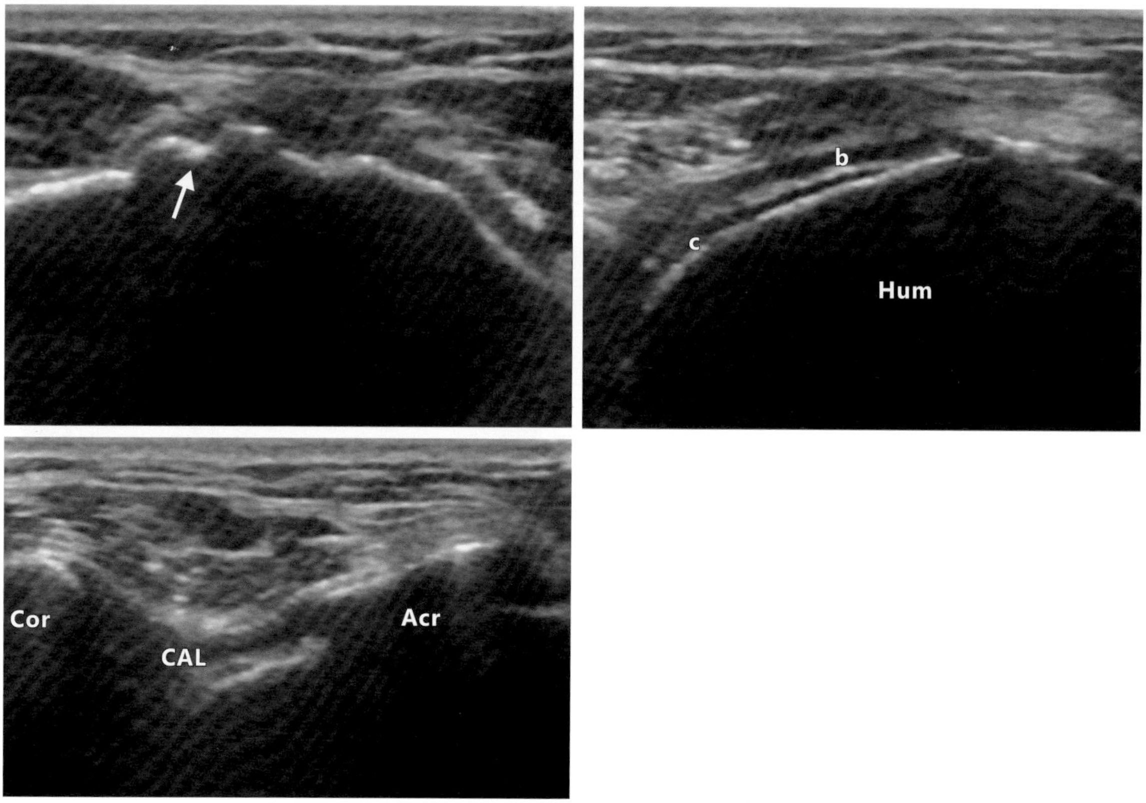

a b c

Axial US images over the rotator cuff show bilateral "naked bone" appearance distally (**a**, **b**) with mild cortical irregularity (*arrow*) on one side (**a**). Coracoacromial (**CAL**) view demonstrates absence of the cuff proximally as well (**c**).

Acr	acromion	**Cor**	coracoid process
b	subacromial-subdeltoid bursa	**Hum**	head of humerus
c	cartilage		

Expert note

Note that the overlying deltoid muscle is quite thin as well.

2.83 Supraspinatus tendon rupture in an elderly man who suffered bilateral frozen shoulder after a high-energy trauma

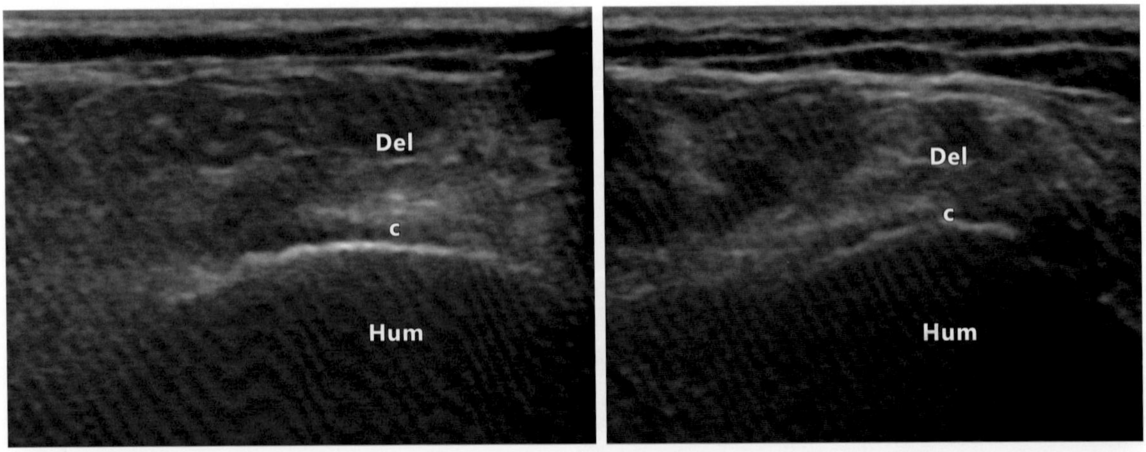

a b

Axial US images over the supraspinatus tendon reveal bilateral massive complete rupture whereby deltoid muscle (**Del**) is covering the "bare bone" (**a**, **b**).

c cartilage
Hum head of humerus

Expert note

In case of complete rotator cuff ruptures, the appearance is termed as "bare" or "naked bone". In young people, the deltoid muscle will have a "starry night" appearance in axial view (bright black, with white septa); in old people the contrast in the images will be less.

Severe rotator cuff tear in a 67-year-old woman with pain and reduced shoulder range of movements (especially abduction) 2.84

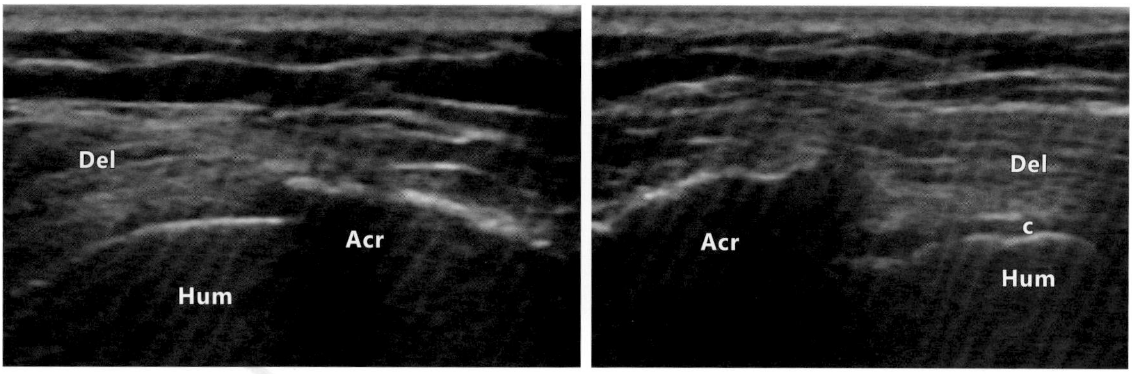

a b

Lateral longitudinal US images demonstrate complete absence of the typical "bird's beak" appearance (**a**, **b**). Accordingly, the humeral heads (**Hum**) seem to almost touch the acromion (**Acr**) due to superior luxation -more overt on the left image (**a**).

c cartilage
Del deltoid

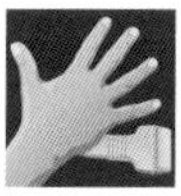

Expert note

While the static images would reveal similar information as compared with the radiographs, dynamic assessment might shed more light into understanding the limited/painful shoulder abduction. For sure, substantial scanning for the tendons can unmask the details of the cuff rupture as well.

2.85 Repaired supraspinatus tendon in an adult after a fall on the shoulder

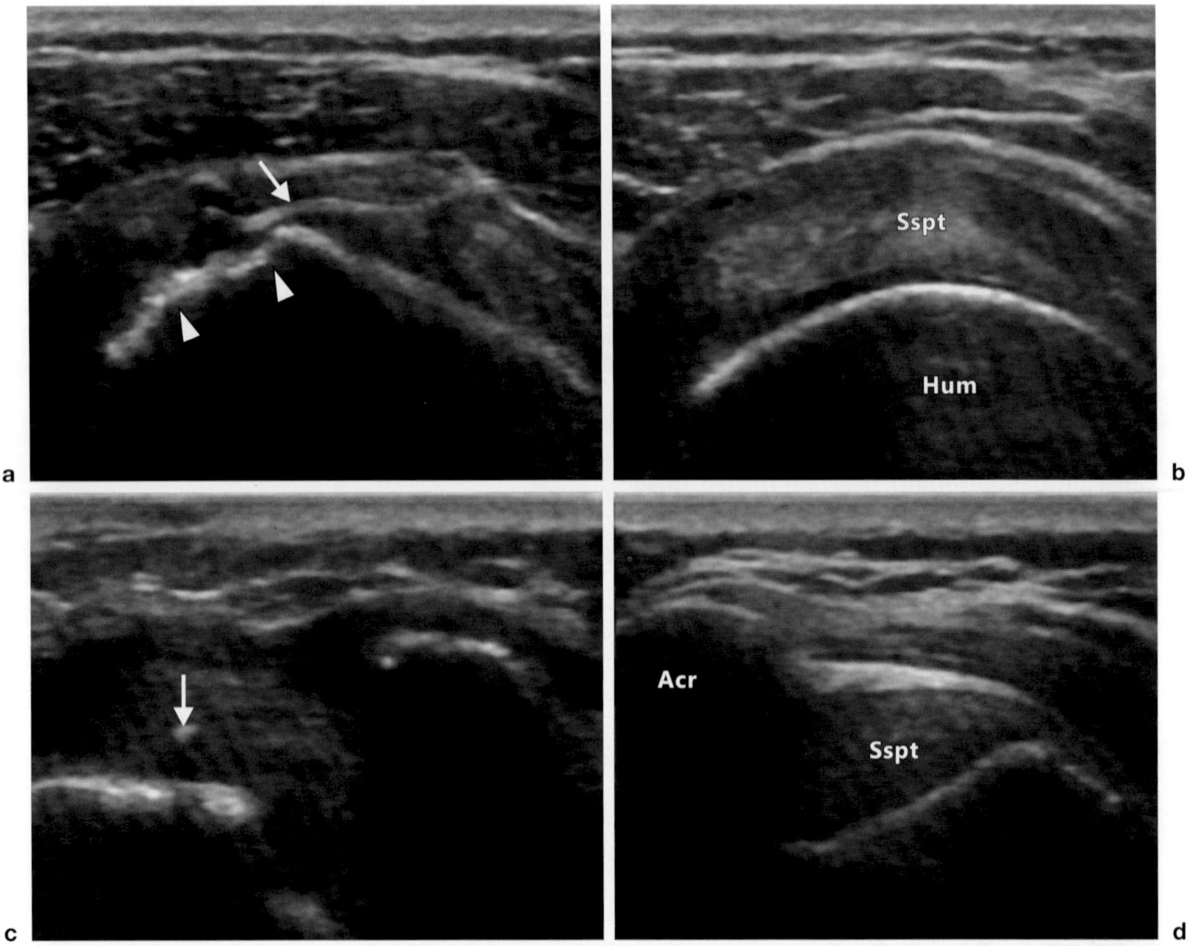

Anterior axial (**a**) and lateral coronal (**c**) US images show cortical irregularities (*arrowheads*) of the humeral head (**Hum**) and hyperechoic suture material (*arrows*) within the irregular supraspinatus tendon (**Sspt**). Normal corresponding images (**b**, **d**).

Acr acromion

Expert note

After repair, the image of a tendon never becomes "perfectly" normal. A single evaluation when postoperative clinical evolution is abnormal, can often be disappointing. Ideally, one should do regular US follow-up during rehabilitation to be able to detect deterioration.

Shoulder

Supraspinatus tendon tear in a 62-year-old man with shoulder pain increasing with abduction and at night **2.86**

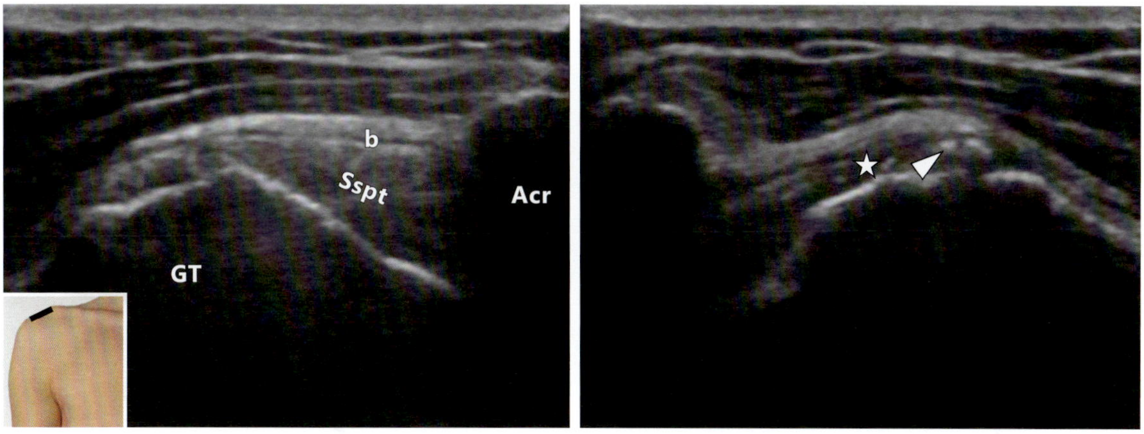

a b

When compared with the normal side (**a**), lateral longitudinal image demonstrates a tear (*star*) at the distal insertion of the supraspinatus tendon (**Sspt**) on the greater tubercle (**GT**) (**b**).
Please note that a small type II calcification (*arrowhead*) is also seen within the distal tendon.

Acr acromion **b** subacromial-subdeltoid bursa

Calcifying supraspinatus tendon in a 55-year-old man with severe disabling pain **2.87**

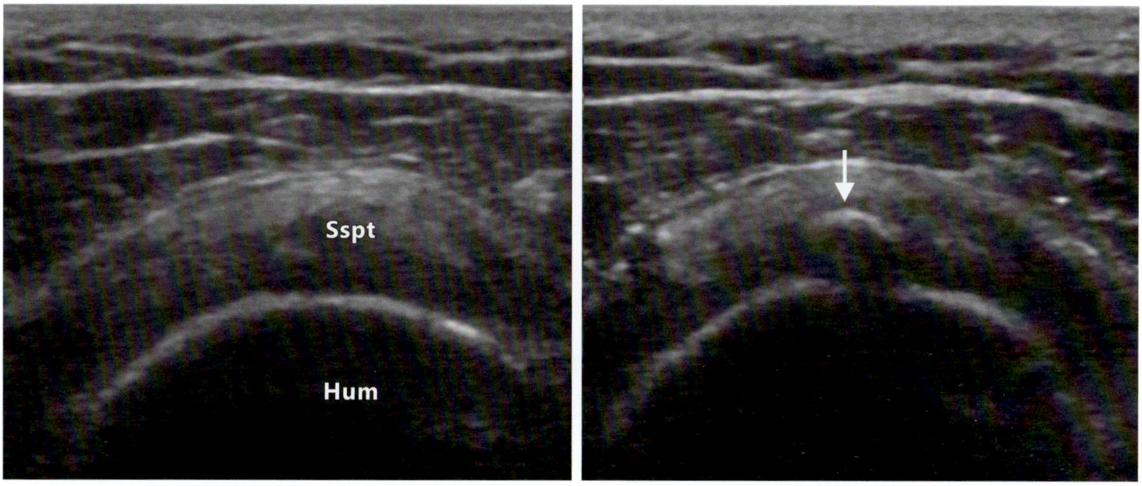

a b

When compared with the normal side (**a**), axial US imaging in Crass position (**b**) shows type I calcification (*arrow*) in the supraspinatus tendon (**Sspt**).

Hum humerus

2.88 Shoulder joint effusion and supraspinatus tendon calcification in a 44-year-old woman

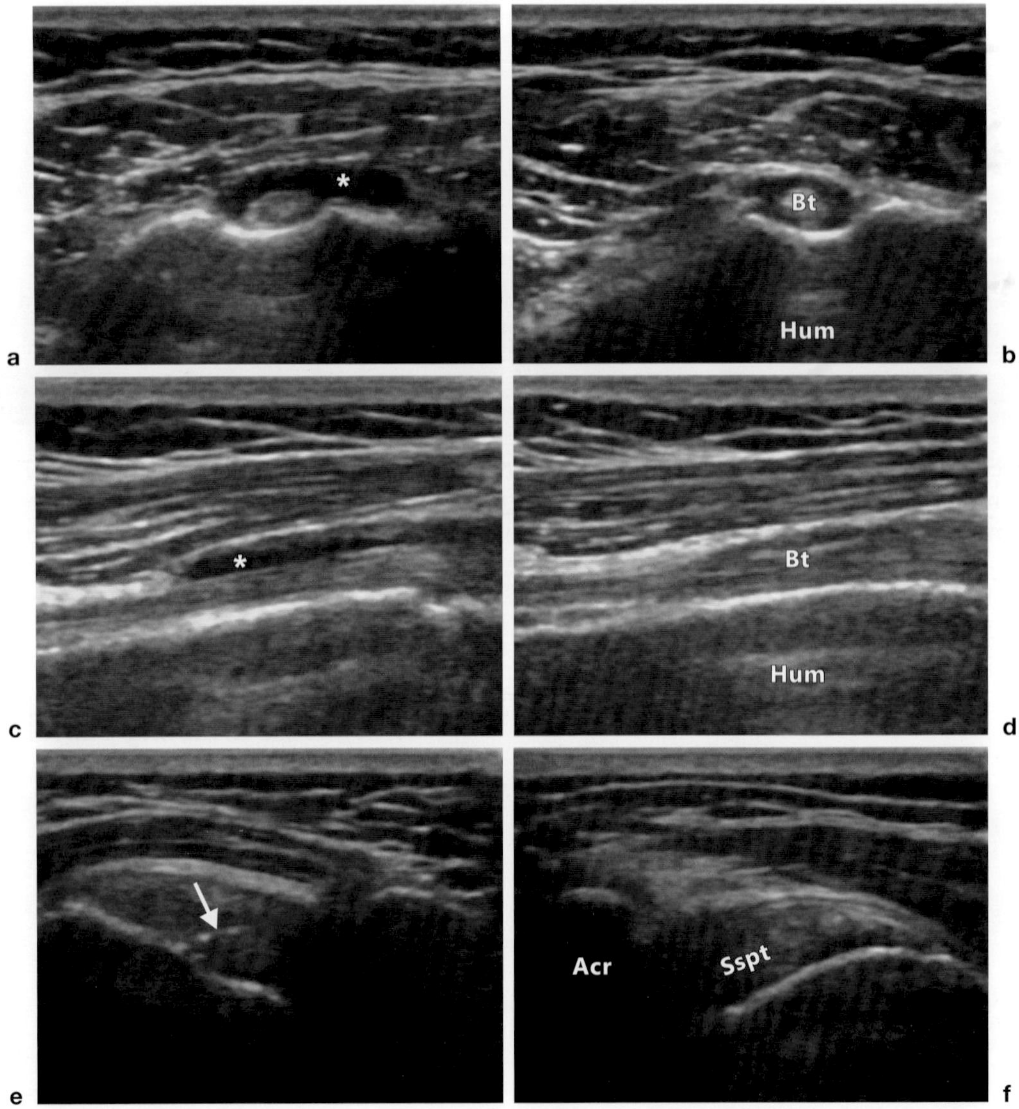

The patient had a 2-month history of intense shoulder pain and tenderness over the medial and posterior parts of her shoulder.

Axial (**a**) and longitudinal (**c**) US images over the humeral head (**Hum**) reveal effusion (*asterisks*) within the biceps tendon (**Bt**) sheath. Lateral longitudinal US image demonstrates a Grade III hyperechoic calcification (*arrow*) within the supraspinatus tendon (**Sspt**) (**e**). Normal corresponding views (**b**, **d**, **f**).

Acr acromion

Calcific supraspinatus tendinitis in a 60-year-old woman who had intermittent shoulder pain **2.89**

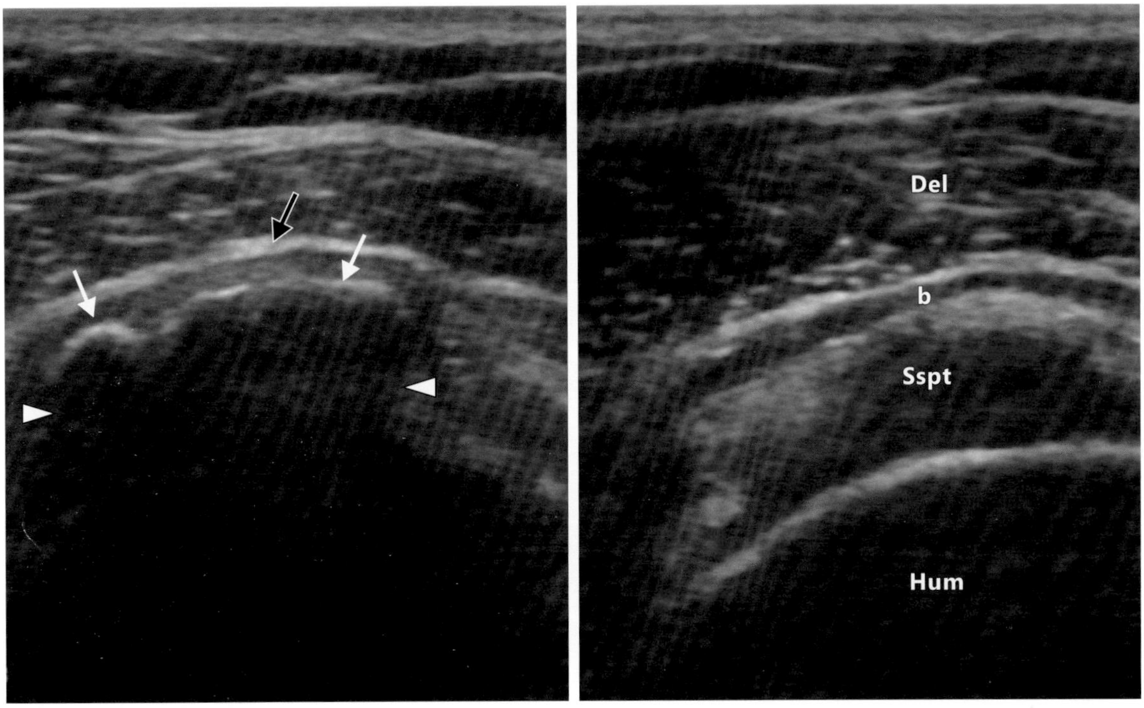

a b

Axial US image (**a**) demonstrates a huge acoustic shadowing (*arrowheads*) obliterating the cortical image of humerus (**Hum**). A large type I calcification (*white arrows*) is seen very close to the subdeltoid fat (*black arrow*) i.e. superficially localized within the supraspinatus tendon (**Sspt**) (**a**). Normal contralateral side (**b**).

b subdeltoid bursa
Del deltoid

Expert note

Although calcifications may be apparent sonographically before they are evident on radiographs, shoulder X-rays can be used to have an overall/better orientation.

2.90 Rotator cuff pathologies in a 54-year-old man with complaints of bilateral chronic shoulder pain

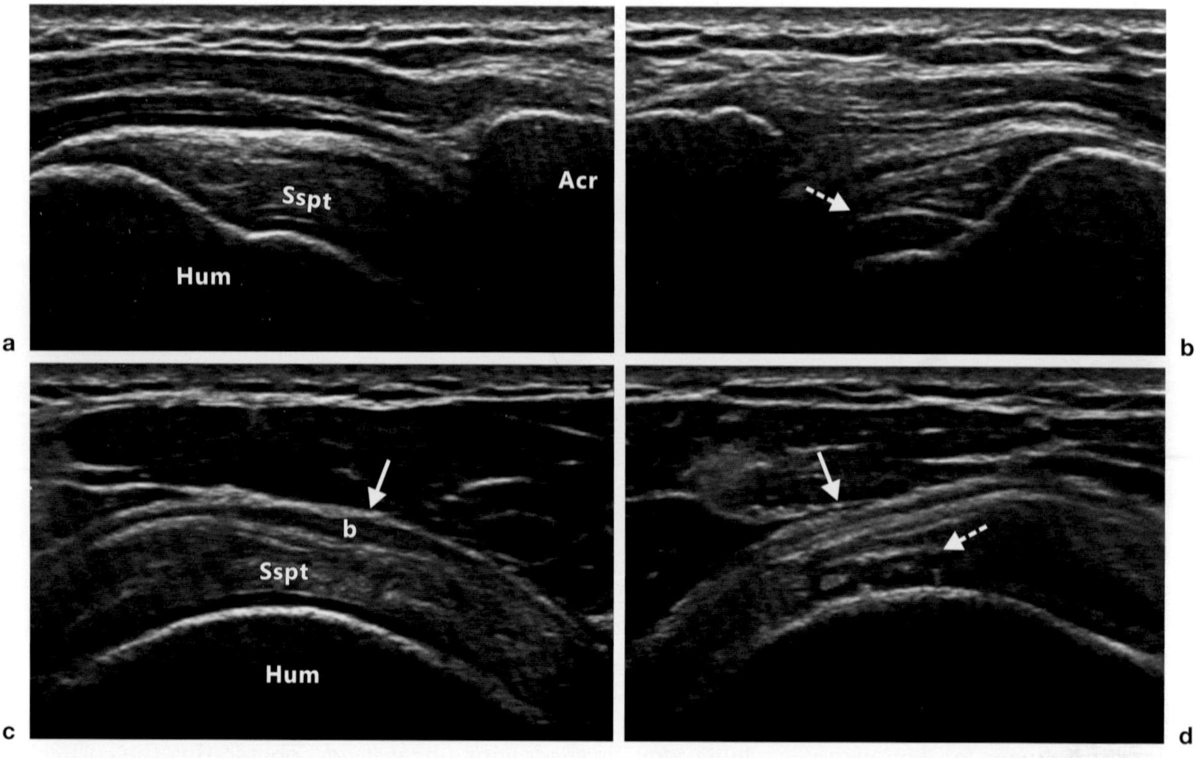

Comparative longitudinal (**a**, **b**) and axial (**c**, **d**) images for supraspinatus tendon (**Sspt**) show bilateral partial-thickness ruptures seen as focal thinning (*arrows*) but also concomitant type III calcific deposits (*dashed arrows*) on one side (**b**, **d**).

Acr acromion
b subdeltoid bursa
Hum humerus

Bilateral calcifying tendinitis of the supraspinatus tendon in a 44-year-old woman **2.91**

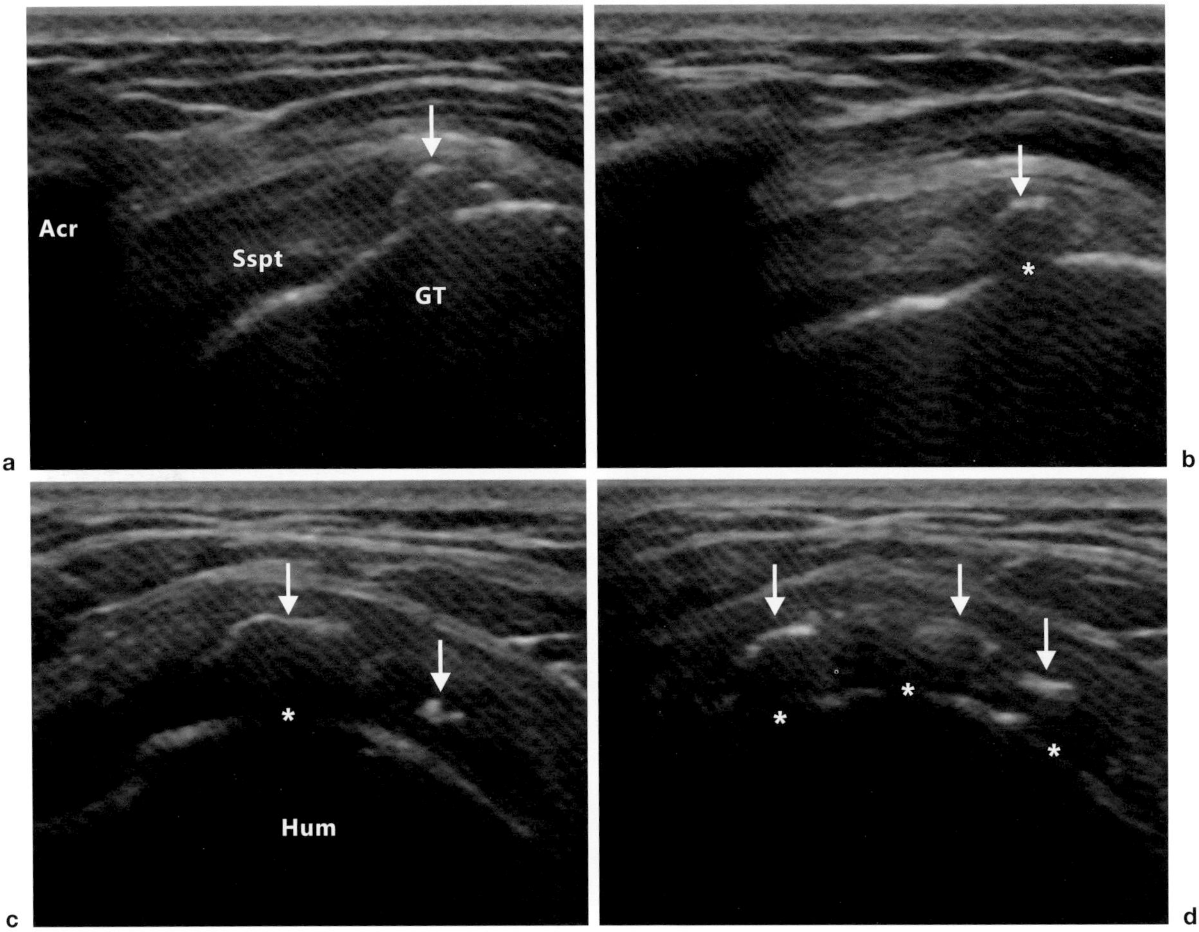

She had 3-month history of intense shoulder pain during abduction of >50°.

Lateral longitudinal (**a**, **b**) and axial (**c**, **d**) US images show type II calcific deposits (*arrows*) within the supraspinatus tendon (**Sspt**) and incomplete posterior acoustic shadowing artifacts (*asterisks*).

Acr	acromion	**Hum**	humerus
GT	greater tubercle		

Expert note

Similar to what is suggested for the evaluation of enthesopathies, axial imaging can better distinguish the multiple lesions (if any) which cannot be readily differentiated while scanning in the long axis.

2.92 Calcifying supraspinatus tendinitis in a 55-year-old woman with limited shoulder movements due to pain and muscle spasm

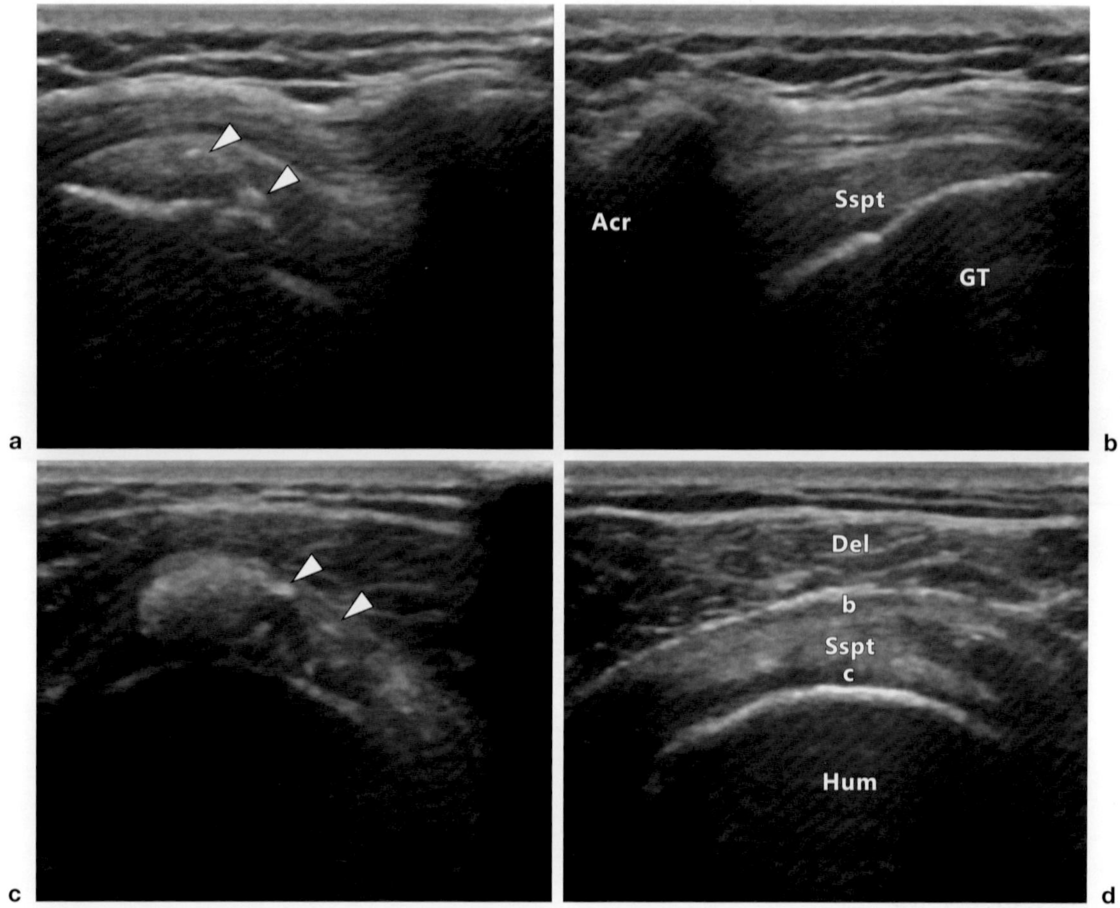

Lateral longitudinal (**a**) and axial (**c**) images reveal swollen appearance and small type II calcifications (*arrowheads*) within the supraspinatus tendon (**Sspt**). Normal side (**b**, **d**).

Acr	acromion	**Del**	deltoid
b	subdeltoid bursa	**GT**	greater tubercle
c	cartilage	**Hum**	humerus

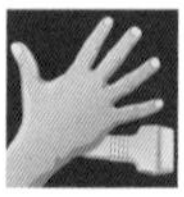

Expert note

The "cloudy" aspect in figure **c** and its superficial location can be signs of disintegration and migration of the calcification into the bursa (which might also cause severe exacerbation of the symptoms).

Calcific supraspinatus tendinitis and subdeltoid bursitis in a 56-year-old man with polymyalgia rheumatica 2.93

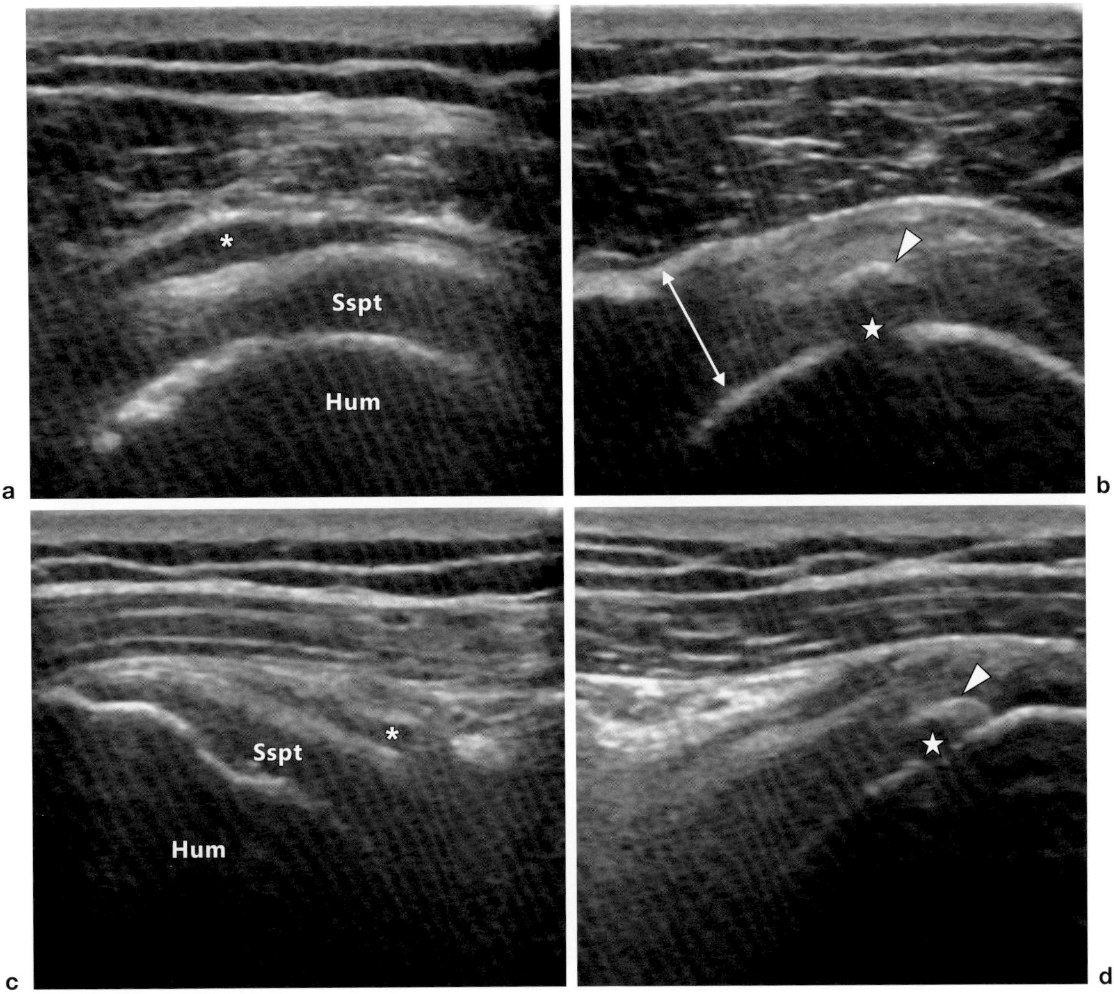

Axial (**a**) and longitudinal (**c**) views demonstrate a small amount of fluid (*asterisks*) in the subdeltoid bursa with relatively normal supraspinatus tendon (**Sspt**). Contralateral side reveals mild thickening of the tendon (*double arrow*) with a small type II calcification (*arrowheads*) (**b**, **d**). Note the incomplete posterior acoustic shadowing artifact (*stars*) deep to the calcification.

Hum humerus

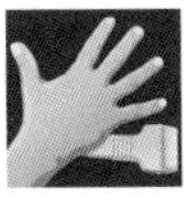

Expert note

The possibility that the supraspinatus tendon is focally thinner (flatter) in figure **a** can be confirmed with compression of the tendon. Compressibility might help diagnose a partial thickness tear.

2.94 Calcifying supraspinatus tendon in a 35-year-old woman with severe shoulder pain after a slip and fall injury

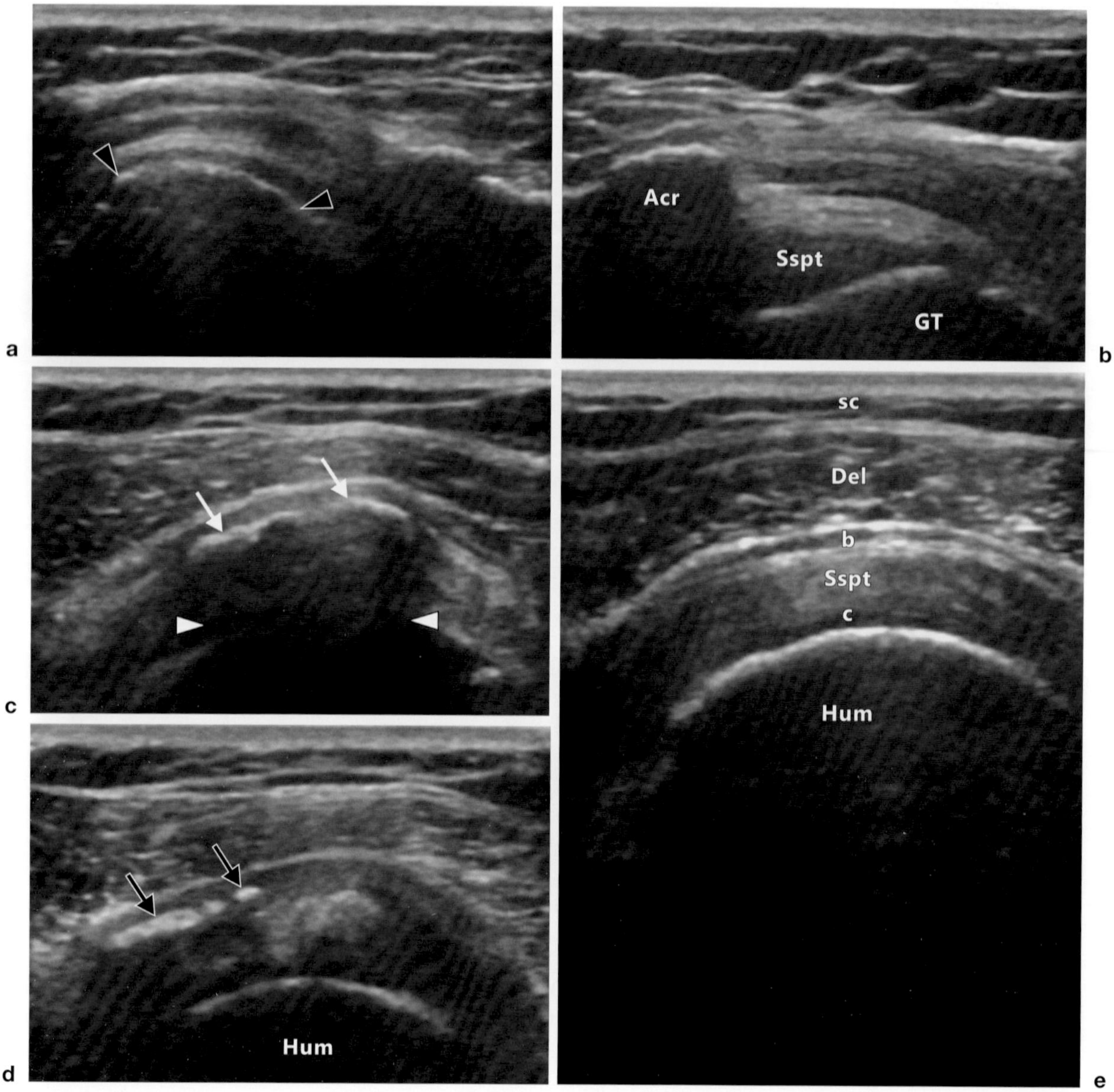

Video 2

Lateral longitudinal US image (**a**) shows a large, type I calcific deposit (*black arrowheads*) within the supraspinatus tendon (**Sspt**). Normal side (**b**). Axial image confirms the posterior acoustic shadowing (*white arrowheads*) caused by the type I calcific deposit (*arrows*) (**c**). Type II calcific deposits (*black arrows*) are also seen in a different view (**d**). Normal side (**e**).

Acr	acromion	**c**	cartilage	**Hum**	humerus
b	subacromial bursa	**Del**	deltoid	**sc**	subcutaneous tissue

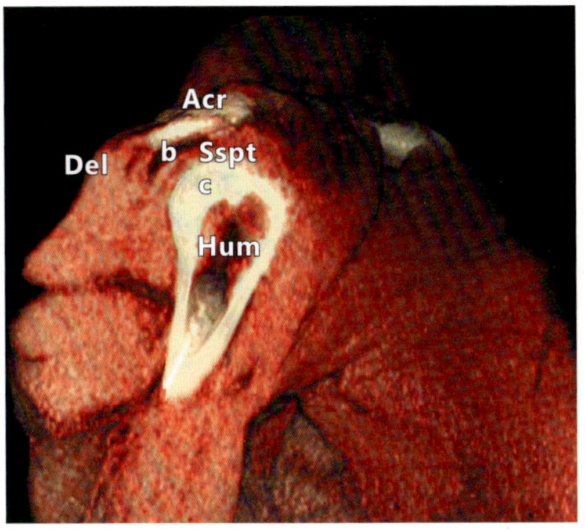

Expert note

Rotator cuff calcifications appear as intratendinous hyperechoic foci in three main types based on the amount of calcium in the deposit [2]. Type I calcifications appear as hyperechoic foci with complete shadowing and they correspond to the formative phase of calcium deposition accounting for approximately 80% of cases. Type II and type III calcifications can be classified as "slurry calcifications" with incomplete (type II) or absent (type III) shadowing and they correspond to the resorptive phase. Of note, slurry deposits have been demonstrated to be nearly liquid and can be successfully aspirated.

2.95 Supraspinatus and subscapularis calcific tendinopathies in a 41-year-old woman

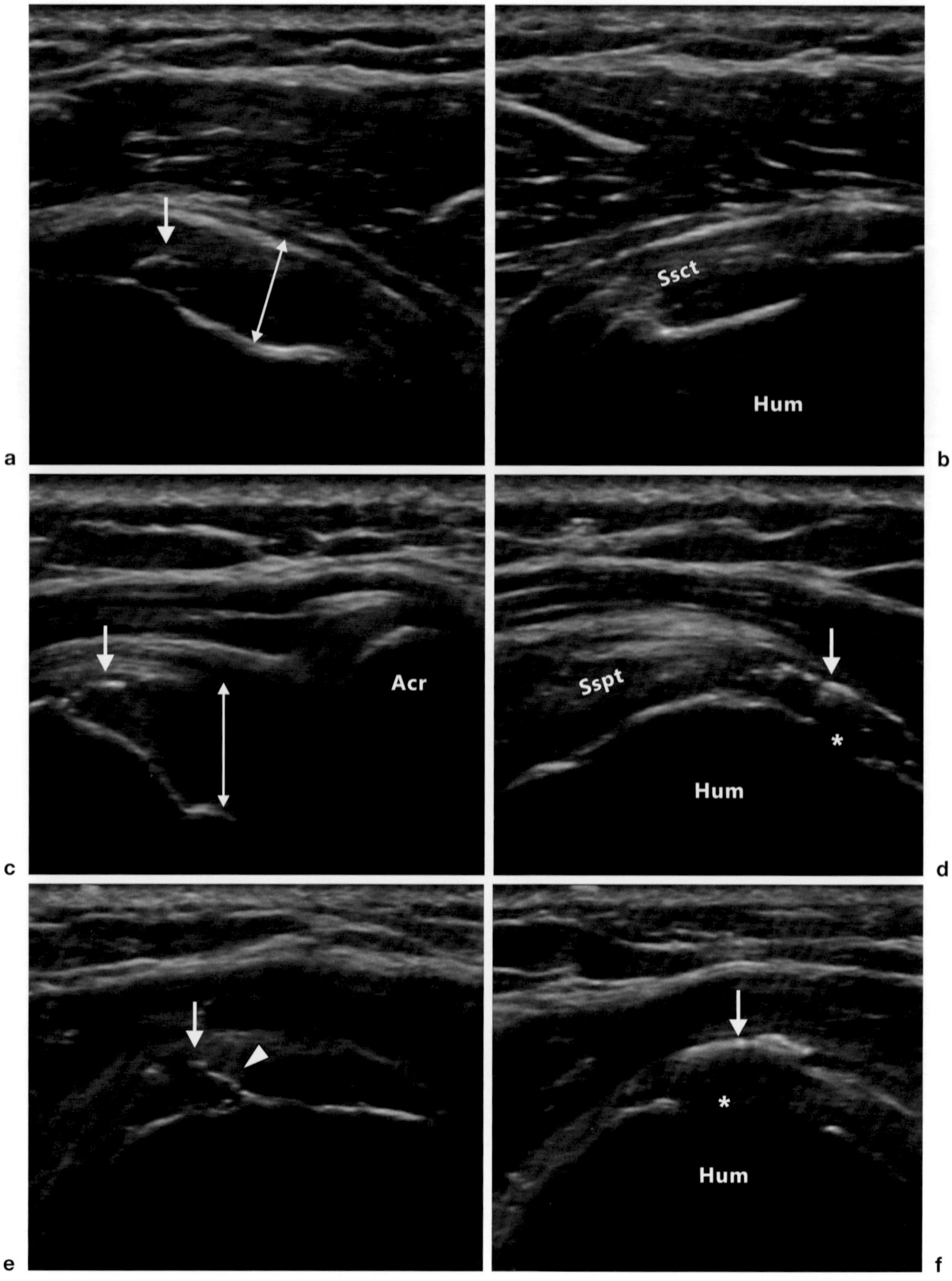

Longitudinal US image over the subscapularis tendon (**Ssct**) shows edematous and hypoechoic appearance (*double arrow*) and a small type III calcification (*arrow*) (**a**). Normal side (**b**).
Lateral longitudinal US image over the supraspinatus tendon (**Sspt**) demonstrates a swollen tendon (*double arrow*) and a distal type III calcification (*arrow*) (**c**). Contralateral side illustrates a relatively normal tendon echotexture but a linear type II calcification (*arrow*) on the distal side with an incomplete posterior acoustic shadowing artifact (*asterisk*) (**d**). Axial views confirms the calcific (*arrows*) and cortical (*arrowhead*) pathologies (**e**, **f**).

Acr acromion
Hum humerus

Expert note

When the calcifications are irregular and close to the cortex, it might sometimes be quite difficult to distinguish them from bony spurs. Again, thorough scanning in different planes would be contributory. For instance, in this case, the axial image (**e**) shows that both are present. Figure **d** is also a good example of how the same calcification can give or not a posterior shadowing.

2.96 Bilateral calcifying supraspinatus tendon in a 36-year-old man

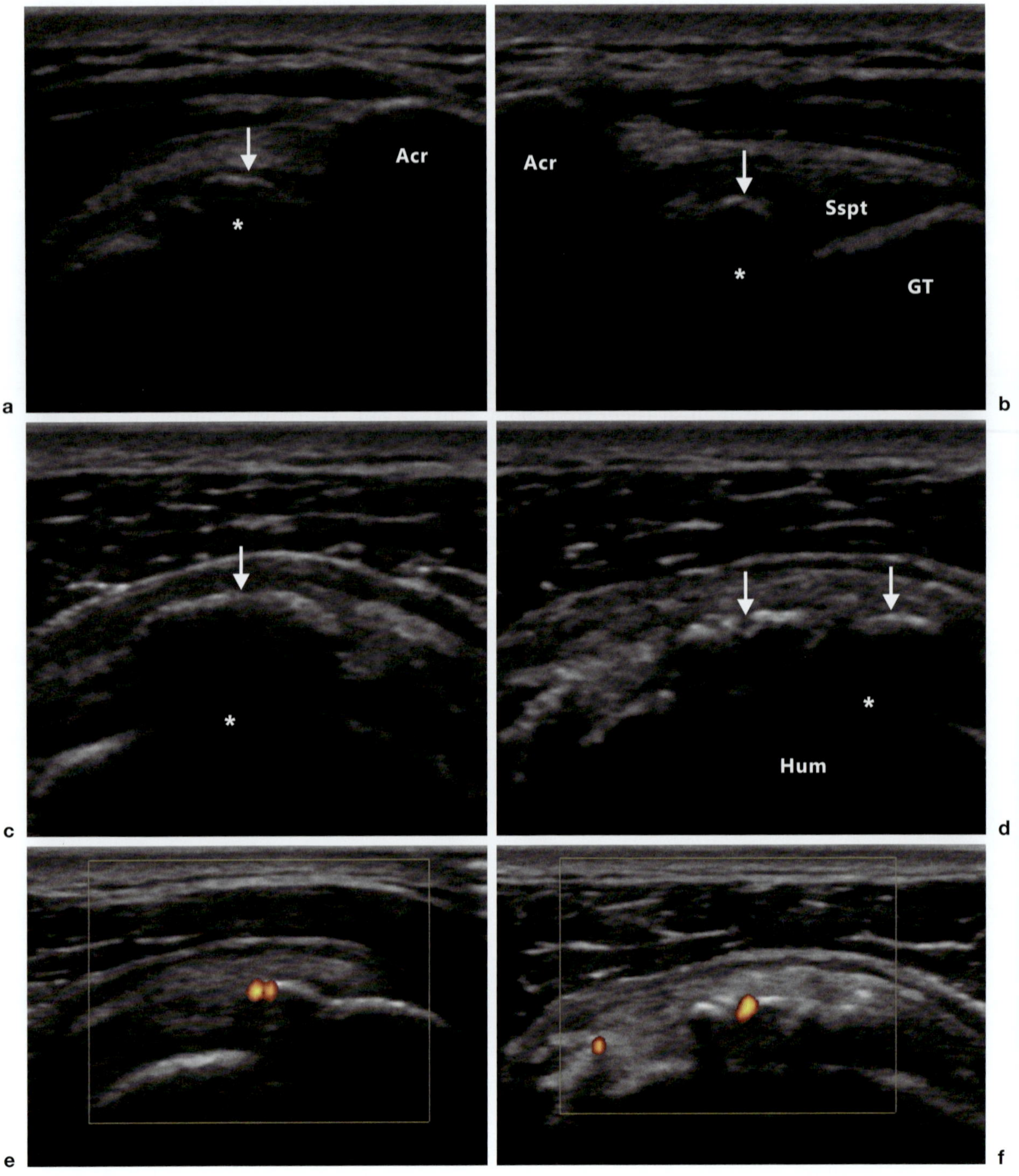

a b c d e f

The patient reported bilateral shoulder pain which was exacerbated on arm elevation and abduction.

Longitudinal (**a**, **b**) and axial (**c**, **d**) US images over the supraspinatus tendon (**Sspt**) demonstrate posterior acoustic shadowing artifacts (*asterisks*) due to type I calcifications (*white arrows*). Axial images show blood flow signals in the tendon as well (**e**, **f**).

Acr acromion
GT greater tubercle
Hum humerus

Expert note

Doppler US may differentiate between the formative and resorptive phases of the calcification [3]. In the resorptive phase, the hyperemia/neovascularization within the tendon demonstrates a perfect correlation with the symptoms [12].

2.97 Bilateral calcifying supraspinatus tendons in a diabetic woman

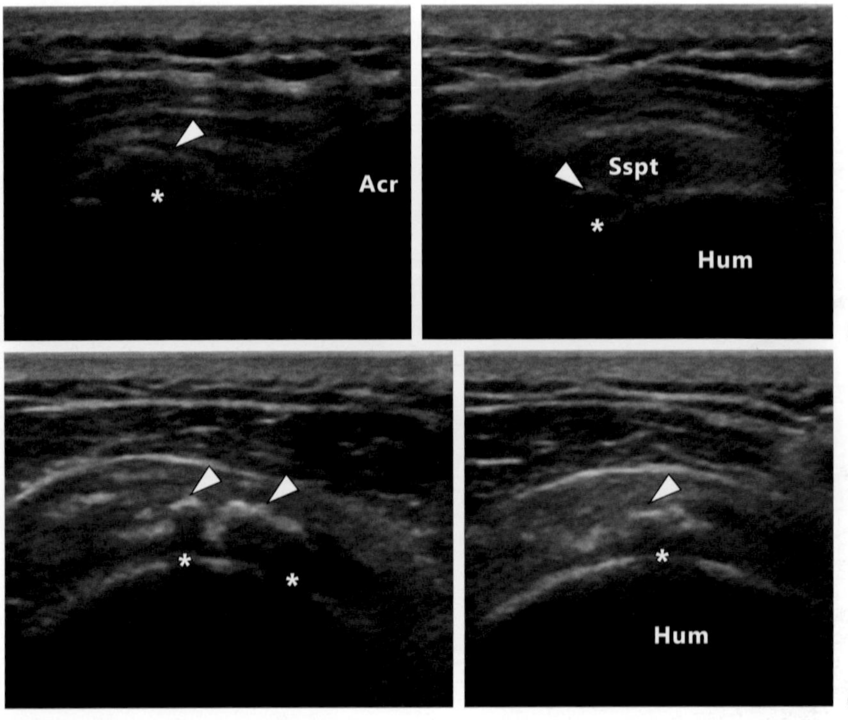

The patient had pain relief with physical therapy and a short course of nonsteroidal anti-inflammatory drugs.

Longitudinal (**a**, **b**) and axial (**c**, **d**) US images over the supraspinatus tendon (**Sspt**) show hyperechoic foci (*arrowheads*) inside the tendon with incomplete posterior acoustic shadowing artifacts (*asterisks*) reflecting type II calcifications.

Acr acromion

Hum humerus

Video 3

Expert note

As elsewhere, confirmation of the pathology in two perpendicular planes is always a preq-uisite. In this case, due to absence of the humerus in long axis, it would otherwise be impossible to distinguish this image from that of a superiorly dislocated humeral head.

Herein, another reason that makes US superior for the assessment of calcifications would be the availability of real-time dynamic imaging during shoulder movements. Yet, especially in case of big calcifications, it is not uncommon to discover that the actual cause of impingement is the calcification itself. For sure, detection of this likely scenario -exactly when the patient experiences the painful sensation during the maneuver- is an invaluable finding and also proves once again that US imaging should be the extension of physical examination.

One should also keep in mind that pain is not always proportionate with the size of the calcification.

Rotator cuff tendinopathies in a 53-year-old woman with shoulder pain and focal tenderness **2.98**

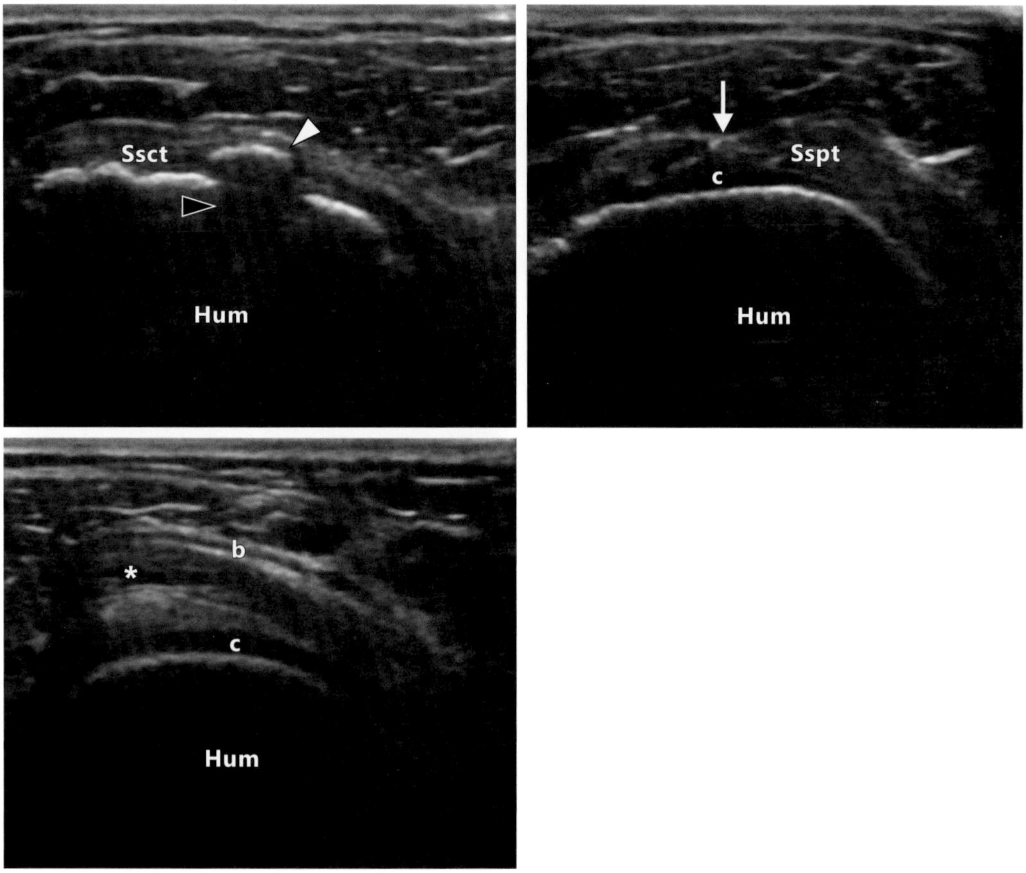

a b c

Anteromedial US image (**a**) shows a small type I calcific deposit (*white arrowhead*) inside the subscapularis tendon (**Ssct**) with posterior acoustic shadowing (*black arrowhead*). Imaging for the supraspinatus tendon (**Sspt**) shows its compressibility (*arrow*) (**b**) and upon release, the partial-thickness tear (seen as a small hypoechoic defect) (*asterisk*) is observed to be intratendinous (**c**).

b subdeltoid bursa
c cartilage
Hum humerus

Expert note

As seen in this case, several tendon pathologies may coexist in the rotator cuff. Again, substantial imaging -also in light of the clinical findings- should remain as the prerequisite.

2.99 Glenohumeral joint instability in a subject with chronic hemiplegia

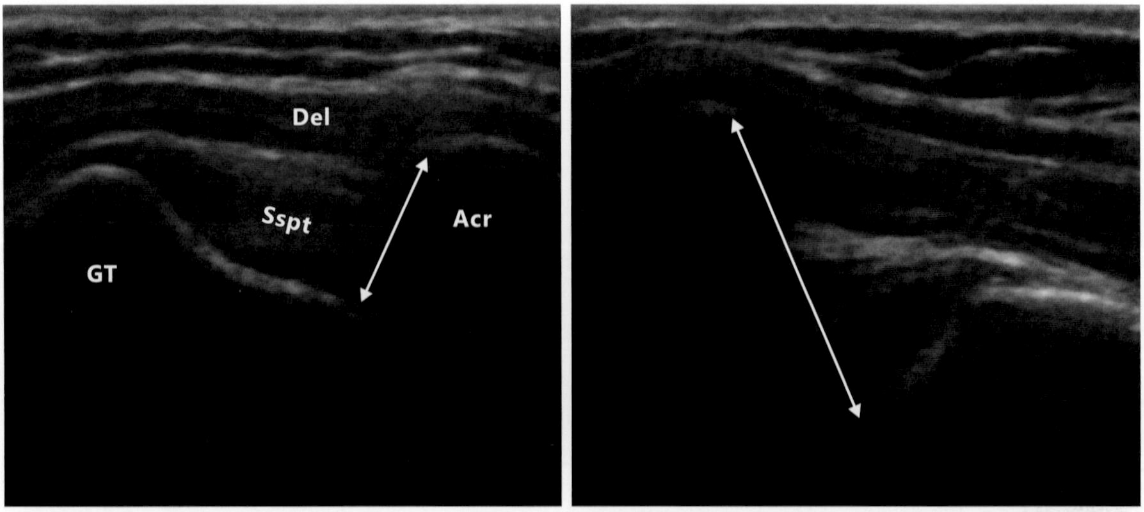

a b

The patient had complaints of pain and weakness in the affected shoulder with a positive sulcus sign.

When compared with the normal side (**a**), lateral longitudinal US image demonstrates an increased distance between the acromion (**Acr**) and the greater tuberosity (**GT**), consistent with joint subluxation (**b**).

Del deltoid
Sspt supraspinatus tendon

Expert note

Although different methods have been described how/where to quantify the distance in between, simple comparative measurements (as shown in the figures) at exactly the same place and shoulder positioning will definitely be conclusive [13].

Subcutaneous lipoma in a 53-year-old woman with a painless mass for about two years **2.100**

a 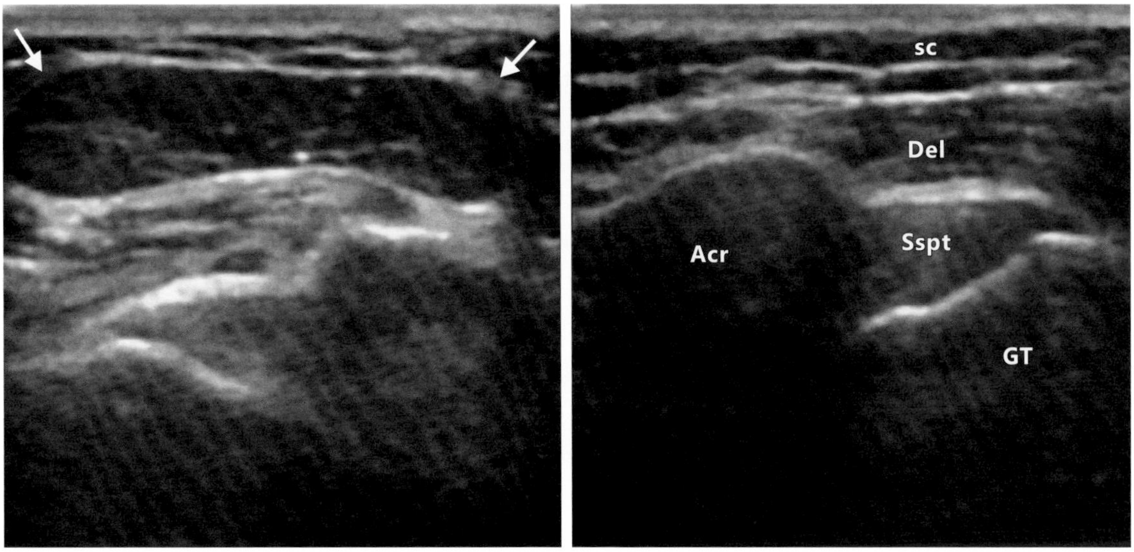 b

Comparative lateral longitudinal US image obtained over the supraspinatus tendon (**Sspt**) demonstrates a large hypoechoic mass with well-defined margins (*arrows*) (**a**). Normal side (**b**).

Acr	acromion	**GT**	greater tubercle
Del	deltoid	**sc**	subcutaneous tissue

Expert note

While the diagnostic accuracy of benign subcutaneous lesions with US imaging has been reported as 82.0%, sensitivity and specificity for the diagnosis of lipomas are 100% for both [14].

2.101 US-guided peritendinous platelet-rich-plasma injection for partial-thickness supraspinatus tendon tear

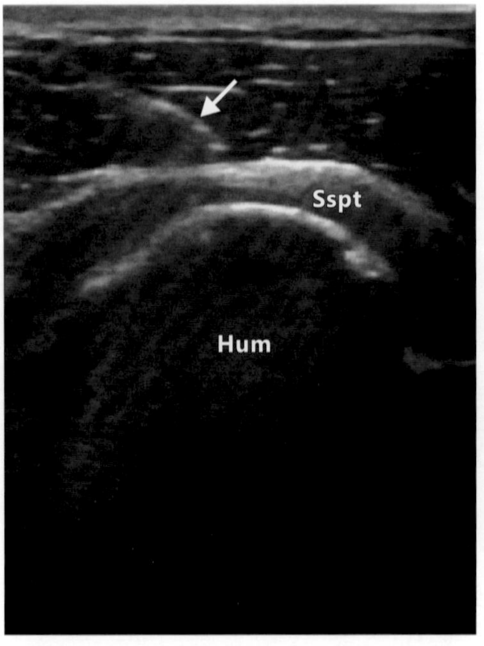

Axial US imaging in Crass position shows the hyperechoic needle (*arrow*) approaching the zone of partial rupture in the supraspinatus tendon (**Sspt**).

2.102 US-guided platelet-rich plasma injection for supraspinatus tendinopathy in a 37-year-old man

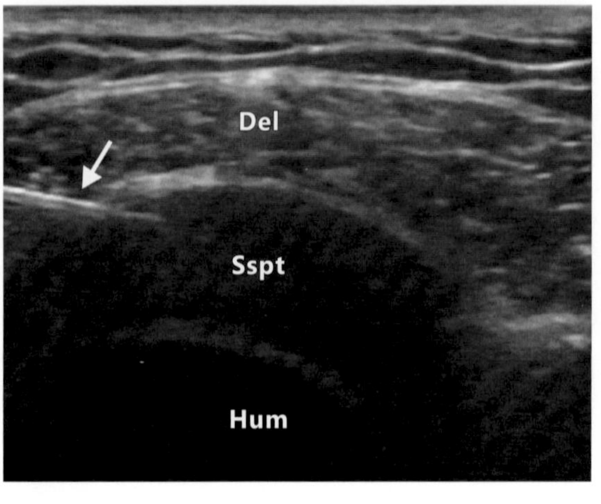

The patient had severe shoulder pain for the last three months.

Axial US image in Crass position shows that the supraspinatus tendon (**Sspt**) is abnormally thickened and hypoechoic in appearance. The needle tip (*arrow*) is placed inside the tendon during direct in-plane technique.

Del deltoid
Hum humerus

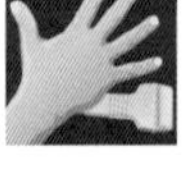

Expert note
Depending on the substantial imaging findings of the lesion, the clinician can easily tailor the details of the procedure i.e. where, how and what to inject [7, 15].

Postoperative shoulder imaging in a 65-year-old worker

2.103

The patient had to be operated for persistent/worsening shoulder pain despite conservative treatment alternatives.

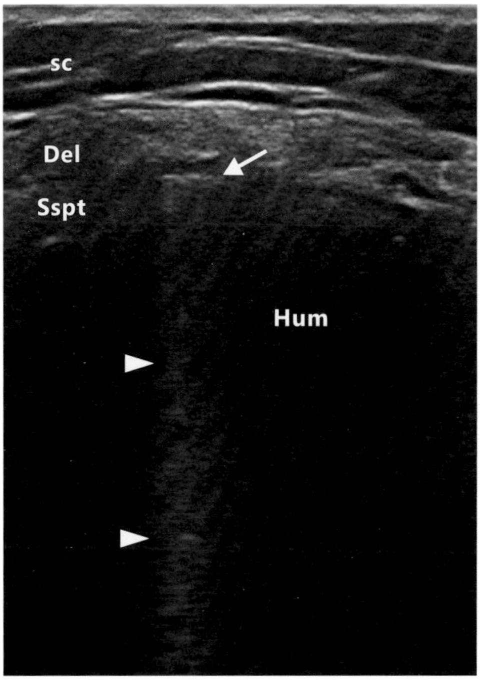

Axial US imaging in Crass position shows the comet-tail artifact (*arrowheads*) pertaining to the surgical (screw) material (*arrow*) on the humerus (**Hum**).

Del deltoid
sc subcutaneous tissue
Sspt supraspinatus tendon

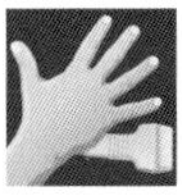

Expert note

While scanning patients who had been operated, the sonographer must have information as regards the details of surgery. Yet, the current scenario can be significantly different on the US screen and the imaging findings might easily/otherwise be misinterpreted.

2.104 Normal posterior shoulder view in a healthy man

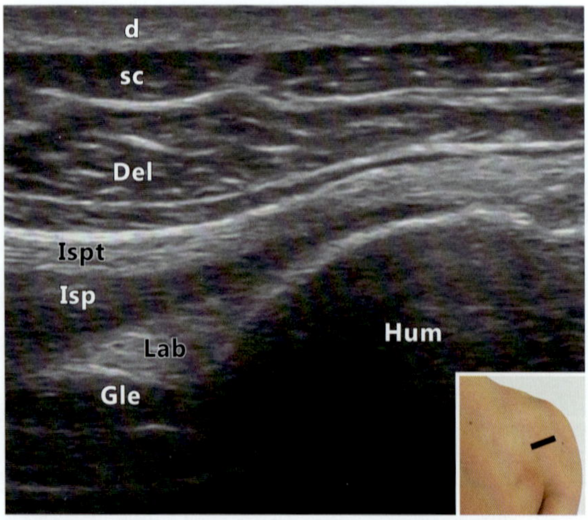

Posterior axial US image illustrates normal appearance of the glenohumeral joint.

d dermis
Del deltoid
Gle glenoid
Hum humerus
Isp infraspinatus
Ispt infraspinatus tendon
Lab labrum
sc subcutaneous tissue

2.105 Shoulder osteoarthritis in an elderly man with pain during activities and worsening at night

Video 4

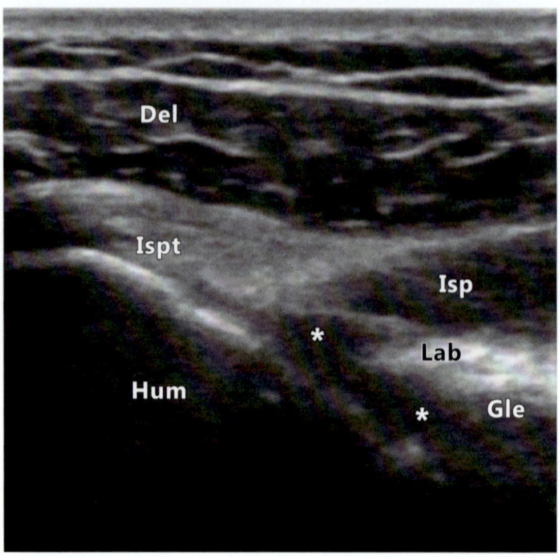

Posterior US imaging demonstrates effusion (*asterisks*) in the shoulder joint.

Expert note

This image was captured at the end of external rotation. Yet, in case of mild fluid, its displacement (i.e. displaying an irregular shape) might be the only hint for precise detection.

Shoulder joint effusion in a 50-year-old woman with rheumatoid arthritis **2.106**

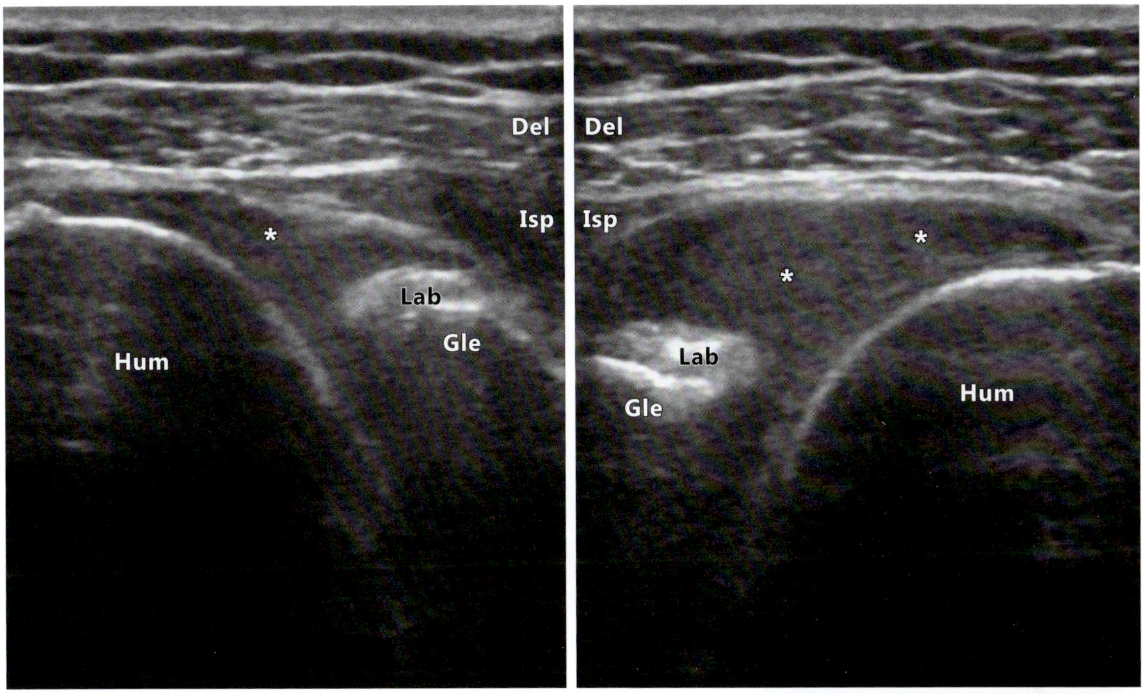

a b

Posterior axial US images demonstrate bilateral effusion (massive on the right side) (*asterisks*) distending the posterior recess of the shoulder joint.

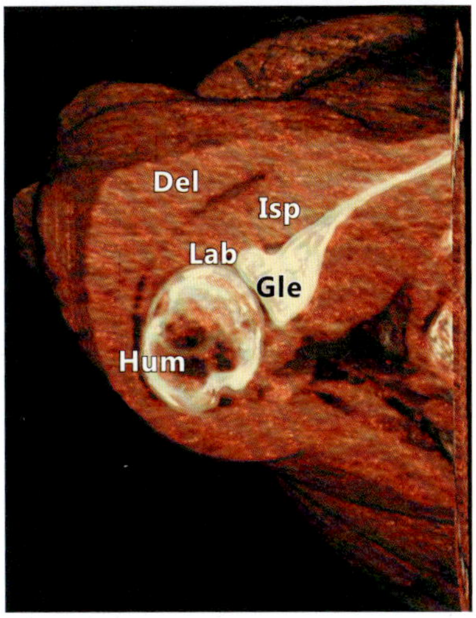

Del deltoid
Gle glenoid
Hum humerus
Isp infraspinatus
Lab labrum

Expert note

For exploring fluid in the shoulder joint, anterior view for the bicipital tendon sheath is definitely the first examination area. Usually, the posterior view (as illustrated in this case) has the second priority. Especially, dynamic assessment with internal/external rotations (showing also the displacement of fluid) would simply be confirmatory.

2.107 Repaired labral tear in a 38-year-old swimmer with pain worsening with overhead activities (before surgery)

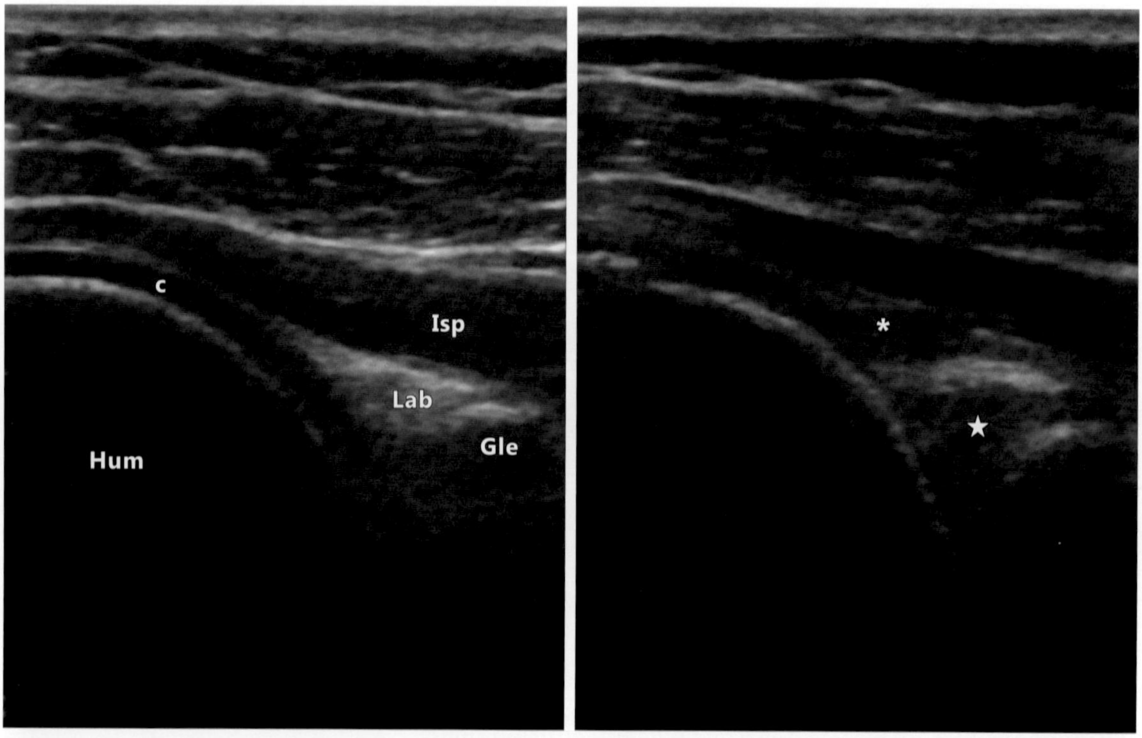

a b

When compared with the normal side (**a**), axial US image over the posterior shoulder shows hypoechoic, edematous (*star*) posterior glenoid labrum (**Lab**) and mild effusion in the joint (*asterisk*) (**b**).

c cartilage
Gle glenoid
Hum humerus
Ispt infraspinatus tendon

Expert note

While its very difficult to scan the anterior labrum, posterior imaging is quite straightforward especially when performed under dynamic assessment. Any structural and deformational injury of the labrum can be thoroughly scanned during rotations of the shoulder joint.

Infraspinatus tendinitis in a 50-year-old woman **2.108**

a 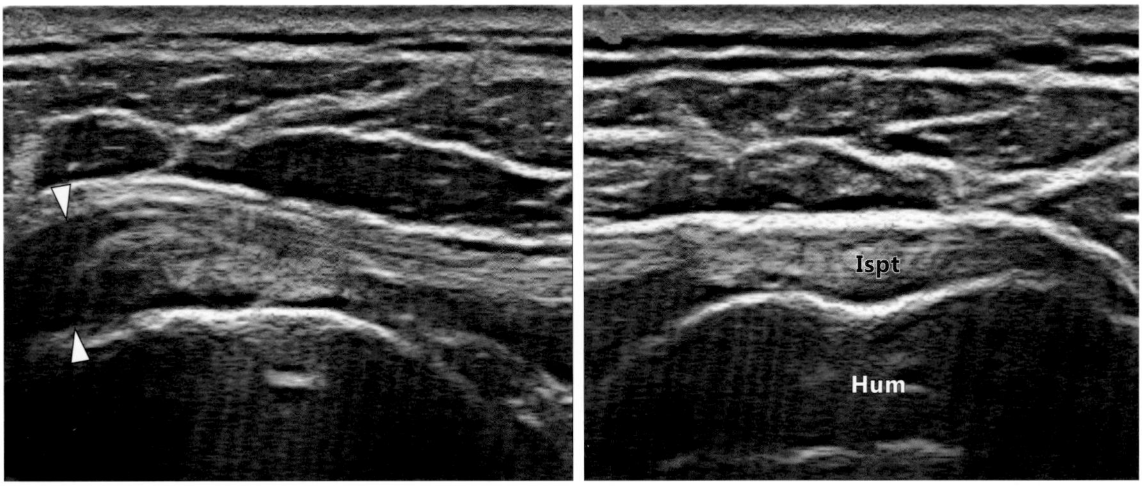 b

The patient had 3-month history of intense posterior shoulder pain after a fall on her lateral shoulder.

Posterior axial US imaging shows a markedly thickened (*arrowheads*) infraspinatus tendon (**Ispt**) with heterogeneous echogenicity (**a**). Normal side (**b**).

Hum humerus

Expert note

Isolated infraspinatus tendon lesions are actually quite rare; however particular traumas (like this one) might ensue and should not be overlooked in an otherwise normal shoulder US examination. Herewith, it is noteworthy that US evaluation of the shoulder does necessitate a thorough imaging i.e. regardless of the suspected diagnosis, all planes should be scanned in each and every patient [1, 2].

2.109 Degenerative osteoarthritis of the acromioclavicular joint in a 51-year-old man

a 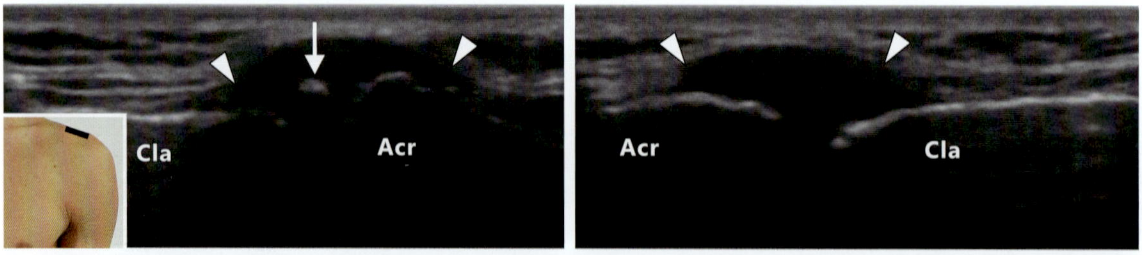 b

He had tenderness on sono-palpation and positive cross-arm adduction test.

Longitudinal US images of the acromioclavicular joints reveal bilateral hypoechoic fluid collections distending the joint capsules (*arrowheads*) (**a**, **b**) and decreased joint spaces with a small osteophyte (*arrow*) on one side (**a**).

Acr acromion
Cla clavicle

Expert note

Owing to the very superficial localization of the joint, US imaging is quite simple -also making the joint easily accessible. Likewise, even a very small (insulin) injector can be used to intervene without damaging the intraarticular meniscus.

2.110 Acromioclavicular joint pain in a 55-year-old man after he fell down from the stairs on his shoulder 3 months ago

a 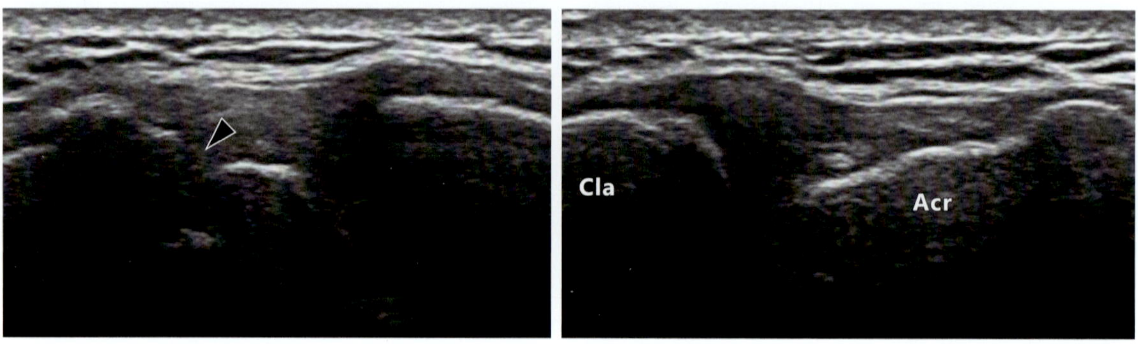 b

Longitudinal US image over the acromioclavicular joint demonstrates a cortical defect (*arrowhead*) on the distal acromion (**Acr**) (**a**). Normal contralateral side (**b**).

Acromioclavicular joint injury (after a motorbike accident) in a 32-year-old man with restricted and painful shoulder adduction

2.111

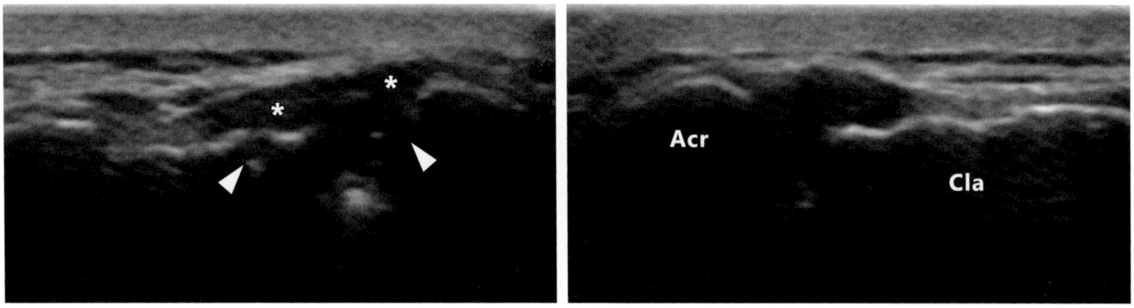

a b

Longitudinal US image obtained over the superior aspect of the acromioclavicular joint exhibits mild fluid within the joint cavity (*asterisks*) and cortical irregularities at the joint surfaces (*arrowheads*) (**a**). Normal side (**b**).

Acr acromion
Cla clavicle

Expert note

Eventually, one can do stress testing (giving a weight to carry) and compare diastasis.

2.112 Bilateral degenerative osteoarthritis of the acromioclavicular joints in a 65-year-old man who suffered pain during overhead activities

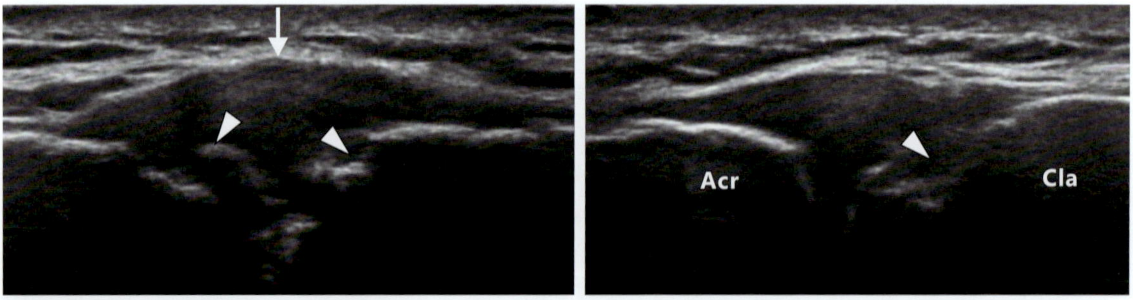

a b

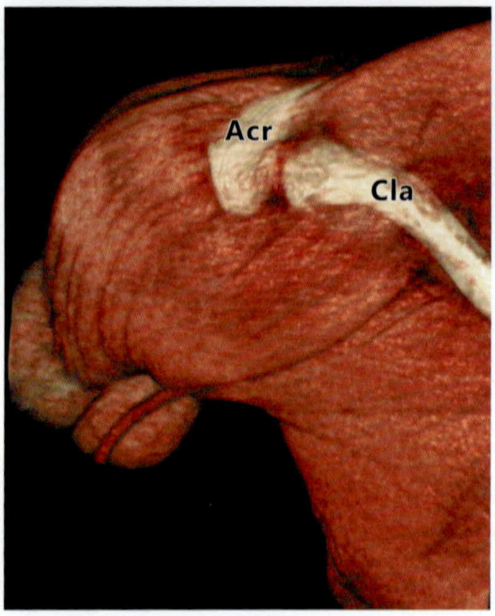

Longitudinal US images over the acromioclavicular joints reveal bilateral apparent cortical irregularities/osteophyte on the joint surfaces (*arrowheads*) (**a**, **b**). Please note that there is also mild distension of the joint capsule (*arrow*) on one side (**a**).

Acr acromion
Cla clavicle

Expert note

Sono-palpation has proven to be the most reliable indicator of acromioclavicular joint inflammation [2].

REFERENCES

1. Özçakar L, Kara M, Chang KV, Tekin L, Hung CY, Ulaülı AM, et al. EURO-MUSCULUS/USPRM basic scanning protocols for shoulder. Eur J Phys Rehabil Med. 2015; 51: 491-6.
2. De Muynck M, Sabbe W. Ultrasound evaluation of the shoulder. In: Özçakar L, De Muynck M, editors. Musculoskeletal ultrasound in physical and rehabilitation medicine. Milan: Edi.Ermes; 2014. p. 37-58.
3. Dasgupta B, Cimmino MA, Kremers HM, et al. 2012 Provisional classification criteria for polymyalgia rheumatica: A European League Against Rheumatism/American College of Rheumatology collaborative initiative. Arthritis Rheum. 2012; 64: 943-54.
4. Schmidt WA, Schmidt H, Schicke B, Gromnica-Ihle E. Standard reference values for musculoskeletal ultrasonography. Ann Rheum Dis. 2004; 63: 988-94.
5. Bianchi S, Martinoli C. Shoulder. In: Bianchi S, Martinoli C, editors. Ultrasound of the musculoskeletal system. Berlin: Springer; 2007. p. 190-324.
6. Hollister MS, Mack LA, Patten RM, Winter TC 3rd, Matsen FA 3rd, Veith RR. Association of sonographically detected subacromial/subdeltoid bursal effusion and intraarticular fluid with rotator cuff tear. AJR Am J Roentgenol. 1995; 165: 605-8.
7. Özçakar L, Onat ŞŞ, Gürçay E, Kara M. Are blind injections ethical or historical? Think twice with ultrasound. Am J Phys Med Rehabil. 2016; 95: 158-60.
8. Chang KV, Şahin Onat Ş, Lee CW, Kara M, Hung CY, Özçakar L. EURO-MUSCULUS/USPRM basic scanning protocols revisited in children. Eur J Phys Rehabil Med. 2016; 52: 887-901.
9. Ptasznik R. Sonography of the shoulder. In: Van Holsbeeck M, Introcaso JH, editors. Musculoskeletal ultrasound. 2nd ed. St Louis: Mosby; 2001. p. 463-516.
10. Gold RH, Seger LL, Yao L. Imaging shoulder impingement. Skeletal Radiol. 1993; 22: 555-61.
11. Tekin L, Kara M, Özçakar L. When the parrot's beak becomes the crocodile's mouth: a story on shoulder ultrasound. Rheumatol Int. 2013; 33: 2447-8.
12. Chiou HJ, Chou YH, Wu JJ, Hsu CC, Huang DY, Chang CY. Evaluation of calcific tendonitis of rotator cuff: role of color Doppler ultrasonography. J Ultrasound Med. 2002; 21: 289-95.
13. Akkaya N. Ultrasound imaging in rehabilitation settings. In: Özçakar L, De Muynck M, editors. Musculoskeletal ultrasound in physical and rehabilitation medicine. Milan: Edi.Ermes; 2014. p. 185-97.
14. Hwang EJ, Yoon HS, Cho S, Park HS. The diagnostic value of ultrasonography with 5-15-MHz probes in benign subcutaneous lesions. Int J Dermatol. 2015; 54: e469-75.
15. Chang KV, Wu CH, Wang TG. Ultrasound imaging for musculoskleletal interventions. In: Özçakar L, De Muynck M, editors. Musculoskeletal ultrasound in physical and rehabilitation medicine. Milan: Edi.Ermes; 2014. p. 241-58.

Arm 3

- **Subcutaneous tissue**

3.1 Lymphedema of the arm in a 37-year-old woman with a history of breast cancer

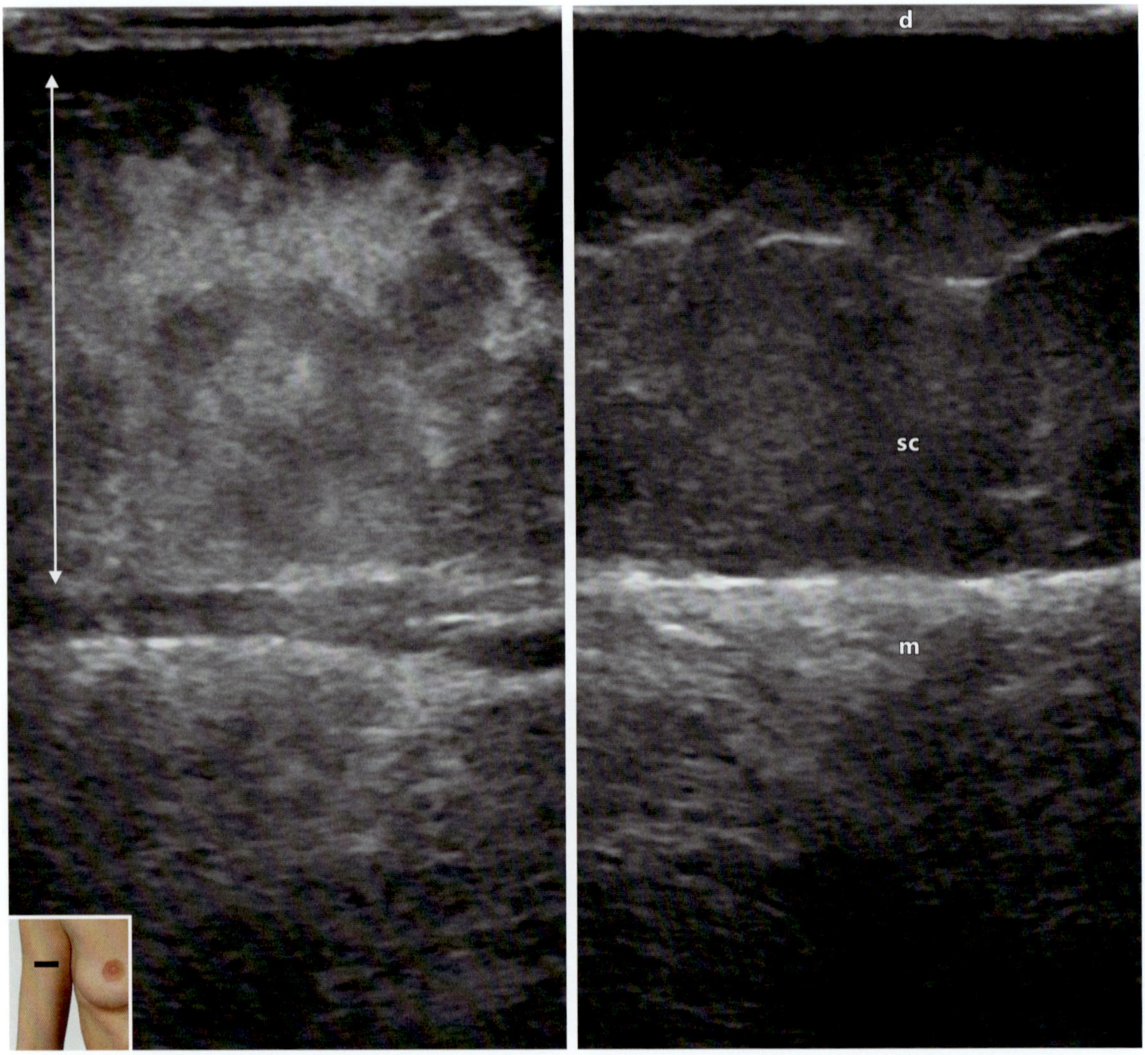

a b

Longitudinal US images demonstrate lymphedema in the subcutaneous tissue (*double arrow*) with diffuse and irregular hyperechoic appearance of fat lobules (**a**). Normal side (**b**).

d	dermis
m	muscle
sc	subcutaneous tissue

Subcutaneous lipoma in an elderly man with a painless lump on the anterolateral aspect of the shoulder **3.2**

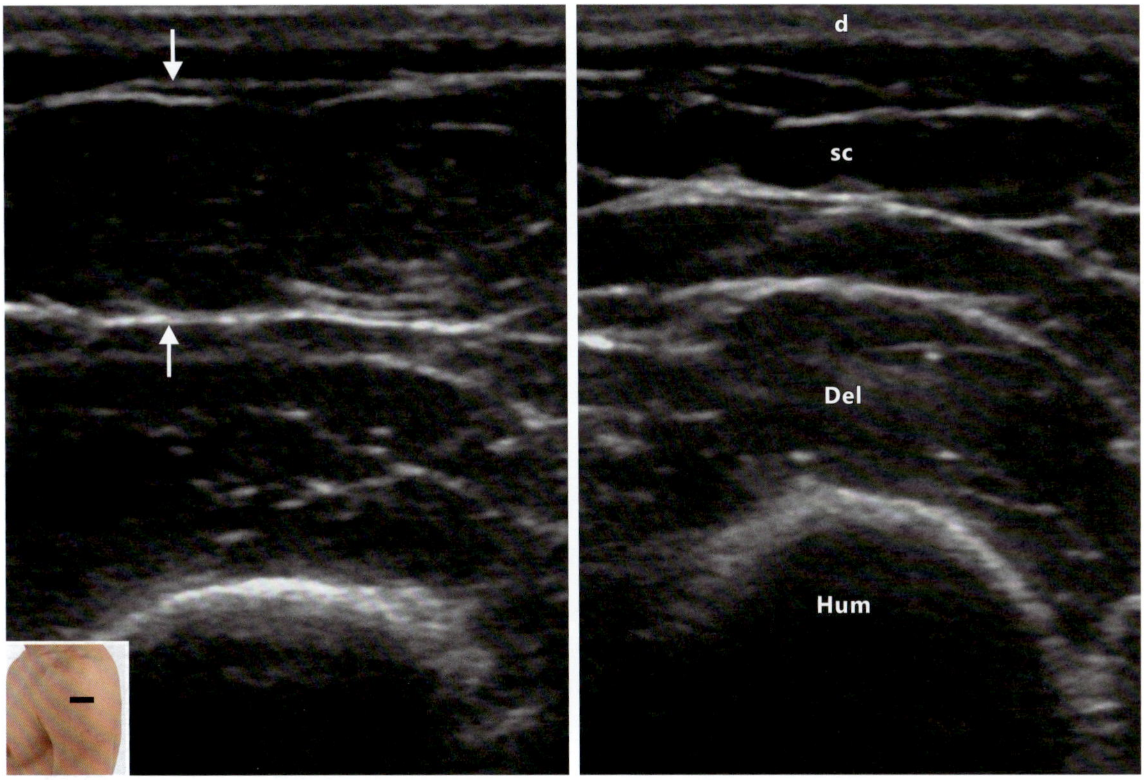

a b

Axial US image reveals a large solid mass localized in the subcutaneous tissue (*arrows*), consistent with a lipoma (**a**). Contralateral side (**b**).

d dermis
Del deltoid
Hum humerus
sc subcutaneous tissue

Expert note

Uncovering the exact anatomic localization -in other words, tissue of origin- US generally gives idea about the pathology of these mass lesions.
Lipomas can be hyper/iso/hypoechoic when compared with the surrounding subcutaneous tissue and they are usually more or less circumscribed.

3.3 Lipoma in a 55-year-old man located at the extensor surface of the upper arm

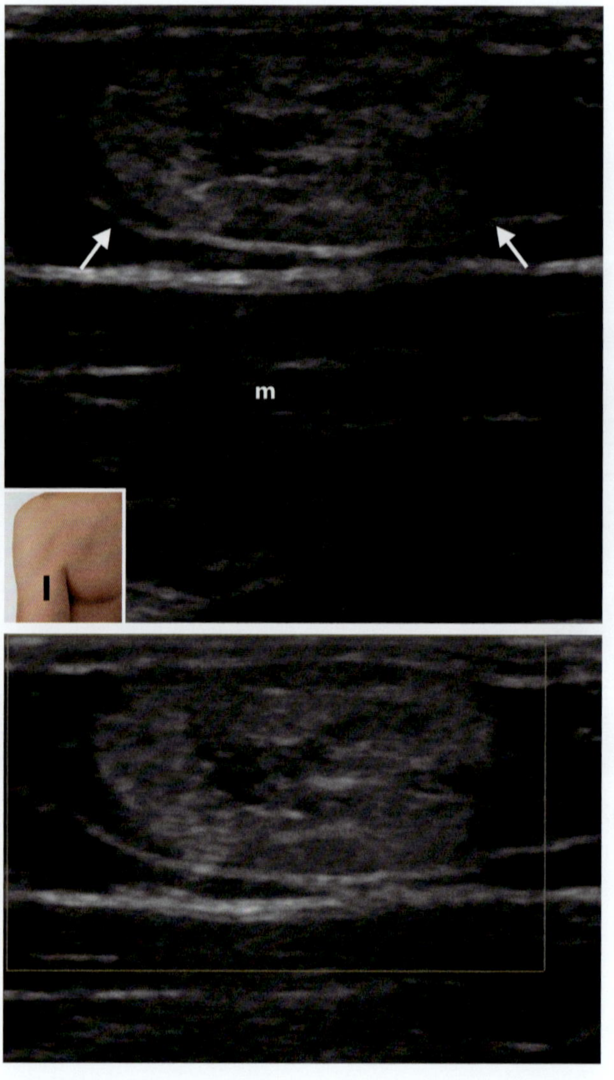

a

b

Longitudinal US image shows an elliptical and well-demarcated hyperechoic mass (*arrows*) confined to the subcutaneous tissue (**a**). Power Doppler imaging shows no signal (**b**).

m muscle

Nodular fasciitis (fascial type) in the arm of a 26-year-old woman with a sudden onset, palpable and painless mass **3.4**

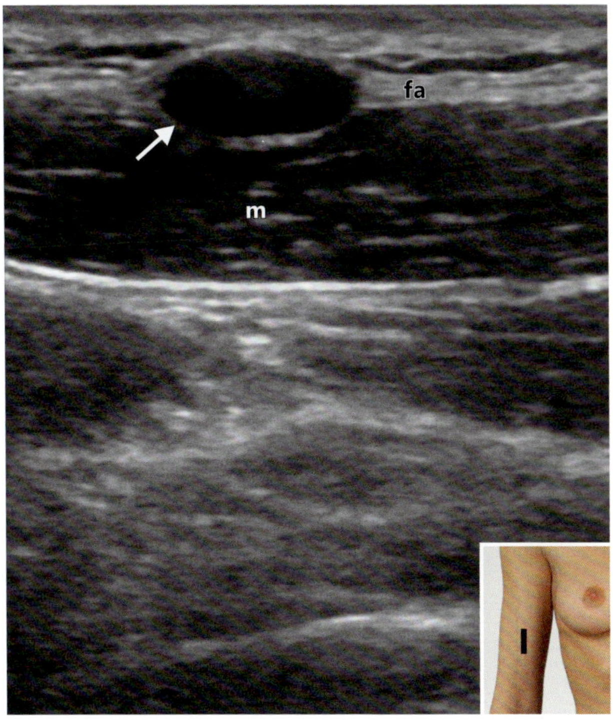

Longitudinal US image reveals a hypoechoic well-defined cystic lesion (*arrow*) expanding inside the fascia.

fa fascia
m muscle

Expert note

Exact localizations of nodular fasciitis can easily be ascertained with US imaging [1].

3.5 Nodular fasciitis in a 47-year-old woman with anterior arm pain

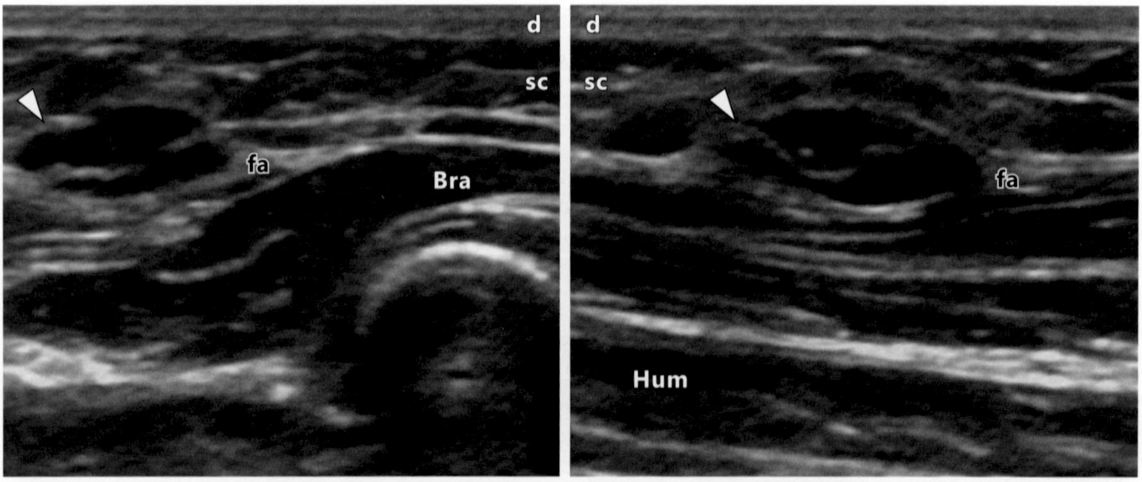

a b

Axial (left) and longitudinal (right) US imaging show an anechoic mass lesion (*arrowheads*) with intrinsic septae inside the outer fascia (**fa**) of the brachialis (**Bra**) muscle.

d dermis
Hum humerus
sc subcutaneous tissue

Expert note

For sure, the clinical history needs to be taken into consideration when interpreting the US images. Otherwise, commenting on the size, margins and the vascularity of a mass lesion might ofttimes not suffice to conclude for a specific diagnosis. On the other hand, the aforementioned three features do guide for differentiating benign *vs.* malignant lesions.

REFERENCES

1. Lee KJ, Jin W, Kim GY, Rhee SJ, Park SY, Park JS, et al. Sonographic features of superficial-type nodular fasciitis in the musculoskeletal system. J Ultrasound Med. 2015; 34: 1465-71.

Arm

Elbow 4

- **Humeroradial joint**
- **Olecranon fossa**
- **Olecranon bursa**
- **Biceps tendon** - Distal
- **Common extensor tendon**
- **Common flexor tendon**
- **Medial collateral ligament**
- **Subcutaneous tissue**

4.1 Effusion in the anterior elbow joint secondary to a fall on the outstretched hand

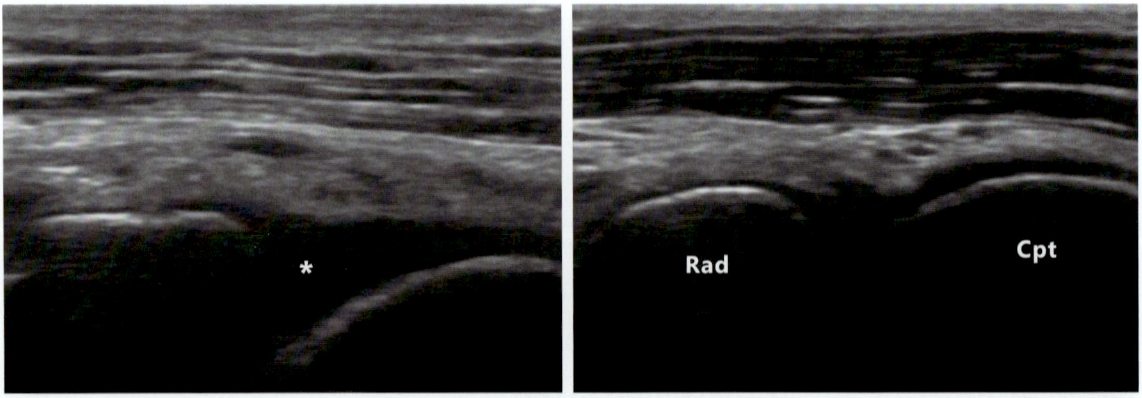

a b

Anterior longitudinal US imaging of the radiocapitellar joint shows anechoic fluid (*asterisk*) (**a**). Normal side (**b**).

Cpt capitulum
Rad head of radius

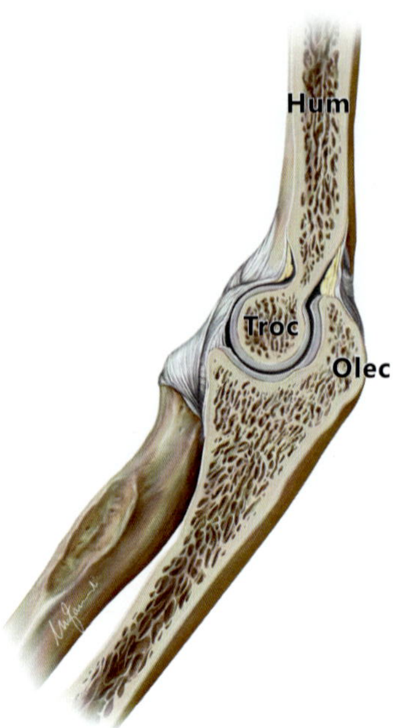

Expert note

Although anterior elbow joint fluid tends to accumulate initially in the proximal (radial and coronoid) fossae; in case of large effusions, fluid might be observed bulging the joint capsule and/or overflowing distally as well [1, 2].

Elbow joint effusion in man with rheumatoid arthritis **4.2**

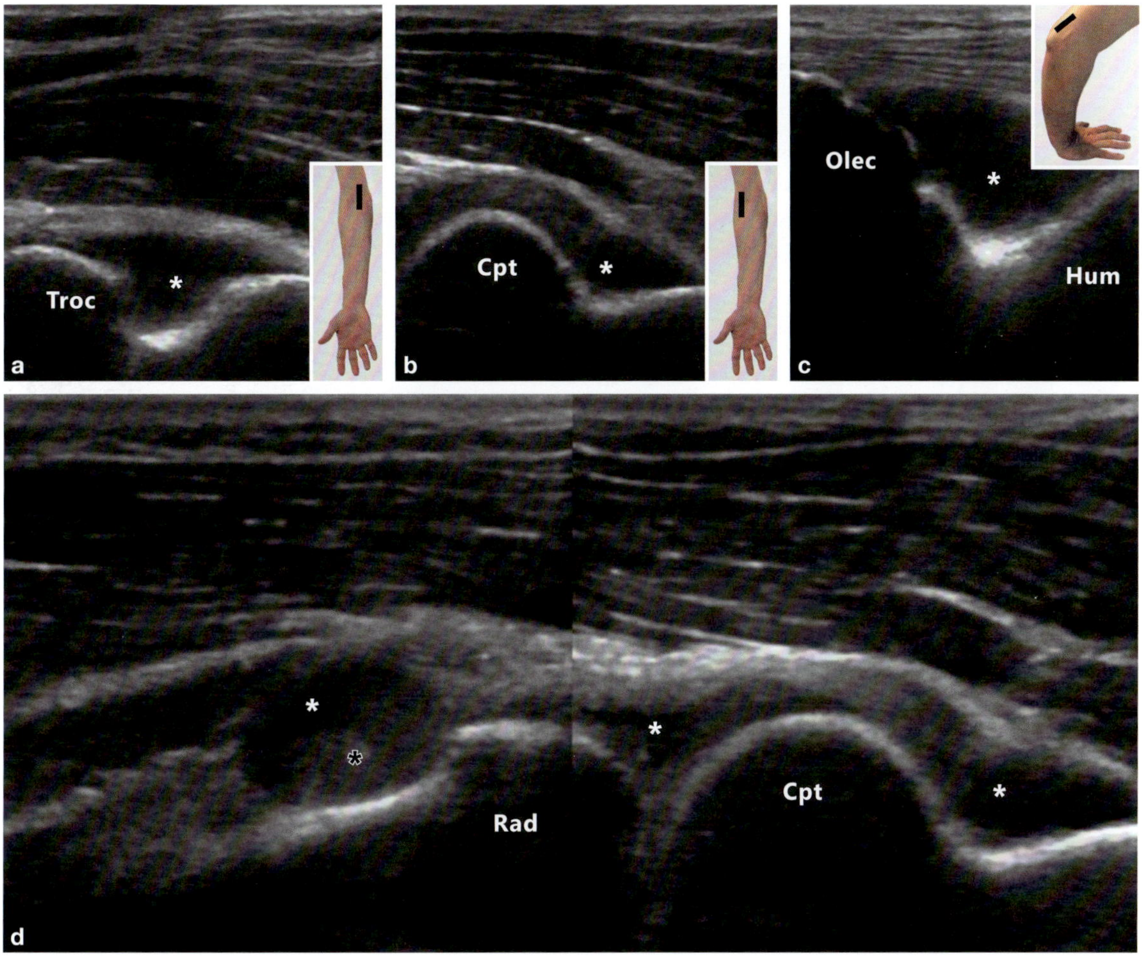

Longitudinal US images obtained over the anterior (**a**, **b**) and posterior (**c**) recesses demonstrate effusion (*white asterisks*) in the joint. Corresponding split-screen view of the radiocapitellar joint shows synovial hypertrophy (*black asterisk*) and effusion (*white asterisks*) that overflow to proximal and distal fossae (**d**).

Cpt	capitulum	**Olec**	olecranon
Hum	humerus	**Rad**	head of radius
ME	medial epicondyle	**Troc**	trochlea

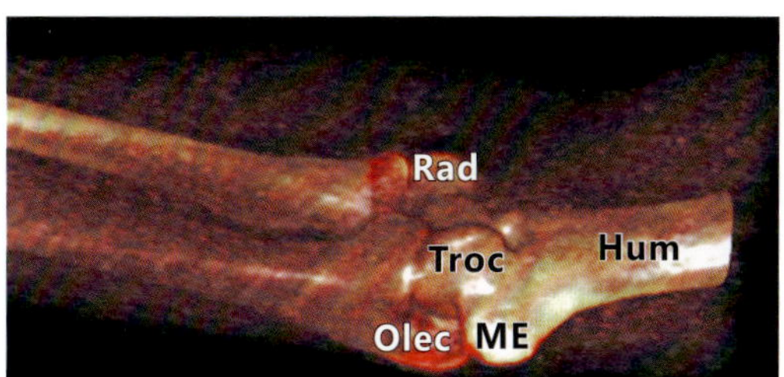

4.3 Hemophilic arthropathy of the elbow joint in a 13-year-old boy with severe hemophilia A

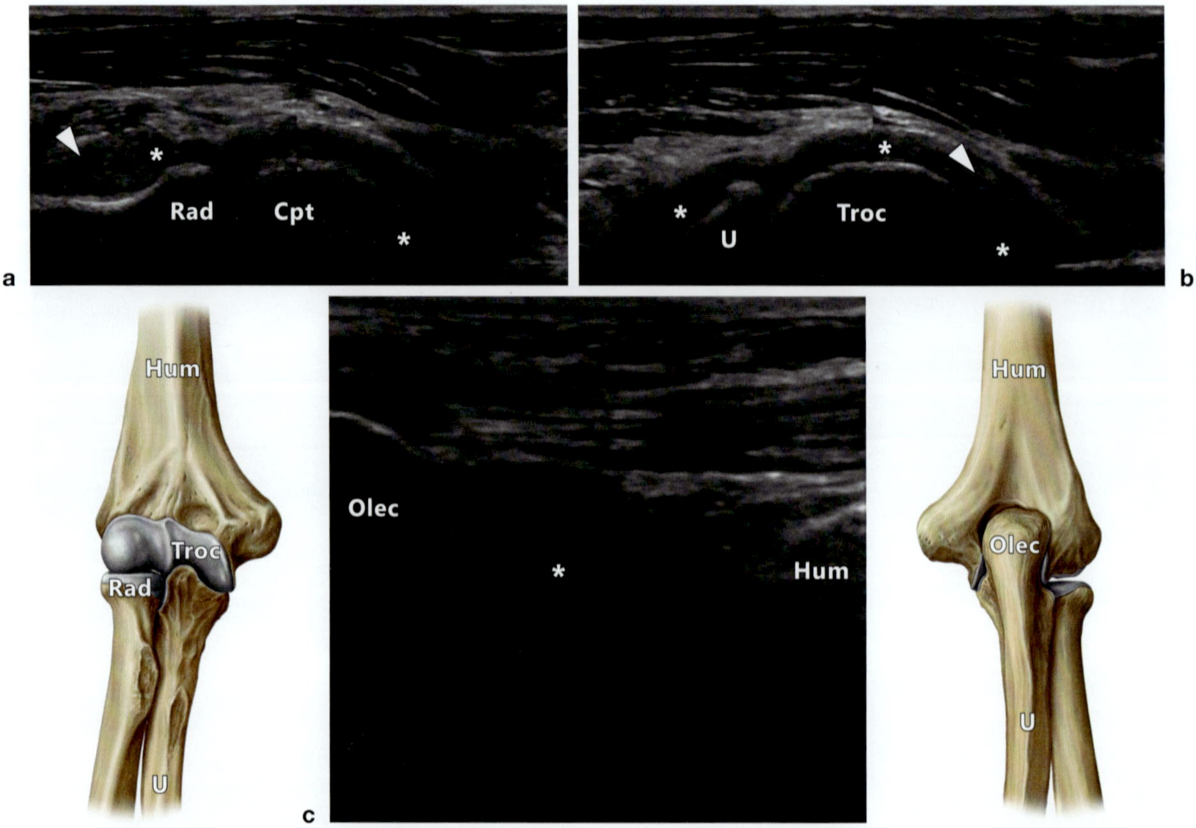

Longitudinal US images on the anterior (**a**, **b**) and posterior aspects (**c**) of the elbow joint reveal hemorrhagic effusion (*asterisks*) and hypertrophied synovium (*arrowheads*) containing scattered areas of fibrin clots within the synovial cavity.

Cpt	capitulum	**Rad**	head of radius
Hum	humerus	**Troc**	trochlea
Olec	olecranon	**U**	ulna

Expert note

Although US imaging can never replace synovial biopsy or fluid cultures, particular appearances of joint effusion might serve as significant clues for the diagnosis. In other words, when joint fluid is detected, the sonographer needs to tell further about the nature of fluid (e.g. simple effusion, infection, synovitis, hemorrhage). For instance, it would not be atypical if US findings (hyperechoic air bubbles) would suggest in favor of an anaerobic infection. Above all, guiding the physician about the possibility of aspiration is even very important. Yet, displaced fluids (with compression) usually indicate that drainage is likely.

Chronic synovitis in a 65-year-old woman with chronic rheumatoid arthritis **4.4**

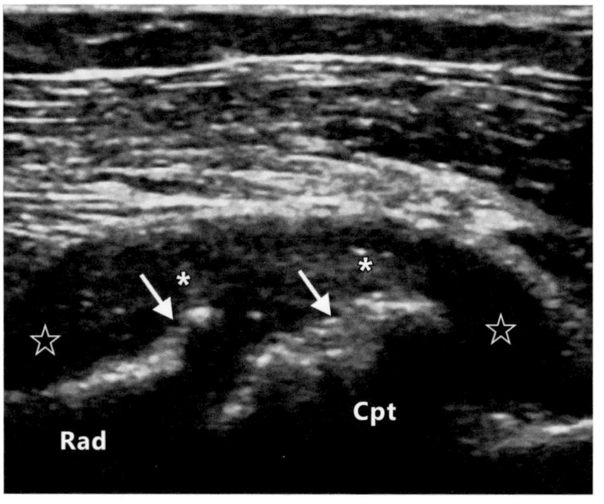

Longitudinal US image on the anterior aspect of the elbow shows distended joint capsule by hypoechoic effusion (*stars*) and synovial hypertrophy (*asterisks*). Please note the cortical irregularities (*arrows*) on both articular sides.

Cpt capitulum
Rad head of radius

4.5 Effusion in the posterior fossa in a footballer after the match

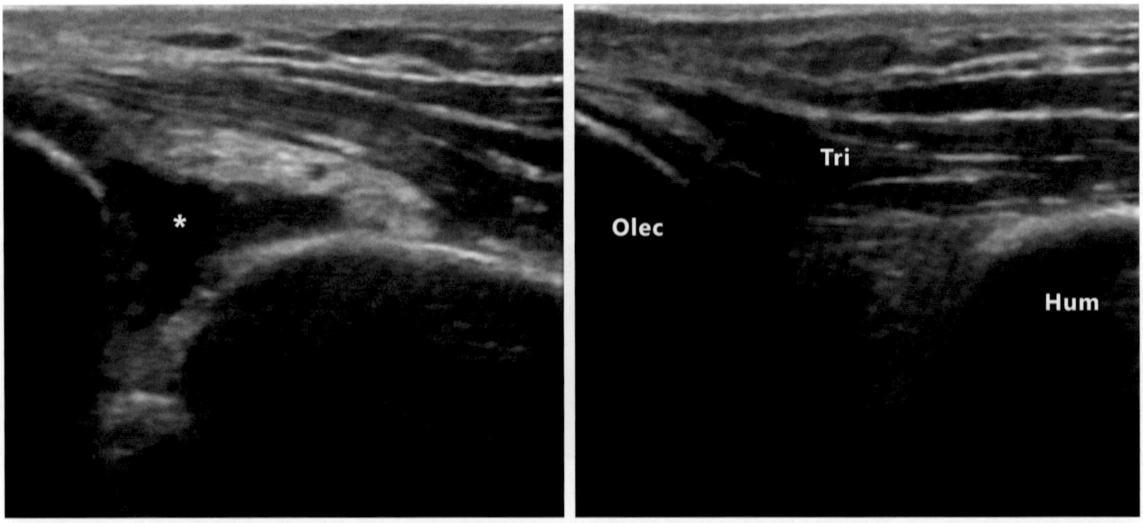

a b

Posterior longitudinal US image demonstrates anechoic fluid (*asterisk*) deep to the triceps (**Tri**) muscle (**a**). Normal side (**b**).

Hum humerus
Olec olecranon

Expert note

While there is a preference view to look for fluid in the hip, knee and shoulder joints; for elbow this is less strict. It is important to evaluate the posterior fossa as well as the anterior ones on the radial or ulnar sides.

Effusion in the elbow joint after a fall episode on the elbow 4.6

Posterior longitudinal US imaging of the olecranon fossa shows a large effusion (*white asterisks*) distending the hyperechoic fat pad (*black asterisks*).

Hum humerus
Tri triceps brachii

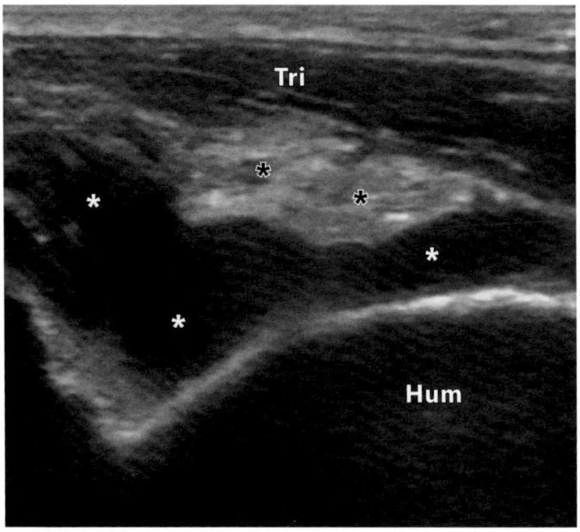

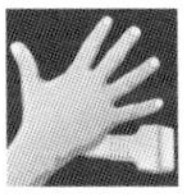

Expert note

Olecranon fossa is the main area to search for elbow joint fluid on the posterior side. Herewith, positioning of the elbow is quite strategic for optimum soft tissue imaging; yet small amount of fluid might be shifted to the anterior recesses in case imaging is undertaken in flexion and pronation (shoulder in abduction and internal rotation). Instead, imaging with the US probe kept from below while the arms are forwarded to the sonographer could be preferred to also benefit from gravity [3].

Direct in-plane posterior approach for injection into the elbow joint 4.7

Longitudinal US image demonstrates anechoic fluid (*asterisks*) and the hyperechoic needle (*arrows*) within the olecranon (**Ole**) fossa.

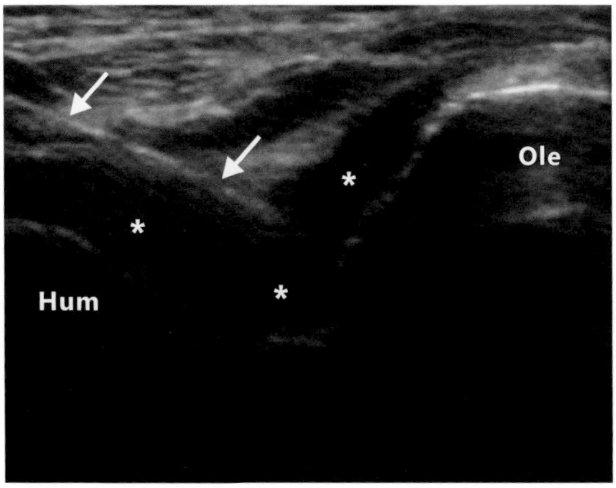

4.8 Olecranon bursitis in a 55-year-old man with local swelling and pain

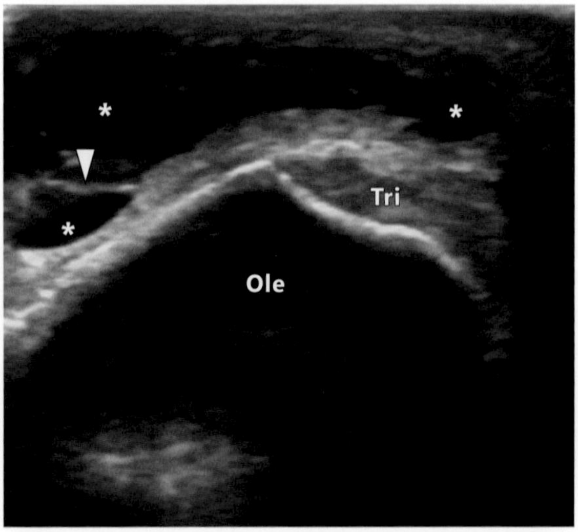

Longitudinal US image over the olecranon (**Ole**) demonstrates distended bursa containing anechoic effusion (*asterisks*) with a thick septum (*arrowhead*).

Tri triceps brachii

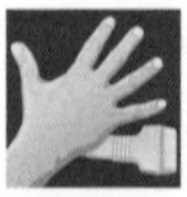

Expert note

As in other superficially located effusions, the sonographer should pay attention not to compress hard -to avoid displacement of the fluid and misdiagnosis accordingly.

4.9 Chronic traumatic olecranon bursitis in a 72-year-old man with painful elbow movements

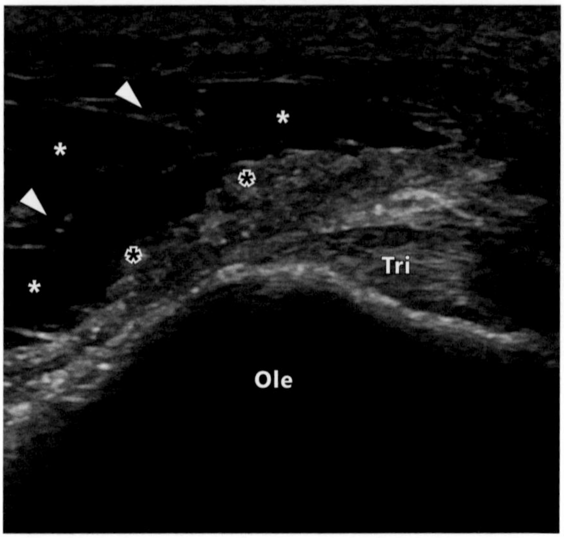

Longitudinal US image of the posterior elbow shows filling of the bursa with fluid (*white asterisks*), septa (*arrowheads*) and significant synovial hypertrophy (*black asterisks*).

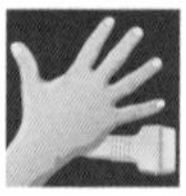

Expert note

When synovial hypertrophy is present, its activity can be assessed using power Doppler imaging. Indisputably, this remains to be the prerequisite in inflammatory conditions, not only for the diagnosis but also for the treatment governance.

Distal biceps tendinopathy in a patient with antecubital pain **4.10**

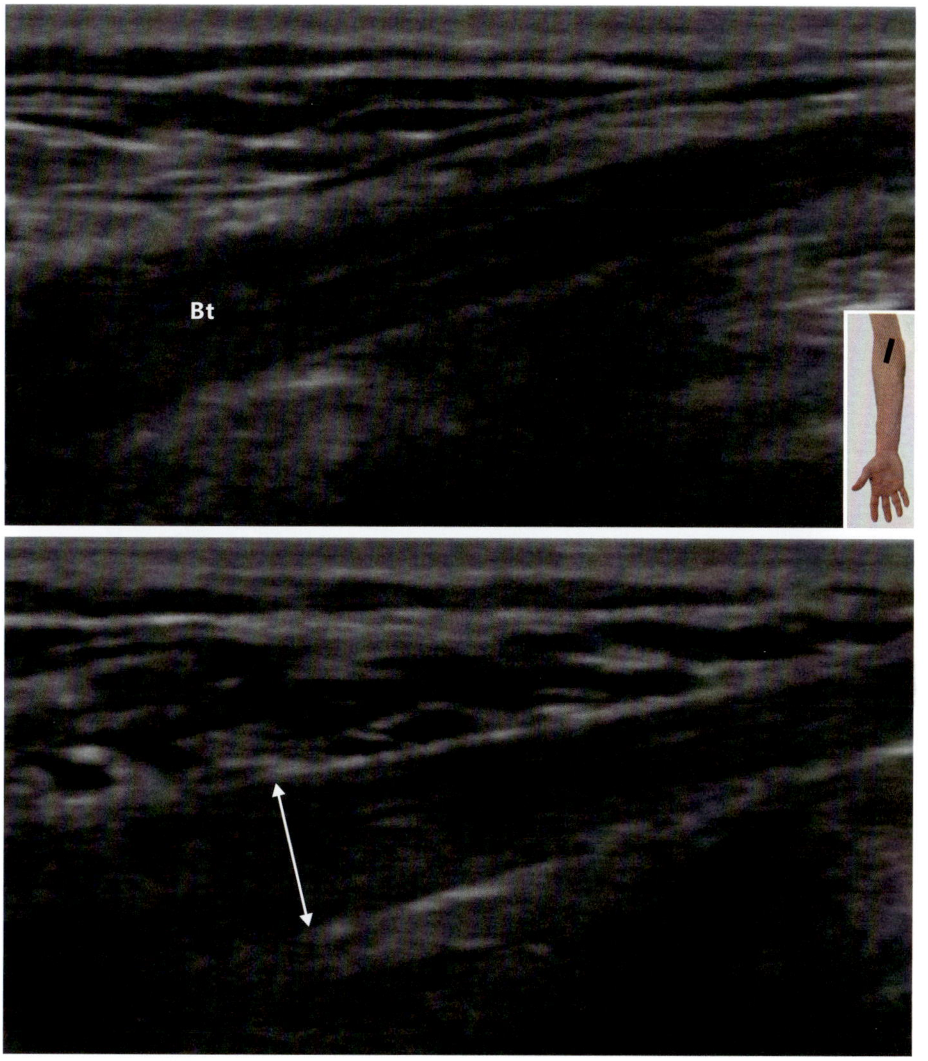

a

b

When compared with the normal side (**a**), longitudinal US imaging displays mild thickening in the distal biceps tendon (**Bt**) (*double arrow*) (**b**).

Expert note

The distal biceps tendon is best evaluated on longitudinal axis with the patient's forearm in maximal supination to bring the tendon insertion into view on the radial tuberosity [4].

4.11 Lateral epicondylitis in a 45-year-old patient with complaints of fatigue and pain at the elbow after strenuous activities

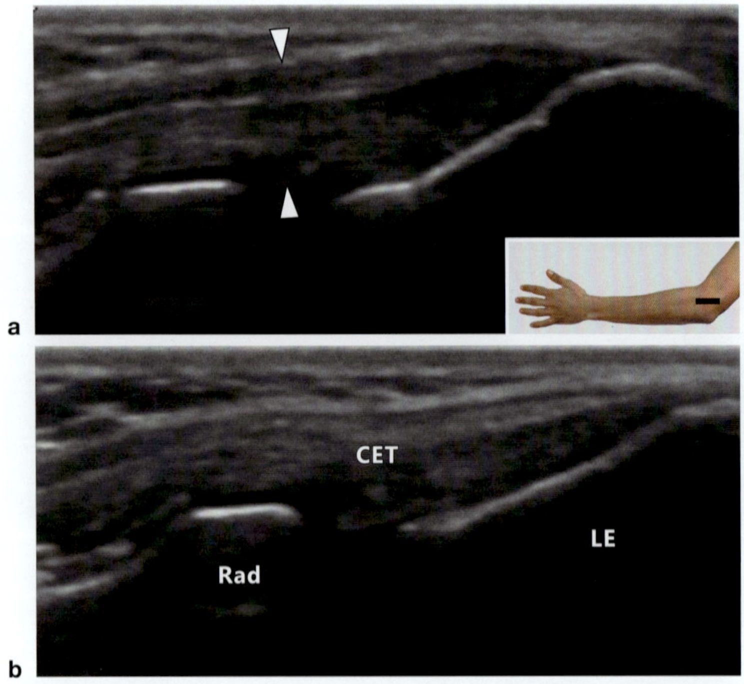

Longitudinal US image of the common extensor tendon (**CET**) demonstrates only mild thickening and hypoechogenicity (*arrowheads*) (**a**). Normal side (**b**).

LE lateral epicondyle
Rad head of radius

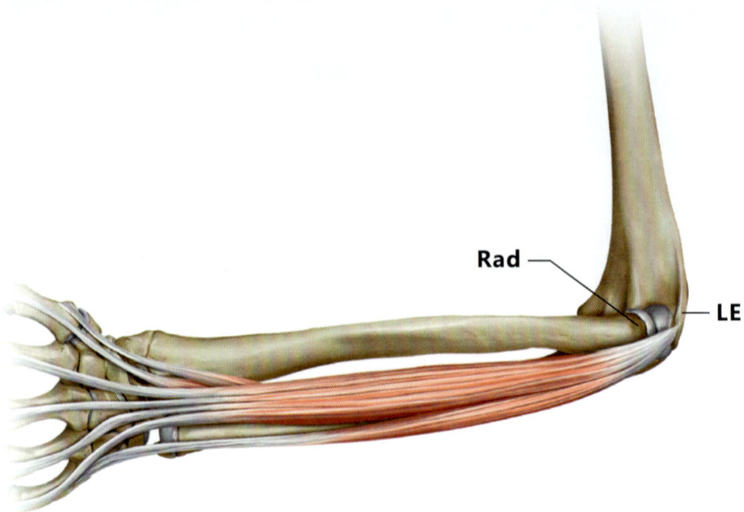

Lateral epicondylitis in a 40-year-old woman with elbow pain radiating to her wrist **4.12**

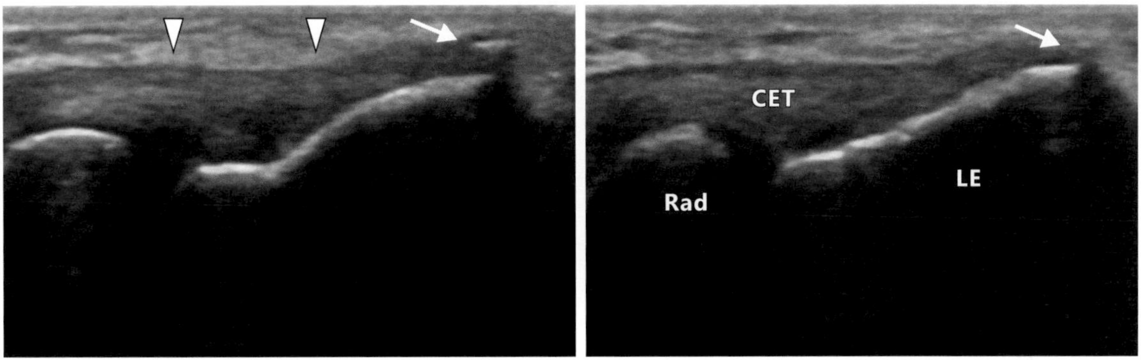

a b

Longitudinal US imaging illustrates the upper border (*arrowheads*) of the common extensor tendon (**CET**) and a prominent spur (*arrow*) (**a**). Asymptomatic side with a small spur (*arrow*) (**b**).

LE lateral epicondyle
Rad head of radius

Expert note

When evaluating entheseal regions, it is important to proceed systematically.
First, look at the cortex of the underlying bone: is it sharp? Are there spurs or erosions? Is there any "pseudo-interruption" or acoustic shadowing artifact?
Second, check for fluid (mainly for tendons surrounded by a synovial sheeth).
Finally, evaluate the tendon (soft tissue): is it present? If not, completely torn, luxated or any anatomical variant? Then, assess its shape (focal or global thickening or thinning?) and echogenicity (sharp borders and fibrillar aspect? Hypo/hyperechoic? Homogenous or not?).
Doppler imaging would definitely/also be important to explore the vascularity.
As illustrated in the figure, it is important to compare both sides; thickness and aspect of tendons very much depends on age, gender and physical structure. It is not uncommon to find spurs on the (currently) asymptomatic sides of the patients after certain ages or whereby the overuse is bilateral. Herein, it is noteworthy that "interactive imaging" as regards their findings can readily be performed during US imaging-for reassurance and protection as well. Indisputably, sonopalpation can be used to gently make the patients "feel" their spurs.

4.13 Lateral epicondylitis in a 32-year-old housemaid with chronic elbow pain

a 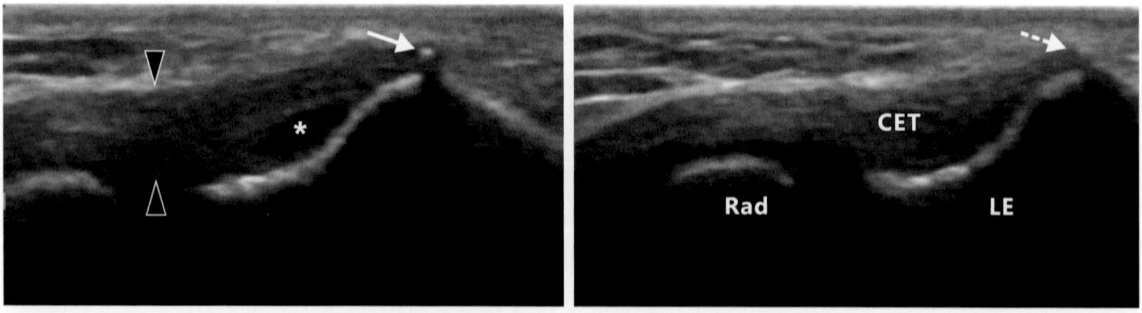 b

Longitudinal US imaging of the common extensor tendon (**CET**) demonstrates hypoechoic and thickened appearance (*arrowheads*) with a focal intratendinous tear (*asterisk*) and a proximal spur (*arrow*) formation (**a**). Please note the indefinite spur formation (*dashed arrow*) on the asymptomatic side (**b**).

LE lateral epicondyle
Rad head of radius

Expert note

Like in other scenarios of enthesopathy, US imaging for lateral epicondylitis necessitates assessment of the cortical and tendinous sides alike. Especially in chronic cases, or after inappropriate corticostreoid injections imaging should also entail a diligent look for the tendon integrity. In case of a focal hypoechoic area, US might not always allow to differentiate between a partial rupture/focal inflammation or degeneration. Looking for compressibility and trying to illustrate retraction during stretching/contraction may be helpful.

Lateral epicondylitis in a 45-year-old man with lateral elbow pain worse during daily activities 4.14

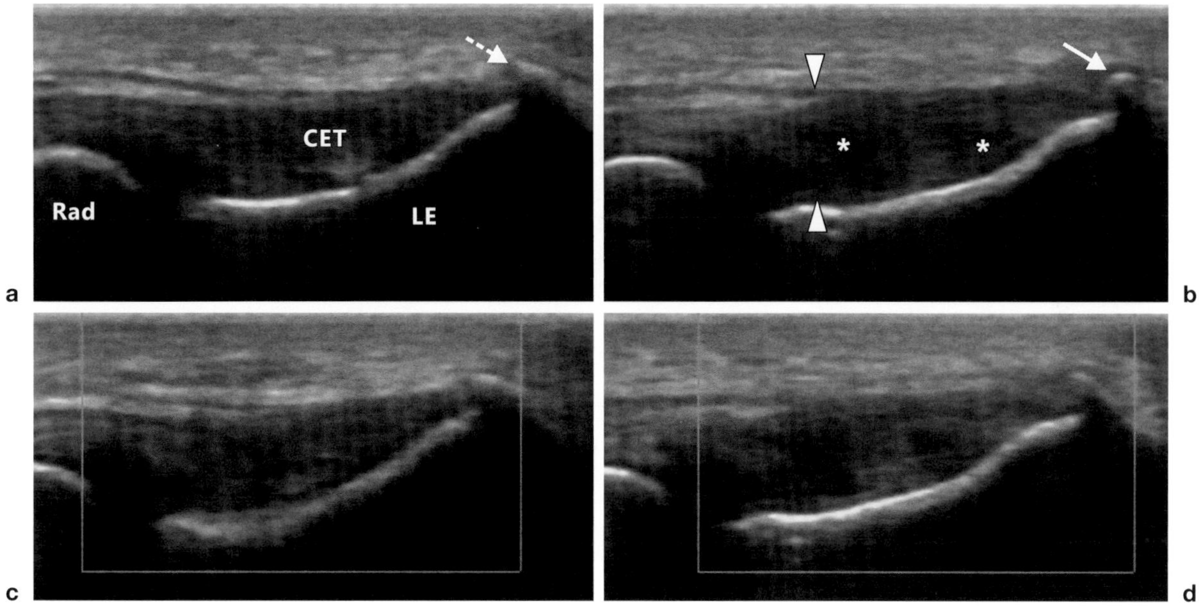

Longitudinal US image over the common extensor tendon (**CET**) reveals only a bony spur (*dashed arrow*) on the asymptomatic side (**a**). Hypoechogenecity (*asterisks*) and swelling of the tendon (*arrowheads*) in addition to spur formation (*arrow*) are seen on the symptomatic side (**b**). Power Doppler images demonstrate no flow signal (**c**, **d**).

LE lateral epicondyle
Rad head of radius

Expert note

Indisputably, power Doppler imaging would help better understand the condition (acute vs chronic) or in case epicondylitis is associated with inflammatory diseases. This could also be paramount in case the patient is planned to undergo a local injection i.e. whether to attempt to supress inflammation or induce regeneration.

4.15 Lateral epicondylitis in a 55-year-old man with elbow pain

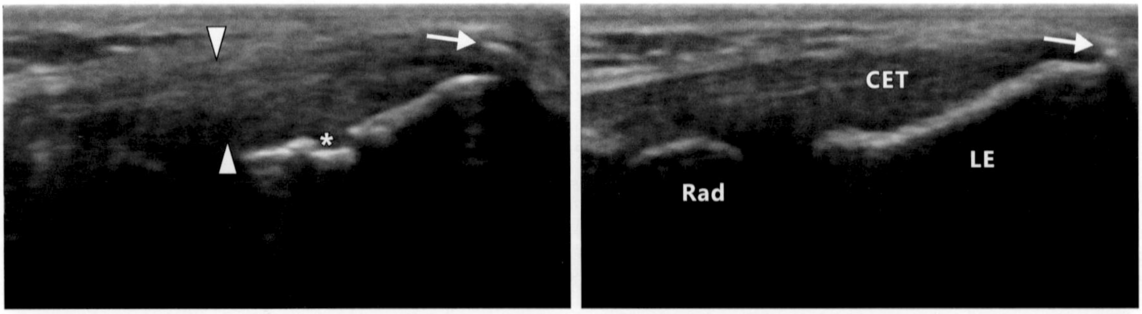

a b

Passive flexion and resistive extension of his wrist were painful.

Longitudinal US image illustrates abnormal thickening (*arrowheads*) of the common extensor tendon (**CET**) and cortical irregularity (*asterisk*) of the lateral epicondyle (**LE**) (**a**). Please note the bony spurs (*arrows*) on both sides (**a**, **b**).

Rad head of radius

Expert note

By far, spurs are the most common cortical irregularities in lateral epicondylitis; however their presence does not preclude extra findings which would actually be alerting especially in rheumatic diseases.

4.16 Lateral epicondylitis in a 35-year-old secretary with localized elbow pain and tenderness

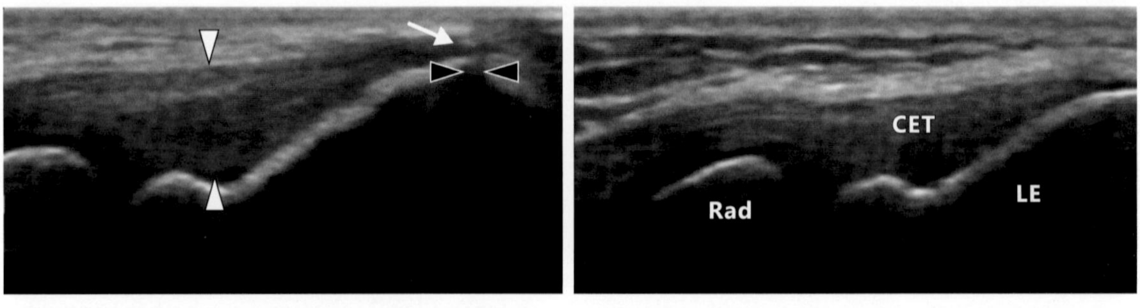

a b

Longitudinal US image depicts abnormal thickening and mild hypoechoic appearance (*white arrowheads*) of the common extensor tendon (**CET**; **a**). Normal side (**b**).
Please note that the existence of the bony spur (*arrow*) can be detected also by the presence of posterior acoustic shadowing artifact (*black arrowheads*) through the bony cortex.

Expert note

Fine movements of the probe might help distinguish such a spur from a calcification. While the former can be visualized in continuity with the bony cortex, the latter is usually not.

Lateral epicondylitis in a 46-year-old man with forearm weakness and pain during gripping activities **4.17**

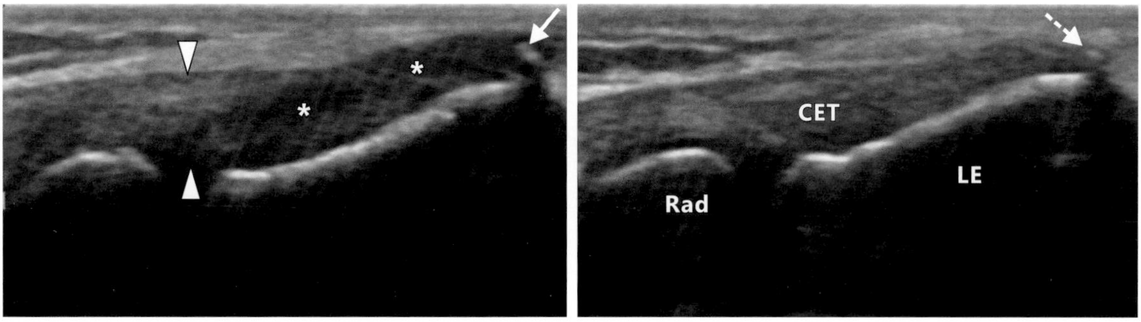

a b

Longitudinal US image demonstrates edematous (*asterisks*) and thickened (*arrowheads*) common extensor tendon (**CET**) and a hyperechoic bony spur (*arrow*) (**a**). Normal tendon echogenicity with a small spur formation (*dashed arrow*) (**b**).

LE	lateral epicondyle	**Rad**	head of radius

Expert note

Compressibility of the extensor tendon can be tested by applying pressure with the probe while subtle tears are to be explored.

Lateral epicondylitis in a 48-year-old man who described gradual progression of painful symptoms culminating in intense pain **4.18**

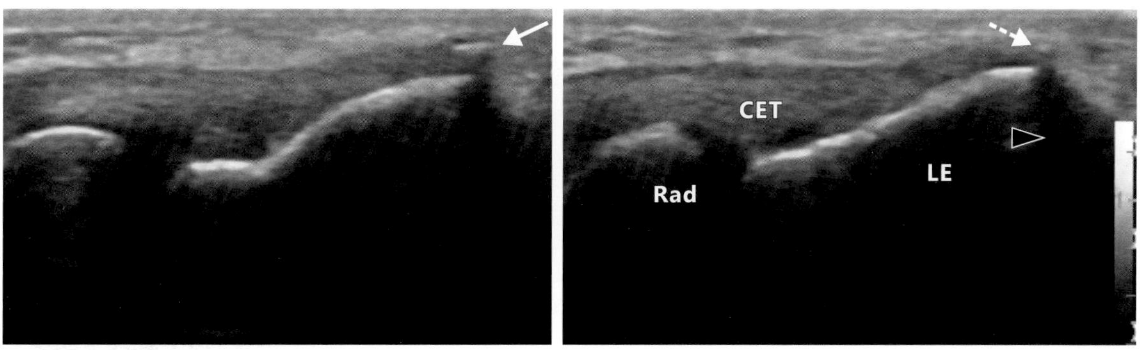

a b

Longitudinal US image over the common extensor tendon (**CET**) illustrates a thin, linear spur (*arrow*) (**a**). Asypmtomatic side with an unclear spur formation (*dashed arrow*) reflecting posterior acoustic shadowing (*arrowheads*) (**b**).

Expert note

Disproportionate clinical and US findings in relevant cases help the physician reallocate the symptomatology and explore other likely causes.

4.19 Chronic lateral epicondylitis in a 57-year-old woman after blunt trauma to the elbow

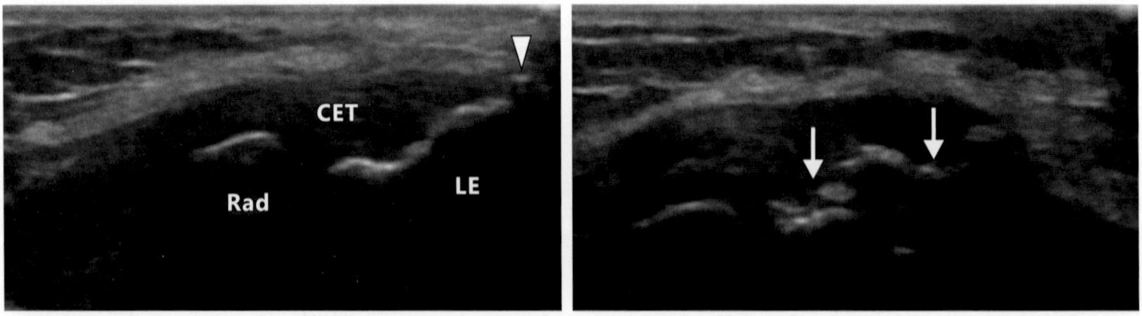

a b

When compared with the asymptomatic side (**a**), longitudinal US image illustrates abnormal irregular thickening of the common extensor tendon (**CET**) with prominent cortical irregularities (*arrows*) (**b**). Please note a small spur on the asymptomatic side (*arrowhead*).

LE lateral epicondyle **Rad** head of radius

4.20 Calcification and tear of the common extensor tendon in a 45-year-old man after sudden heavy lifting

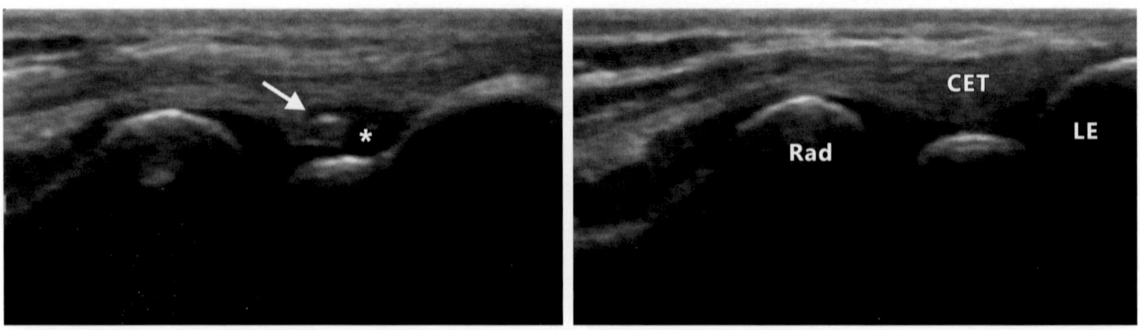

a b

Longitudinal US imaging over the common extensor tendon (**CET**) identifies a small immature calcification (*arrow*) a neighboring tear (*asterisk*) involving the deep fibers (**a**). Normal contralateral side (**b**).

Expert note

While findings like calcifications might indicate chronicity, they might also guide the onward treatment plan/procedure including barbotage, shock wave etc. Further, US imaging can definitely/conveniently be used for close follow-up of these lesions.

Bilateral lateral epicondylitis in a recreational tennis player with a history of chronic lateral elbow pain **4.21**

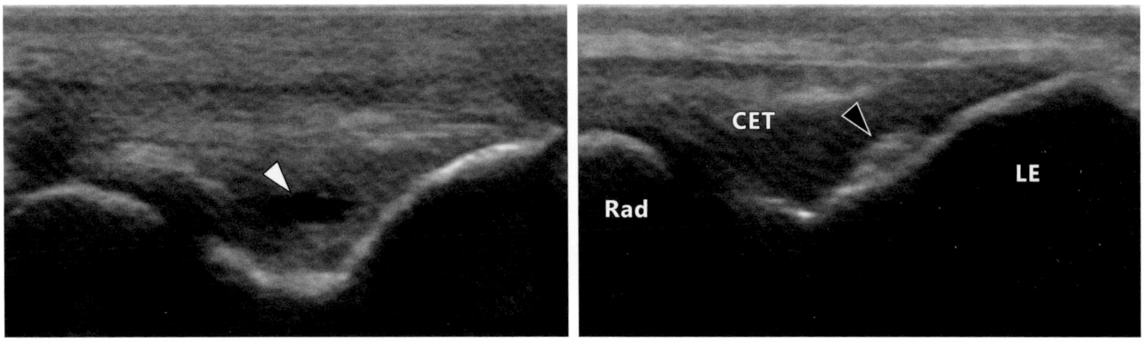

a b

Longitudinal US images identify thickened common extensor tendon (**CET**) with blurred borders and a tear involving the deep fibers (*white arrowhead*) (**a**), and abnormal echotexture associated with an immature calcification (*black arrowhead*) without acoustic shadowing (**b**).

LE lateral epicondyle **Rad** head of radius

Calcifying tendinopathy of the common extensor tendon in a 75-year-old woman who suffered pain for the last six months **4.22**

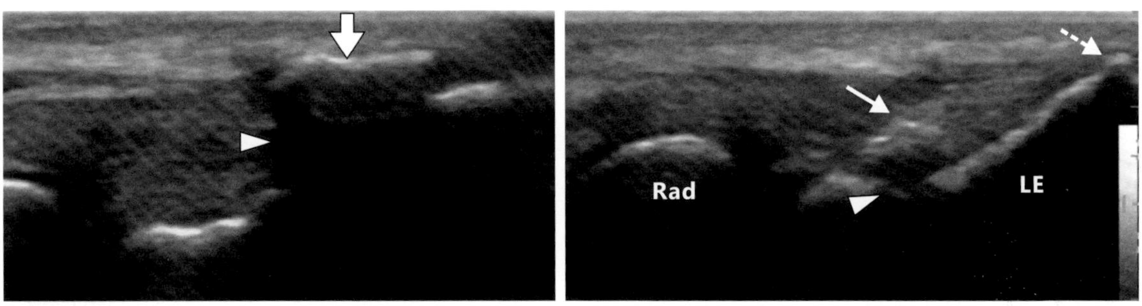

a b

Longitudinal US image of the common extensor tendon illustrates a large calcification within the tendon (*thick arrow*) (**a**). Contralateral side also reveals an intratendinous calcification (*thin arrow*), and a small bony spur (*dashed arrow*) (**b**). Please note the posterior acoustic shadowings pertaining to the calcifications (*arrowheads*).

Expert note

While US is proven very sensitive in early/small calcifications, an overall imaging/orientation for bigger lesions like in this case would better be provided by radiographs.

The big, dense calcifications (**a**) are rare; the aspect and location of the small calcification (**b**) are more frequent. Intratendinous calcifications may also be seen as part of crystal deposition diseases [5].

4.23 Severe lateral epicondylitis in a 53-year-old woman with refractory lateral elbow pain

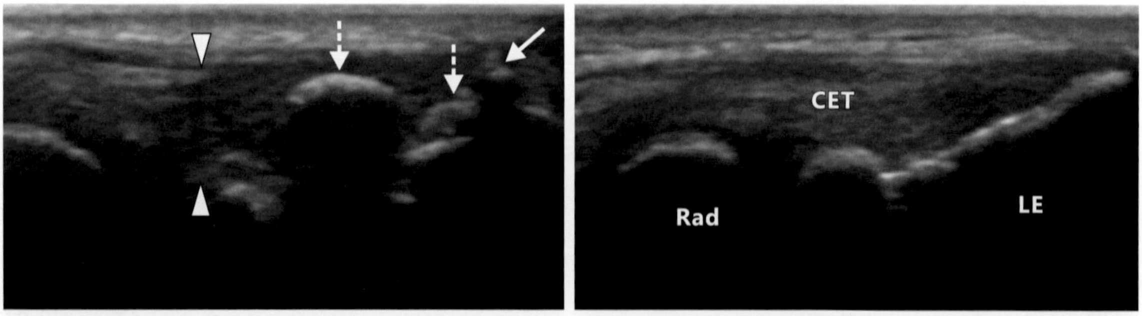

a b

Longitudinal US image reveals edematous and thickened (*arrowheads*) common extensor tendon (**CET**) with calcifications (*dashed arrows*) and a spur (*thin arrow*) (**a**). Normal contralateral side (**b**).

LE lateral epicondyle
Rad head of radius

Medial epicondylitis in a 45-year-old woman who had tenderness and pain radiating into the forearm **4.24**

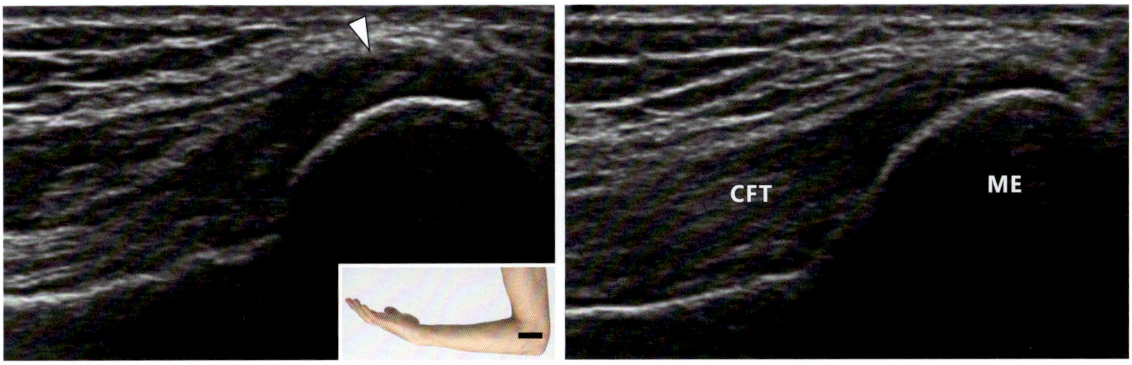

a b

Longitudinal US image obtained over the common flexor tendon (**CFT**) shows thickened and hypoechoic appearance (*arrowhead*) at the proximal attachment (**a**). Normal side (**b**).

ME medial epicondyle

Expert note
Tendon borders are again blurred and the nice fibrillar pattern is lost. The underlying cortex appears to be more echogenic due to acoustic enhancement.

Medial epicondylitis in a 47-year-old man with elbow pain during resisted wrist flexion **4.25**

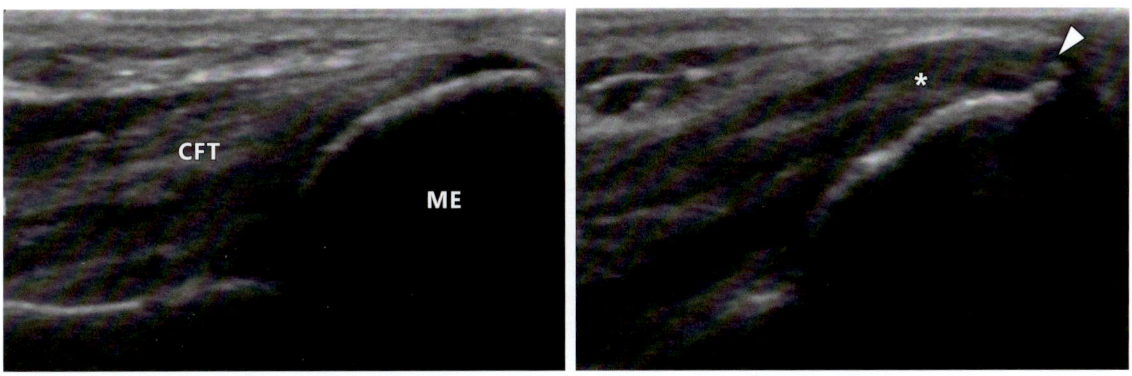

a b

When compared with the normal side (**a**), longitudinal US image reveals edematous and hypoechoic common flexor tendon (**CFT**) (*asterisk*) with a small hyperechoic spur (*arrowhead*) (**b**).

Expert note
In medial epicondylitis, the swelling will almost always be very proximally situated.

4.26 Bilateral medial epicondylitis in a 52-year-old woman with elbow pain due to repetitive heavy lifting

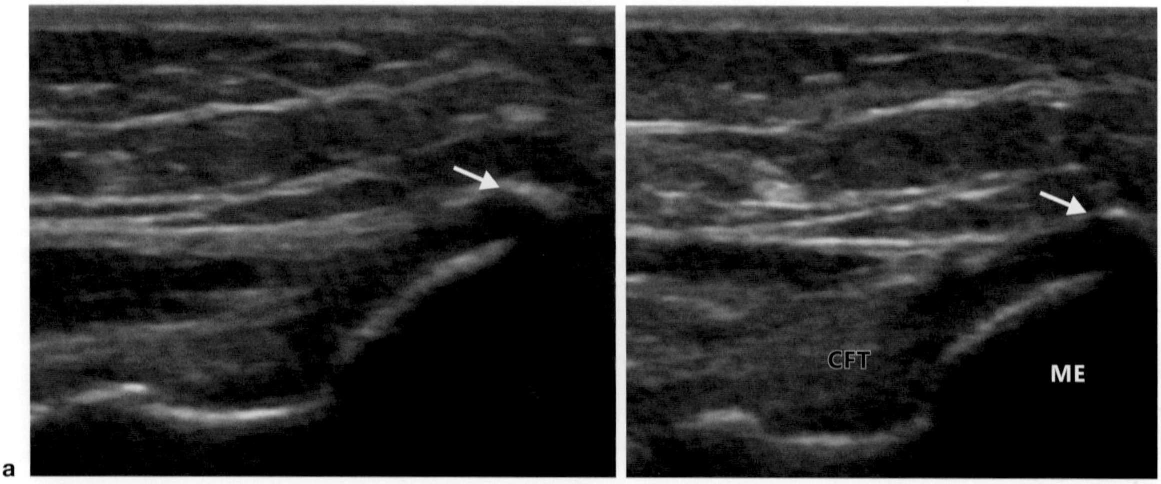

Longitudinal US images reveal bony spurs (*arrows*) at the common flexor tendon (**CFT**) insertion on both sides.

ME medial epicondyle

4.27 Medial epicondylitis in a patient with dull pain at the elbow which started after intensive gardening activity

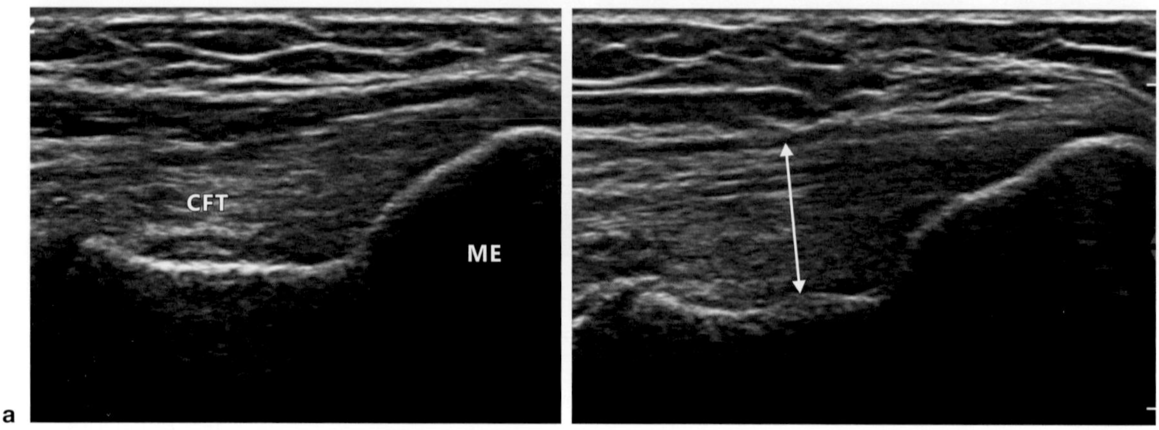

When compared with the normal side (**a**), longitudinal US image demonstrates an edematous and thickened common flexor tendon (**CFT**) (*double arrow*) (**b**).

Medial epicondylitis in a painter with aggravated pain on wrist flexion and pronation **4.28**

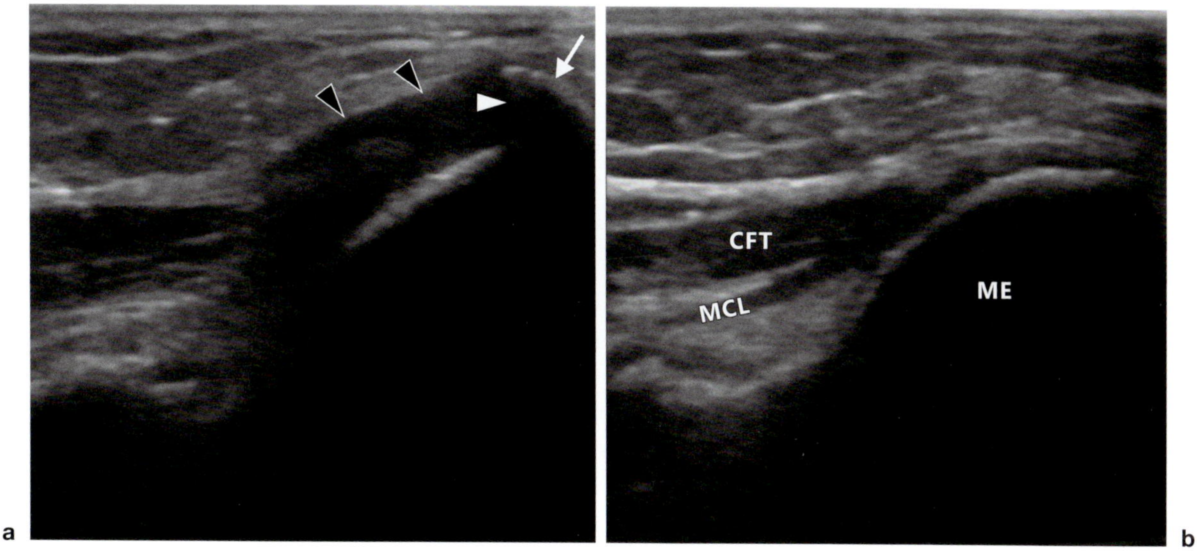

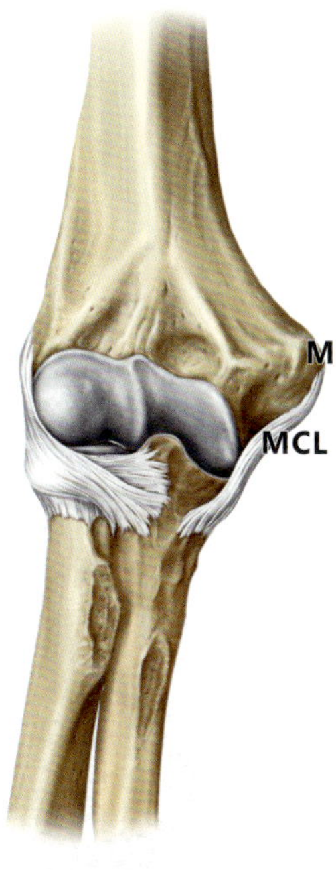

Longitudinal US image reveals a swollen (*black arrowheads*) common flexor tendon (**CFT**) with a large spur formation (*arrow*) giving posterior accoustic shadowing (*white arrowhead*) (**a**). Normal side (**b**).

MCL medial collateral ligament
ME medial epicondyle

4.29 Medial collateral ligament injury in 65-year-old man with medial elbow pain

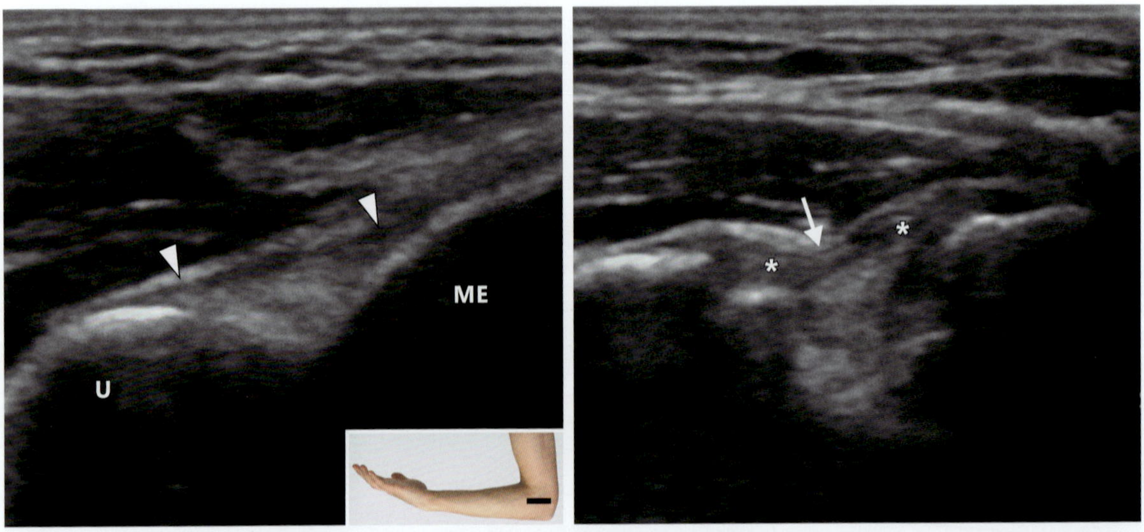

a b

When compared with the normal side (*arrowheads*) (**a**), longitudinal US imaging demonstrates intact but thickened (*asterisks*) and bowed medial collateral ligament (*arrow*) (**b**).

ME medial epicondyle
U ulna

Expert note

Like in other ligament lesions, passive or active dynamic imaging would definitely unmask the details of the structural damage if any.

Rheumatoid nodules in a patient with longstanding rheumatoid arthritis 4.30

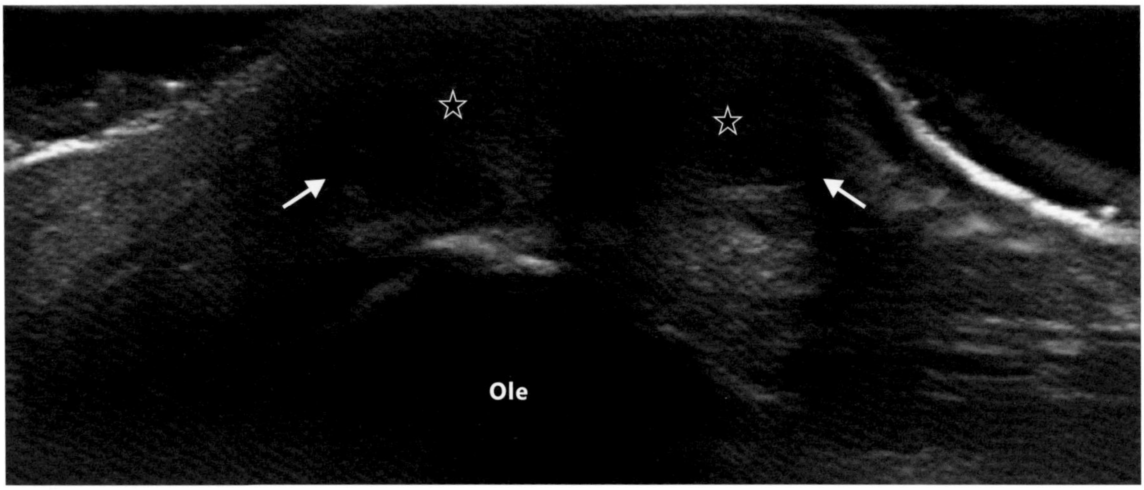

Posterior longitudinal US image over the olecranon (**Ole**) shows the subcutaneous nodules (*arrows*) with heterogenous echogenicities (*stars*).

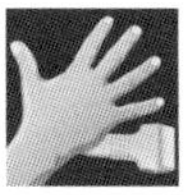

Expert note

While rheumatoid nodules are in hypoechoic appearance with well-defined borders and containing no or few Doppler signals; gouty tophi appear as hyperechoic, cloudy structures, occasionally containing calcifications with posterior acoustic shadowing [6].

REFERENCES

1. Özçakar L, Kara M, Chang KV, Hung CY, Tekın L, Ulaşlı AM, et al. EURO-MUSCULUS/USPRM basic scanning protocols for elbow. Eur J Phys Rehabil Med. 2015; 51: 485-9.
2. Schmidt WA, Schmidt H, Schicke B, Gromnica-Ihle E. Standard reference values for musculoskeletal ultrasonography. Ann Rheum Dis. 2004; 63: 988-94.
3. Finlay K, Ferri M, Friedman L. Ultrasound of the elbow. Skeletal Radiol. 2004; 33: 63-79.
4. De Cock K, Sabbe W. Ultrasound evaluation of the elbow. In: Özçakar L, De Muynck M, editors. Musculoskeletal ultrasound in physical and rehabilitation medicine. Milan: Edi.Ermes; 2014. p. 59-72.
5. Bianchi S, Martinoli C. Elbow. In: Bianchi S, Martinoli C, editors. Ultrasound of the musculoskeletal system. Berlin: Springer; 2007. p. 348-405.
6. Nalbant S, Corominas H, Hsu B, Chen LX, Schumacher HR, Kitumnuaypong T. Ultrasonography for assessment of subcutaneous nodules. J Rheumatol. 2003; 30: 1191-5.

Forearm 5

- **Subcutaneous tissue**
- **Nerve** - Volar side

5.1 Subcutaneous edema and bullous lesions in a 43-year-old woman

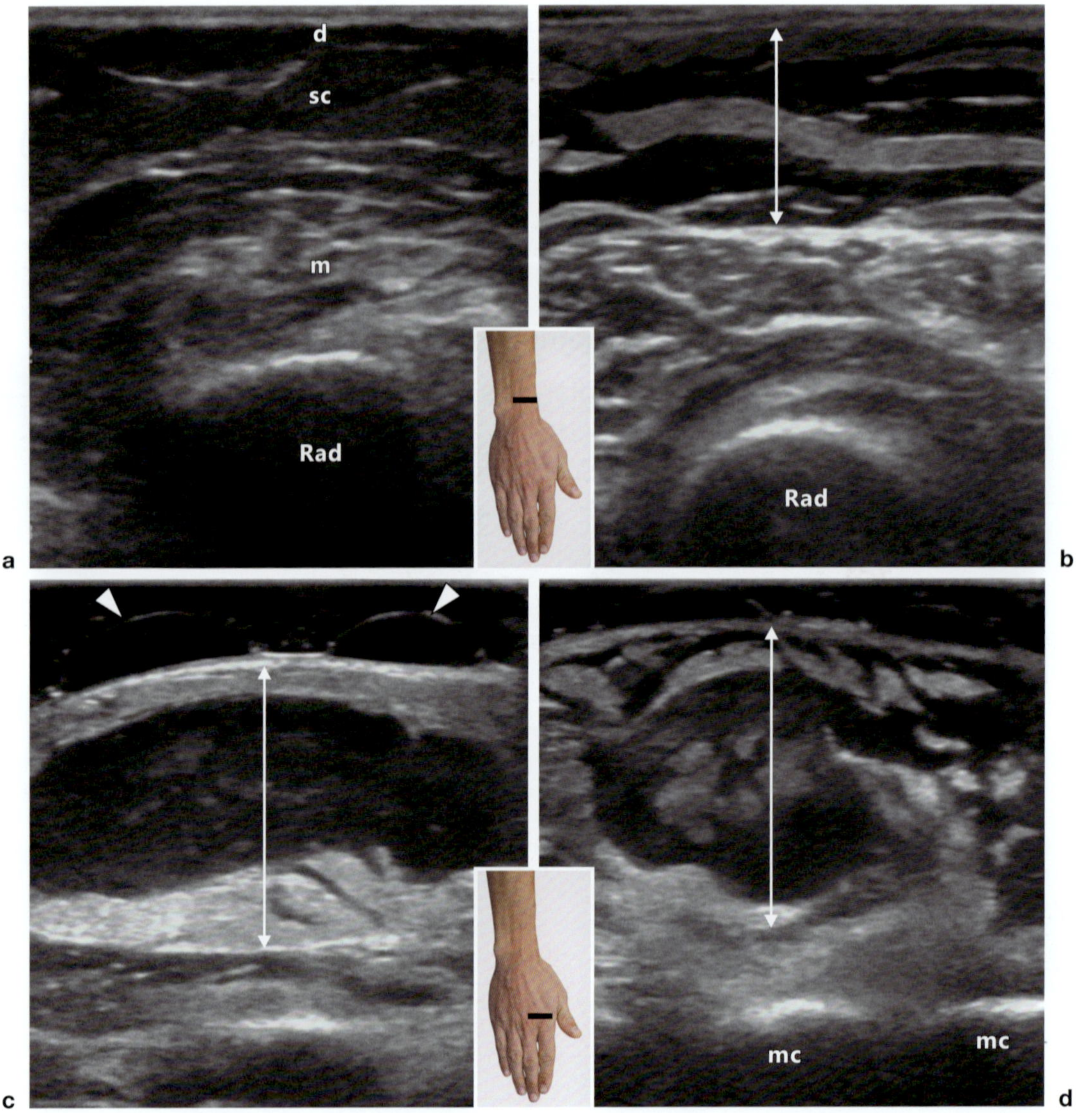

US imaging was performed 1-day after the computed tomography scan during which she suffered extravasation of the contrast material.

When compared with the normal side (**a**), axial US images obtained over the dorsal forearm (**b**) and hand (**c**, **d**) demonstrate various degrees of subcutaneous (**sc**) edema (*double arrows*) and bullous formations (*arrowheads*) in the epidermis.

d	dermis	**mc**	metacarpal bone
m	muscle	**Rad**	radius

Schwannoma in a 46-year-old man with a progressively enlarged mass in the forearm

5.2

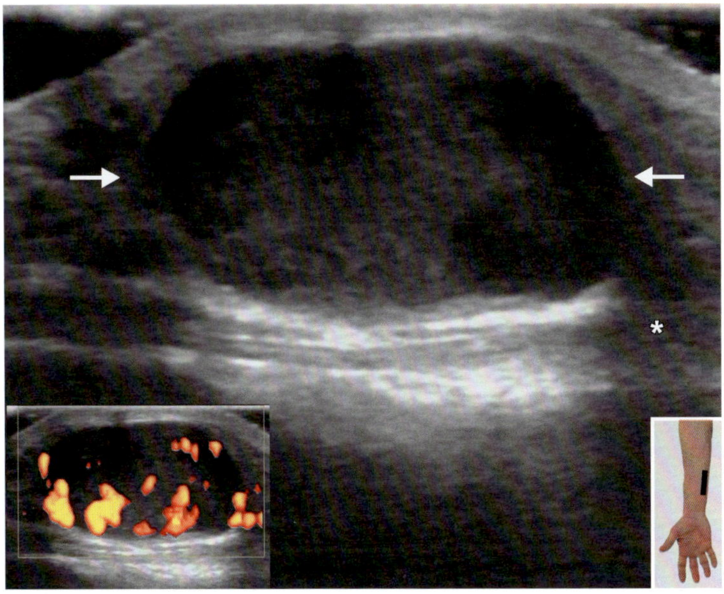

Longitudinal US image obtained over the volar aspect of the distal forearm demonstrate a large, encapsulated, hypoechoic and globoid mass (*arrows*) arising from the ulnar nerve. Significant vascular flow is seen at power Doppler imaging (*small figure*).

Expert note

Despite its being well-marginated, this much flow pattern should always raise suspicion as regards malignant peripheral nerve sheath tumor.
A vacuolar aspect and posterior enhancement are more typical for schwannomas than for other nerve tumors (but of course not 100% specific or conclusive).

5.3 Neurofibromatosis type 1 in a 19-year-old woman with a painless swelling in the forearm

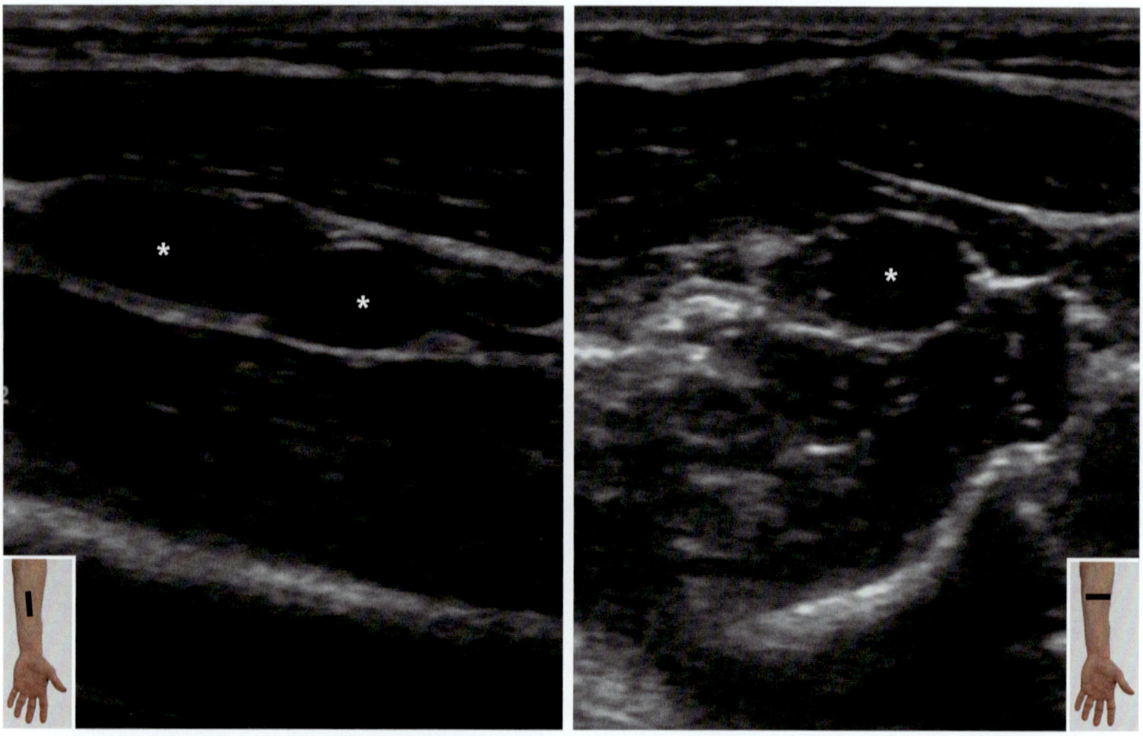

a b

Longitudinal (**a**) and axial (**b**) US images over the volar forearm demonstrate hypoechoic swellings of different sizes (*asterisks*) arising from the median nerve.

Expert note

Substantial US imaging of the (symptomatic and asymptomatic) peripheral nerves is very convenient and informative as regards the type and extent of involvement in neurofibromatosis [1]. Especially in pediatric population, the role of US imaging can further be appreciated [2].

REFERENCES

1. Kara M, Yilmaz A, Ozel S, Özçakar L. Sonographic imaging of the peripheral nerves in a patient with neurofibromatosis type 1. Muscle Nerve. 2010; 41: 887-8.
2. Kara M. Ultrasound imaging for peripheral nerve problems. In: Özçakar L, De Muynck M, editors. Musculoskeletal ultrasound in physical and rehabilitation medicine. Milan: Edi.Ermes; 2014. p. 141-60.

Forearm

6

Wrist and Hand

- Radiocarpal joints
- Triangular fibrocartilage complex
- Extensor tendon compartments
- Flexor carpi radialis tendon
- Flexor digitorum superficialis tendon
- Flexor carpi ulnaris tendon
- First carpometacarpal joint
- Flexor pollicis longus tendon
- Subcutaneous tissue
- Lumbrical muscle
- Flexor digitorum superficialis/profundus tendons
- Extensor tendons
- Metacarpophalangeal joint
- Nail

6.1 Synovitis in a patient with rheumatoid arthritis suffering from wrist pain and stiffness

a

b

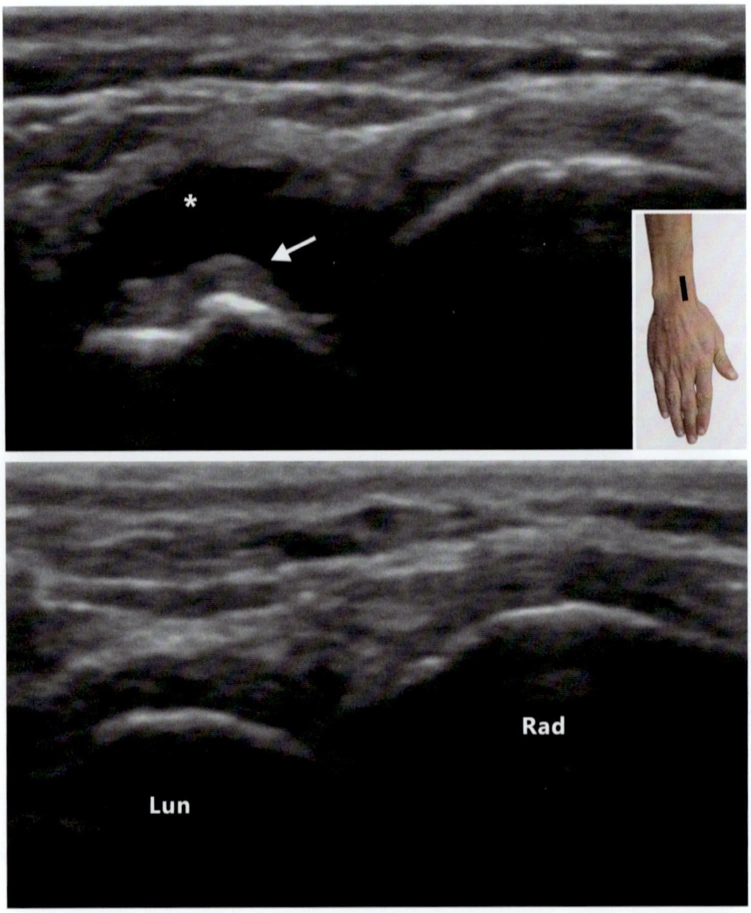

Dorsal longitudinal US imaging over the radiolunate joint demonstrates anechoic fluid collection (*asterisk*) and Grade II synovial hypertrophy (*arrow*) within the joint space (**a**). Normal side (**b**).

Lun lunate
Rad radius

Expert note

Please see Table 6.2 (pag. 248) for the grading of synovitis in B-mode imaging.

Chronic synovitis in a 35-year-old patient **6.2**

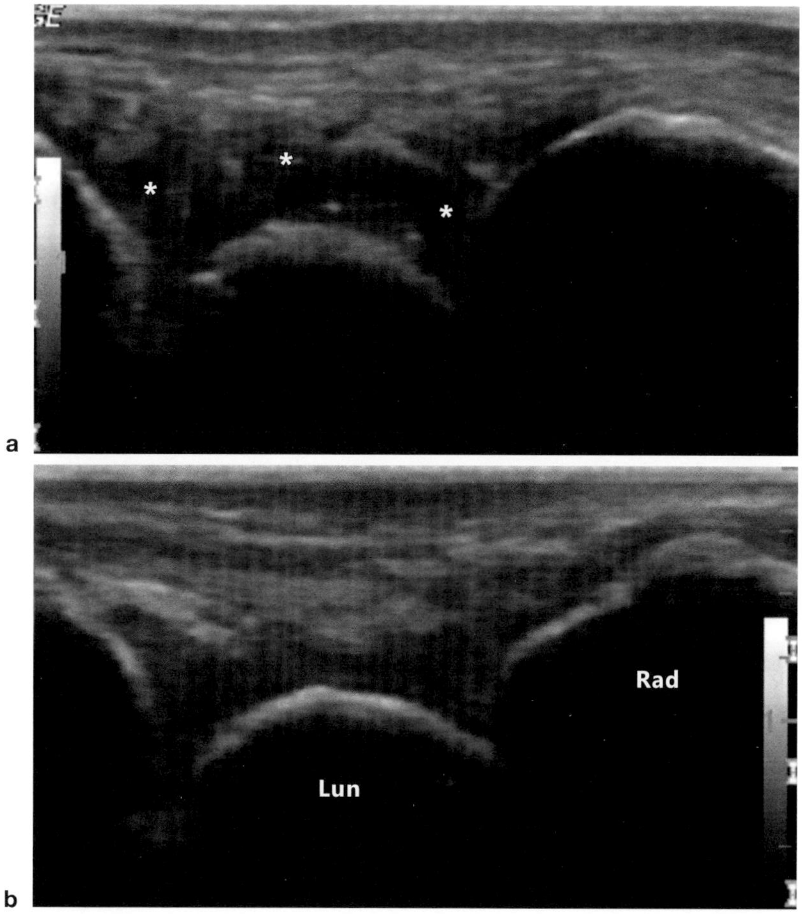

The patient complained of increasing pain and local inflammatory symptoms for the last one month.

Longitudinal US imaging over the dorsal aspect of the wrist joint demonstrates heterogenous Grade II effusion/synovitis (*asterisks*) inside the radio-lunate joint (**a**). Asymptomatic side (**b**).

Lun lunate
Rad radius

6.3 Synovitis in a 48-year-old woman with advanced rheumatoid arthritis

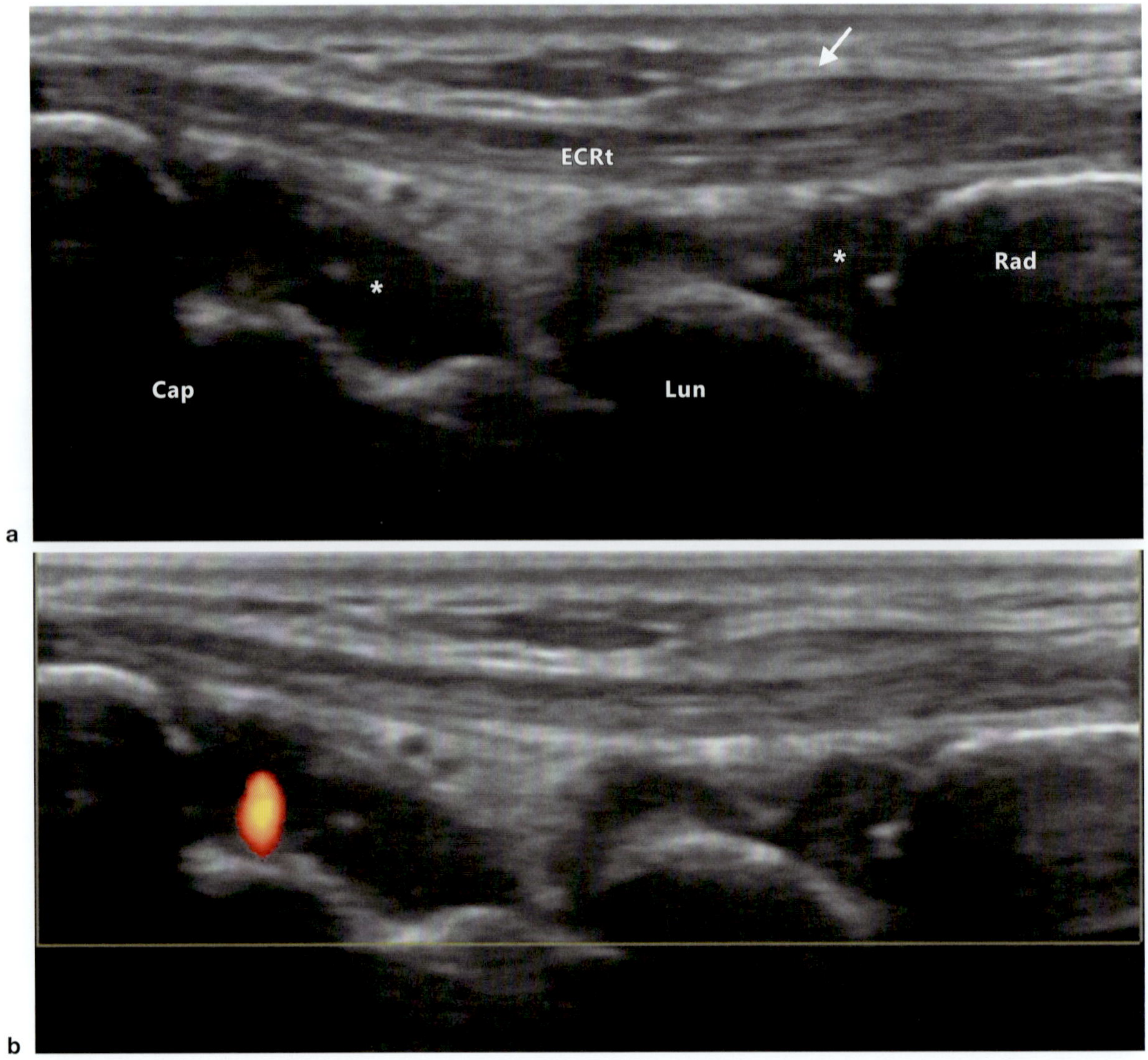

Longitudinal B-mode (**a**) and power Doppler (**b**) images over the dorsal aspect of the wrist illustrate Grade II synovial hypertrophy (*asterisks*) with a single signal (Grade I). Please note the hump view above the extensor carpi radialis tendon (**ECRt**) indicating the thickening of the extensor retinaculum (*arrow*).

Cap capitate
Lun lunate
Rad radius

Wrist involvement in chronic severe rheumatoid arthritis 6.4

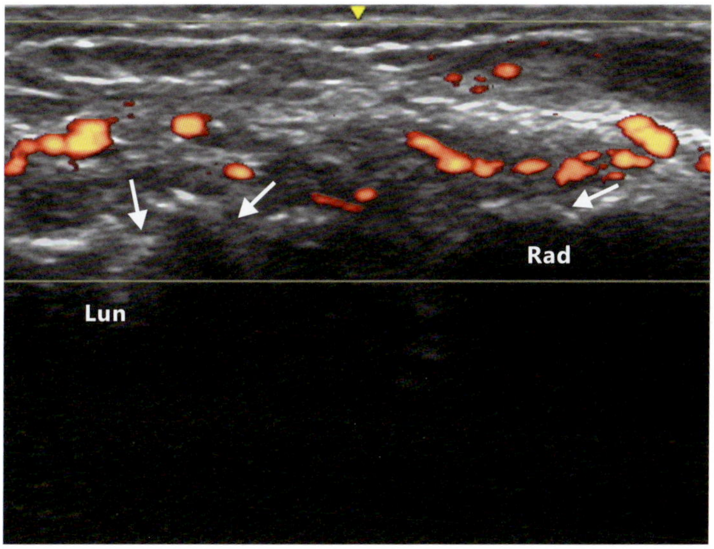

Power Doppler imaging of the wrist joint shows Grade II synovial hyperemia and extensive erosive changes on the articular surfaces of the radiolunate joint (*arrows*).

Lun lunate
Rad radius

6.5 Synovitis in a 53-year-old woman with rheumatoid arthritis

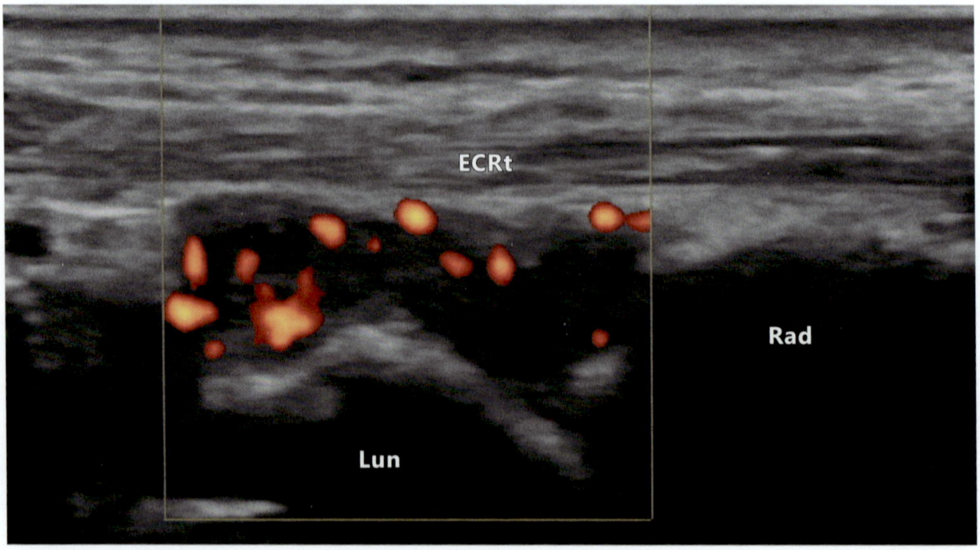

Longitudinal power Doppler US imaging over the dorsal wrist joint shows active synovitis (Grade II).

ECRt extensor carpi radialis tendon
Lun lunate
Rad radius

Expert note

Either in the (very) early period or during the follow up of patients with rheumatic problems, the use of gray scale and power Doppler imaging have been well established in the literature. While the early detection of erosions is diagnostic and guiding rapid treatment, convenient/prompt assessment of the disease activity is of great importance for monitoring therapeutic outcome as well [1].

Synovitis in a 40-year-old woman with active rheumatoid arthritis 6.6

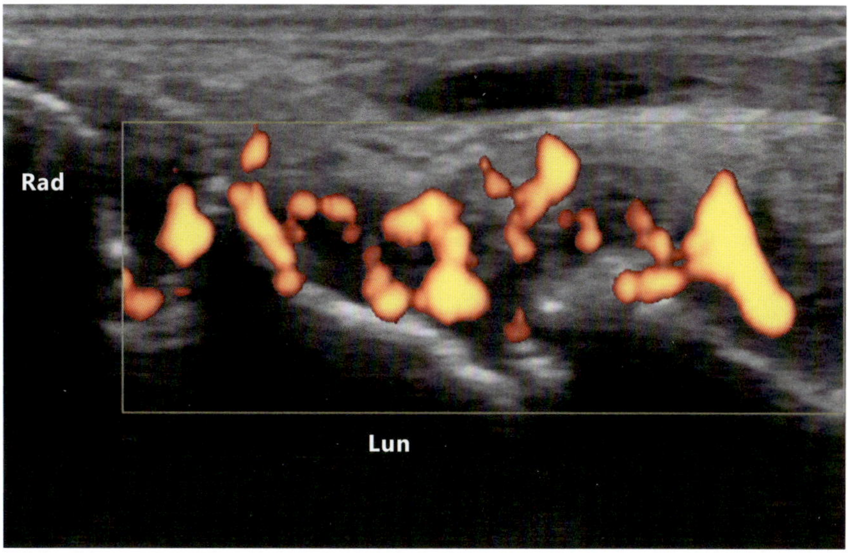

Longitudinal power Doppler US imaging shows active synovitis characterized by Grade III hypervascular pattern.

Lun lunate
Rad radius

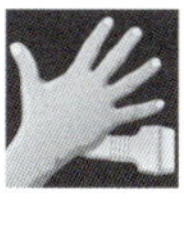

Expert note

Doppler signals being present in more than 50% of the area of interest (synovial hypertrophy) corresponds to Grade III [2].

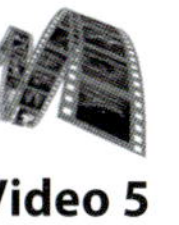

Table 6.1

Grade	Signal
0	No flow
I	Single flow signal(s)
II	Confluent signals but less than 50% of the area of interest
III	Signals more than 50% of the area of interest

6.7 Hand and wrist involvement in a 37-year-old woman with long standing rheumatoid arthritis

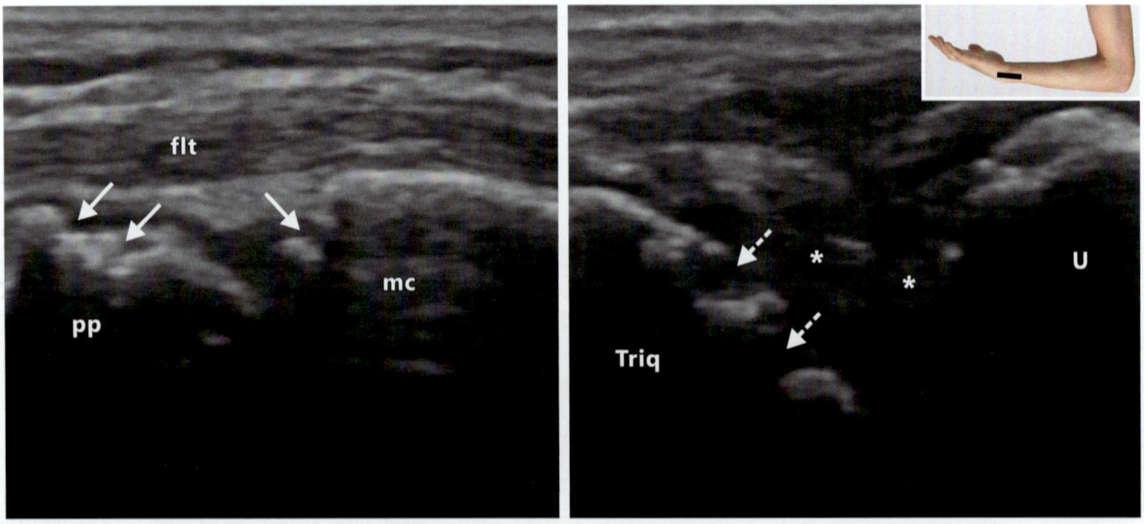

a b

Palmar longitudinal US image demonstrates erosions (*arrows*) affecting both articular surfaces of the 2nd metacarpophalangeal joint (**a**). Medial longitudinal US image of the radiocarpal joint shows thickened synovium (*asterisks*) with erosions (*dashed arrows*) on the triquetrum (**Triq**) (**b**).

flt flexor tendon
mc metacarpal bone
pp proximal phalanx
U ulna

Expert note

The challenge while exploring erosions on the metacarpophalangeal joints would be the inability to have access to certain portions of the joints. As such, during routine scanning the relevant protocols tend to include the 2nd and 5th metacarpal heads around which the US probe can be better positioned/surrounding.

Chronic synovitis in rheumatoid arthritis 6.8

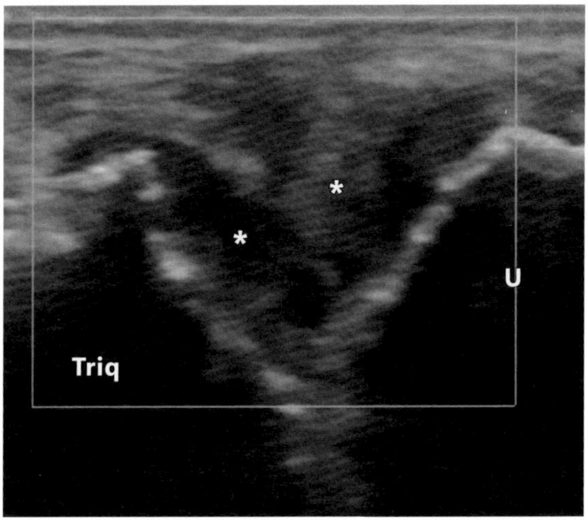

Medial longitudinal US image over the wrist reveals synovial effusion and hypertrophy (*asterisks*) without hyperemia at power Doppler imaging.

Triq triquetrum
U ulna

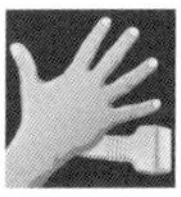

Expert note

The ulnar side of the wrist is a typical area of involvement that needs to be checked while scanning for rheumatoid arthritis.

6.9 Pseudogout in a 82-year-old woman with pain, tenderness and swelling at the wrist joint

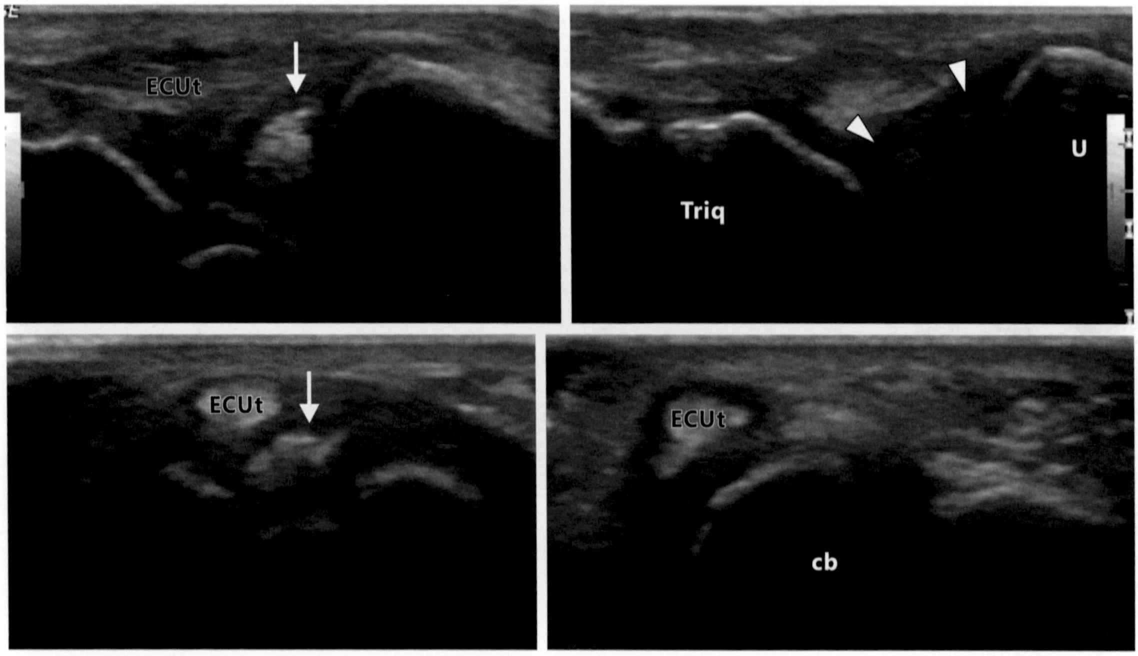

Longitudinal (**a**) and axial (**c**) US images show calcific deposition (*arrows*) within the triangular fibrocartilage complex deep to the extensor carpi ulnaris tendon (**ECUt**). Normal triangular fibrocartilage complex (*arrowheads*) on the contralateral side (**b**, **d**).

cb carpal bones
Triq triquetrum
U ulna

Expert note

In patients with pseudogout, regardless of the currently involved joint(s); areas like triangular fibrocartilage or symphysis pubis can always be scanned for a substantial/complete examination.

A 30-year-old athlete with a history of fall on the extended hand 6.10

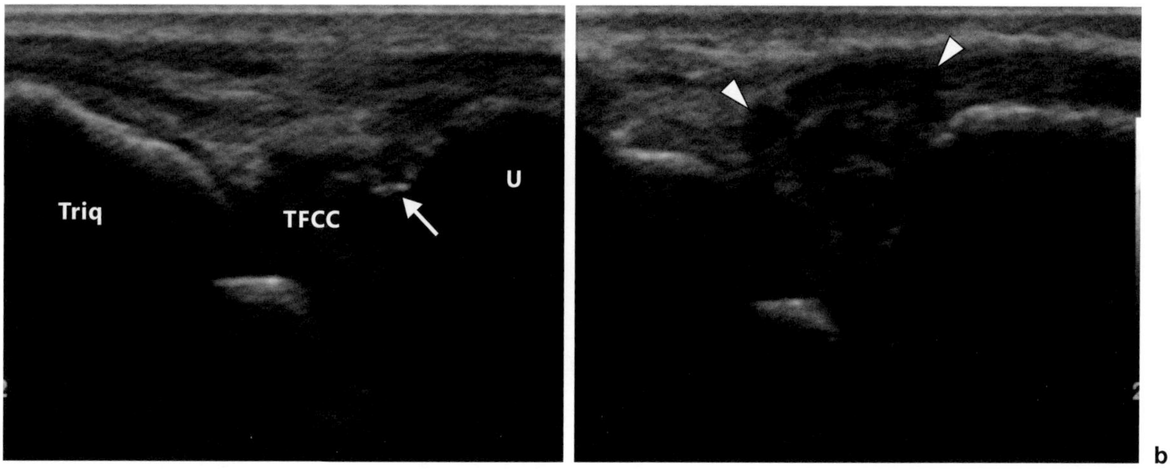

When compared with the asymptomatic side with a small spur (*arrow*) on the distal ulna (**a**), longitudinal US image shows swollen triangular fibrocartilage complex (**TFCC**) with heterogenous appearance (*arrowheads*) (**b**).

Triq triquetrum
U ulna

6.11 Lipedema in a 25-year-old woman with painful swelling of the distal forearm

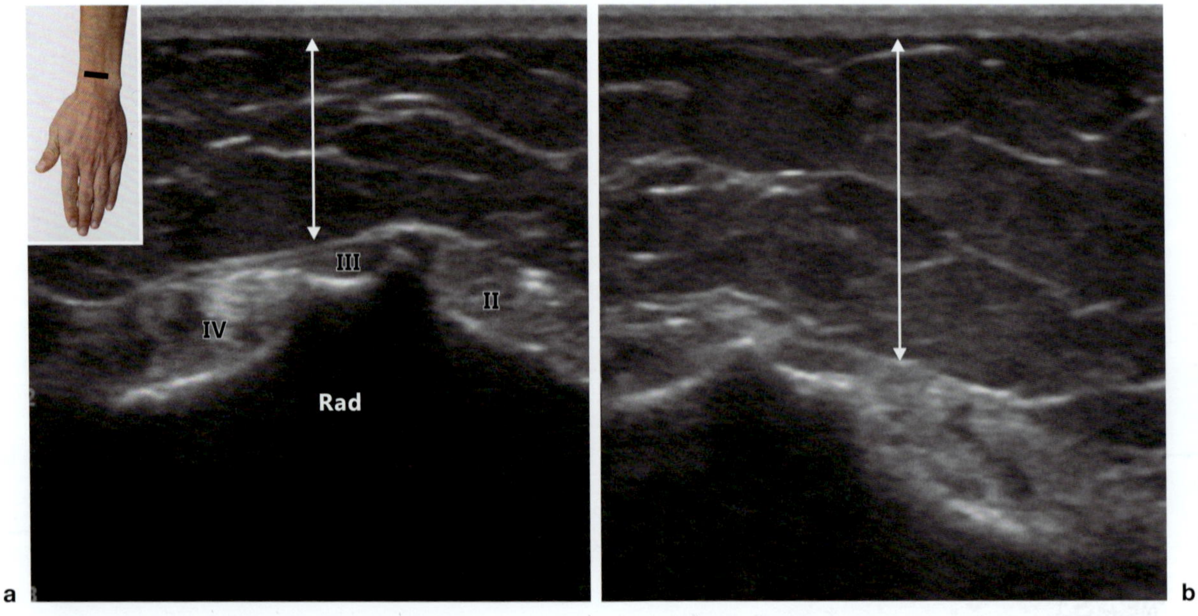

Dorsal axial US imaging reveals lipedema in the subcutaneous/adipose tissue (*double arrows*) over the extensor tendon compartments II-IV on both wrists (**a**, **b**).

Rad radius

Occult dorsal ganglion cyst of the wrist in a young woman **6.12**

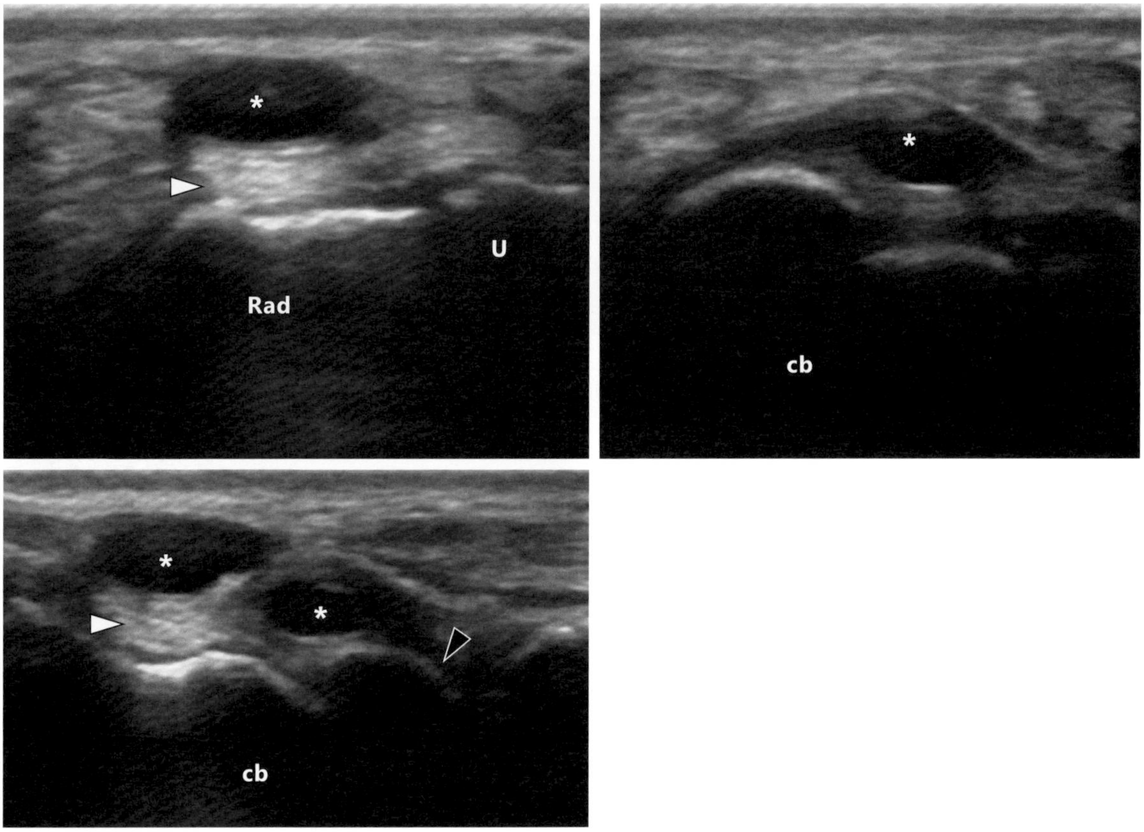

a b c

Dorsal US images reveal a lobulated an/hypoechoic fluid-filled mass (*asterisks*) with enhanced through transmission artifact (*white arrowheads*). Axial images at different levels (**a**, **b**). Longitudinal image (**c**) shows its possible origination from the joint (*black arrowhead*).

cb carpal bones
Rad radius
U ulna

Expert note

It is not always possible to see the "stem" of a cyst; giving compression with the probe sometimes widens it.

6.13 De Quervain tenosynovitis in a 34-year-old woman with tenderness and pain over the radial styloid process

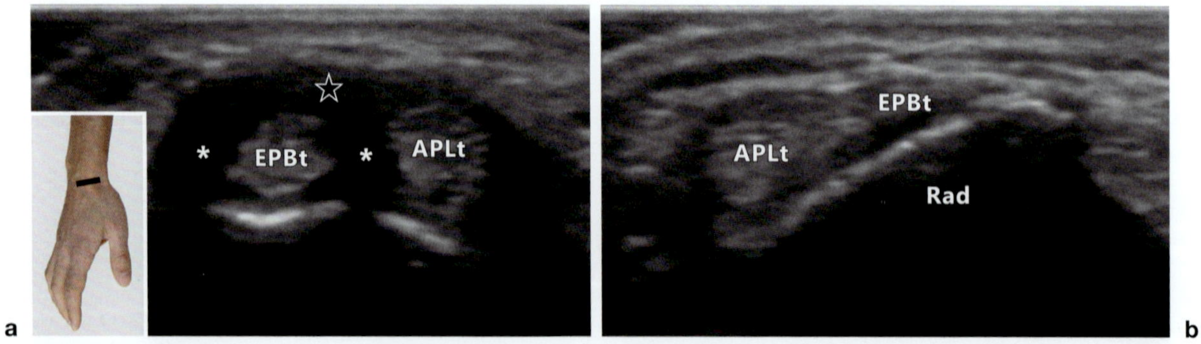

Axial US imaging of the first extensor tendon compartment identifies sheath effusion (*asterisks*) and hyperechoic retinaculum thickening (*star*) (**a**). Contralateral normal side (**b**).

APLt abductor pollicis longus tendon
EPBt extensor pollicis brevis tendon
Rad radius

De Quervain tenosynovitis in a 33-year-old man with local pain, particularly during ulnar deviation

6.14

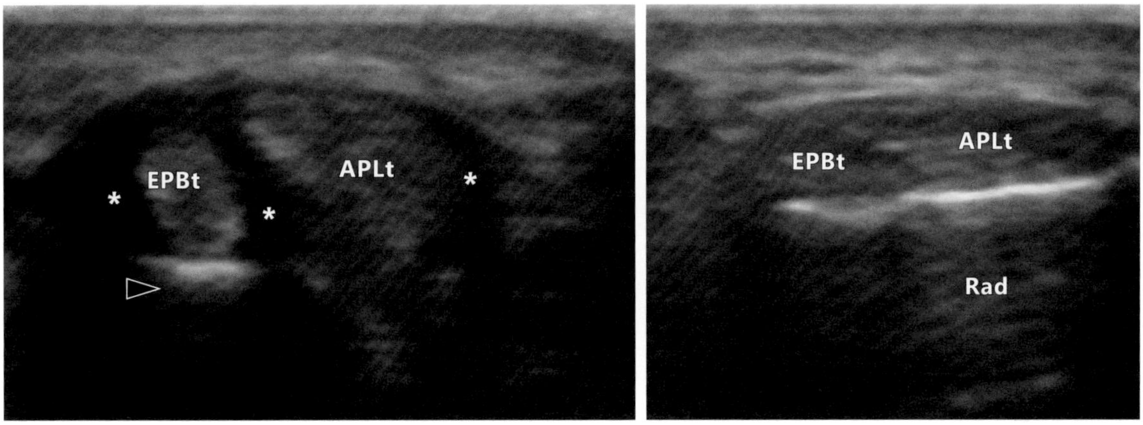

a b

Axial US image illustrates fluid (*asterisks*) around the edematous extensor pollicis brevis (**EPBt**) and abductor pollicis longus (**APLt**) tendons (**a**). *Arrowhead* reveals enhanced through transmission artifact. Contralateral normal side (**b**).

Rad radius

Expert note

In this case, in contrast to the fluid accumulation, the tendons seem to be rather less affected i.e. normal size and normal shape. As regards echogenicity, they appear as better demarcated due to the enhanced through transmission artifact.

6.15 De Quervain tenosynovitis in a new mother who had difficulty in holding her baby's head

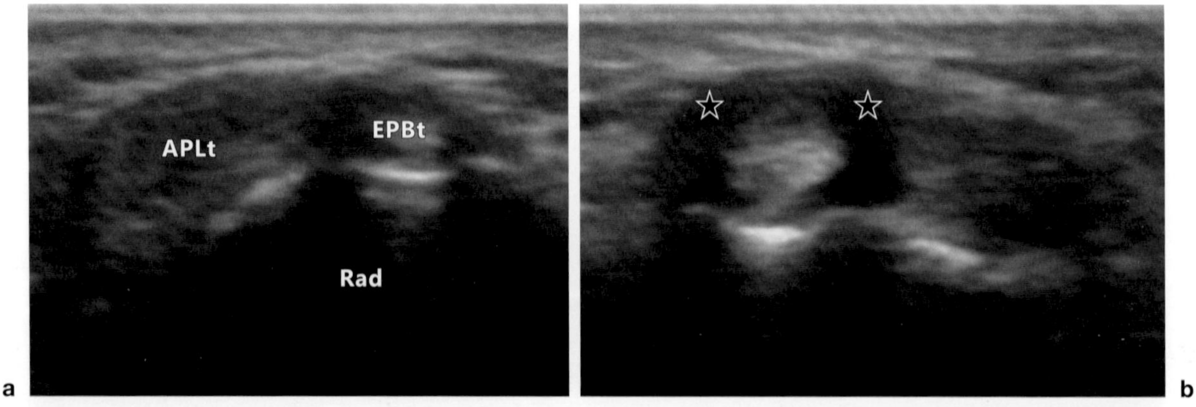

When compared with the normal side (**a**), axial (**b**) US imaging over the 1st extensor tendon compartment reveals global hypoechoic swollen retinaculum (*stars*) around the thickened extensor pollicis brevis tendon (**EPBt**).

APLt abductor pollicis longus tendon **Rad** radius

6.16 De Quervain tenosynovitis in a young woman with pain during grasping objects and positive Finkelstein test

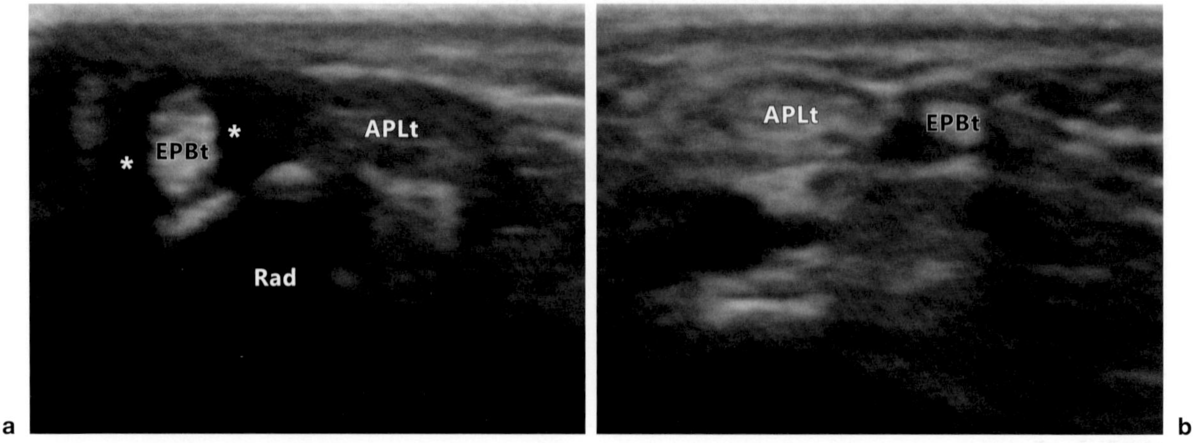

Axial US image illustrates the presence of anechoic synovial effusion (*asterisks*) inside the extensor pollicis brevis tendon (**EPBt**) sheath and edematous abductor pollicis longus tendon (**APLt**) (**a**). Normal findings of the 1st extensor compartment (**b**).

Rad radius

De Quervain tenosynovitis and subcompartmentalization of the extensor tendons in a 55-year-old man with dorsal wrist pain 6.17

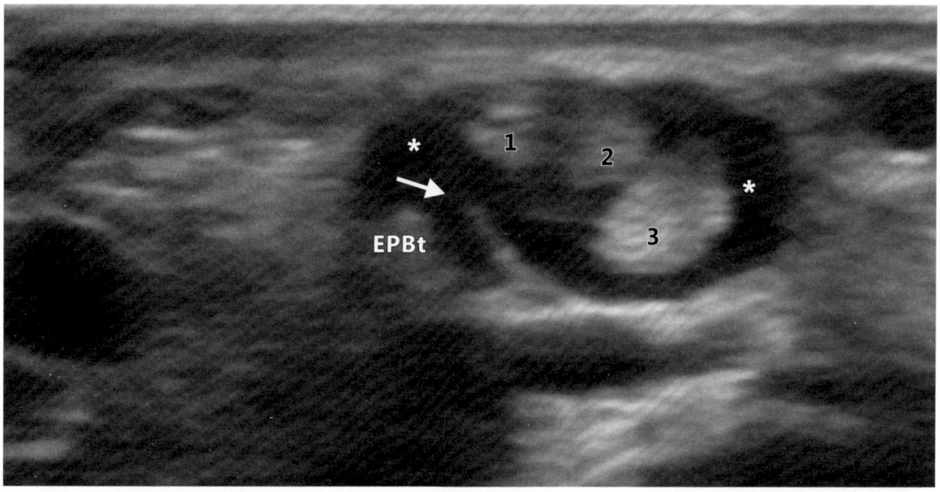

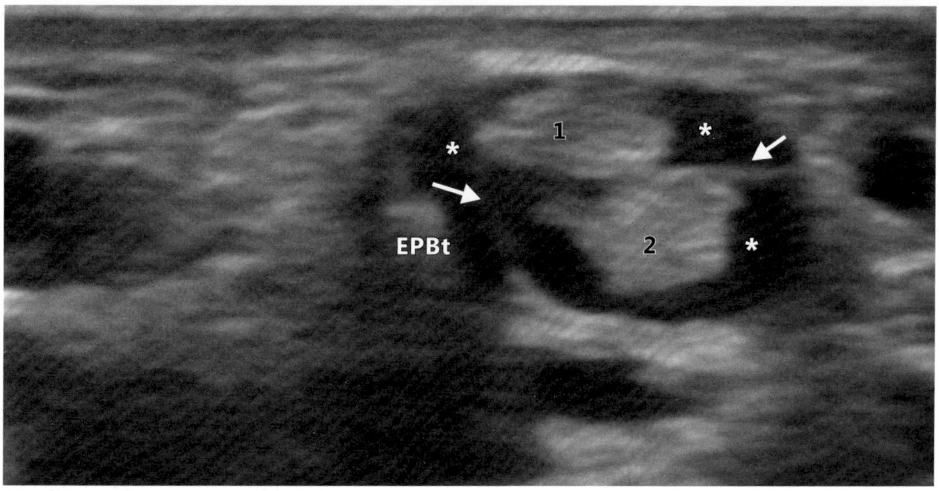

Axial US images demonstrate fluid (*asterisks*) and septae (*arrows*) inside the first extensor compartment of the extensor pollicis brevis tendon (**EPBt**) on both sides. The abductor longus pollicis tendon is found to split into three (**a**) and two (**b**) pieces.

Expert note

The two tendons in the 1st extensor compartment have variations as regards their sheath anatomy (separate or common). Further, there might also be subcompartmentalization, more frequent on the abductor pollicis longus side. Both conditions are important during a substantial examination for De Quervain tenosynovitis. While they might be informative for the diagnosis (overuse, friction), US imaging for understanding the exact scenario is even more important for a precise/effective injection [3-6].

6.18 De Quervain tenosynovitis and subcompartmentalization

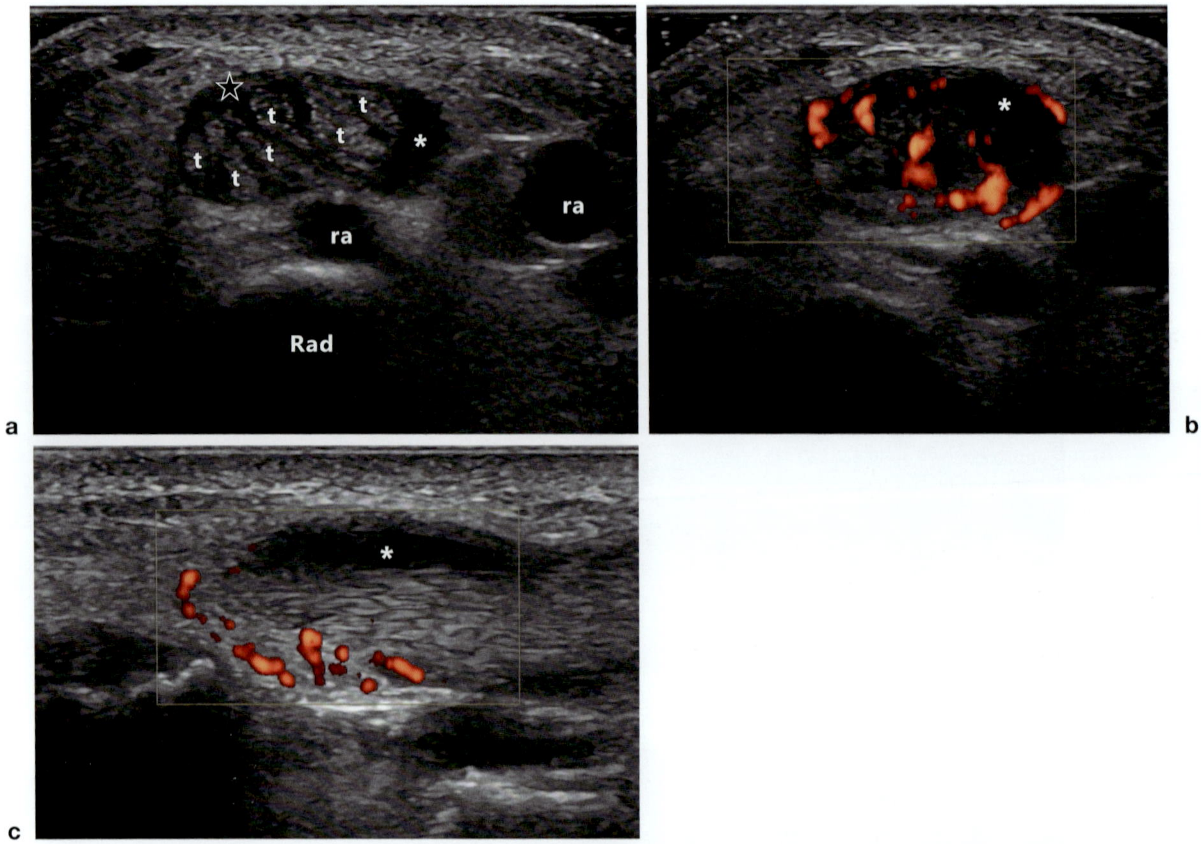

Axial (**a**, **b**) and longitudinal (**c**) US images demonstrate the subcompartmentalization of abductor pollicis longus and extensor pollicis brevis tendons (**t**) with effusion inside the tendon sheath (*asterisks*) and thickening of the retinaculum (*star*). Power Doppler imaging shows Grade II blood flow signals (**b**, **c**).

ra branches of radial artery
Rad radius

Intersection syndrome in a 45-year-old man with dorsal wrist pain **6.19**

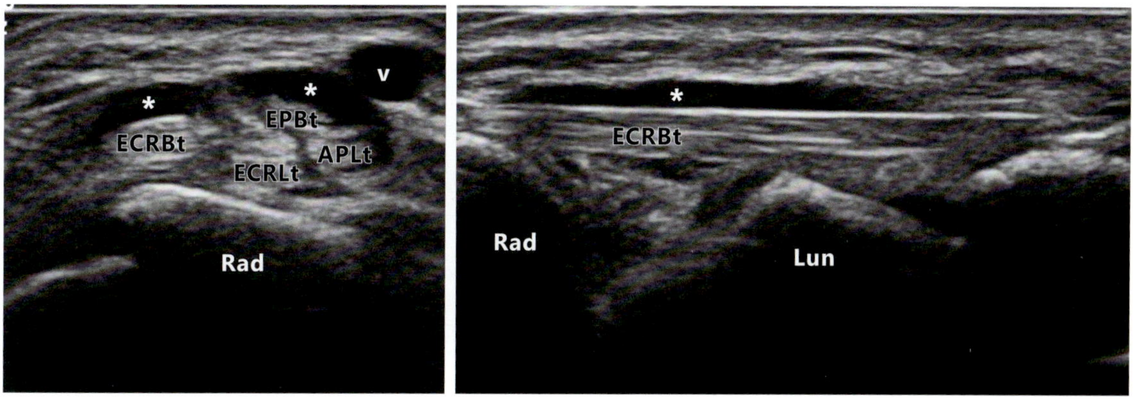

a b

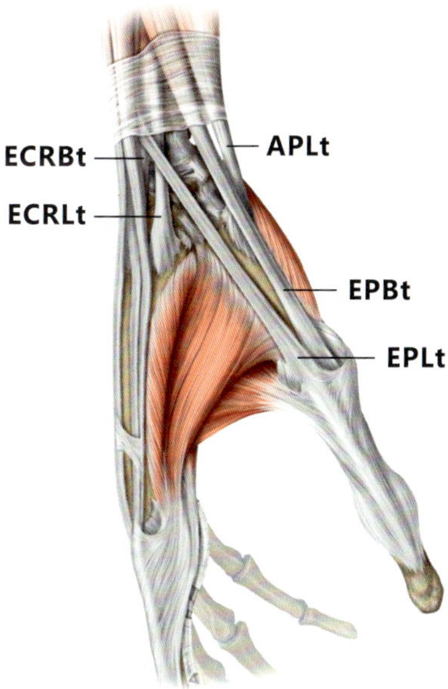

Axial (**a**) and longitudinal (**b**) US images demonstrate effusion of the extensor tendons (*asterisks*) where the 1st extensor compartment crosses over the 2nd one. Note that the tendons display normal size, shape and echogenicity.

APLt	abductor pollicis longus tendon
ECRBt	extensor carpi radialis brevis tendon
ECRLt	extensor carpi radialis longus tendon
EPBt	extensor pollicis brevis tendon
EPLt	extensor pollicis longus tendon
Lun	lunate
Rad	radius
v	vein

Expert note

Either by medical history or physical examination alone, it is usually difficult to distinguish involvement of the individual extensor compartments. However, especially with the use of sono-palpation, it would be quite easy and straightforward.
Intersection syndrome can ensue in two types i.e. proximal (while APL and EPB tendons cross over the second compartment) and distal (while EPLt crosses over the 2nd compartment) [4].

6.20 Extensor tenosynovitis in a patient with long-standing rheumatoid arthritis

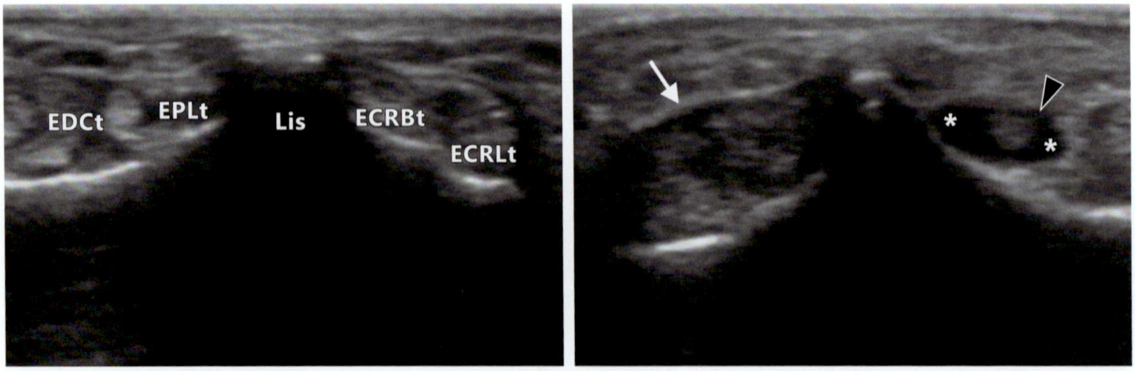

a b

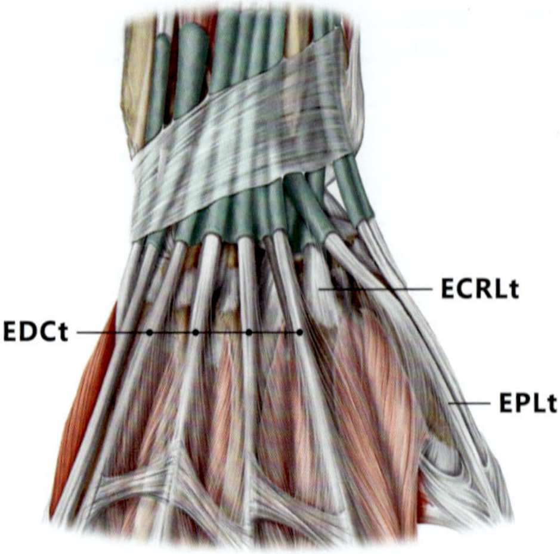

When compared with the normal side (**a**), dorsal axial view shows irregular and edematous 2nd extensor tendon compartment (*arrow*) and synovial effusion (*asterisks*) inside the 3rd extensor compartment (*arrowhead*) (**b**).

ECRBt extensor carpi radialis brevis tendon
ECRLt extensor carpi radialis longus tendon
EDCt extensor digitorum communis tendons
EPLt extensor pollicis longus tendon
Lis Lister's tubercle on radius

Cortical defects in a young woman with a fall history on her wrist **6.21**

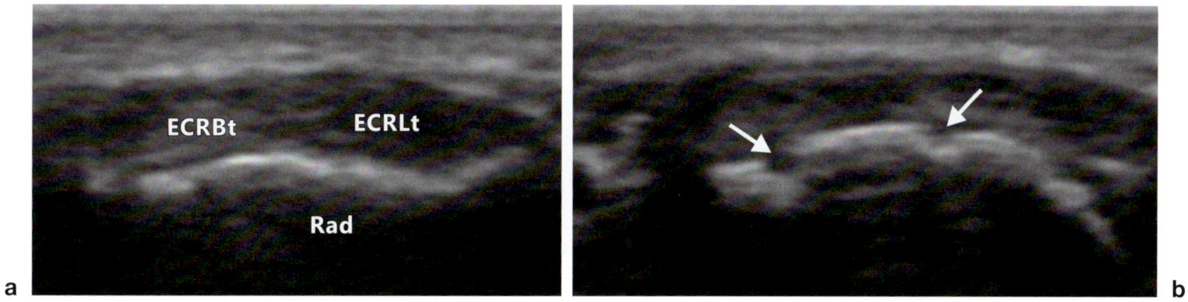

When compared with the normal side (**a**), axial image reveals focal disruptions of the hyperechoic cortical line (*arrows*) at the distal part of the radius (**b**).

ECRBt extensor carpi radialis brevis tendon
ECRLt extensor carpi radialis longus tendon
Rad radius

Extensor carpi ulnaris tenosynovitis in a middle-aged woman with wrist pain **6.22**

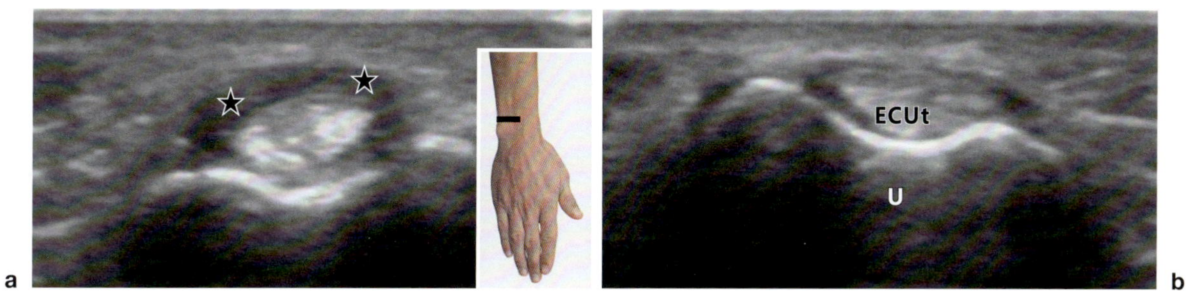

Axial US imaging reveals an hypoechoic synovial effusion (*stars*) surrounding the oval tendon (**a**). Normal side (**b**).

ECUt extensor carpi ulnaris tendon
U ulna

6.23 Extensor carpi ulnaris tenosynovitis in a middle-aged woman with multiple sclerosis

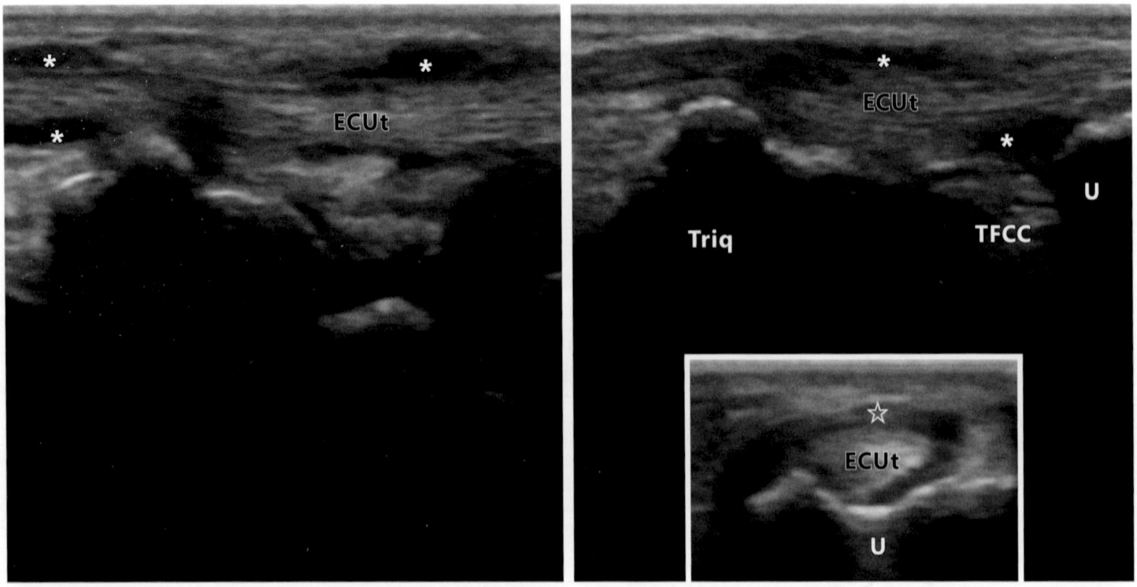

Longitudinal US images (**a**, **b**) over the wrists show mild effusion in the synovial sheath (*asterisks*) of the extensor carpi ulnaris tendon (**ECUt**). While the hypoechoic tendon is nicely seen in the longitudinal image (**b**), thickening of the retinaculum (*star*) is better visualized in the axial view (*small image*).

TFCC triangular fibrocartilage complex
Triq triquetrum
U ulna

Extensor carpi ulnaris tenosynovitis in a 42-year-old woman after wrist trauma 6.24

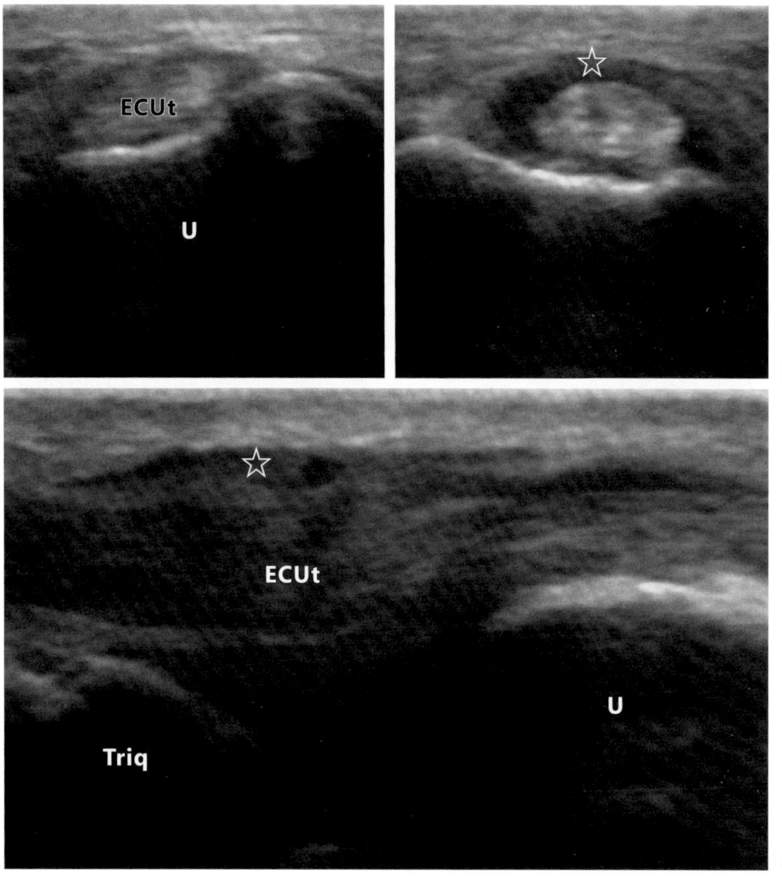

When compared with the normal side (**a**), axial (**b**) and longitudinal (**c**) images reveal thickening of the retinaculum (*stars*) and the extensor carpi ulnaris tendon (**ECUt**).

Triq triquetrum
U ulna

6.25 Extensor digitorum communis tenosynovitis in a patient with an initial diagnosis of ganglion cyst

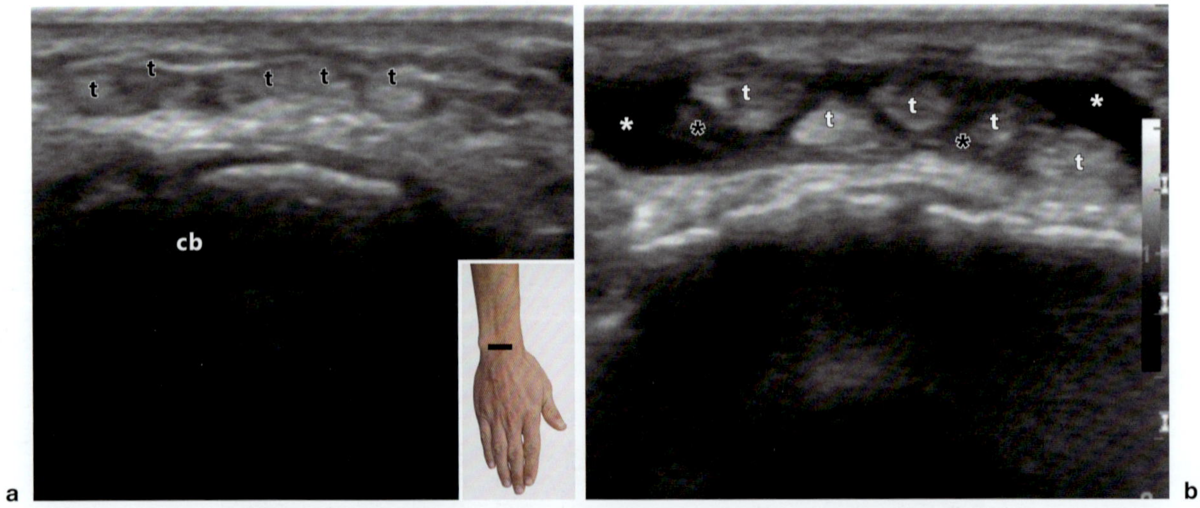

When compared with the normal side (**a**), axial US imaging of the dorsal wrist (**b**) demonstrates anechoic fluid (*white asterisks*) and hypoechoic synovial thickening (*black asterisks*) surrounding the extensor tendons (**t**) which also seem to be edematous.

cb carpal bones

Extensor digitorum communis tenosynovitis in a young woman

6.26

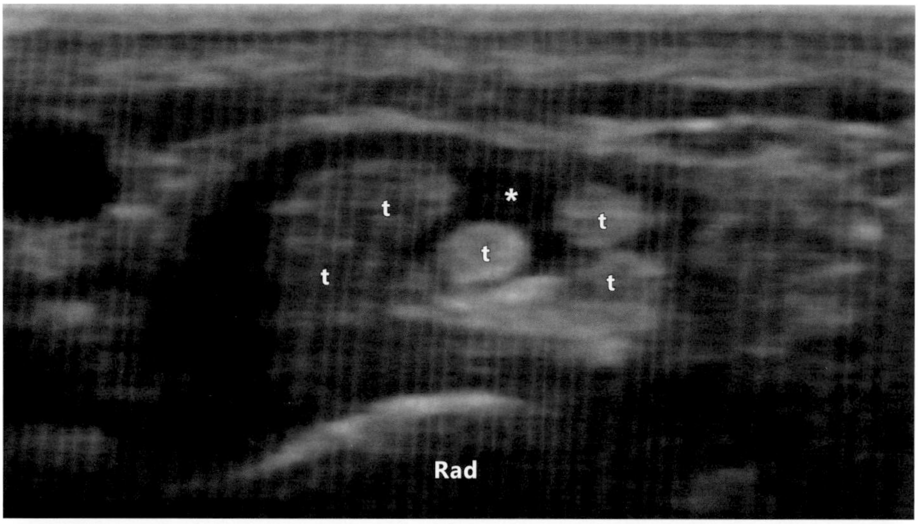

a

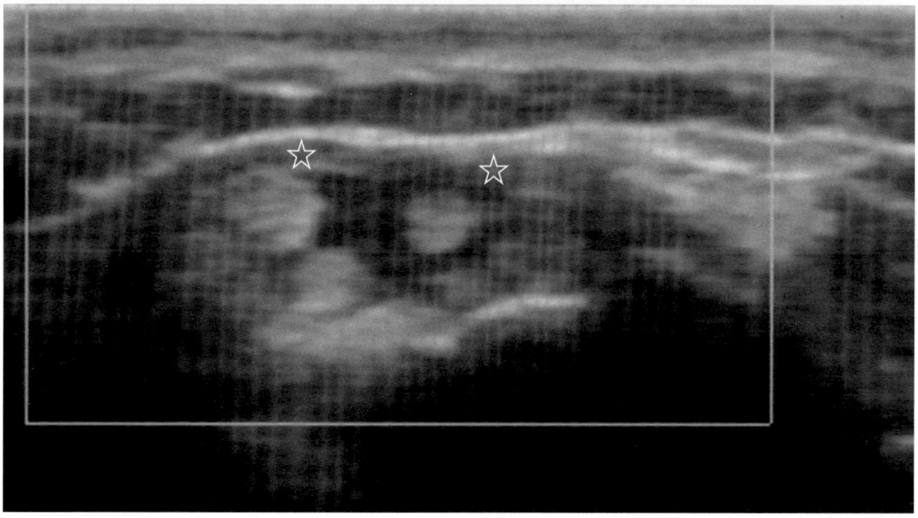

b

The patient had a previous trauma at the dorsal hand and inability to perform hand grip.

Axial US images of the extensor digitorum tendons (**t**) obtained over the distal radius (**Rad**) illustrate mild fluid (*asterisk*) and thickened retinaculum (*stars*) without any flow signal (**a**, **b**).

6.27 Extensor digitorum communis tenosynovitis in a 27-year-old woman with prior hand sprain

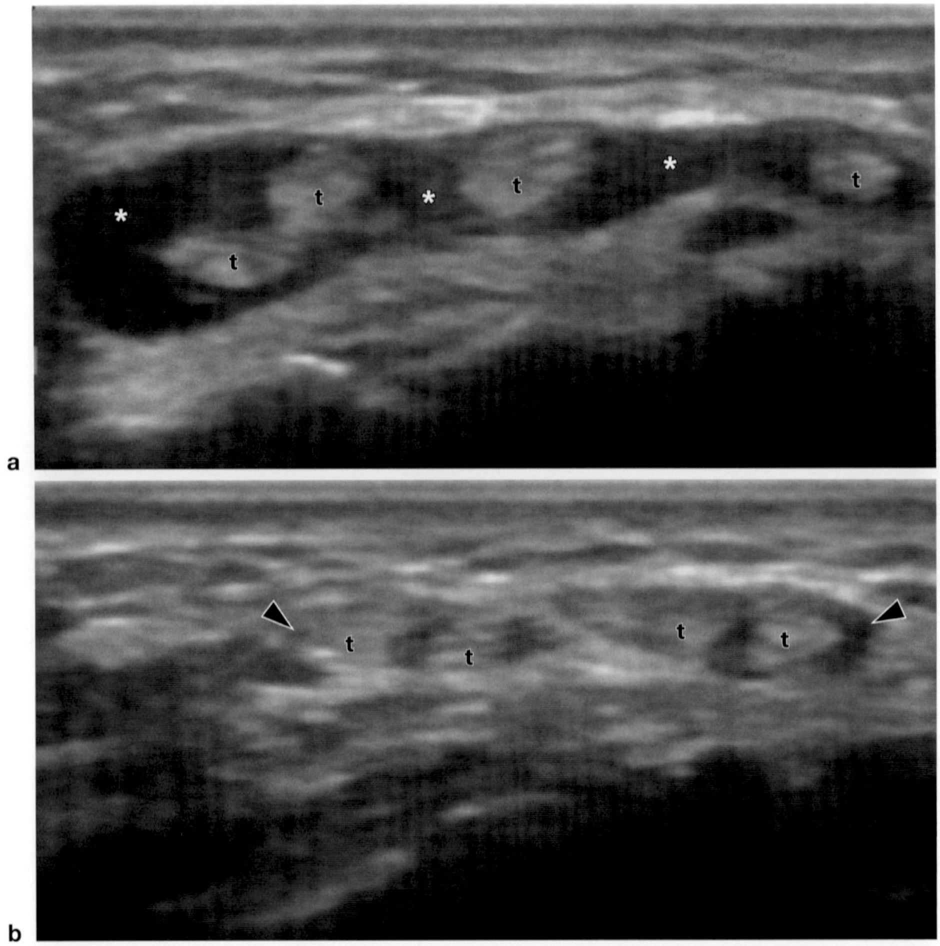

Axial US imaging demonstrates fluid collection (*asterisks*) separating the tendons (**t**) within the 4th extensor compartment (**a**). The borders of the normal compartment are indicated by *arrowheads* (**b**).

Ganglion cyst in a 60-year-old woman with painful mass on the volar wrist 6.28

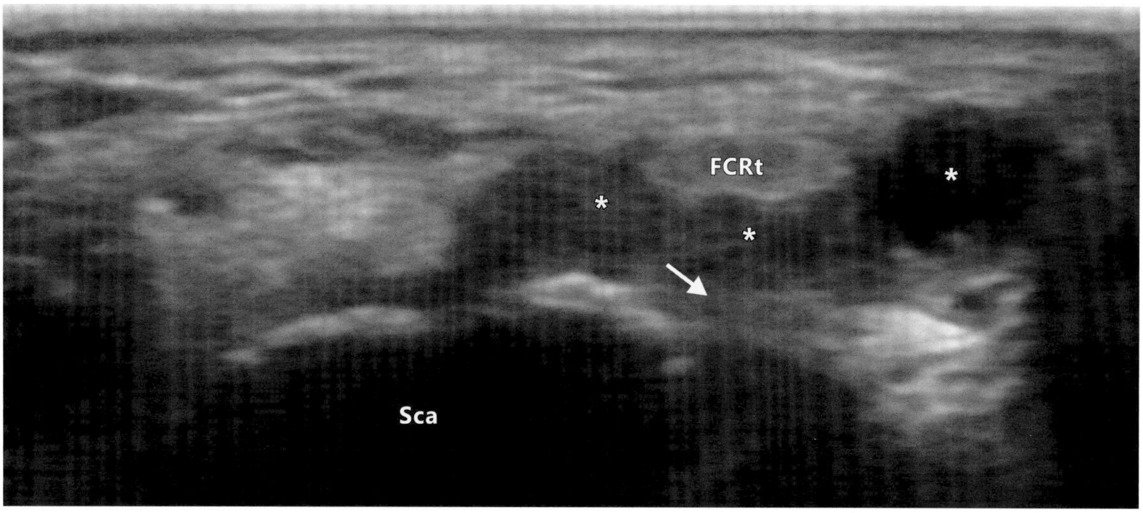

Axial US imaging exhibits a ganglion cyst with heterogenous echoes (*asterisks*) located deep/adjacent to the flexor carpi radialis tendon (**FCRt**). The ganglion is likely to communicate with the scapho-trapezium joint by a pedicle (*arrow*).

Sca scaphoid

6.29 Flexor carpi radialis tendinopathy in a middle-aged woman with pain and local lump

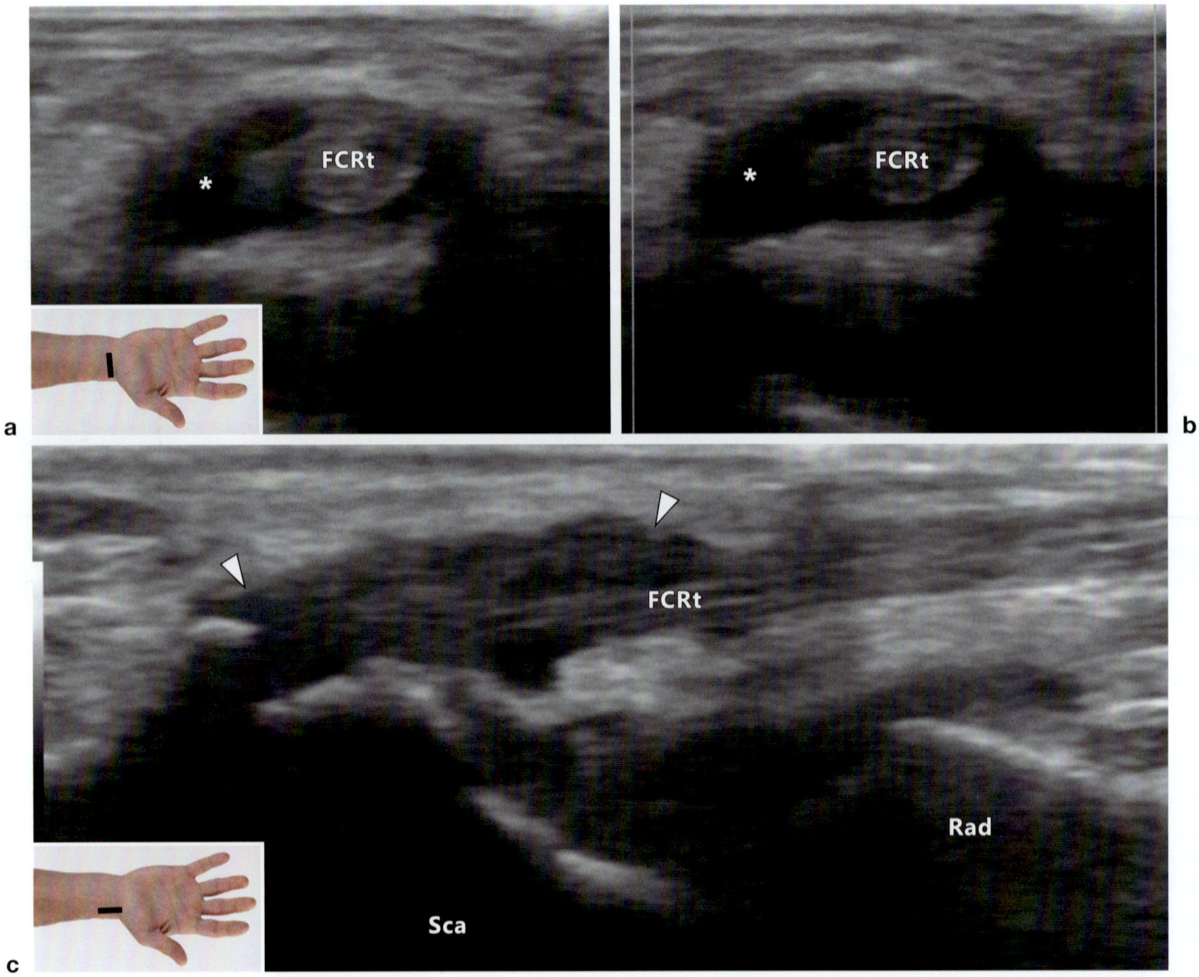

Axial (**a**, **b**) and longitudinal (**c**) US images at the wrist demonstrates distension of the flexor carpi radialis tendon (**FCRt**) sheath by hypoechoic fluid (*asterisks*) and synovial tissue proliferation (*arrowheads*). Power Doppler imaging is unremarkable (**b**).

Rad radius
Sca scaphoid

Expert note

Since there is a mesotenon -a fold between the visceral and parietal layers of synovium- around these tendons, one should be cautious not to misinterpret while assessing small synovial thickenings.

Flexor carpi radialis tendinopathy in a 45-year-old woman with a painful lump **6.30**

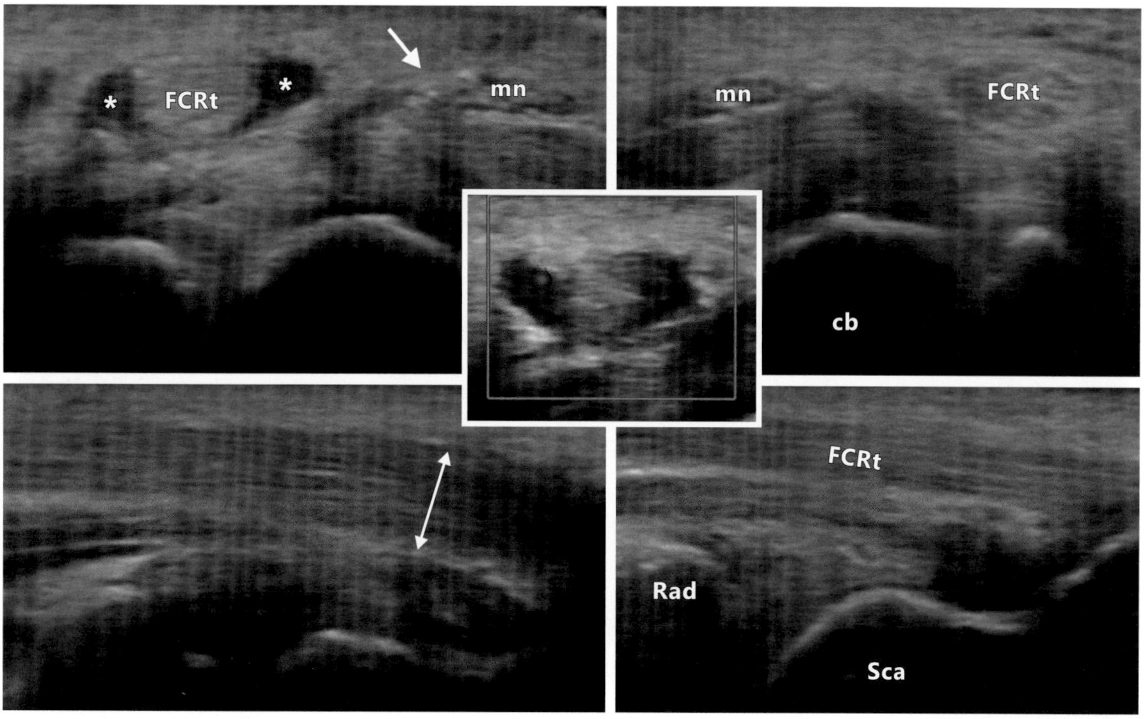

a b c d

Axial (**a**) and longitudinal (**c**) US imaging shows hypoechoic effusion (*asterisks*) surrounding the thickened (*double arrow*) flexor carpi radialis tendon (**FCRt**). Normal side (**b**, **d**). Power Doppler imaging (*middle*) shows mild synovitis.
Please note the relationship among the FCRt, flexor retinaculum (*arrow*) and the median nerve (**mn**).

cb carpal bones
Rad radius

Expert note

While scanning on the volar side, the flexor tendons do not display separate compartments similar to the extensor side. Except FCRt (and palmaris longus when present), they can be found altogether in the carpal tunnel beneath the flexor retinaculum. Therefore, FCRt can easily be distinguished from the other flexors as a large tendon on the radial side overlying the retinaculum.

6.31 Flexor tendon repair after a traumatic injury

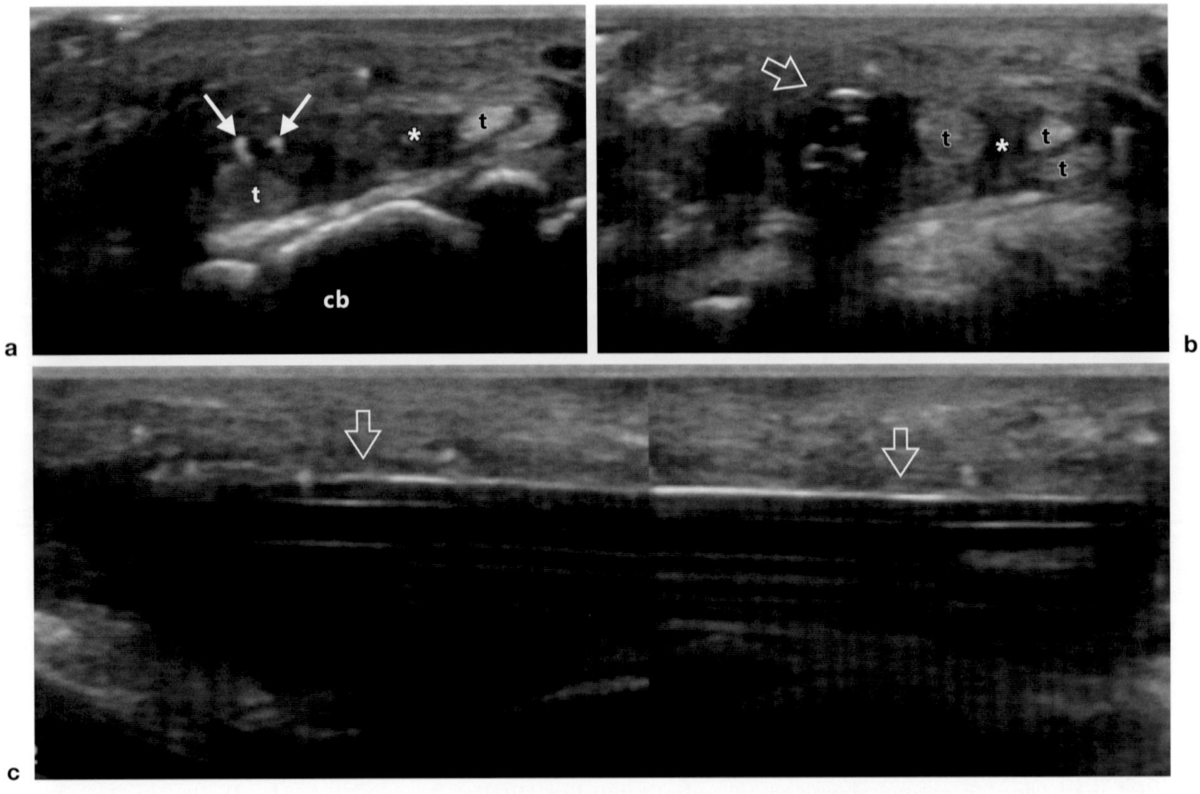

Axial images demonstrate the flexor tendons (**t**), suture materials (*arrows*), spacer (*void arrow*) and synovial tissue proliferation (*asterisks*) (**a**, **b**). Split-screen longitudinal view on the spacer (*void arrows*) with its huge artifact (**c**).

cb carpal bones

Expert note

Either before or after surgery for tendon injuries, US imaging provides a wide range of advantages [7]. Especially, the ability to perform repeat/dynamic assessment with delicate passive/active movements of the different finger joints readily displays specific/important information guiding the management of the patients (rehabilitation, re-operation etc.).

Flexor carpi ulnaris tendinopathy in a young man with wrist pain **6.32**

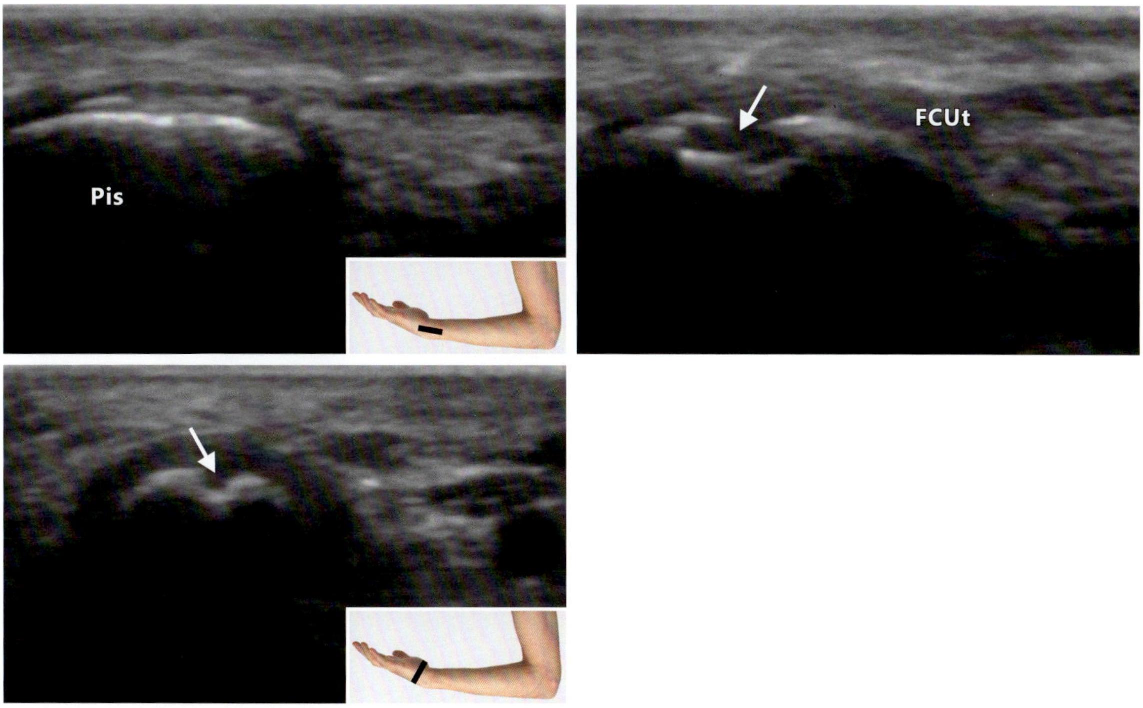

a b c

When compared with the normal side (**a**), longitudinal (**b**) and axial (**c**) US image demonstrate mild thickening of the flexor carpi ulnaris tendon (**FCUt**) and focal irregularity on the pisiform (**Pis**) (*arrows*).

6.33 Carpometacarpal joint osteoarthritis in a 55-year-old patient with thumb pain during grip activities

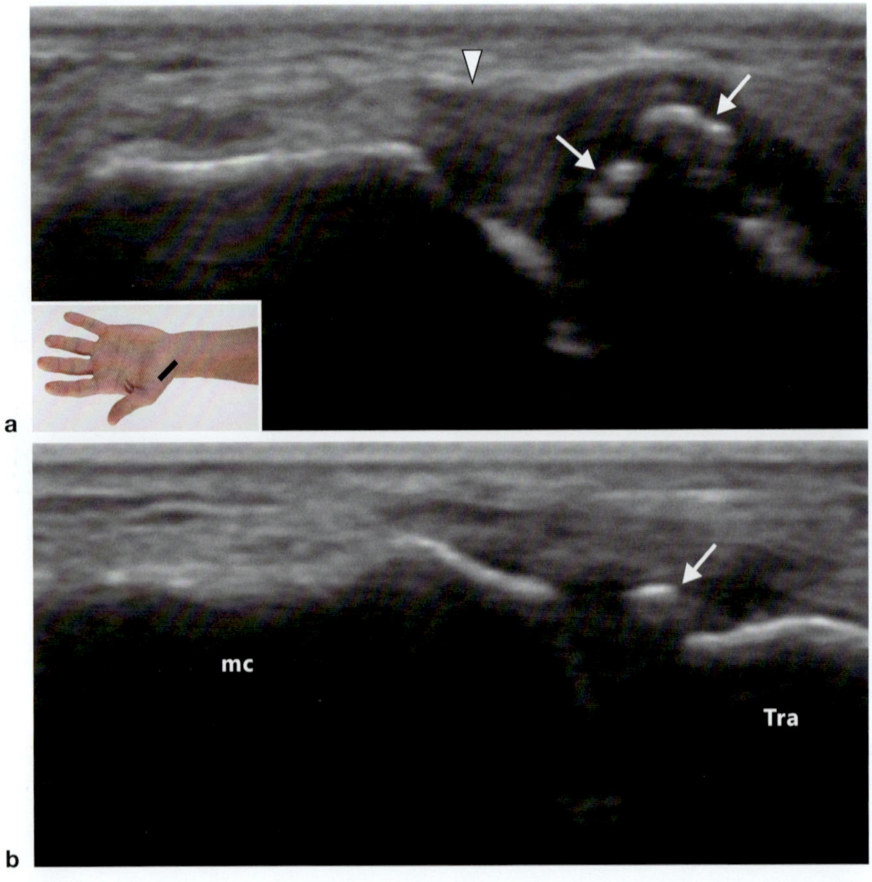

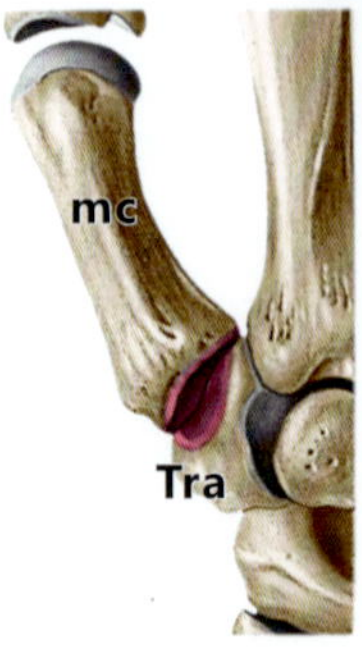

Longitudinal US image demonstrates distended joint capsule (*arrowhead*) and cortical irregularities on the trapezium (**Tra**) (*arrows*) (**a**). A small osteophyte formation (*arrow*) can also be seen on the asymptomatic side (**b**).

mc metacarpal bone

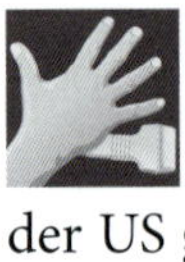

Expert note

While carpometacarpal joint osteoarthritis can easily be diagnosed with clinical examination; in case an onward intervention is planned, it can safely/comfortably be done under US guidance i.e. with the possibility of using smaller needles and being able to avoid irregular bony surfaces.

Bilateral hand osteoarthritis in a 55-year-old woman with painful and limited finger motions **6.34**

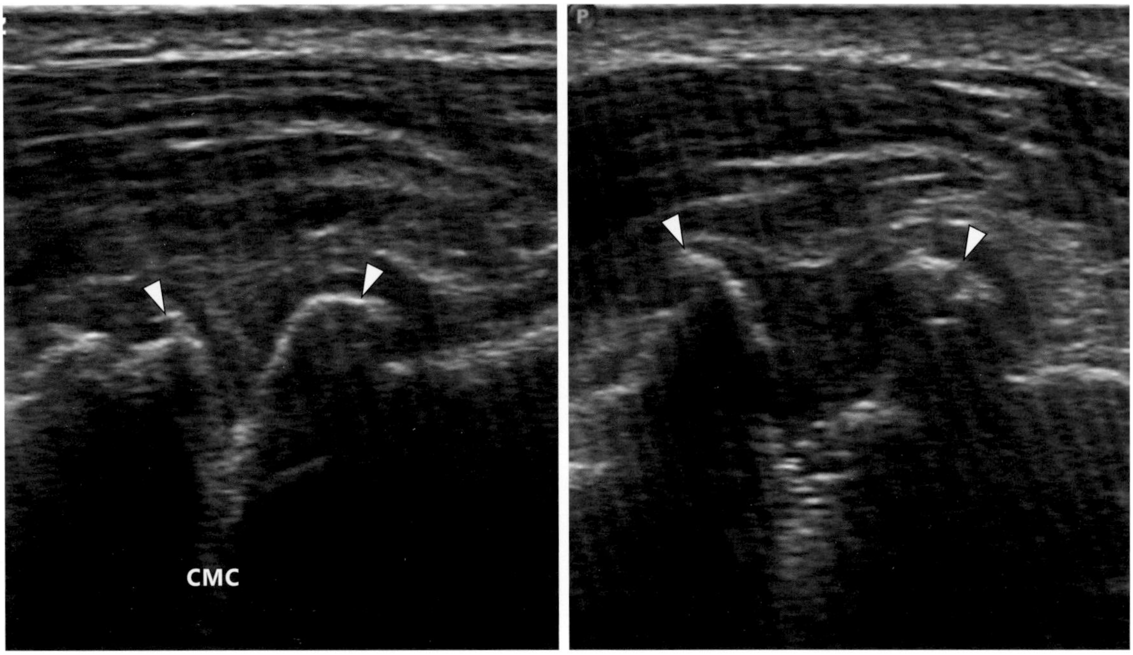

Longitudinal US views reveal joint space narrowing, bony irregularities and large osteophytes (*arrowheads*) at the level of the carpometacarpal joint (**CMC**) on both sides.

6.35 Flexor pollicis longus tendon injury in an active middle-aged man after sports trauma

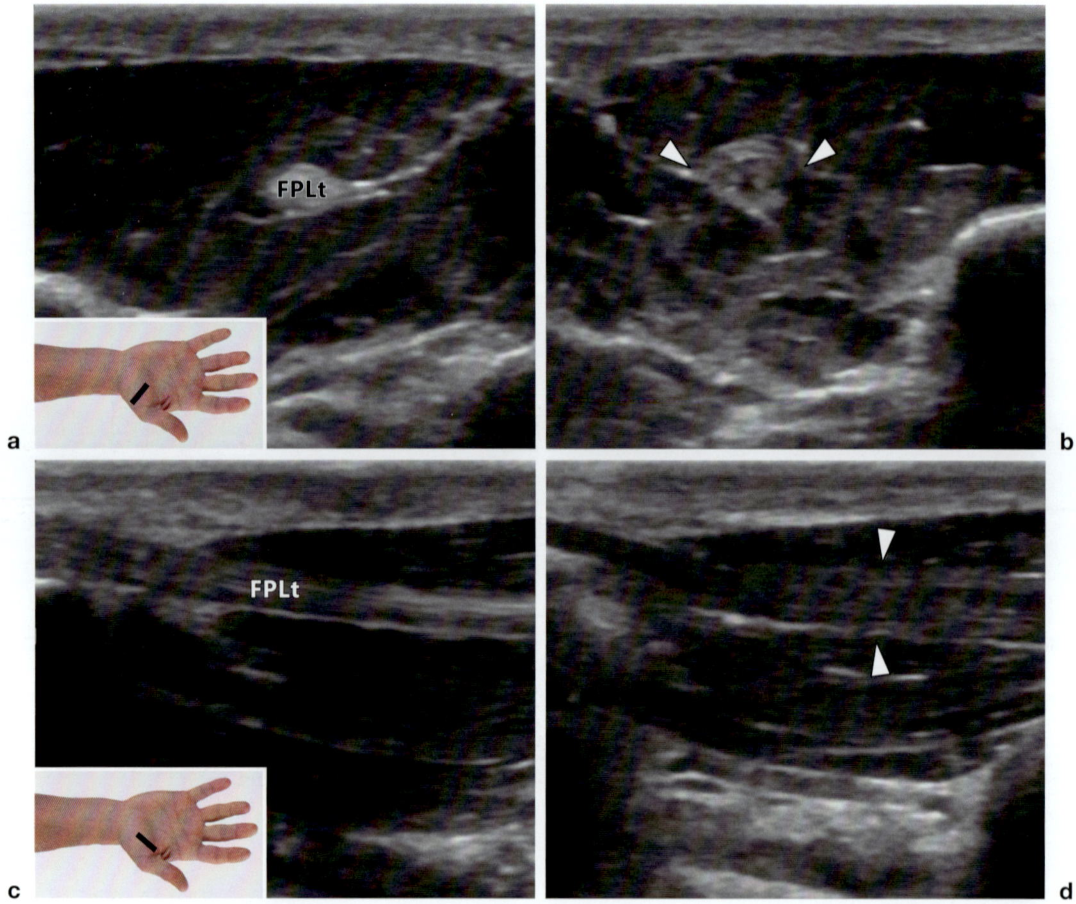

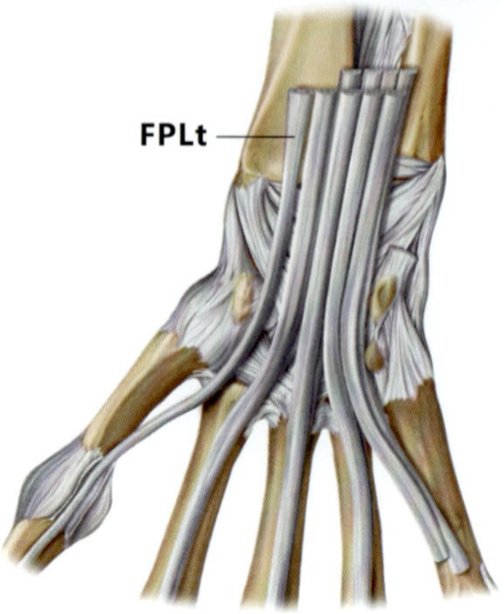

When compared with the normal side (**a**, **c**), axial (**b**) and longitudinal (**d**) US images demonstrate edematous and heterogeneous appearance of the flexor pollicis longus tendon (**FPLt**) (*arrowheads*).

Stenosing tenosynovitis in a woman with painful thumb movements **6.36**

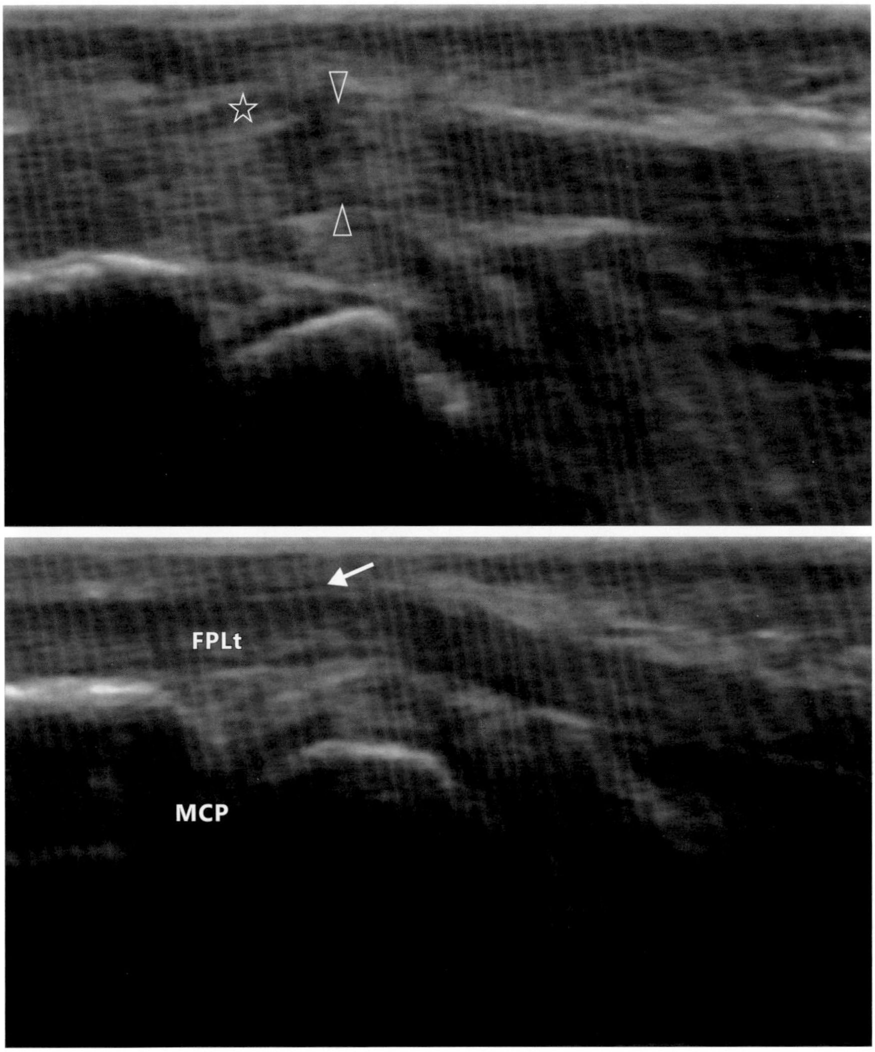

a

b

Longitudinal US image over the metacarpophalangeal joint (**MCP**) identifies intact but swollen tendon (*arrowheads*) with mild irregular thickening of the A1 pulley (*star*) (**a**). Normal flexor pollicis longus tendon (**FPLt**) and A1 pulley (*arrow*) (**b**).

Expert note

In stenosing tenosynovitis, the sonographer should look for hypoechoic thickening of the pulley/retinaculum (with or without positive doppler signal) and/or thickening of the tendon, and changes in the echogenicity of the tendon and/or synovial swelling and peritendinous fluid.

6.37 Flexor tenosynovitis of the thumb in a middle-aged manual worker after strenuous lifting

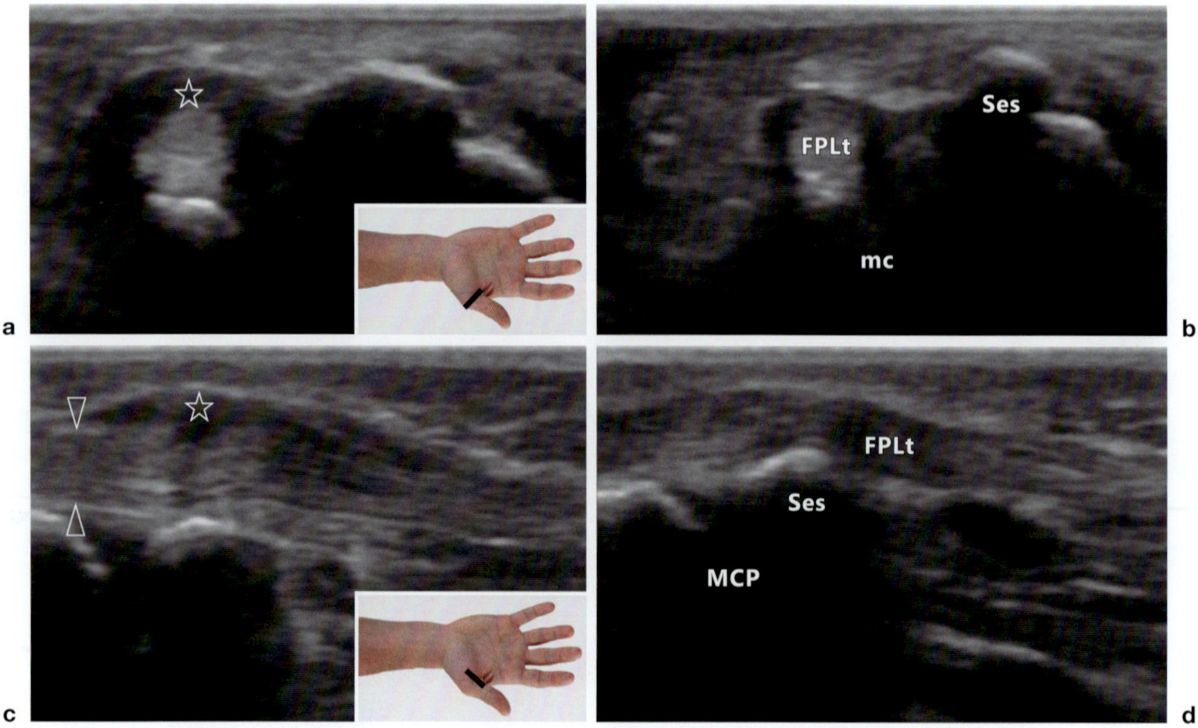

Axial (**a**) and longitudinal (**c**) US images over the metacarpal head of the thumb demonstrate thickened A1 pulley (*stars*) and flexor tendon (*arrowheads*) consistent with tenosynovitis. Normal side (**b**, **d**).

FPLt flexor pollicis longus tendon
mc metacarpal bone
MCP metacarpophalangeal joint
Ses sesamoid bone

Expert note

Moving the interphalangeal joint passively could help to differentiate whether the tendon is moving or stuck under the swollen pulley.

Ganglion cyst in the thumb causing triggering 6.38

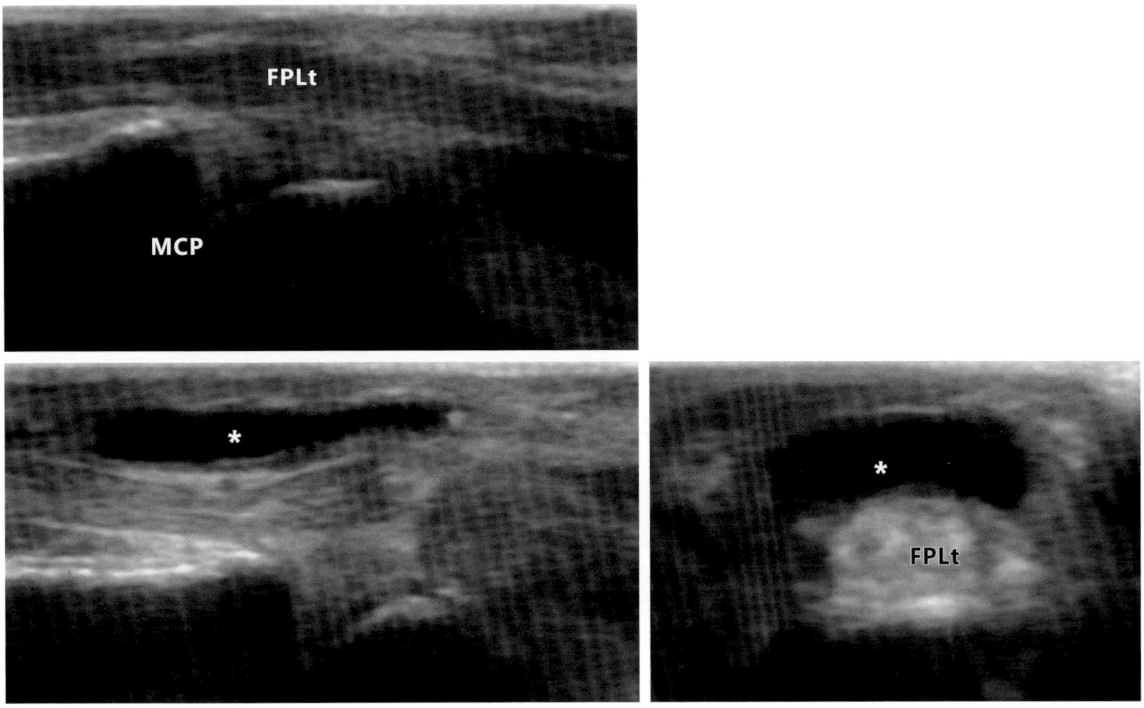

a b c

When compared with the normal side (**a**), palmar longitudinal imaging over the metacarpophalangeal joint (**MCP**) of the thumb reveals anechoic cyst (*asterisks*) corresponding to A1 pulley localization (**b**). Axial imaging is also confirmatory (**c**).

FPLt flexor pollicis longus tendon

Expert note

Compressibility (displacement) of a fluid accumulation might be one of the easiest ways to understand that it is not chronic and can thus/potentially be aspirated.
The significant brightness of the FPLt on the symptomatic side (on both views) is again a nice example of acoustic enhancement due to the overlying anechoic cyst.

6.39 1st metacarpophalangeal joint osteoarthritis in a 65-year-old man

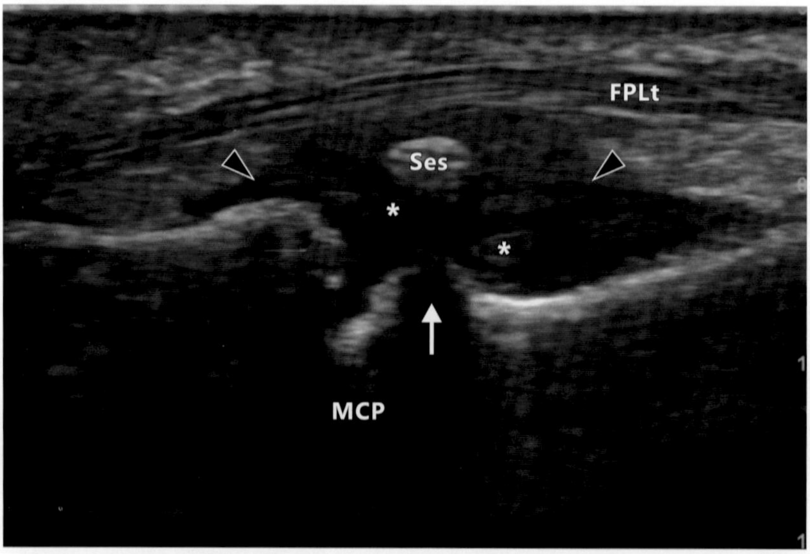

Longitudinal US image over the palmar aspect of the first metacarpophalangeal joint (**MCP**) reveals distension of the joint capsule (*arrowheads*), effusion and synovial hypertrophy (*asterisks*). The overlying flexor pollicis longus tendon (**FPLt**) and the sesamoid bone (**Ses**) are also viewed with normal size and echotexture. Please note that the cortical defect (*arrow*) stems from the acoustic shadowing of the sesamoid bone.

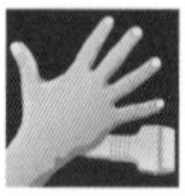

Expert note

In case the artifact of the sesamoid bone needs to be distinguished from a likely erosion, imaging at different joint angles or views might be necessary/confirmatory.

Repaired flexor pollicis longus tendon in a 34-year-old woman after a glass injury

6.40

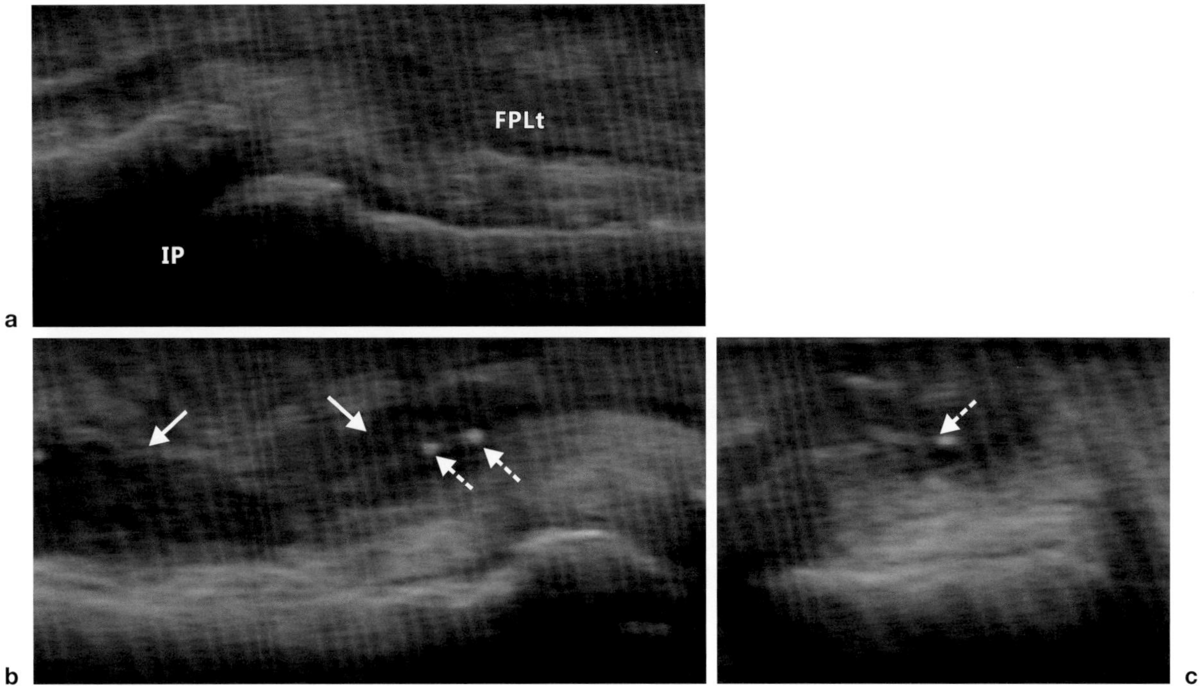

When compared with the normal side (**a**), longitudinal (**b**) and axial (**c**) US images over the palmar aspect of the thumb demonstrate the irregular and edematous tendon (*arrows*) in which the surgical stitches (*dashed arrows*) can also be observed.

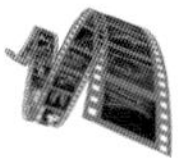

Video 6

FPLt flexor pollicis longus tendon
IP interphalangeal joint

6.41 Lymphedema on the dorsum of the hand in a 45-year-old woman with history of breast cancer/surgery

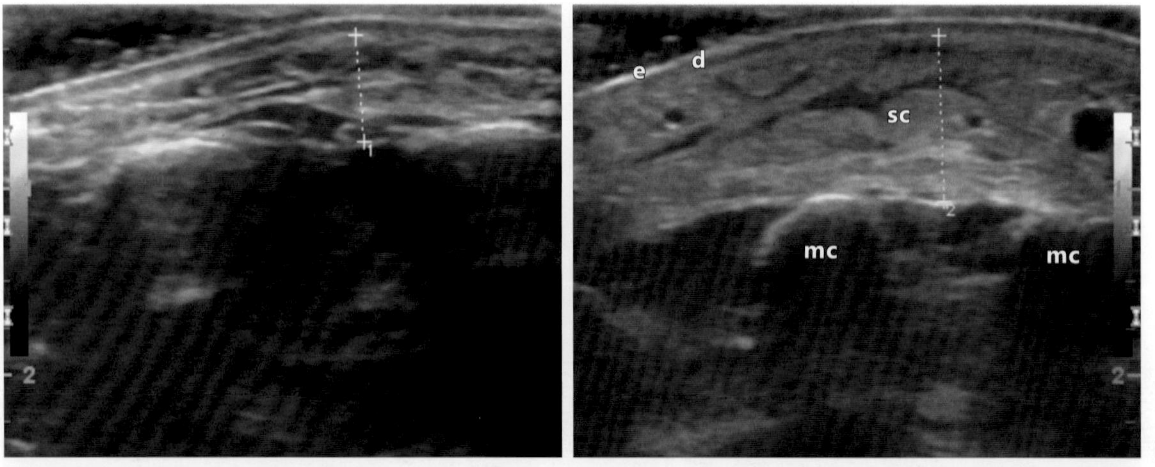

a b

When compared with the normal side (**a**), dorsal axial US image over the metacarpal bones (**mc**) demonstrates swollen subcutaneous tissue (**sc**) which can also be compared quantitatively (**b**). Note that epidermis (**e**) and dermis (**d**) are not involved on either side.

Subcutaneous edema in a man with lung cancer during intravenous infusion (due to extravasation) 6.42

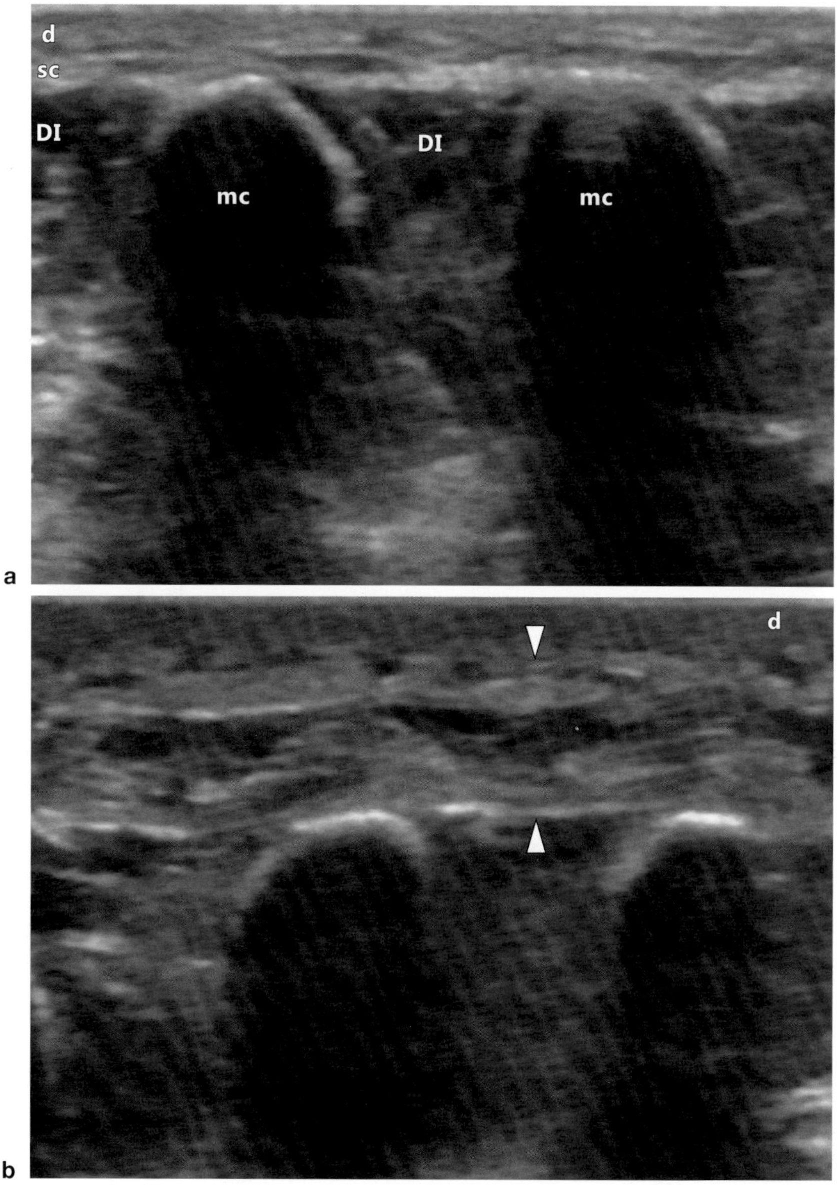

When compared with normal side (**a**), axial US image over the dorsal hand demonstrates increased echogenicity of fat lobules and fluid distention (*arrowheads*) reflecting subcutaneous edema (**b**). Please note that the border between the layers of dermis (**d**) and subcutaneous tissue (**sc**) is blurred.

DI dorsal interosseous muscle
mc metacarpal bone

6.43 Organizing hematoma in a 4-year-old child with a superficial lump

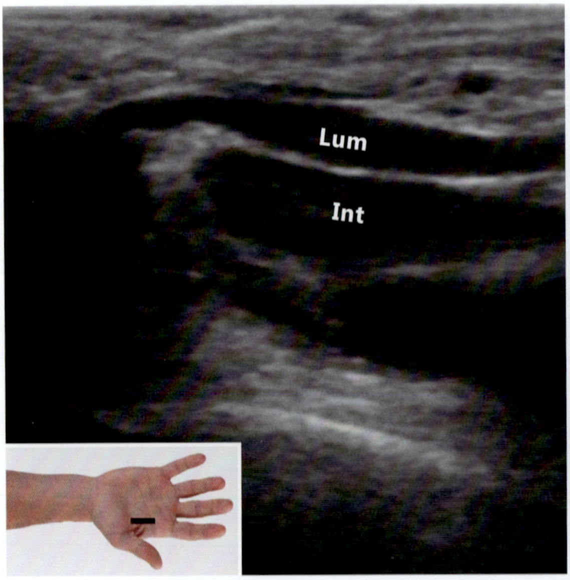

a

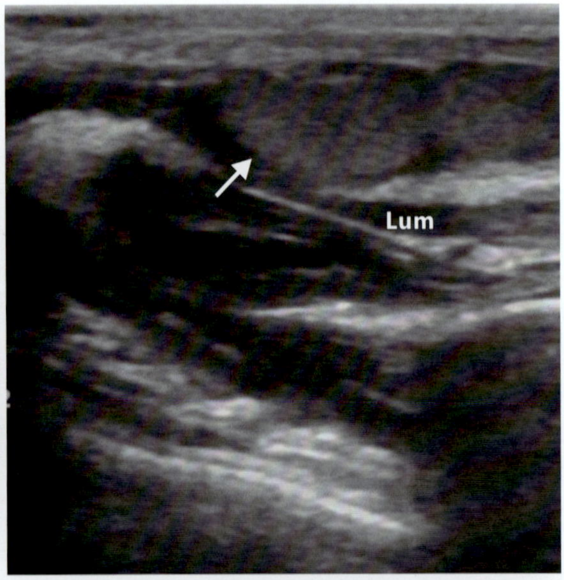

b

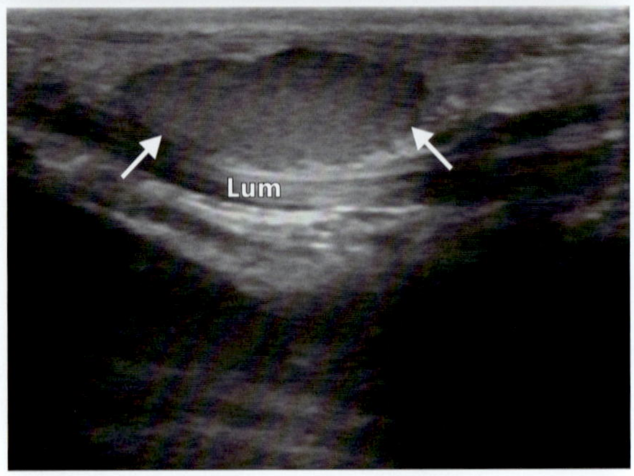

c

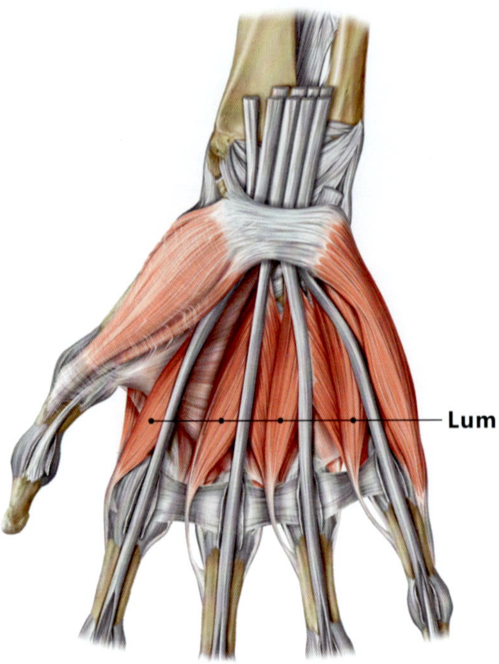

When compared with the normal side (**a**), longitudinal US images (**b**, **c**) reveal a lobulated hyperechoic mass (*arrows*) consistent with an organizing hematoma which compresses the lumbrical muscle (**Lum**) (**c**).

Int interosseous muscle

An elderly woman with trigger finger **6.44**

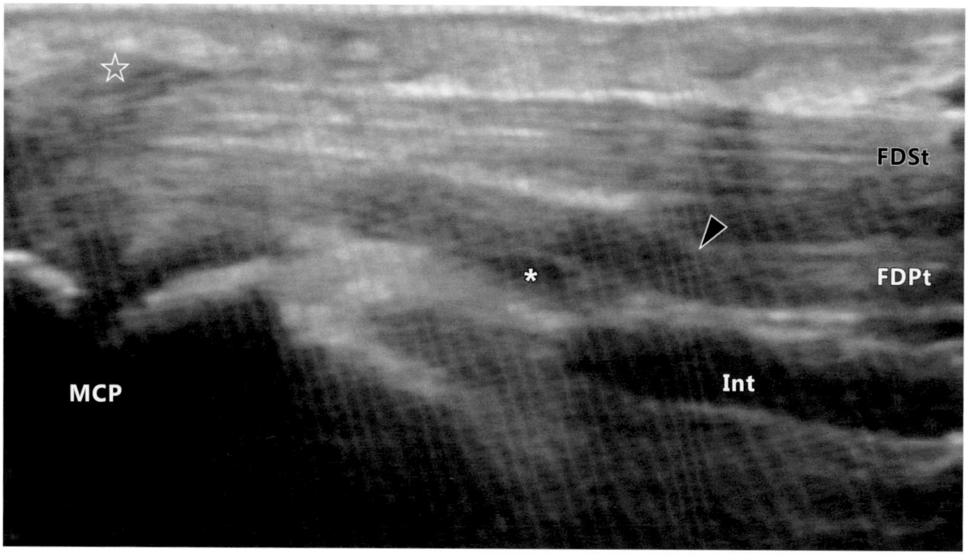

Longitudinal US imaging shows a small effusion (*asterisk*) within the tendon sheath and bowing (*arrowhead*) of the flexor digitorum profundus tendon (**FDPt**). Please note the mild thickened A1 pulley (*star*).

FDSt flexor digitorum superficialis tendon
Int interosseous muscle
MCP metacarpophalangeal joint

Expert note

Although one might think that the diagnosis of trigger finger is quite easy with medical history and clinical examination, the dynamic and real-time imaging during selective passive movements of the flexor tendons definitely yield more information [8]. Not only can the underlying cause or exact place of triggering be ascertained (which is usually more proximal than what physical examination suggests) but also the onward interventions would better be planned.

Video 7

6.45 Flexor tenosynovitis in a 43-year-old man

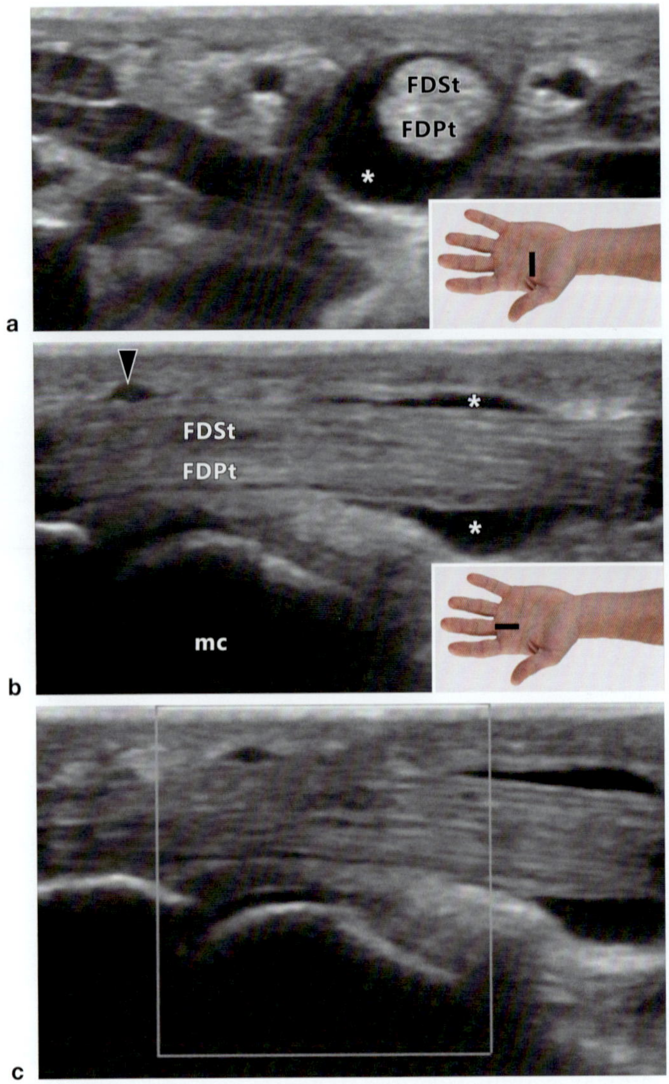

This patient (with seronegative arthritis) had pain and stiffness in the fingers.

Axial (**a**) and longitudinal (**b**) US images demonstrate thickened A1 pulley (*arrowhead*) and fluid collection (*asterisks*) inside the tendon sheath. The flexor tendons seem to be normal in B-mode (**a**, **b**) and power Doppler imaging on the painful area (**c**).

FDPt flexor digitorum profundus tendon
FDSt flexor digitorum superficialis tendon
mc metacarpal bone

Trigger finger in a housewife with painful finger motions **6.46**

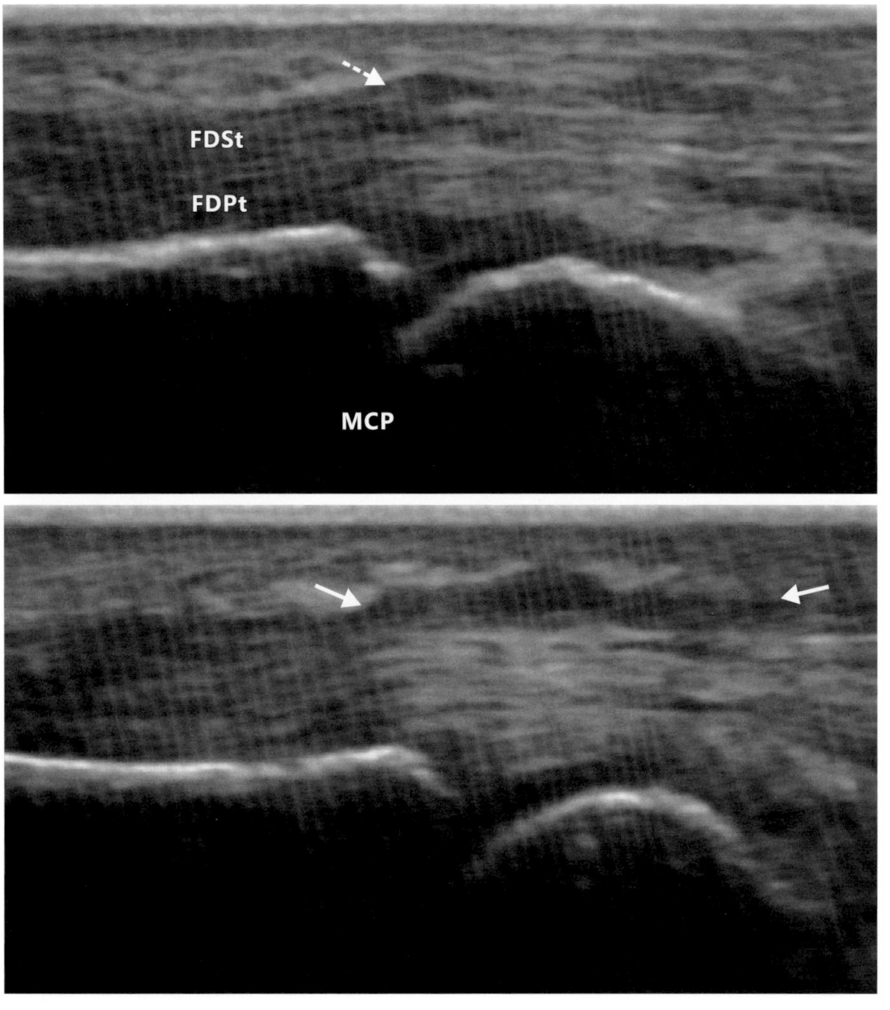

a

b

When compared with the normal A1 pulley (*dashed arrow*) (**a**), longitudinal US image presents thickened and irregular A1 pulley (*arrows*) (**b**).

FDPt flexor digitorum profundus tendon
FDSt flexor digitorum superficialis tendon
MCP metacarpophalangeal joint

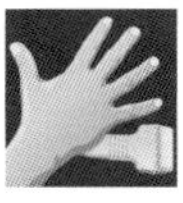

Expert note

In this patient, the exact location of triggering was found to be at the pulley level during dynamic imaging and accordingly injection with corticosteroids was performed under US guidance using a 26 G needle.

6.47 Flexor sheath hematoma in a patient with portal vein thrombosis under anticoagulant treatment

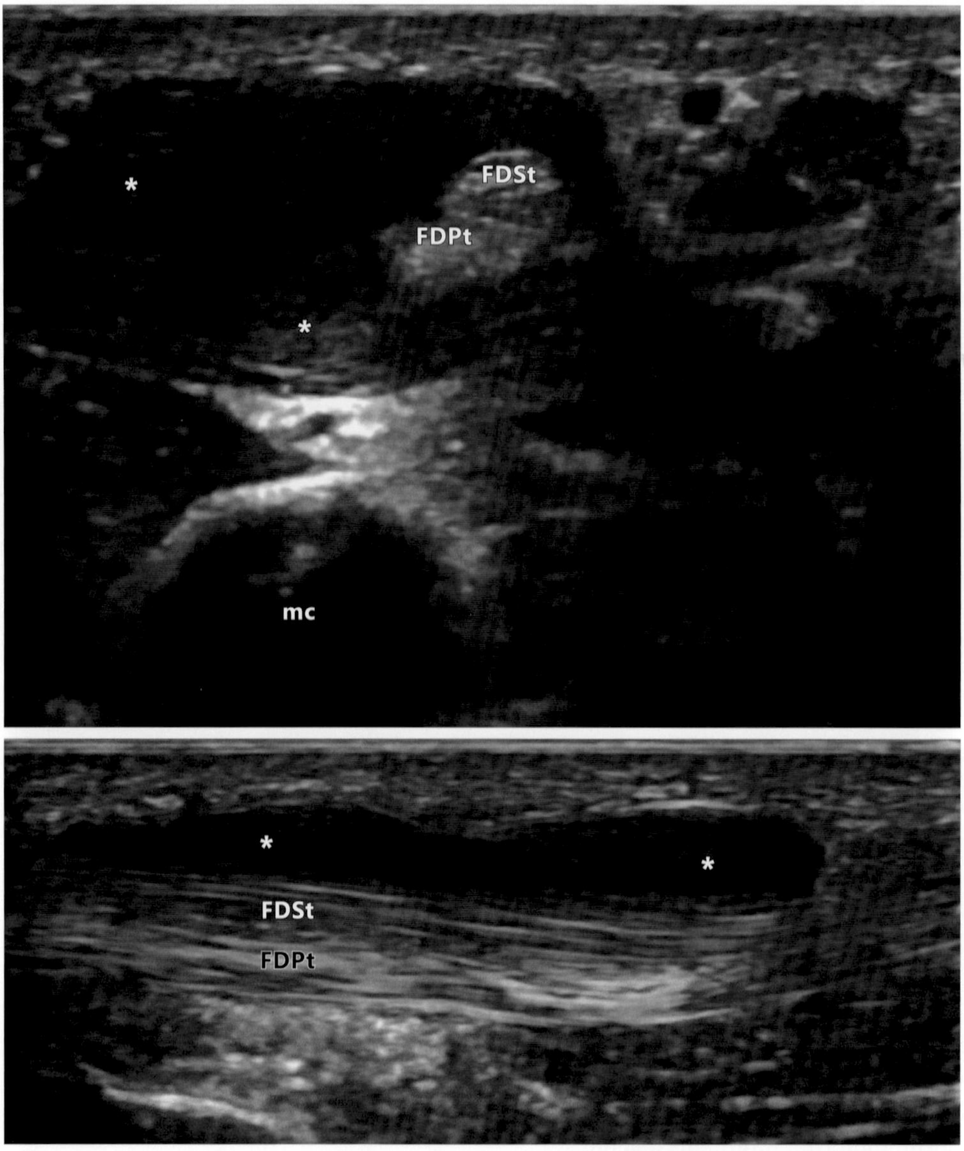

Palmar axial (**a**) and longitudinal (**b**) images show hypoechoic hematoma (*asterisks*) surrounding the flexor tendons.

FDPt flexor digitorum profundus tendon
FDSt flexor digitorum superficialis tendon
mc metacarpal bone

Stenosing tenosynovitis in a patient with painful finger motions 6.48

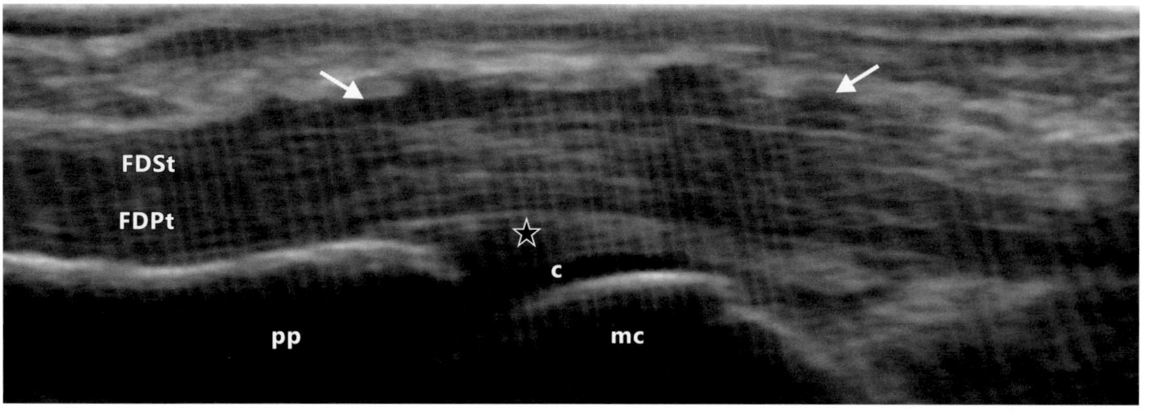

Palmar longitudinal US image over the metacarpophalangeal joint demonstrates irregular, thickened A1 pulley (*arrows*). Please note the different echogenicities of the two adjacent cartilaginous structures i.e. articular (hyaline) cartilage (**c**) and volar plate (fibrocartilage) (*star*).

FDPt flexor digitorum profundus tendon
FDSt flexor digitorum superficialis tendon
mc metacarpal bone
pp proximal phalanx

6.49 Swollen pulleys of the ring finger

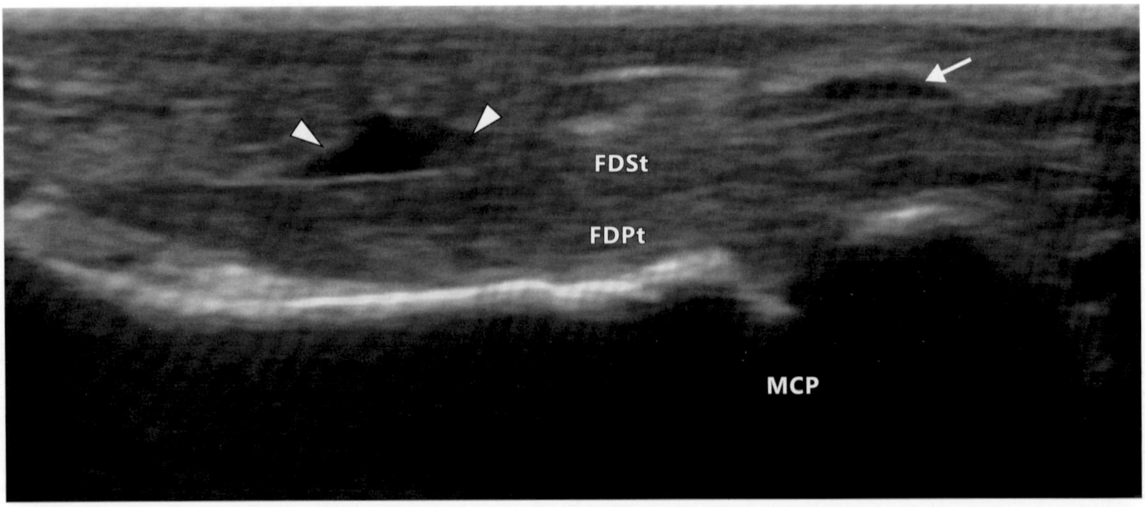

Volar longitudinal US image over the flexor tendons illustrates irregular widening (*arrowheads*) of A1 and A2 pulleys (*arrow*).

FDPt flexor digitorum profundus tendon
FDSt flexor digitorum superficialis tendon
MCP metacarpophalangeal joint

Expert note

For sure, rather than a simple morphological diagnosis; it is more important to understand how the complaints or physical findings of the patient are related with the interactive and dynamic US imaging. Otherwise, not each and every finding on the US scan might be clinically relevant.

Flexor tenosynovitis in a 32-year-old man

6.50

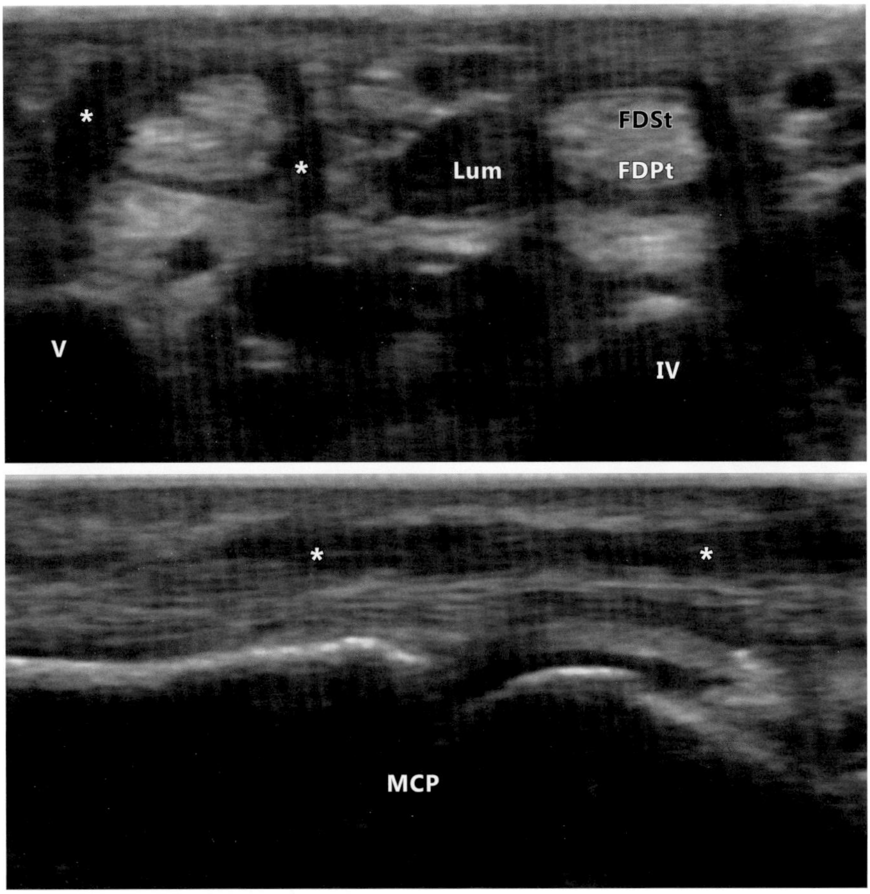

Wrist and Hand

Axial (**a**) and longitudinal (**b**) US images over the palmar aspect of the 5th metacarpophalangeal (**MCP**) joint show hypoechoic effusion (*asterisks*) around the flexor tendons.

IV & V metacarpal bones
FDPt flexor digitorum profundus tendon
FDSt flexor digitorum superficialis tendon
Lum lumbrical muscle

Expert note

Again, this could as well be swelling of the pulley. One should move the probe proximally/distally in transverse view whereby the pulley will be marked by two small "angel wings" reaching medially and laterally. In longitudinal view, the swelling of the pulley will be seen as a focal hypoechoic structure on top of the tendons.

6.51 Trigger finger in a 47-year-old woman with type-2 diabetes mellitus

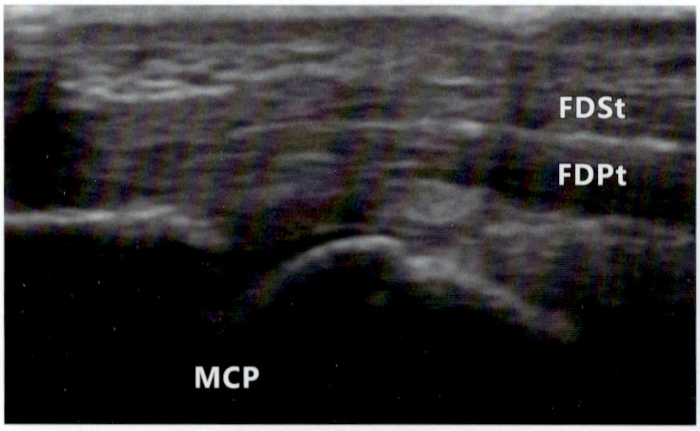

a

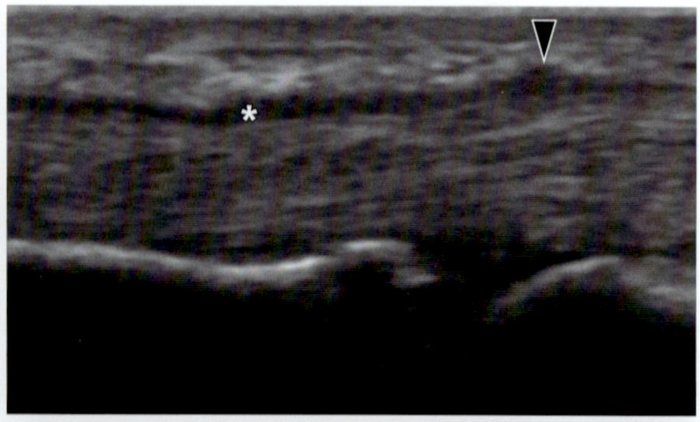

b

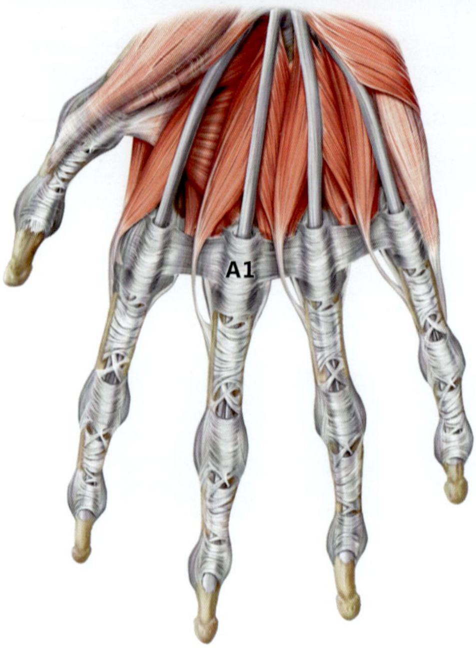

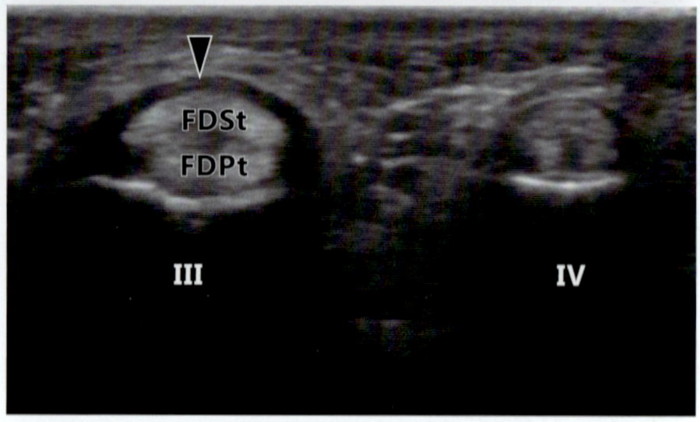

c

When compared with the normal metacarpophalangeal (**MCP**) joint (**a**), longitudinal (**b**) and axial (**c**) US images show swollen A1 pulley (*arrowhead*) and mild fluid (*asterisk*) around the thickened flexor tendons.

III & IV metacarpal bones
FDPt flexor digitorum profundus tendon
FDSt flexor digitorum superficialis tendon

Expert note

In the longitudinal image, you can appreciate the fluid all along the tendon (not a focal hypoechoic area at the site of the pulley).

Diabetes should be kept in mind in patients who suffer frequent limitations in finger mobility (or multiple trigger fingers). The prevalence of trigger finger among diabetics ranges from 10% to 20%, higher than the general population (2-3%) [9, 10].

Acute synovitis in a 48-year-old woman with rheumatoid arthritis 6.52

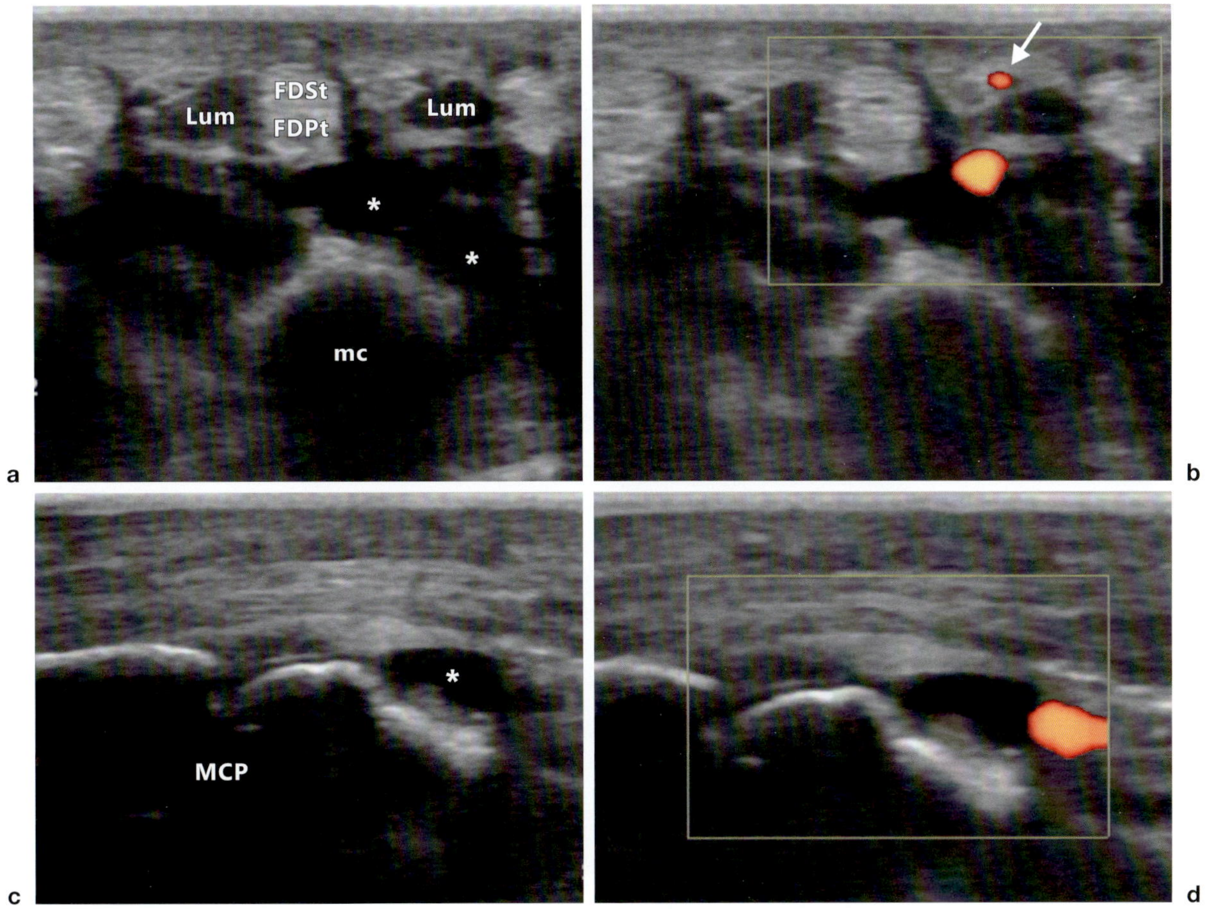

Axial (**a**) and longitudinal (**c**) US views obtained at the metacarpophalangeal joint (**MCP**) level demonstrate anechoic fluid (*asterisks*) in the joint. Corresponding power Doppler images (**b**, **d**) show marked hyperemia above the metacarpal bone (**mc**) in addition to the digital artery (*arrow*).

FDPt flexor digitorum profundus tendon
FDSt flexor digitorum superficialis tendon
Lum lumbrical muscle

6.53 Chronic stenosing tenosynovitis in a 45-year-old woman

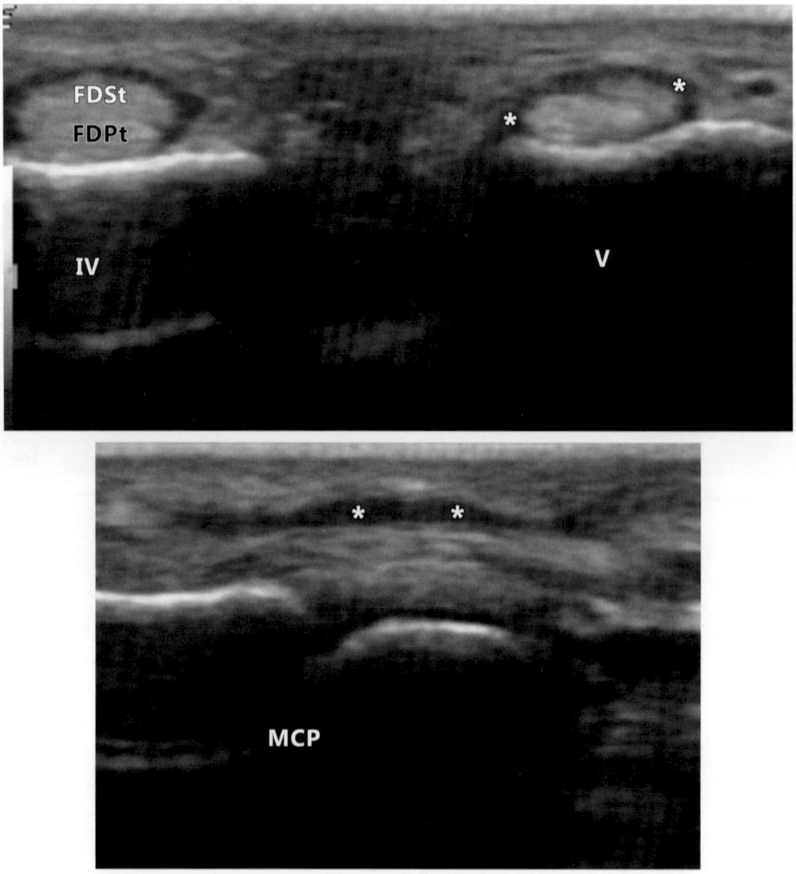

a

b

Axial (**a**) and longitudinal (**b**) US images obtained over the 5th metacarpophalangeal joint (**MCP**) show mild thickening (*asterisks*) of the A1 pulley.

IV & V metacarpal bones
FDPt flexor digitorum profundus tendon
FDSt flexor digitorum superficialis tendon

Ganglion cysts in a patient with localized painful mass lesions **6.54**

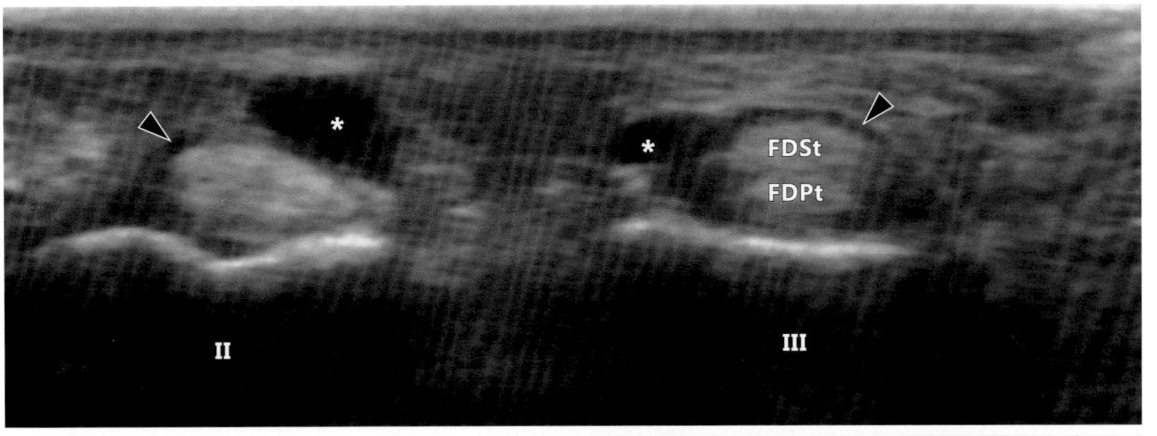

a

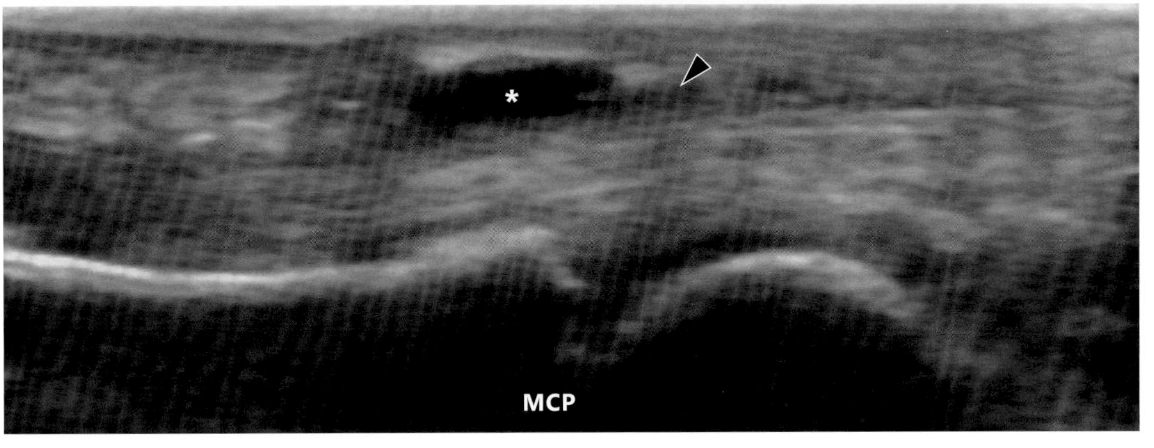

b

Axial (**a**) and longitudinal (**b**) US images at the metacarpophalangeal joint (**MCP**) level reveal anechoic ganglion cysts (*asterisks*) adjacent to the A1 pulleys which seem mildly thickened and hypoechoic (*arrowheads*).

II & III metacarpal bones
FDPt flexor digitorum profundus tendon
FDSt flexor digitorum superficialis tendon

6.55 Trigger finger in a 45-year-old woman

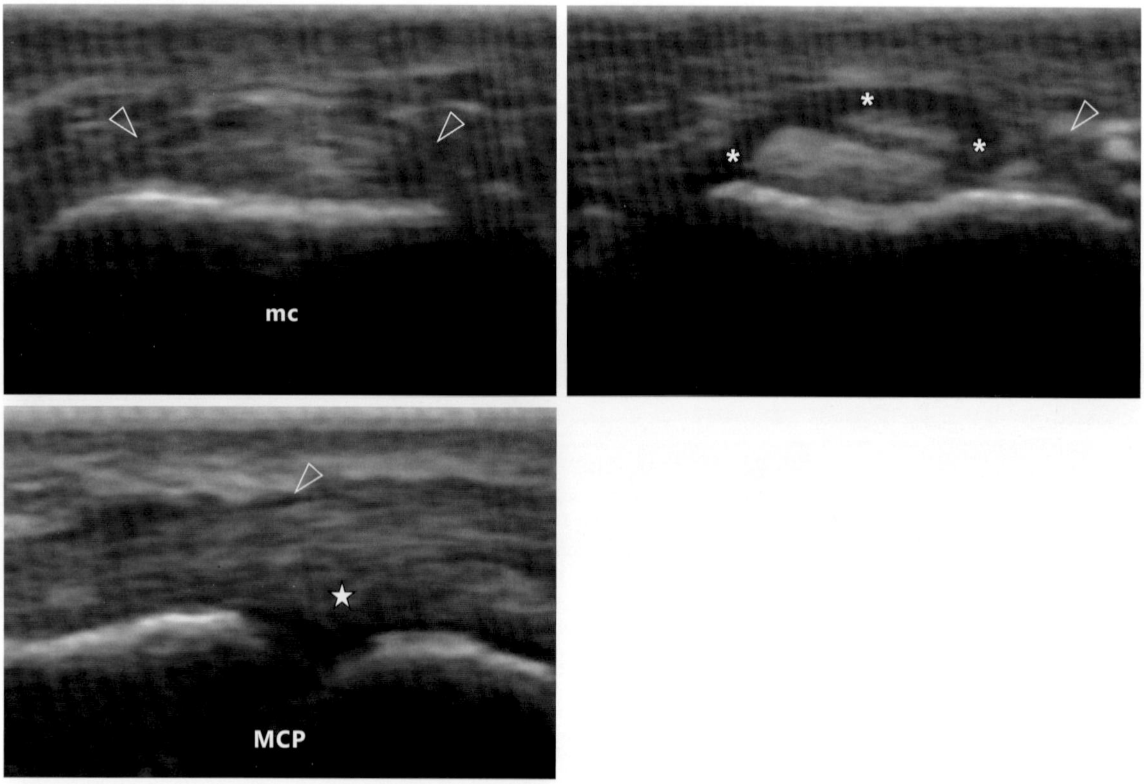

When compared with the normal side (**a**), axial (**b**) and longitudinal US (**c**) images obtained at the 5th metacarpophalangeal joint (**MCP**) level reveal mild fluid in the tendon sheath (*asterisks*). A1 pulleys (*arrowheads*) seem to be normal on both sides. The *star* indicates volar plate.

mc metacarpal bone

Expert note

Thickening and hypoechogenicity of the A1 pulley can be seen in trigger finger. A thickness of 0.5 mm in normal A1 pulleys and increased thickness of 1.8 mm in hypertrophied pulleys were reported on US. Hypervascularization of the A1 pulley on power Doppler imaging was found in 91% of the trigger fingers, in 55% of the peritendinous effusion, in 48% of tendinosis, or in 39% of tendinosis with effusion. The most commonly affected digits are the thumb and ring finger [11].

Dupuytren disease in a 58-year-old woman with type-2 diabetes mellitus 6.56

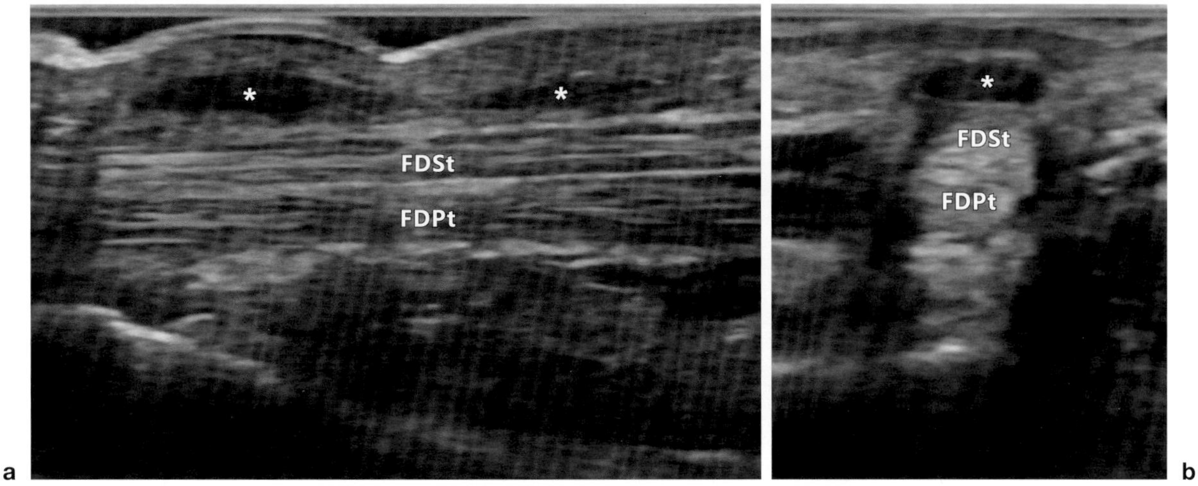

A marked fibrous band (causing flexion contracture) was detected during physical examination.

Longitudinal (**a**) and axial (**b**) US image just proximal to distal palmar crease reveal fusiform hypoechoic lesions (*asterisks*) of the palmar aponeurosis located between the skin and flexor tendons. The very superficial skin deformation shaped in parallel with the morphology of the deeper lesions can also be observed (**a**).

FDPt flexor digitorum profundus tendon
FDSt flexor digitorum superficialis tendon

Expert note

Dupuytren disease is more common in diabetic patients and can also be associated with fibromatosis in the plantar aspect of the foot (Ledderhose disease) in the form of plantar nodules [12]. US can conveniently be used in such cases to simultaneously scan the foot as well.

6.57 Surgical treatment of metacarpal fracture in a young man after a fall on the hand

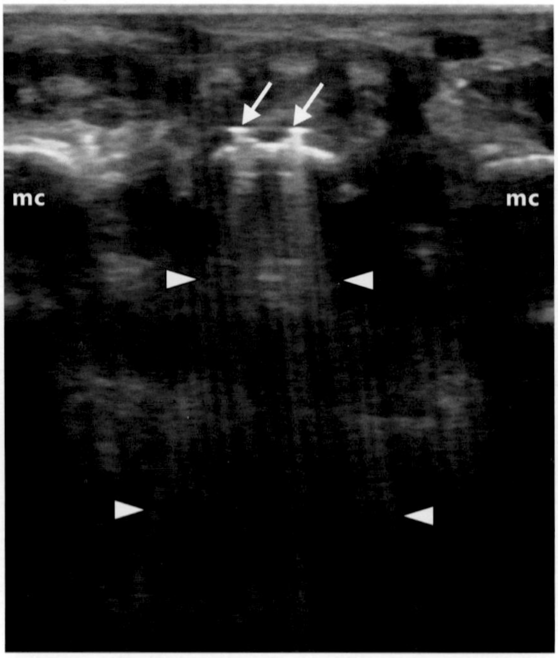

Axial US image over the metacarpal bones (**mc**) demonstrates metallic implants (*arrows*) that give bright specular echoes of typical "comet-tail" artifact (*arrowheads*).

Expert note

Certain artifacts (like "comet-tail") are observed to extend until the end of the screen; otherwise if they do not, one should be cautious to call it an artifact.

Expert note

In a single image, it would definitely be difficult to understand whether osseous structures like this one is a separated cortical fragment or a bony overgrowth. For instance, while the axial images suggest the former, the longitudinal image suggests the latter. In this sense, moving the probe in different planes over the lesion and trying to visualize a bony continuation would be clarifying. This is actually quite similar to the evaluation of enthesopathy elsewhere.

Hand osteoarthritis in a 55-year-old patient six months after trauma **6.58**

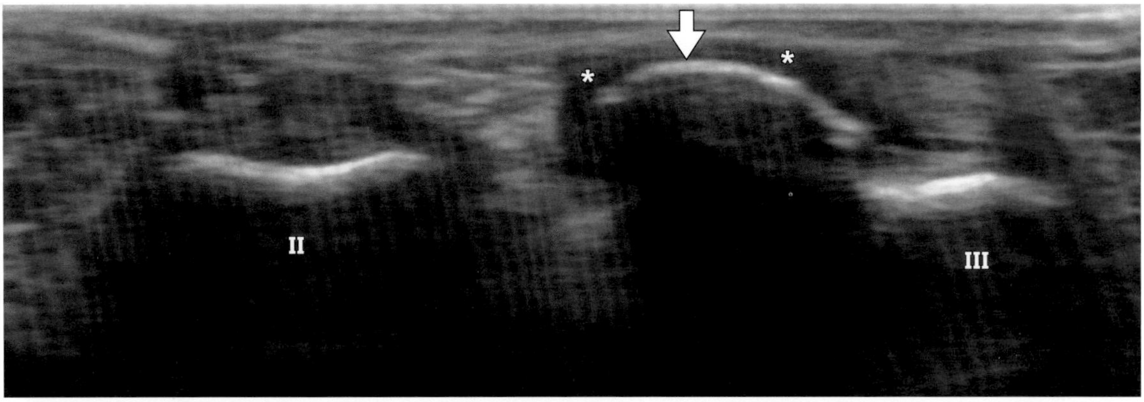

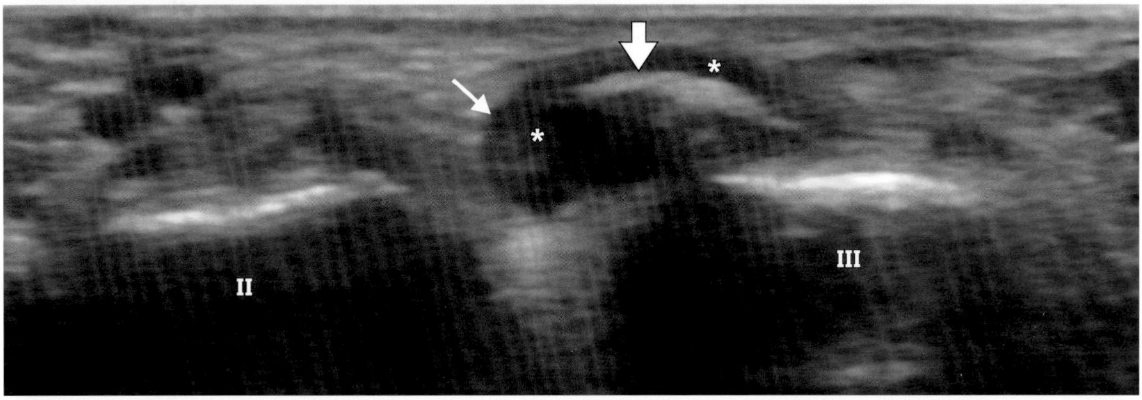

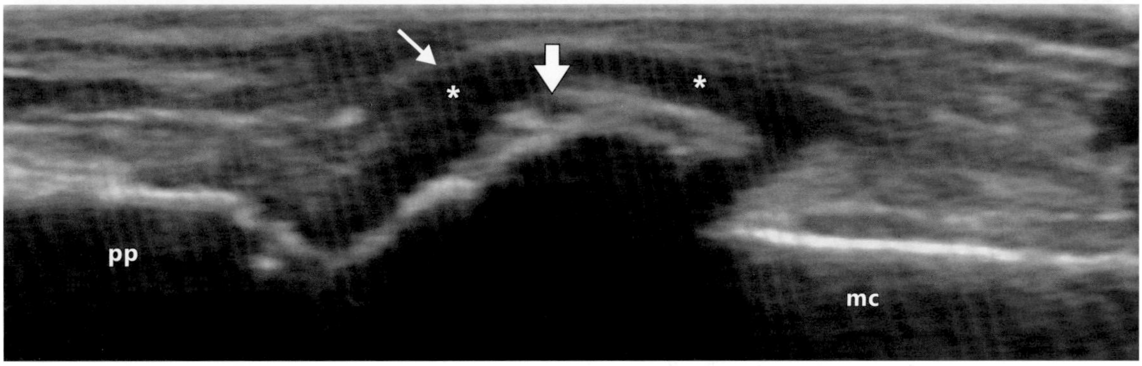

Axial (**a**, **b**) and longitudinal (**c**) US images over the metacarpophalangeal joint level show effusion (*asterisks*) and distended joint capsule (*thin arrows*). Please note the bony overgrowth/spur of the 3rd metacarpal bone (**mc**) at different sections (*thick arrows*) (**a**, **b**).

II & III metacarpal bones
pp proximal phalanx

6.59 Metacarpal erosion in a 47-year-old woman with longstanding rheumatoid arthritis

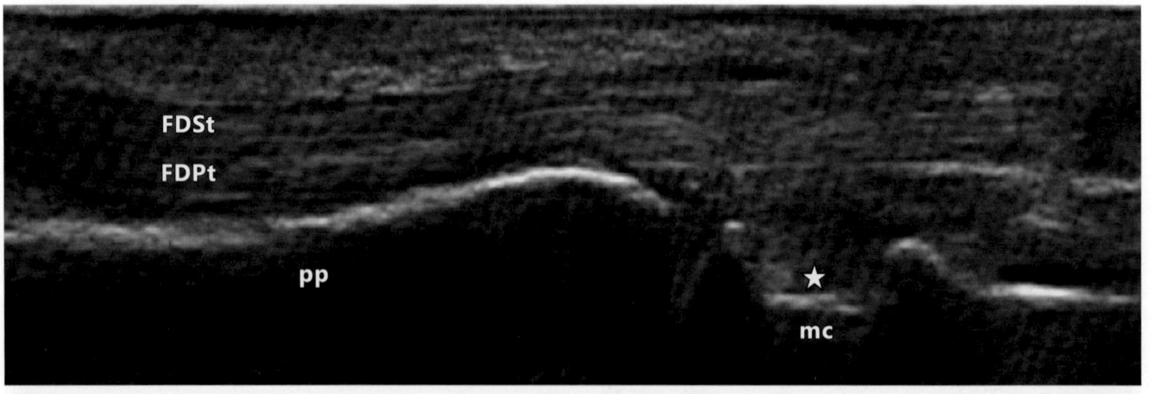

Palmar longitudinal US image demonstrates a well-defined large cortical erosion (*star*) on the metacarpal head (**mc**).

FDPt flexor digitorum profundus tendon
FDSt flexor digitorum superficialis tendon
pp proximal phalanx

Erosive arthritis in an elderly woman with inflammatory night pain **6.60**

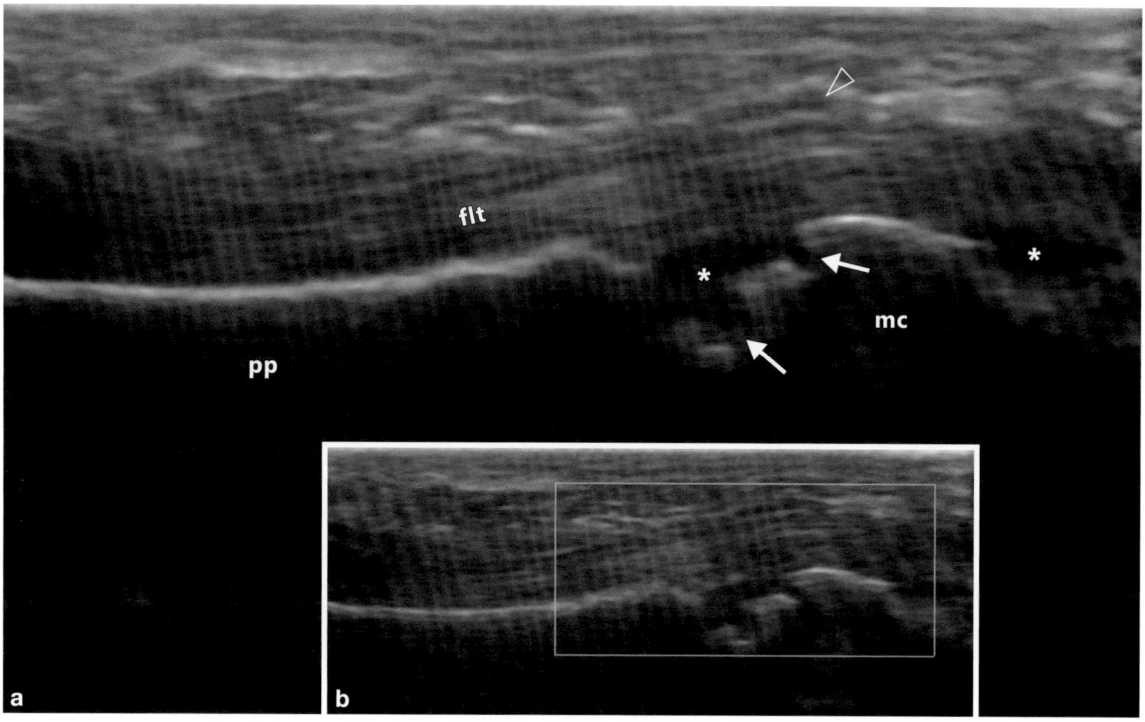

Longitudinal US image over the third metacarpophalangeal joint reveals erosive changes involving the articular surfaces (*arrows*) and mild joint effusion (*asterisks*) also overflowing proximally. Flexor tendons and the A1 pulley (*arrowhead*) look quite normal (**a**). Power Doppler imaging does not show any internal flow signal either (**b**).

flt flexors tendon
mc metacarpal bone
pp proximal phalanx

6.61 Trigger finger in a 35-year-old man after heavy lifting

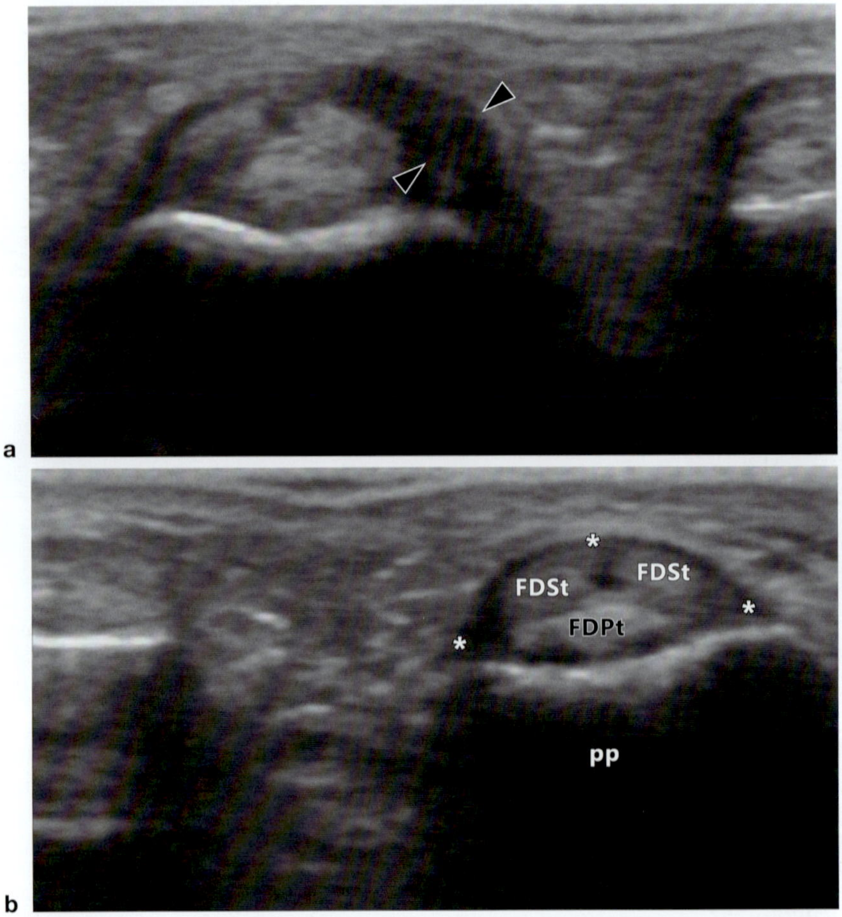

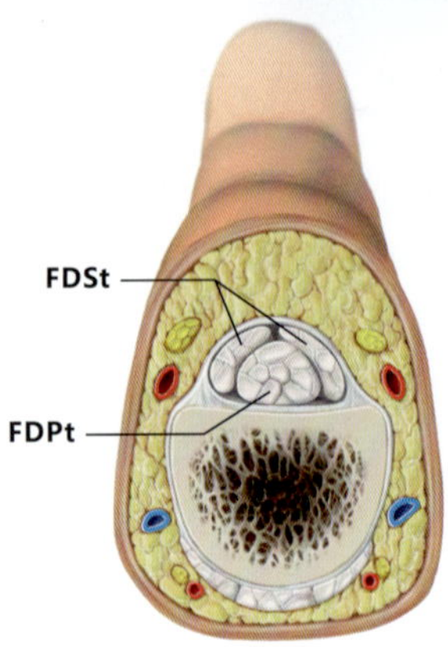

Axial US image over the proximal phalanx (**pp**) illustrates thickened and irregular (*arrowheads*) A3 pulley (**a**). Normal A3 pulley (*asterisks*) on the contralateral side (**b**).

FDPt flexor digitorum profundus tendon
FDSt flexor digitorum superficialis tendon

Pulley lesion in a 33-year-old manual worker after heavy lifting **6.62**

Axial US image over the palmar aspect of the metacarpal bones (**II-III**), shows mild thickening (*arrowheads*) of the A1 pulley on the 3rd finger in comparison with the 2nd.

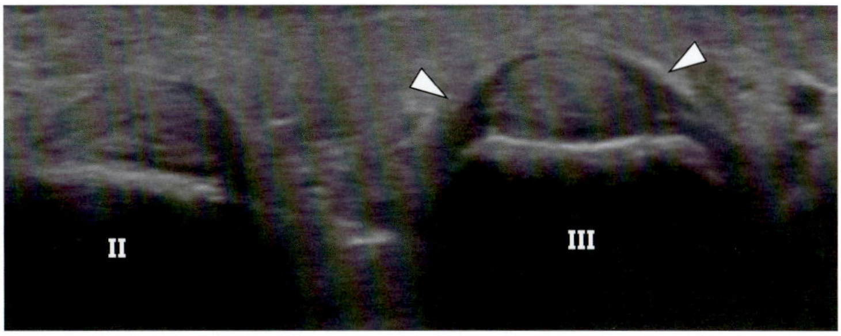

Expert note

Pulley problems can be detected either by observation of a direct lesion on the pulley or by indirect findings like the malalignment of the flexor tendons. For instance, instead of a parallel configuration of the tendon in relation with the underlying phalanx, one might see a straight alignment (like a rope) in pulley ruptures as in climber's finger.

Trigger finger in a middle-aged woman with painful snapping **6.63**

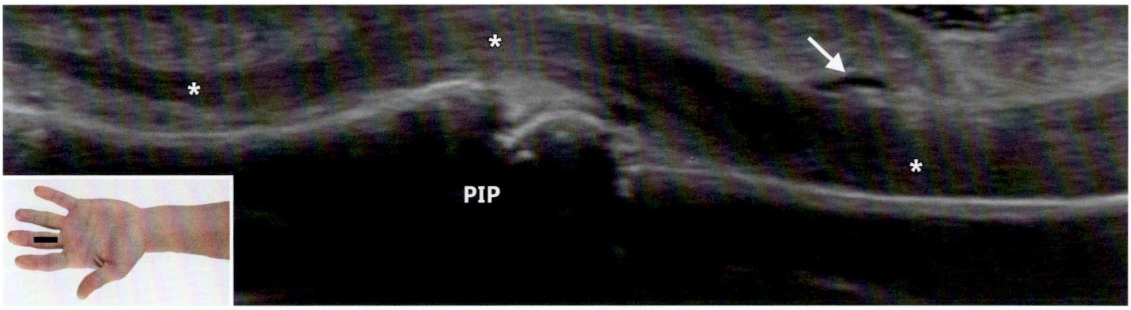

Longitudinal US image obtained over the palmar aspect of the proximal interphalangeal joint (**PIP**) reveals hypoechoic thickening of the A2 pulley (*arrow*). The flexor tendons are otherwise normal (*asterisks*).

Expert note

While assessing the echogenicity of the flexor tendons, caution should remain as the prerequisite. Yet, their alignment will not always be strictly parallel to the long axis of the probe i.e. rather oblique between the interphalangeal joint zones (making them appear hypoechoic) as seen in this figure.

6.64 Mild joint sprain in a young adult man

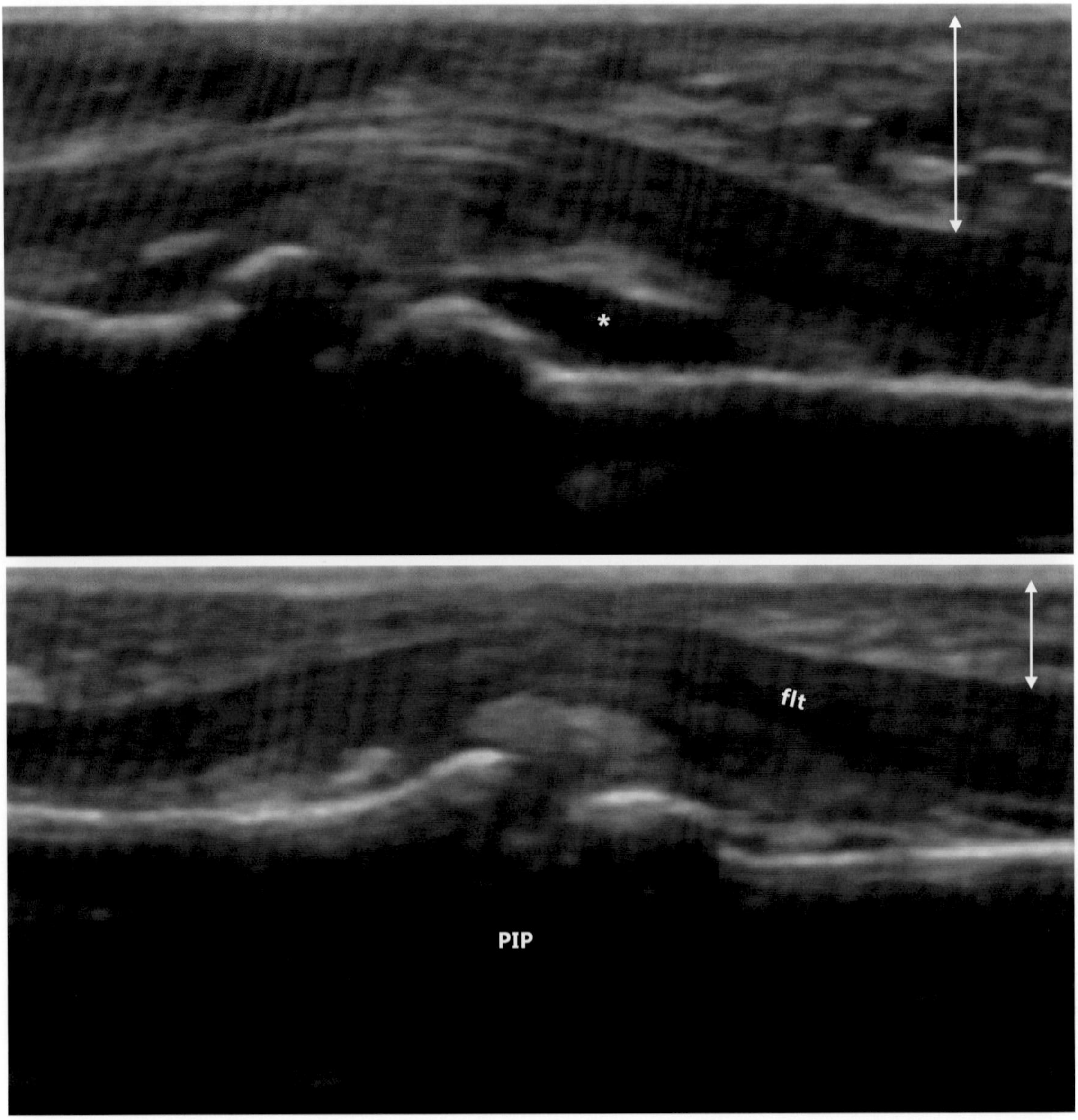

a

b

The patient described to have hit the ring finger to the wall as he tried to protect himself from falling.

Longitudinal US image over the proximal interphalangeal joint (**PIP**) reveals anechoic joint effusion (*asterisk*) and edema in the subcutaneous tissue (*double arrow*) while the flexor tendons (**flt**) seem to be unaffected (**a**). Normal side (**b**).

Foreign body in a 25-year-old man bioengineer with painful local swelling 6.65

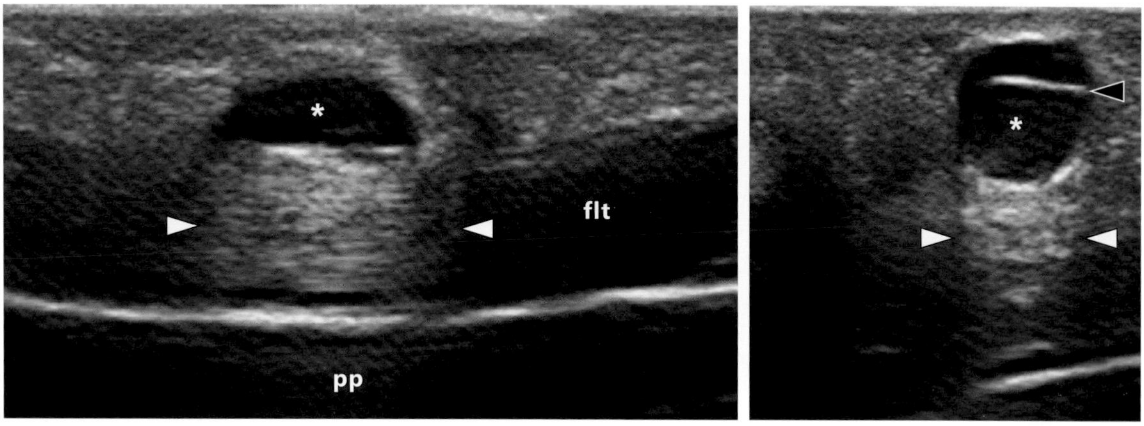

a b

Palmar longitudinal (**a**) and axial (**b**) US images over the 3rd finger demonstrate a hypoechoic well-defined fluid collection (*asterisks*) over the flexor tendons (**flt**). A linear hyperechoic structure consistent with a foreign body (*black arrowhead*) is clearly seen within the collection. Please note the enhanced through transmission artifact (*white arrowheads*) due to the fluid collection.

pp proximal phalanx

Expert note

This patient was "lucky"; the foreign body did not enter the tendon sheath. Yet, this is important to estimate the risks of infection and also for the surgeon.

6.66 Stenosing tenosynovitis of the flexor tendons in a patient with inflammatory arthritis

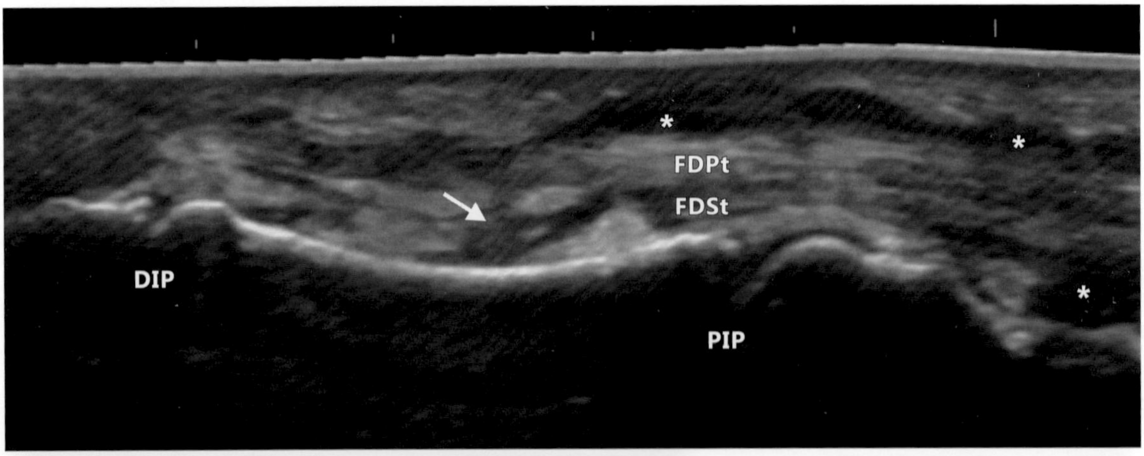

a

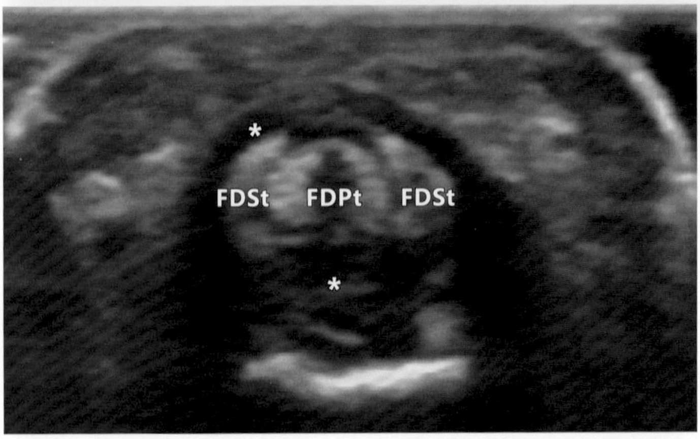

b

Panoramic longitudinal view (**a**) reveals diffuse distension of the flexor tendon sheath by synovial fluid (*asterisks*). The distal axial image of the chiasm is also confirmatory (**b**). Please note the attachment site (*arrow*) of the flexor digitorum superficialis tendon (**FDSt**).

DIP distal interphalangeal joint
FDPt flexor digitorum profundus tendon
PIP proximal interphalangeal joint

Tenosynovitis in a 42-year-old woman with rheumatoid arthritis **6.67**

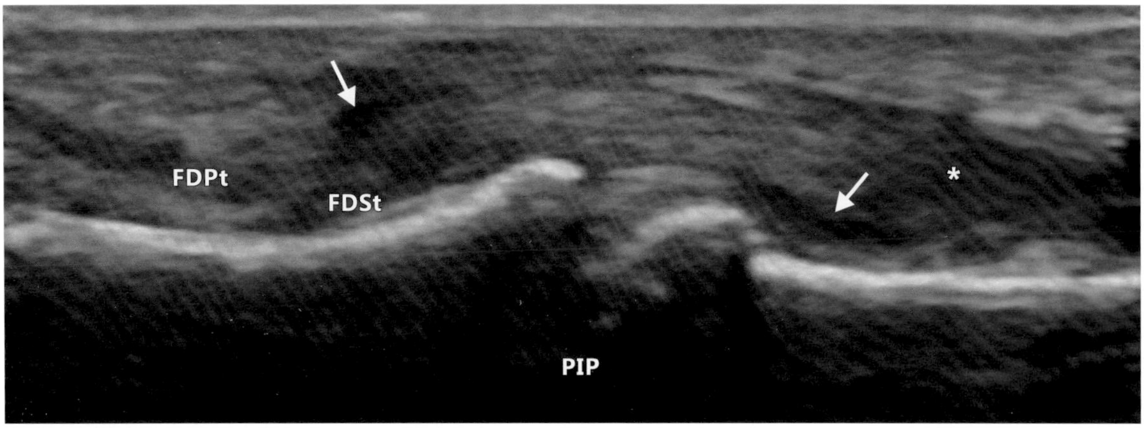

Longitudinal US image identifies edema (*asterisk*) in the proximal parts of the flexor tendons and small amounts of fluid (*arrows*) within their sheath.

FDPt flexor digitorum profundus tendon
FDSt flexor digitorum superficialis tendon
PIP proximal interfalangeal joint

Expert note

Prompt assessment of the flexor tendon echogenicity is difficult in the hand; yet, their alignment is not always straight (parallel to the probe). Therefore, delicate check as regards anisotropy is crucial (in two planes) before one can conclude about hypoechogenicity (i.e. edema or disturbed arrangement of tendon fibers).

6.68 Flexor tenosynovitis in a 23-year-old woman with painful snapping

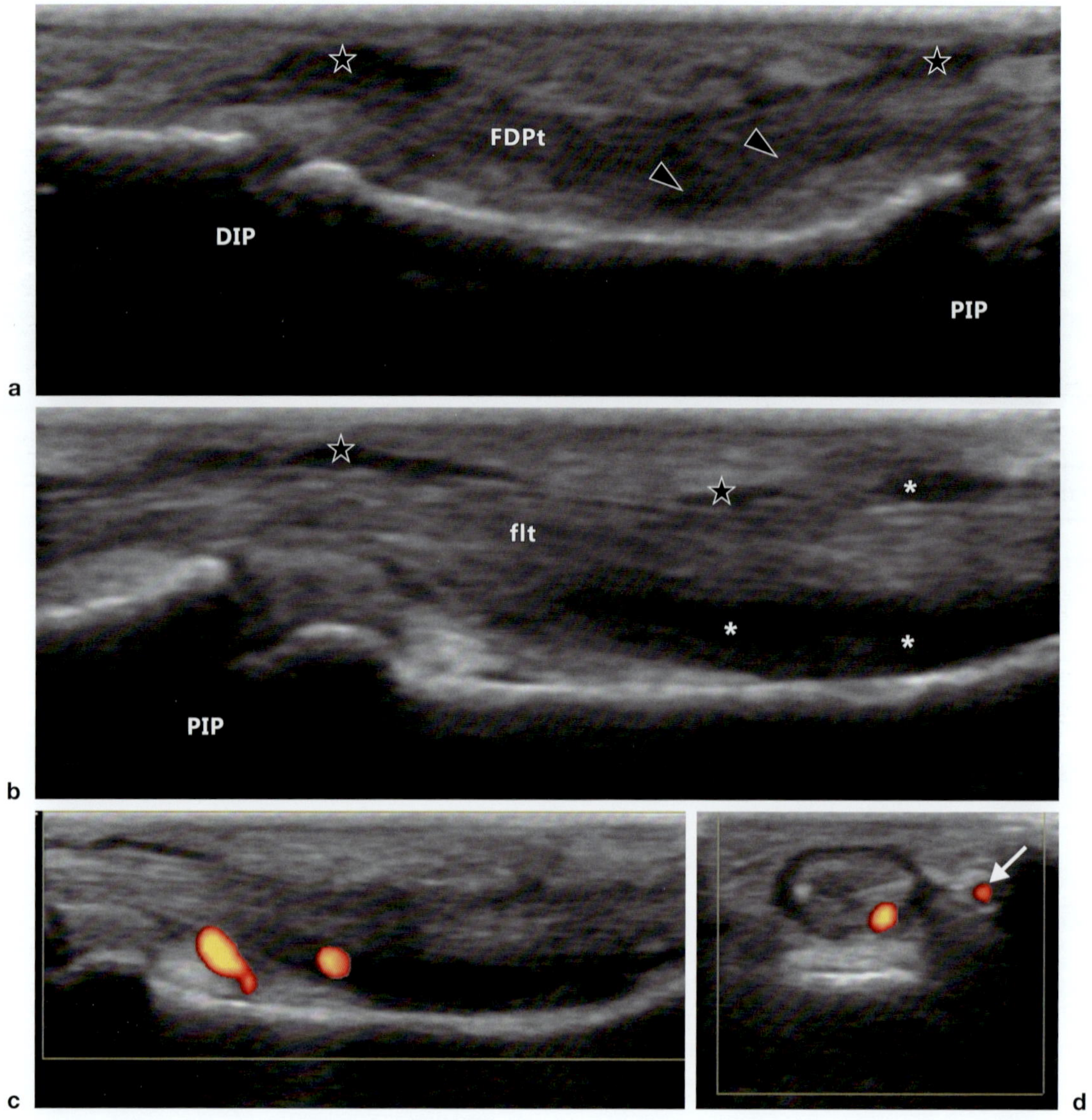

Longitudinal US images obtained at middle (**a**) and proximal (**b**) phalanx levels reveal synovial fluid within the flexor tendon sheath (*asterisks*) and thickening of the pulleys (*stars*). *Arrowheads* present insertion of the flexor digitorum superficialis tendon (**FDSt**). Longitudinal (**c**) and axial (**d**) power Doppler images demonstrate signs of hyperemia in addition to the digital artery (*arrow*).

DIP	distal interphalangeal joint	**flt**	flexor tendons
FDPt	flexor digitorum profundus tendon	**PIP**	proximal interphalangeal joint

Phalangeal spur after a traumatic injury 6.69

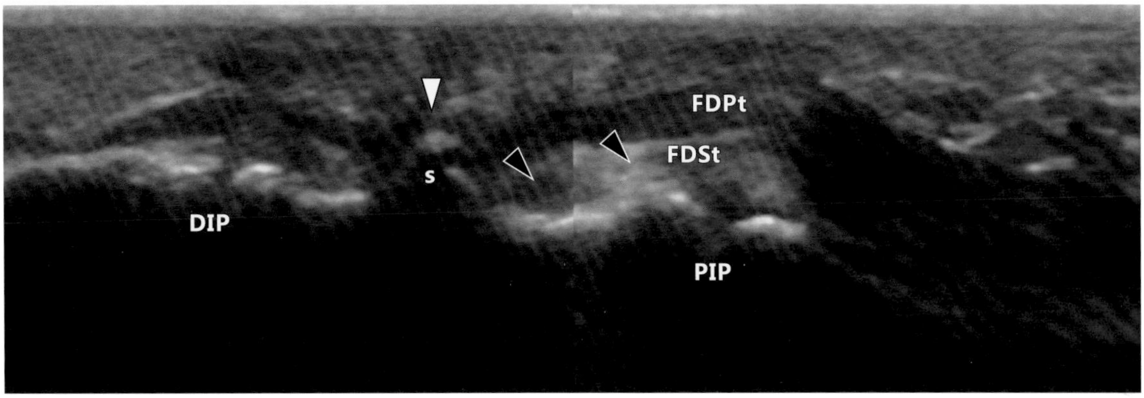

Longitudinal split-screen US image demonstrates a bony spur formation (**s**) that causes impingement (*white arrowhead*) on the flexor digitorum profundus tendon (**FDPt**). Please note the distal insertion (*black arrowheads*) of the flexor digitorum superficialis tendon (**FDSt**).

DIP distal interphalangeal joint
PIP proximal interphalangeal joint

6.70 Dorsal subluxation of the proximal interphalangeal joint in an amateur football player after a ball hit

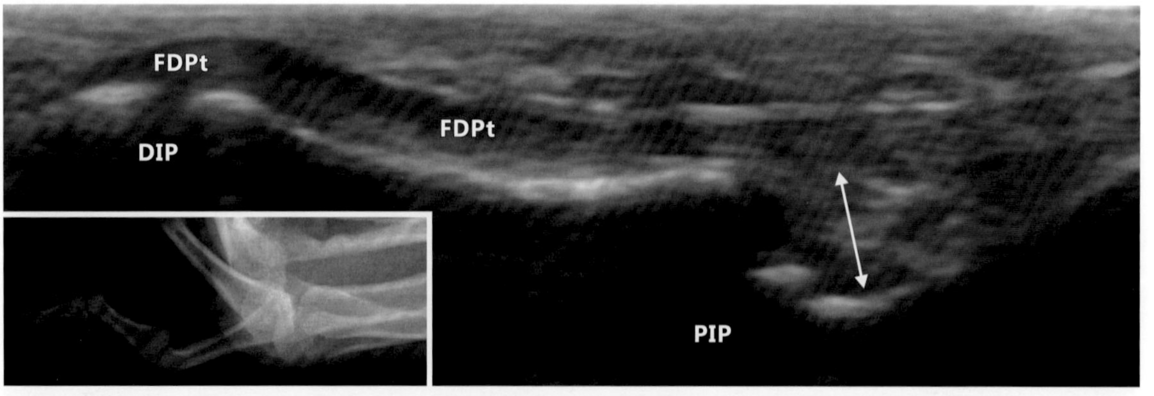

Longitudinal US image demonstrates marked distance (*double arrows*) at the proximal interphalangeal joint (**PIP**) due to the displacement of the proximal phalanx. The flexor digitorum profundus tendon (**FDPt**) seems to be quite normal. Dorsal subluxation of the proximal phalanx resulting in the development of boutonniere deformity is also seen on the lateral radiograph (*small image*).

DIP distal interphalangeal joint

Expert note

Like in many other conditions related with the bones, a radiograph might be more informative in the general/overall sense. However, a possible soft tissue consequence cannot be clearly unmasked unless US is used conveniently.

Extensor digiti minimi tendinopathy in a 48-year-old woman after hyperflexion injury of the wrist/finger **6.71**

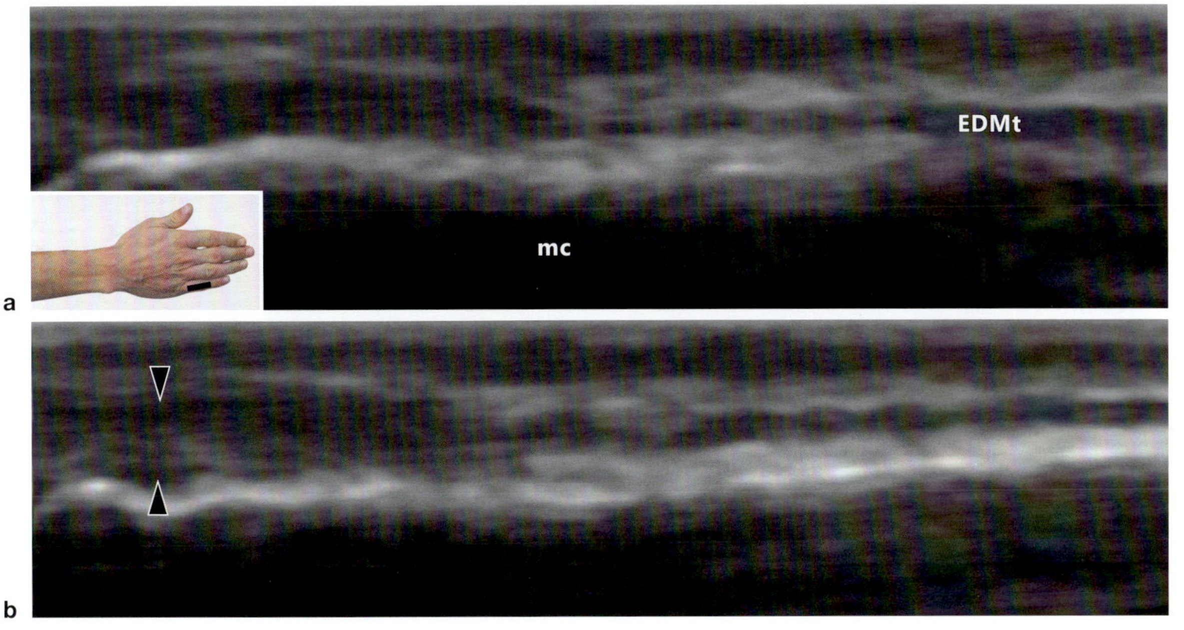

When compared with the normal side (**a**), longitudinal US image identifies irregular and hypoechoic thickening (*arrowheads*) of the extensor digiti minimi tendon (**EDMt**) (**b**).

mc metacarpal bone

6.72 A small foreign object following a penetrating trauma

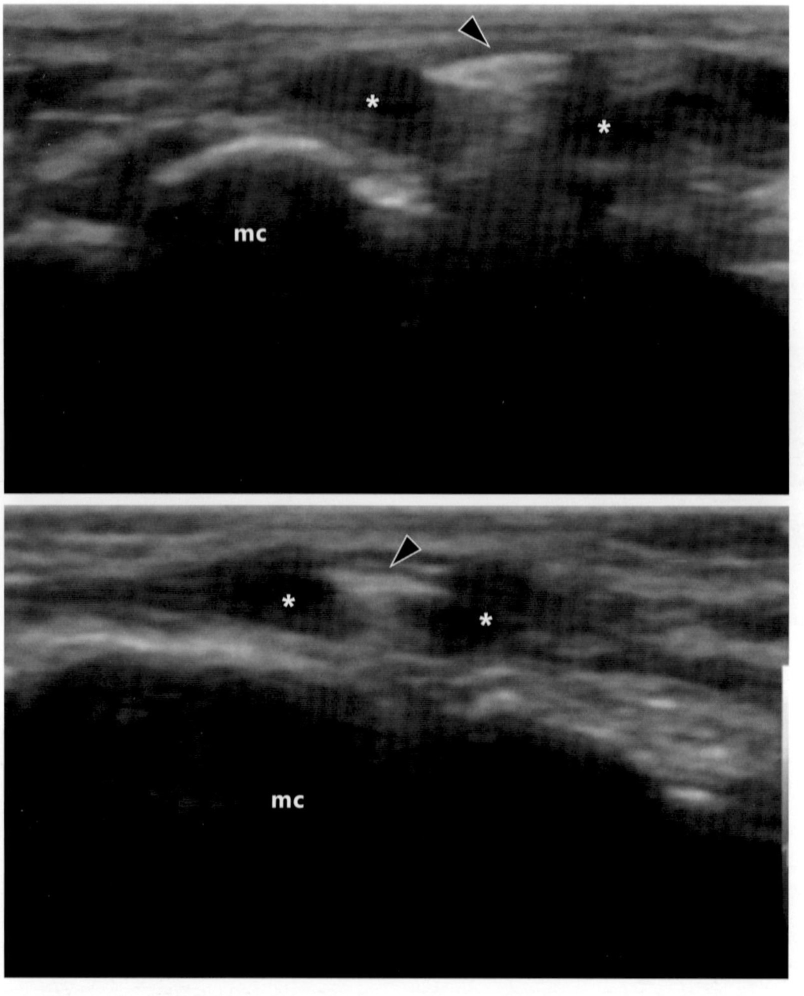

a b

Video 8

Dorsal axial (**a**) and longitudinal (**b**) images over the metacarpal bone (**mc**) shows a well demarcated hyperechoic foreign body (*arrowheads*) surrounded by reactive soft tissue (*asterisks*).

Expert note

For the detection of foreign objects, US is very sensitive. Herewith, if the foreign body is an organic one (wood, plant etc.); it might be resolved by the surrounding tissues in 2-3 weeks. Therefore, the sonographer should be aware of this issue if the examination is performed afterwards. Otherwise, this is not the case for inorganic objects (glass, metal, etc.).
Likewise, it would also be possible to say that there will be more soft tissue reaction (edema, hyperemia) around organic than inorganic materials.

Synovitis in a 35-year-old man due to local overload and work **6.73**

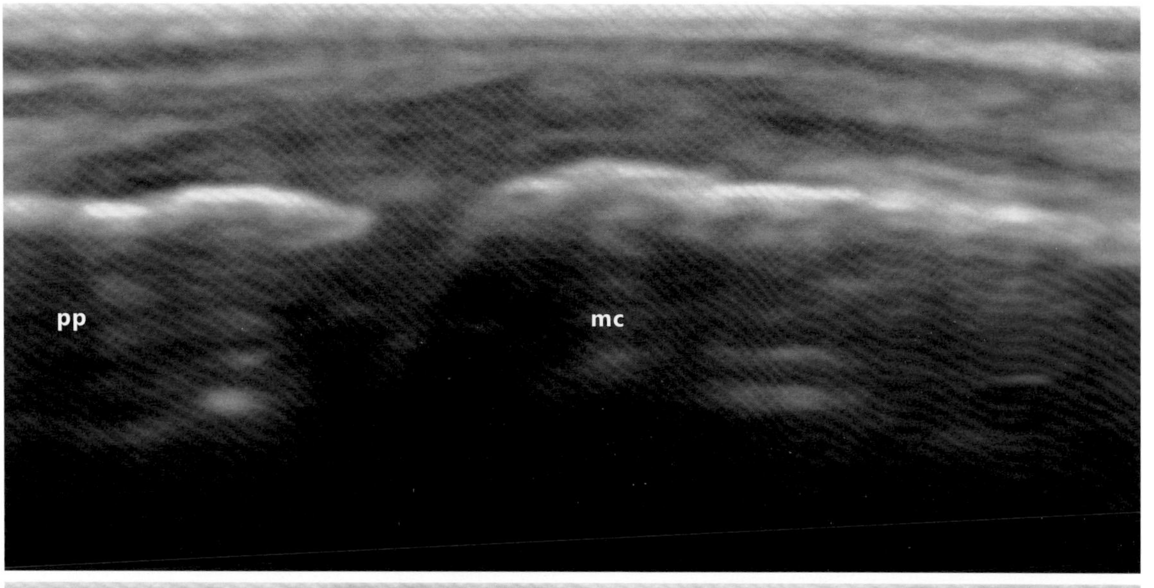

a

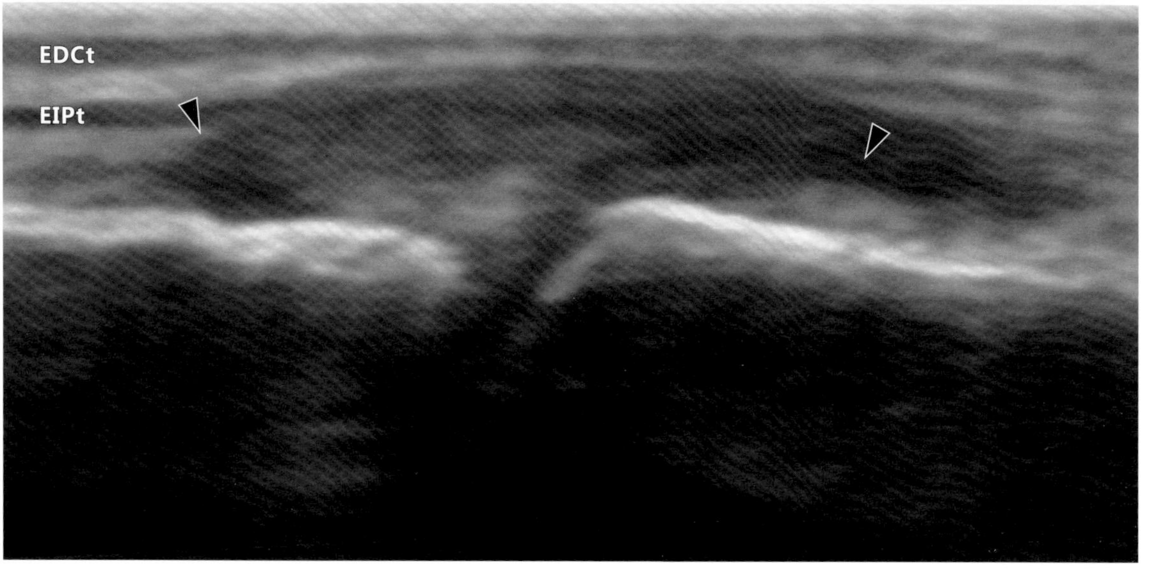

b

When compared with the normal appearance of the 2nd metacarpophalangeal joint (**a**), longitudinal US image shows synovitis causing expansion of the joint capsule (*arrowheads*) (**b**). Note that the overlying extensor tendons look quite normal.

EDCt	extensor digitorum communis tendon	**mc**	metacarpal bone
EIPt	extensor indicis proprius tendon	**pp**	proximal phalanx

6.74 Proximal interphalangeal joint effusion in 55-year-old woman with previous local trauma

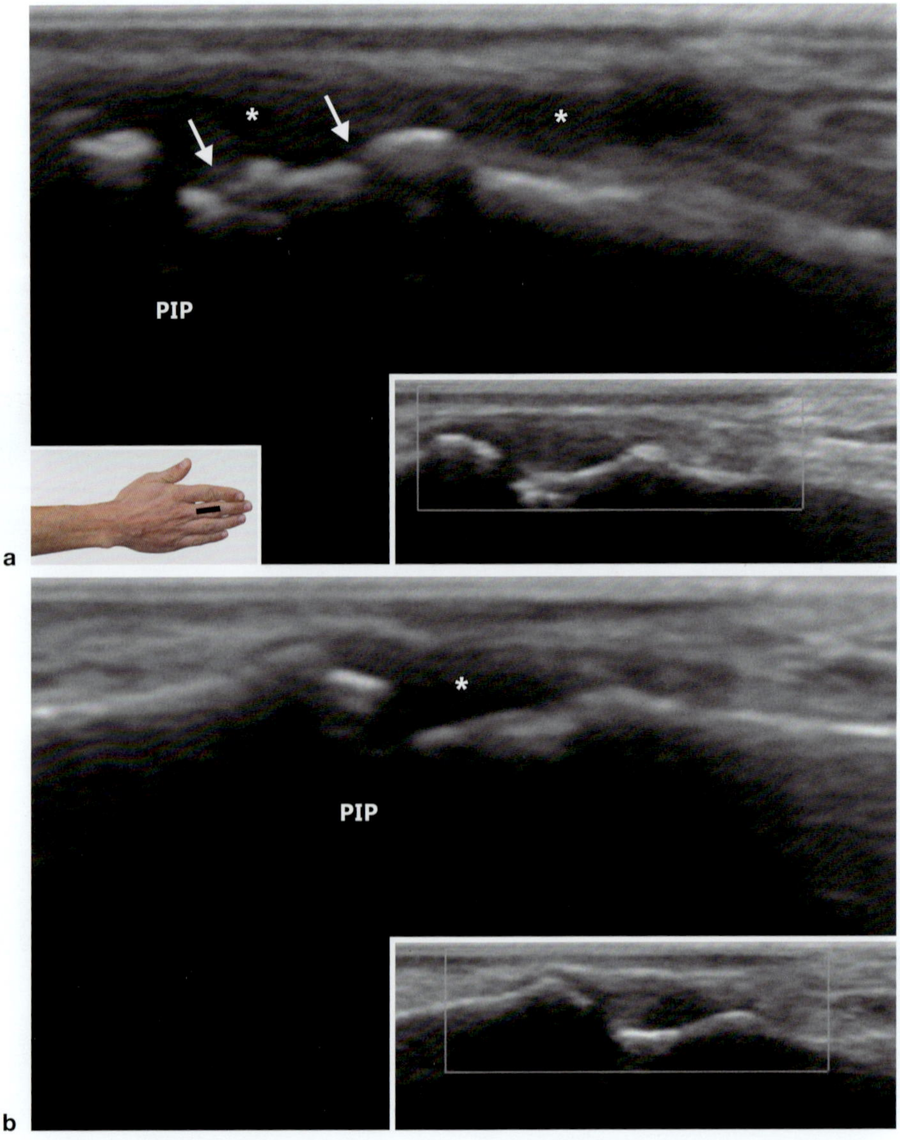

Longitudinal US images obtained over the dorsal aspect of the proximal interphalangeal joint (**PIP**) indicate effusion (*asterisks*) and bony irregularities (*arrows*) (**a**). Normal side with mild effusion (**b**). Corresponding power Doppler images (*small images*) demonstrate no internal flow signal.

Finger sprain in a 25-year-old man with painful movements 6.75

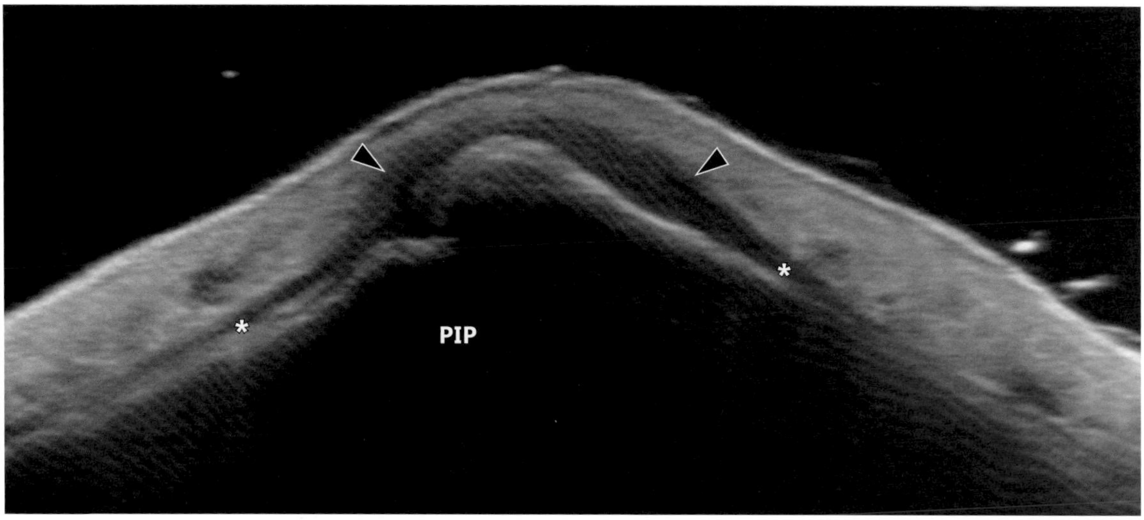

Dorsal longitudinal US imaging over the proximal interphalangeal joint (**PIP**) demonstrates intact but hypoechoic and thickened (*arrowheads*) extensor tendon (*asterisks*).

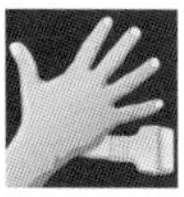

Expert note

Especially while scanning the small portions of the body (with deformities), extra gel or gel pads can be used for better technical view. Other practical ways to provide sufficient medium to transmit enough sound waves over the curved contours of the subject would be to use gloves filled with water (as shown above) or to simply insert the part to be scanned inside water. Historically, when there were only lower-frequency probes in the past, this was also necessary to get the area of interest at a depth of 3-5 cm.

6.76 Extensor tenosynovitis of the 2nd finger in a 40-year-old woman after blunt trauma

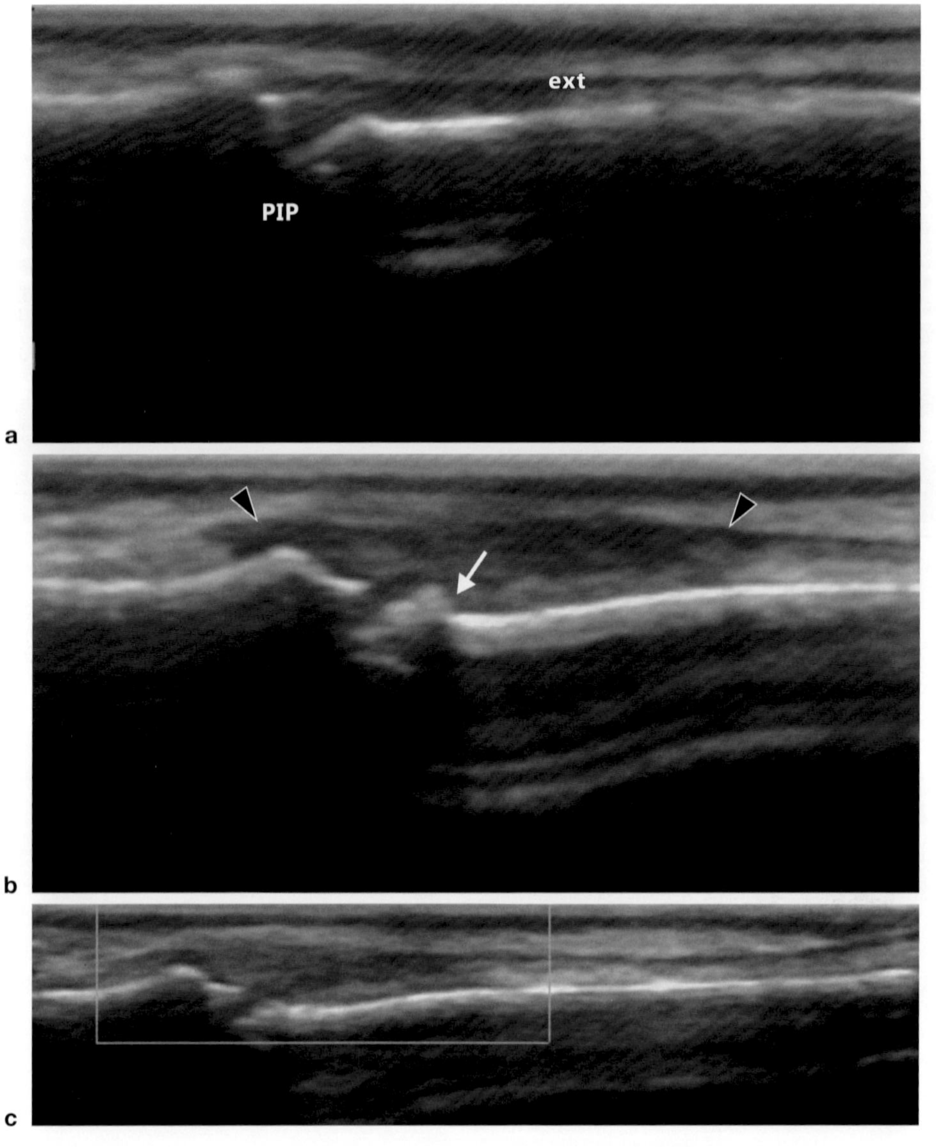

When compared with the normal side (**a**), longitudinal US imaging over the proximal interphalangeal joint (**PIP**) shows marked swelling at the central insertion of the extensor tendon (**ext**) (*arrowheads*) and a small cortical irregularity (*arrow*) of the proximal phalanx (**b**). Correlative power Doppler scan demonstrates no flow signal (**c**).

Fracture of the phalanx in a young patient after heavy manual work

6.77

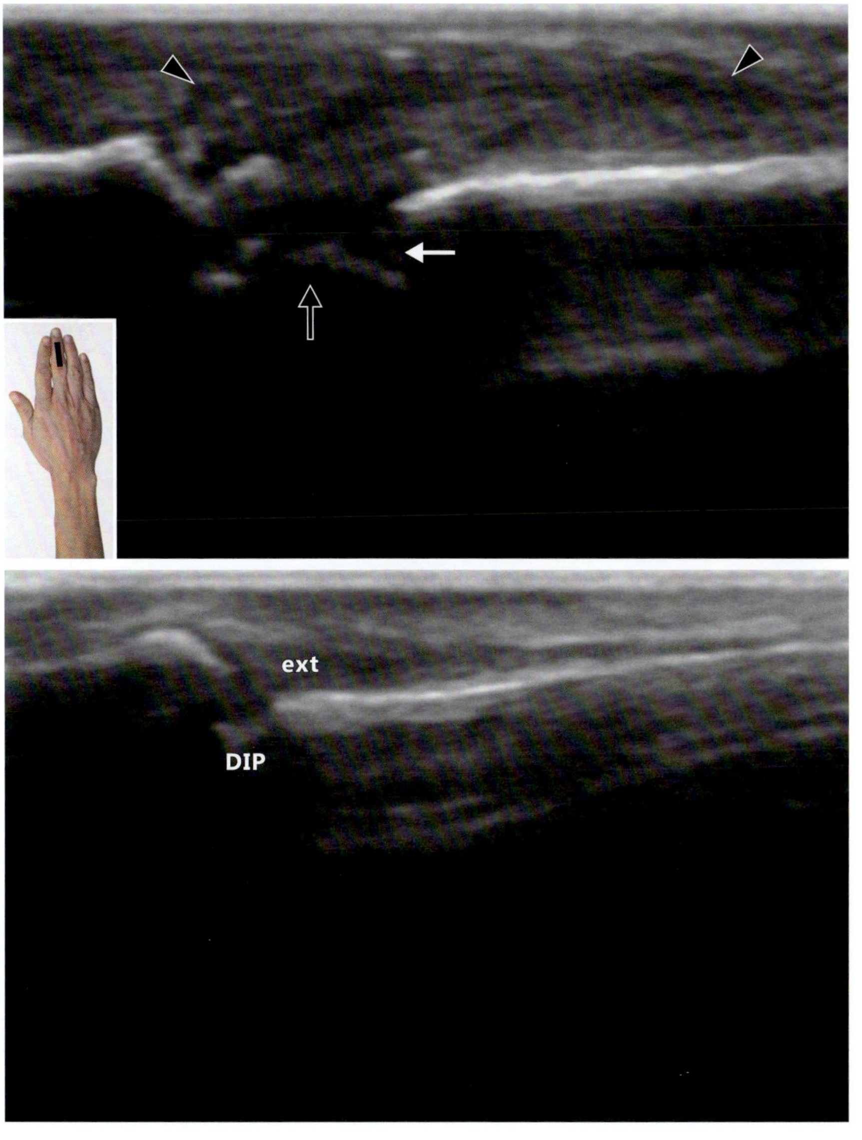

a

b

Longitudinal US image obtained over the dorsal aspect of the distal interphalangeal joint (**DIP**) demonstrates a cortical fracture (*black arrow*) and irregularly thickened but intact extensor tendon (**ext**) (*arrowheads*) (**a**). Please note the "step off" phenomenon (*white arrow*) which is a typical appearance for fractures. Normal side (**b**).

6.78 Degenerative osteoarthritis in a 65-year-old woman with painful and restricted finger movements

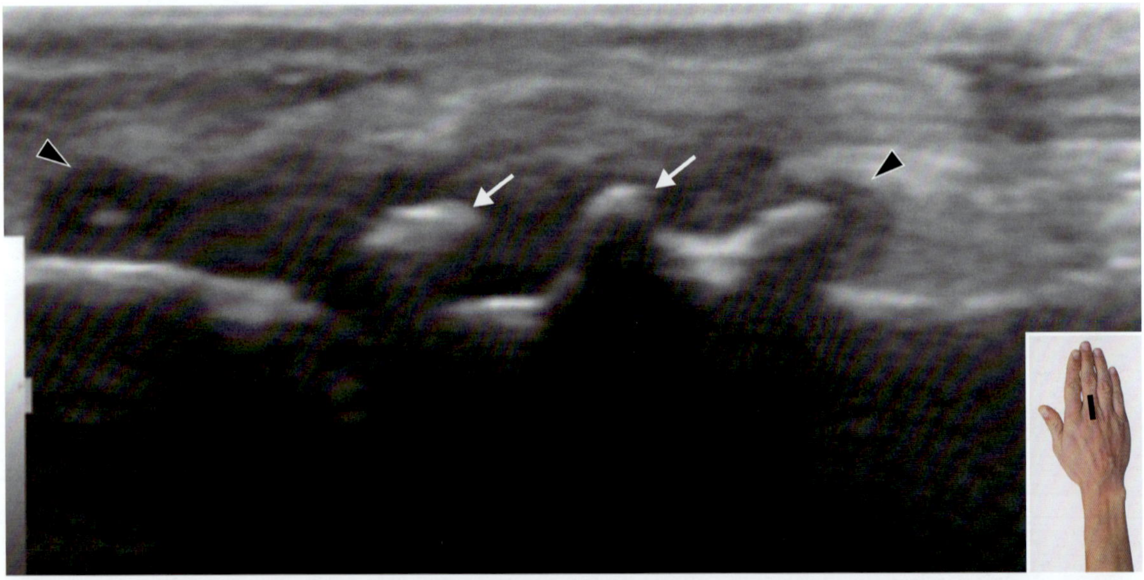

a

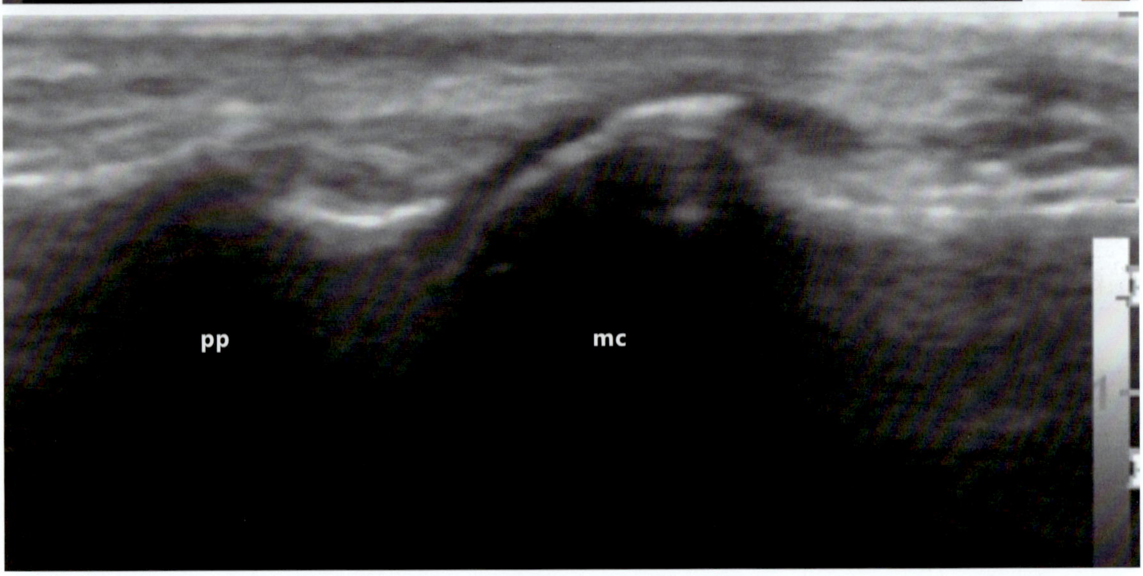

b

Longitudinal US image over the dorsal hand shows capsular distension and large osteophytes (*arrows*) on the metacarpal head (**a**). Normal side (**b**).

mc metacarpal bone
pp proximal phalanx

Degenerative osteoarthritis of the metacarpophalangeal joint in a 55-year-old woman

6.79

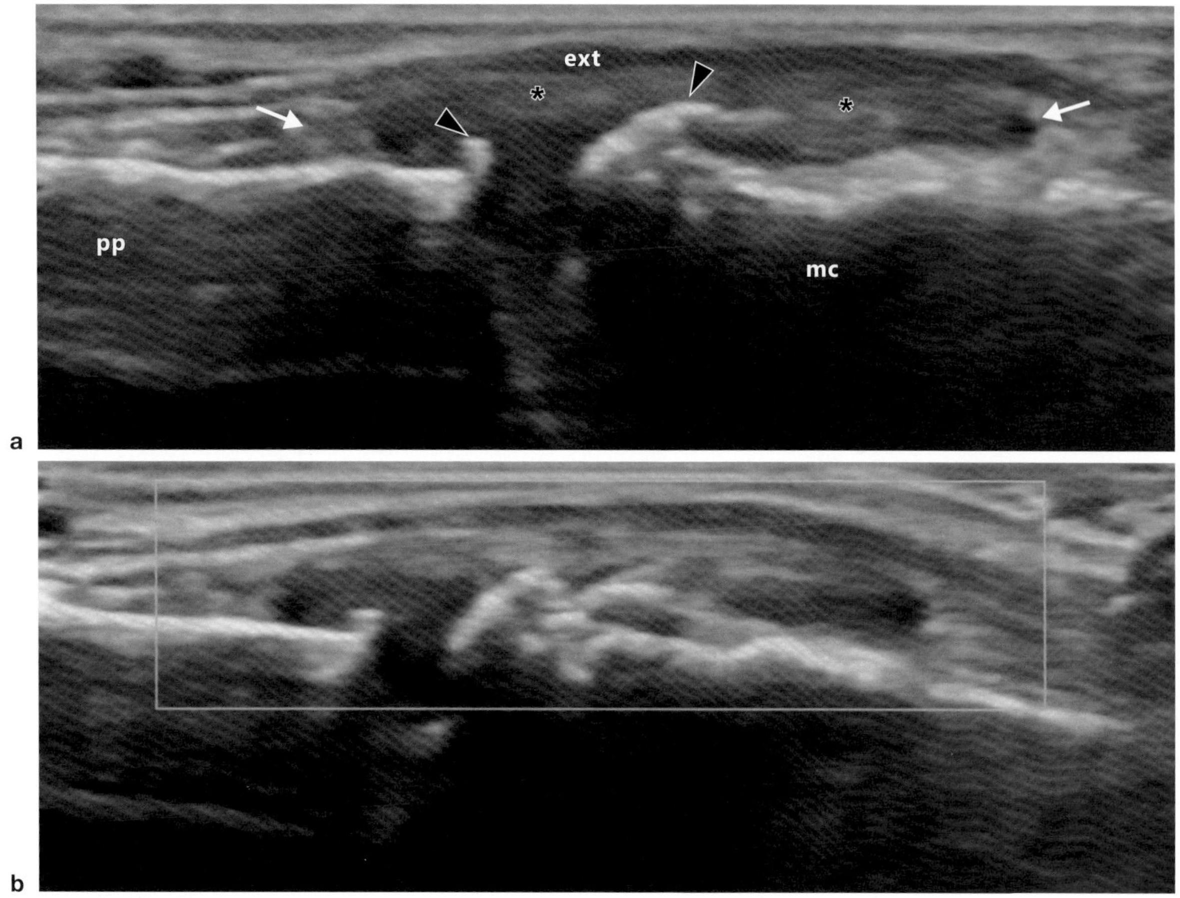

Longitudinal US image demonstrates diffuse thickening of the extensor tendon (**ext**) and Grade III synovial proliferation (*black asterisks*) in the underlying metacarpophalangeal joint. Osteophytes (*arrowheads*) on the articular surfaces and enlarged joint capsule (*arrows*) are also seen (**a**, **b**). Correlative power Doppler image shows no flow signal (**b**).

mc metacarpal bone
pp proximal phalanx

6.80 Metacarpophalangeal joint synovitis in a 45-year-old woman with rheumatoid arthritis

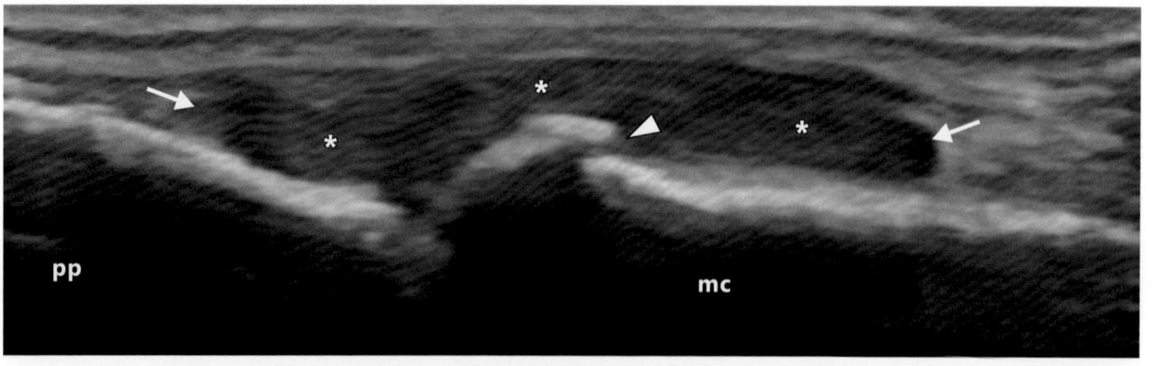

Dorsal longitudinal US image over the 3rd metacarpophalangeal joint shows an erosion (*arrowhead*) on the metacarpal head and Grade III synovitis (*asterisks*) distending the capsular recess (*arrows*).

mc metacarpal bone
pp proximal phalanx

Expert note

Semi-quantitative classification of synovitis is given in Table 6.2 [13].

Table 6.2 Classification of synovitis (Grey Scale)

Grade		Signal
0		Absent
I	mild	A small hypoechoic/anechoic line beneath the joint capsule
II	moderate	The joint capsule is elevated parallel to the joint area
III	severe	A strong distension of the joint capsule

Erosive lesions of the metacarpophalangeal joint in a patient with rheumatoid arthritis 6.81

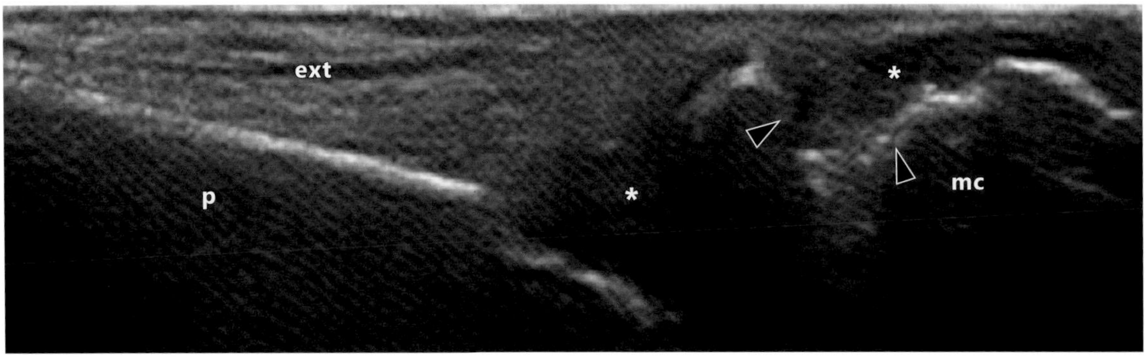

Dorsal longitudinal US image reflects bony erosions (*arrowheads*) of the metacarpal head and synovial effusion (*asterisks*) within the metacarpophalangeal joint.

ext extensor tendon
mc metacarpal bone
p phalanx

Synovial calcification in a young woman with painful finger movements after local trauma 6.82

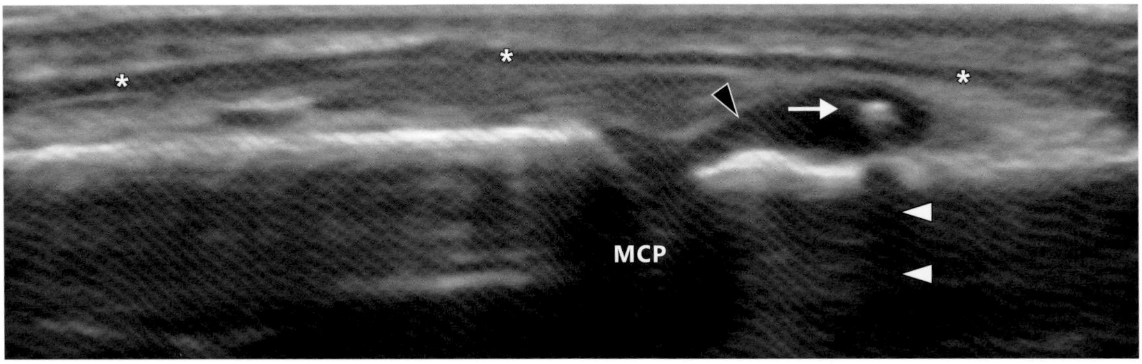

Dorsal longitudinal US image on the metacarpophalangeal joint (**MCP**) reveals mild effusion (*black arrowhead*) and a small type II calcification (*arrow*) inside the joint capsule giving incomplete acoustic shadowing (*white arrowheads*). The overlying extensor tendon (*asterisks*) is normal.

6.83 A young man with pain and reduced finger extension at the level of distal interphalangeal joint

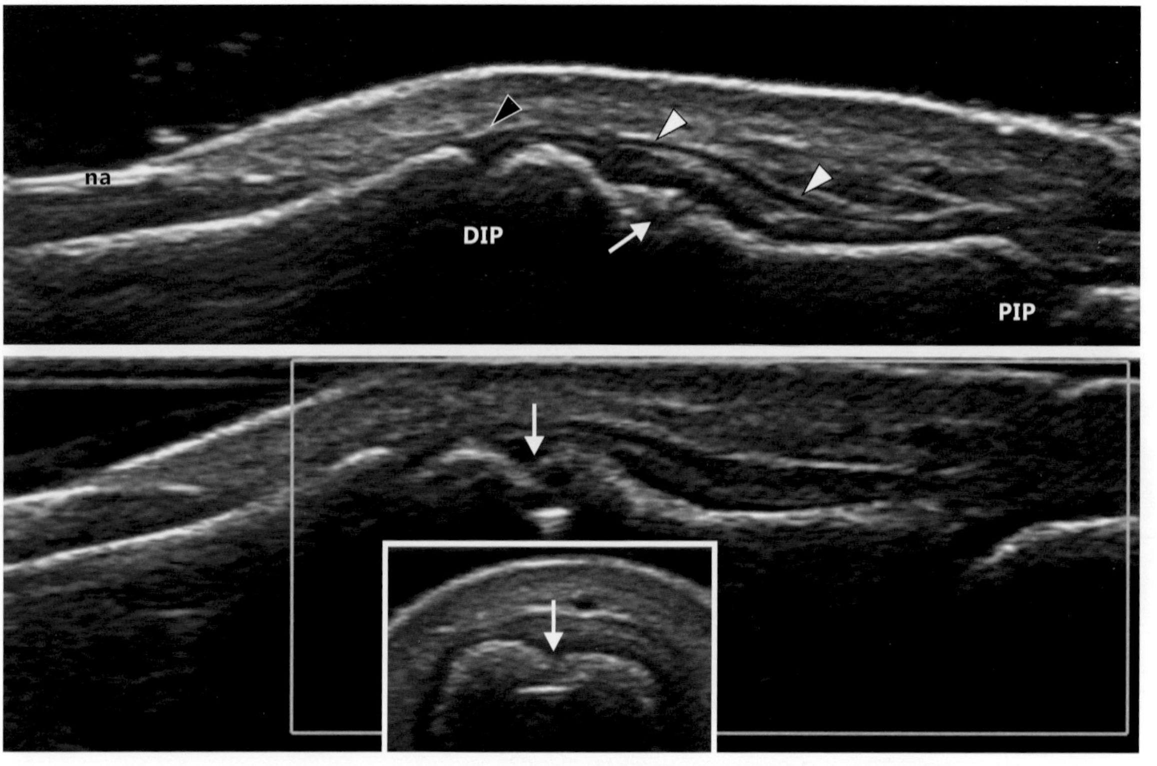

a

b

Longitudinal US image (**a**) shows the normal appearance of the extensor tendon (*white arrowheads*) and its central insertion (*black arrowhead*). Other than the small cortical irregularity (*arrow*), all the soft tissues (including the nail, **na**) seem to be quite normal. While the bony lesion is confirmed on the axial view (*small image*), it did not exhibit any flow signal on power Doppler imaging (**b**).

DIP distal interphalangeal joint
PIP proximal interphalangeal joint

REFERENCES

1. Kılıç E, Akgül Ö, Kılıç G, Özgöçmen S. Ultrasound imaging in rheumatic diseases. In: Özçakar L, De Muynck M, editors. Musculoskeletal ultrasound in physical and rehabilitation medicine. Milan: Edi.Ermes; 2014. p. 161-83.
2. Naredo E, Möller I, Cruz A, Carmona L, Garrido J. Power Doppler ultrasonographic monitoring of response to anti-tumor necrosis factor therapy in patients with rheumatoid arthritis. Arthritis Rheum. 2008; 58: 2248-56.
3. Vuillemin V, Guerini H, Bard H, Morvan G. Stenosing tenosynovitis. J Ultrasound. 2012; 15: 20-8.
4. Ulaşlı AM. Ultrasound evaluation of the wrist and hand. In: Özçakar L, De Muynck M, editors. Musculoskeletal ultrasound in physical and rehabilitation medicine. Milan: Edi.Ermes; 2014. p. 73-86.
5. Tekin L, Tok F, Özçakar L. RE: Ultrasound-guided corticosteroid injection for the treatment of de Quervain's tenosynovitis. Am J Phys Med Rehabil. 2014; 93: 277.
6. Chang KV, Hung CY, Özçakar L. Snapping thumb and superficial radial nerve entrapment in De Quervain Disease: ultrasound imaging/guidance revisited. Pain Med. 2015; 16: 2214-5.
7. Bianchi S, Martinoli C. Wrist. In: Bianchi S, Martinoli C, editors. Ultrasound of the musculoskeletal system. Berlin: Springer; 2007. p. 425-94.
8. Özçakar L, Kara M, Chang KV et al. EURO-MUSCULUS/USPRM Basic scanning protocols for wrist and hand. Eur J Phys Rehabil Med. 2015; 51: 479-84.
9. Vuillemin V, Guerini H, Bard H, Morvan G. Stenosing tenosynovitis. J Ultrasound. 2012; 15: 20-8.
10. Kameyama M, Meguro S, Funae O, Atsumi Y, Ikegami H. The presence of limited joint mobility is significantly associated with multiple digit involvement by stenosing flexor tenosynovitis in diabetics. J Rheumatol. 2009; 36: 1686e90.
11. Guerini H, Pessis E, Theumann N, Le Quintrec JS, Campagna R, Chevrot A, et al. Sonographic appearance of trigger fingers. J Ultrasound Med. 2008; 27: 1407-13.
12. Bianchi S, Martinoli C. Hand. In: Bianchi S, Martinoli C, editors. Ultrasound of the musculoskeletal system. Berlin: Springer; 2007. p. 495-550.
13. Schmidt WA, Schönau V, Reiche BE, Oberdorfer PD, Ohrndorf S, Backhaus M. Grading of ultrasound Doppler signals in synovitis: does it need an update? Rheumatology (Oxford). 2015; 54: 1897-903.

Section 3
LOWER LIMB

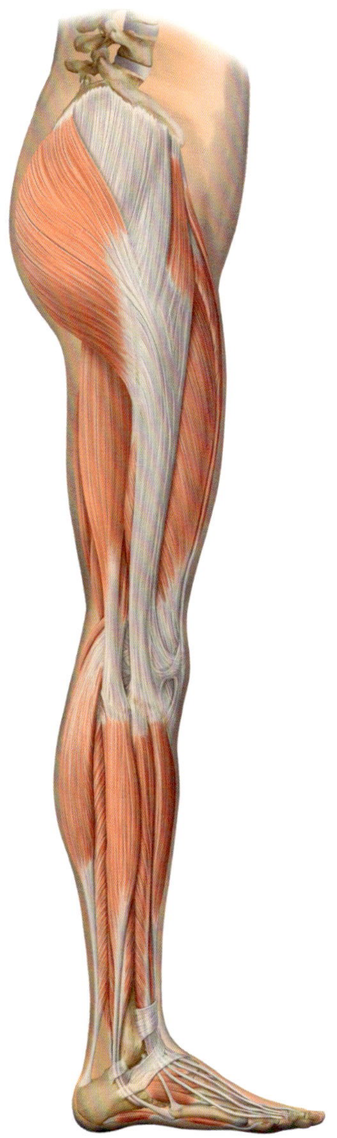

Hip 7

- Femoroacetabular joint
- Acetabular labrum
- Iliopsoas muscle
- Fascia lata
- Greater trochanter
- Pubis

7.1 Postinfection transient synovitis of the hip joint in a 8-year-old boy with sudden hip pain and limping

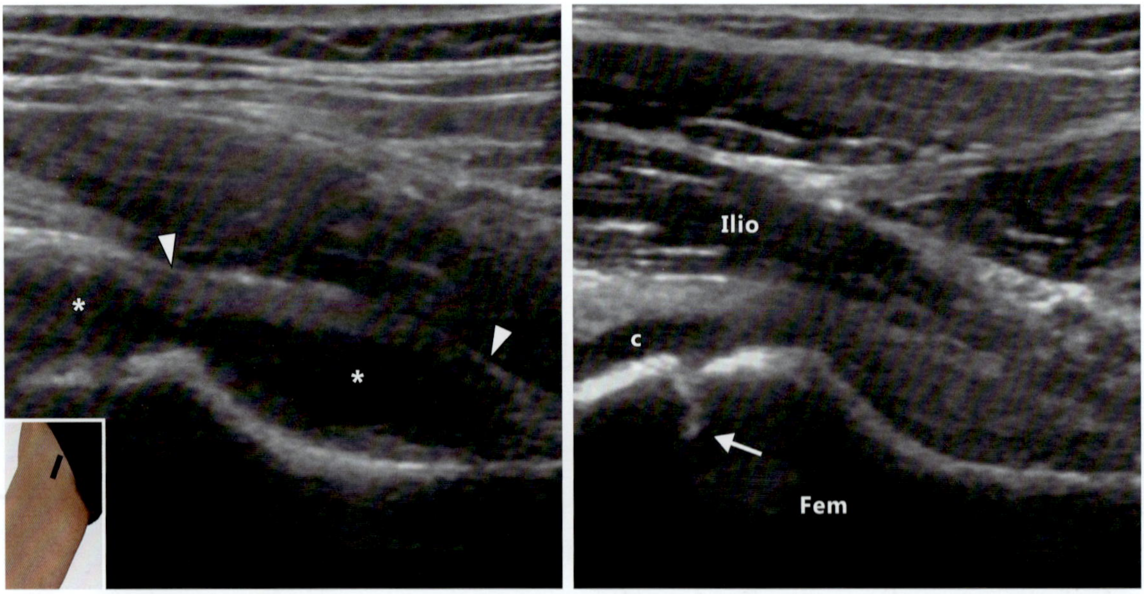

a b

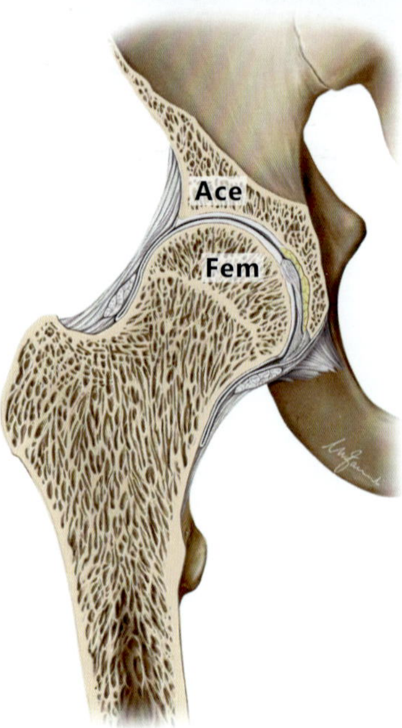

Longitudinal US imaging over the hip joint shows anechoic fluid collection (*asterisks*) distending the anterior joint recess (*arrowheads*) (**a**). Asymptomatic side (**b**). Please also note the growth plate (*arrow*).

Ace	acetabulum	**Fem**	femur
c	cartilage	**Ilio**	iliopsoas

Expert note

Being a deeply seated joint, physical examination of the hip (especially for presence of fluid) is not straightforward like in other joints (e.g. wrist, knee). Further, in children, vague symptoms of hip pain might not always be trustworthy either. As such, particularly in children (where there is less amount of overlying tissues), US imaging of the hip joint would be paramount and highly contributory as well.

One should be very meticulous in positioning the patient. In extension and internal rotation, the capsule can become a little convex in normal hips; whereas in flexion, abduction and external rotation (antalgic position) less fluid might be seen under the capsule.

A time delay between the onset of complaints and positive ultrasound findings is possible; as such if US is inconclusive, repeat exam(s) would always be recommended.

Assessing hip joint effusion in a 50-year-old woman with pain radiating to the anterior thigh 7.2

a 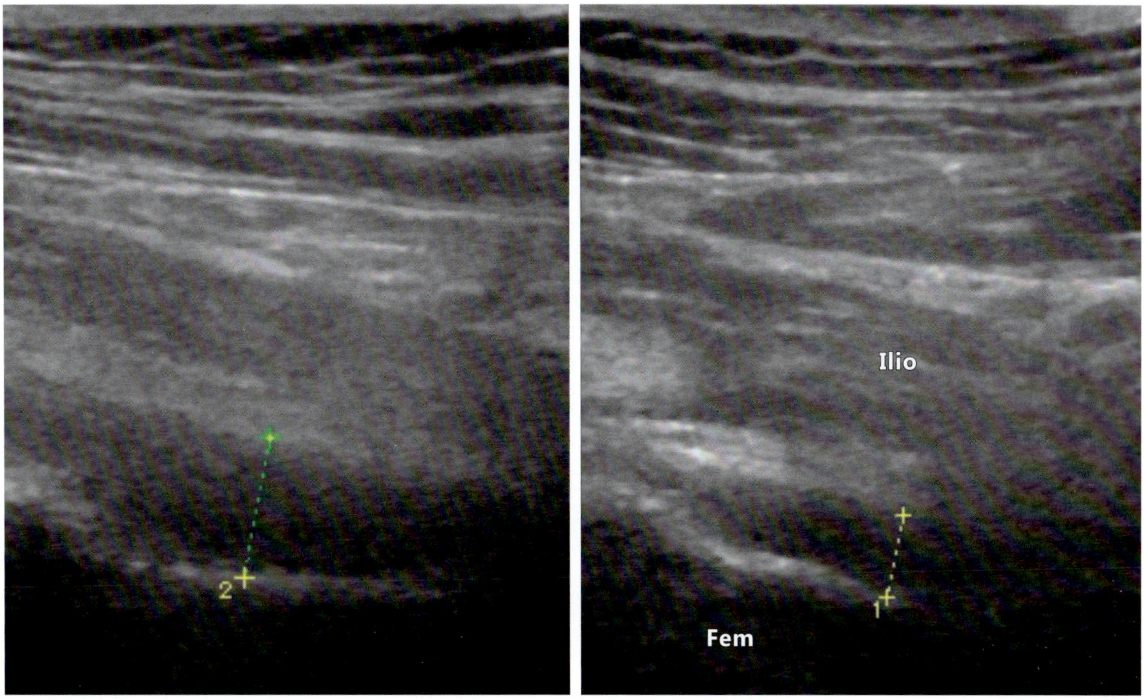 b

Longitudinal US images show the quantitative measurement of the capsular distension which can be used to assess joint fluid. Symptomatic side (**a**). Normal side (**b**).

Fem femur
Ilio iliopsoas

Expert note

While measuring the distance between the femoral neck and the joint capsule, either certain cut-off values (<7 mm) or side-to-side differences (<1 mm) needs to be taken into account [1]. Indisputably, the position of the lower limbs should be symmetrical for optimum comparison and the measurements should be taken at the same areas.

7.3 Synovial effusion in a 60-year-old obese patient with chronic hip pain and limping

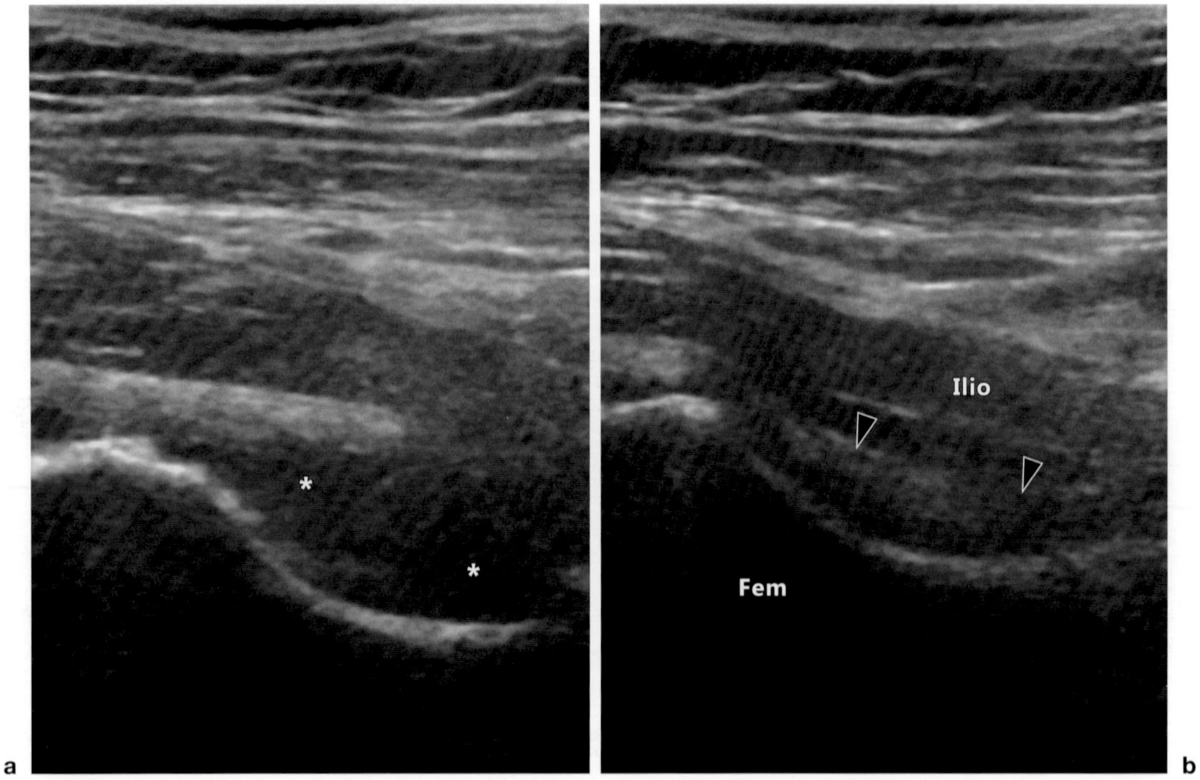

Longitudinal US image shows large amount of fluid collection (*asterisks*) within the hip joint (**a**). Normal anterior synovial recess (*arrowheads*) on the contralateral side (**b**).

Fem femur
Ilio iliopsoas

Intra-articular effusion in a 50-year-old woman with groin pain especially during passive hip internal rotation

7.4

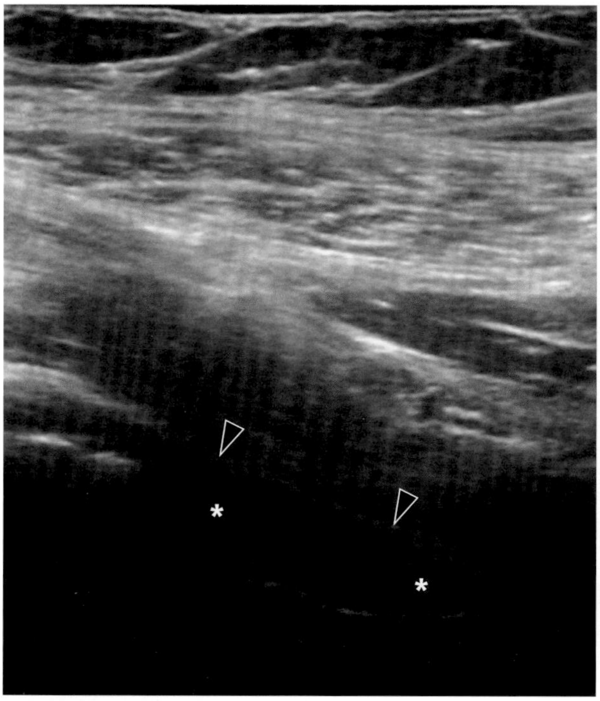

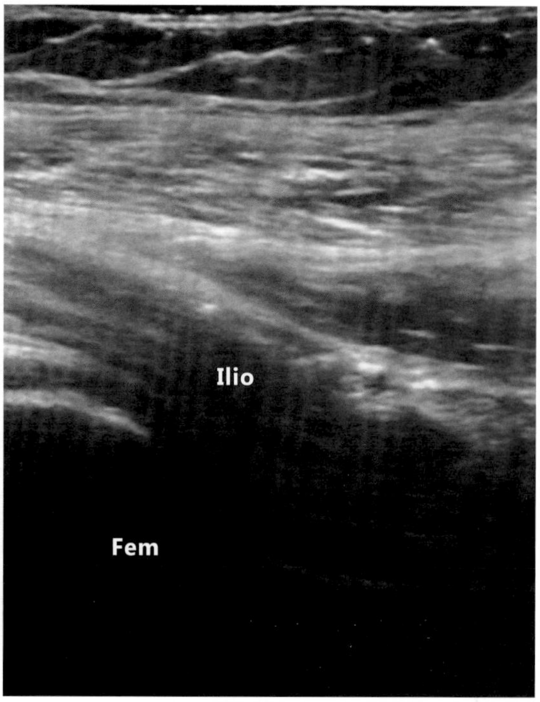

Longitudinal US image obtained over the anterior hip joint reveals increased intra-articular fluid (*asterisks*) distending the anterior synovial recess (*arrowheads*) (**a**). Normal side (**b**).

Fem femur
Ilio iliopsoas

Expert note

It is not always possible to have a sharp image of the cortex; for instance, one can look for a cortical bump, indicative of a Cam-type femoroacetabular impingement.
Although the anterior aspect of the hip joint is best evaluated in supine position (with the legs extended and in mild external rotation), strong correlations were found between magnetic resonance imaging and US measurements especially in 20° internal rotation of the hip joint in patients with Cam-type impingement [2].

Video 9

7.5 Bilateral synovitis of the hip joints in a 82-year-old woman with a diagnosis of polymyalgia rheumatica

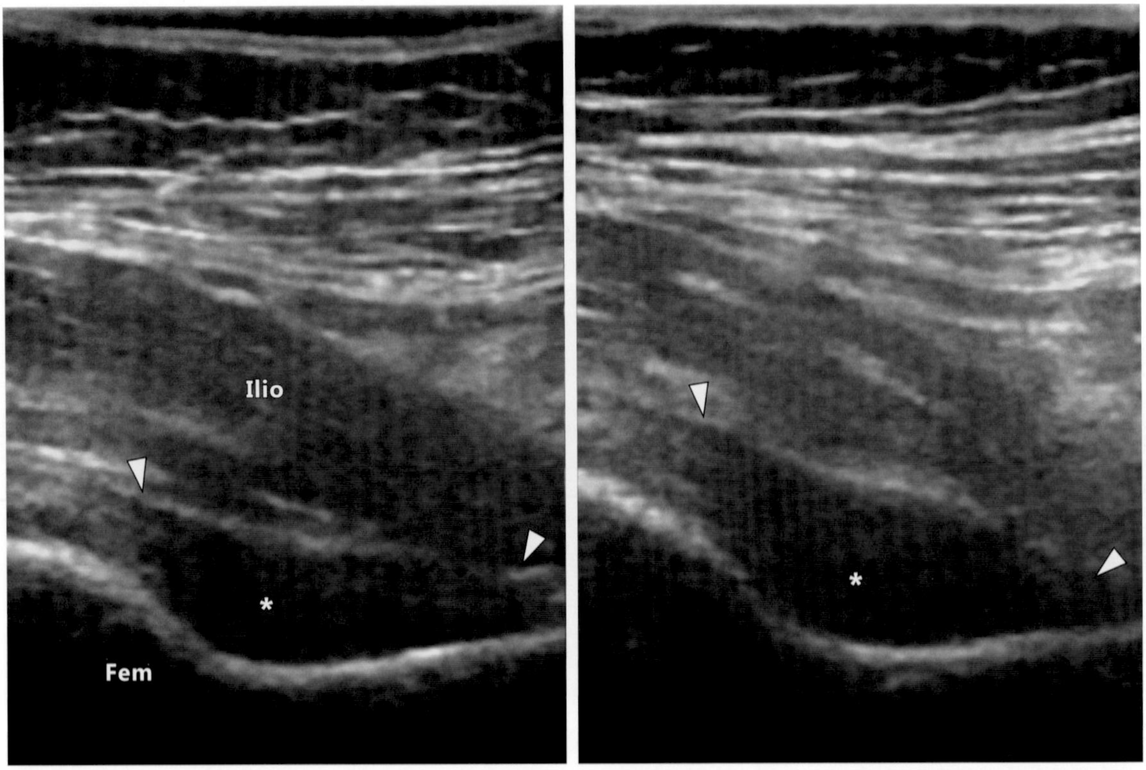

Longitudinal US images demonstrate effusion (*asterisks*) distending the joint capsule (*arrowheads*) more predominant on the right image.

Fem femur
Ilio iliopsoas

Expert note

The challenge for imaging fluid in the hip joint would again be related with its deep localization. While compression would be necessary for better scanning of the deep tissues especially in obese subjects, it would be a little misleading since fluid might be displaced and not well visualized on the femoral neck.

Considering the fact that little is known about normal aging and how much fluid can be present in asymptomatic joints of older people (>70 years); history, clinical exam and US imaging should definitely be interpreted together.

Bilateral hip joint synovitis in a 60-year-old patient with polymyalgia rheumatica 7.6

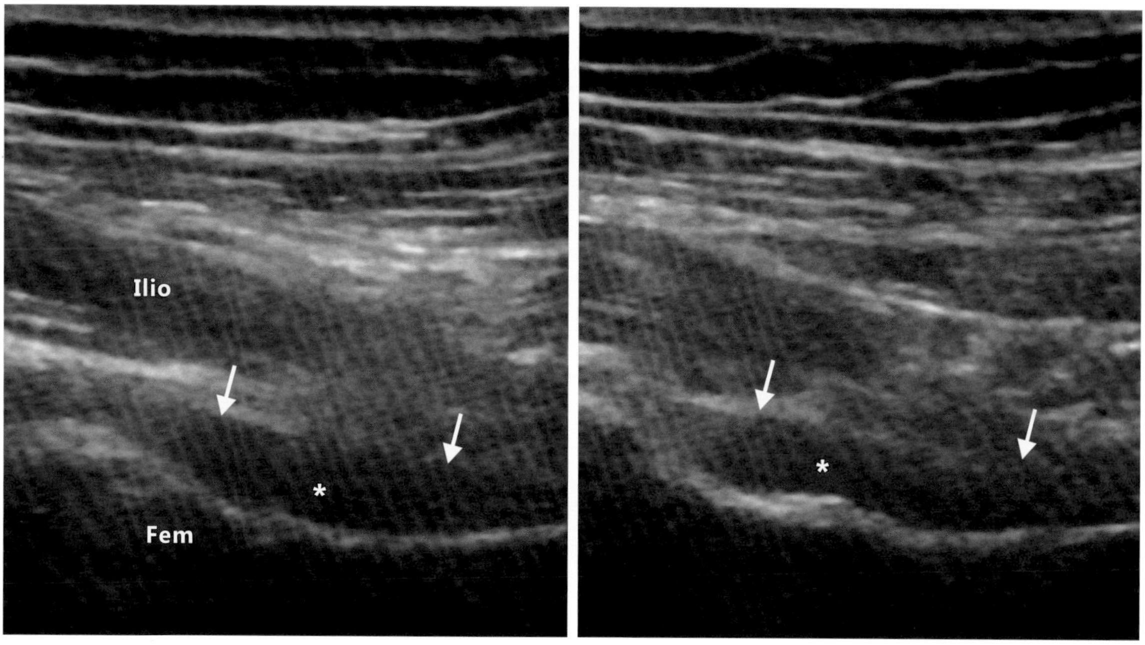

a b

Longitudinal US images show intra-articular effusion (*asterisks*) distending the anterior joint capsules (*arrows*) on both sides.

Fem femur
Ilio iliopsoas

Expert note

In addition to relevant shoulder findings (subdeltoid bursitis, biceps tenosynovitis, glenohumeral synovitis), the presence of hip effusion and/or trochanteric bursitis have been accepted to improve the specificity of the diagnosis in polymyalgia rheumatica [3].

7.7 Degenerative hip joint in a 75-year-old woman with chronic groin pain and limping

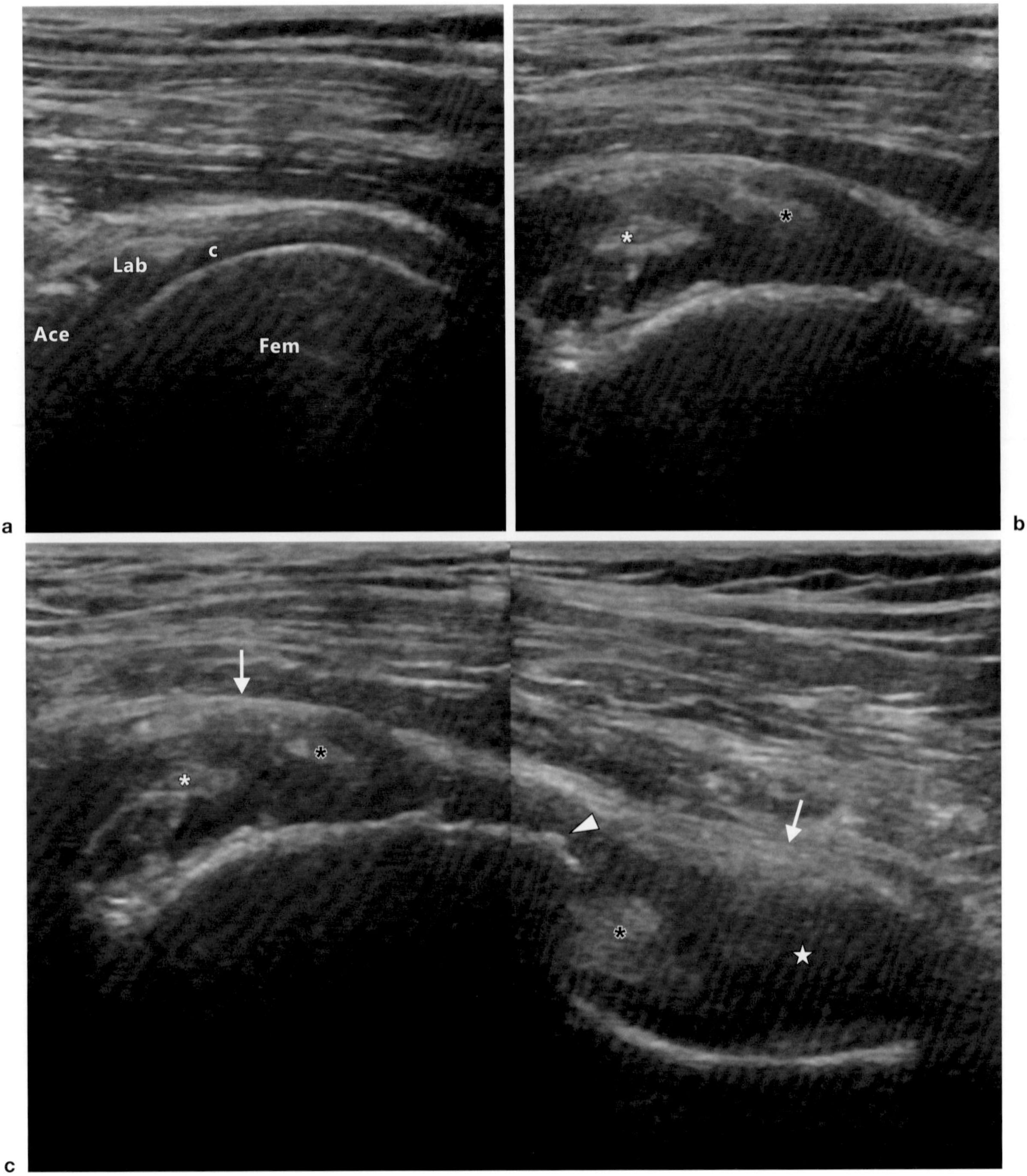

When compared with the normal side (**a**), longitudinal proximal (**b**) and split-screen (**c**) US images show swollen and irregular labrum (*white asterisks*), synovial hypertrophy (*black asterisks*) and hypoechoic effusion (*star*) distending the anterior joint recess (*arrows*).
Also, note that an anterior osteophyte (*arrowhead*) appears as a hyperechoic irregularity between the head and neck of the femur (**Fem**).

Ace acetabulum
c cartilage
Lab labrum

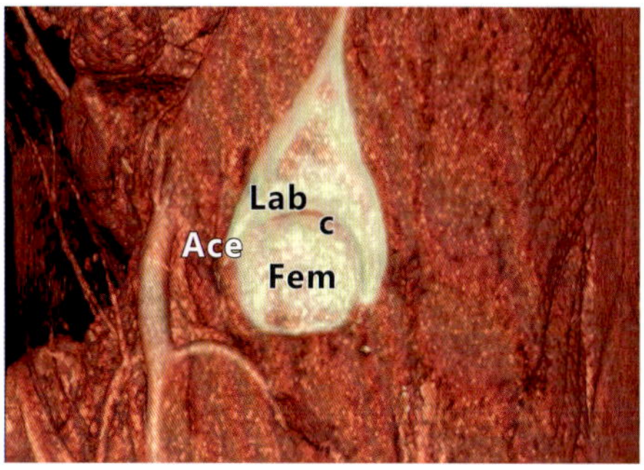

Expert note

Dynamic imaging can be used to evaluate whether the degenerated labrum or the osteophyte causes any impingement during hip movements.

7.8 Hip labral tear in an elite athlete with anterior groin pain radiating to the medial knee

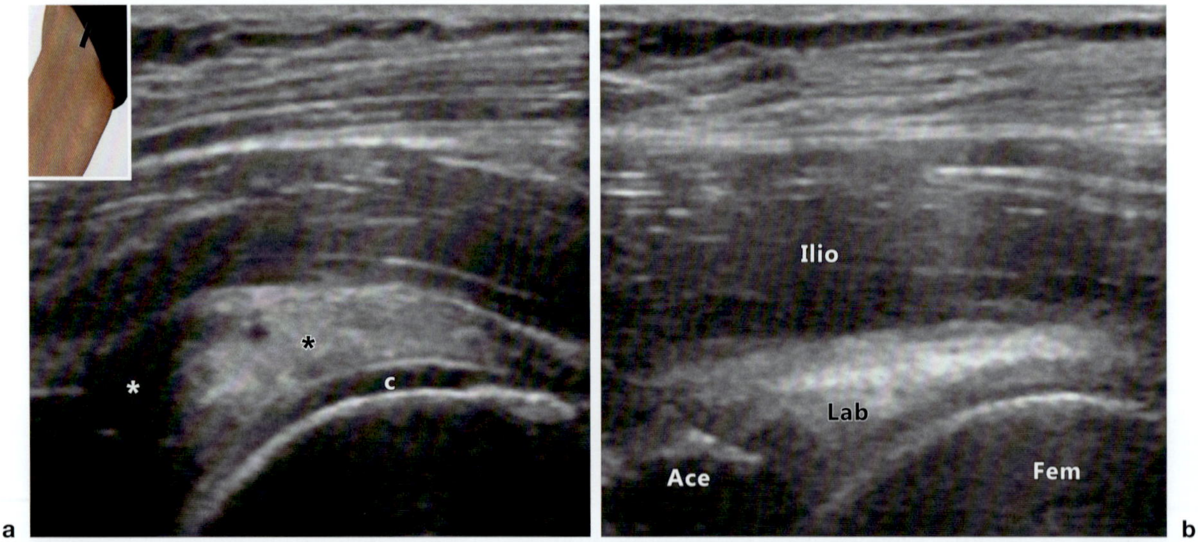

Anterior longitudinal US image demonstrates an enlarged and hypoechoic labrum (**Lab**) (*black asterisk*) with a partial tear (*white asterisk*) at its proximal attachment site (**a**). Normal side (**b**).

Ace acetabulum
c cartilage
Fem femur
Ilio iliopsoas

Acetabular labral tear in a 33-year-old man with groin pain worse after strenuous activities 7.9

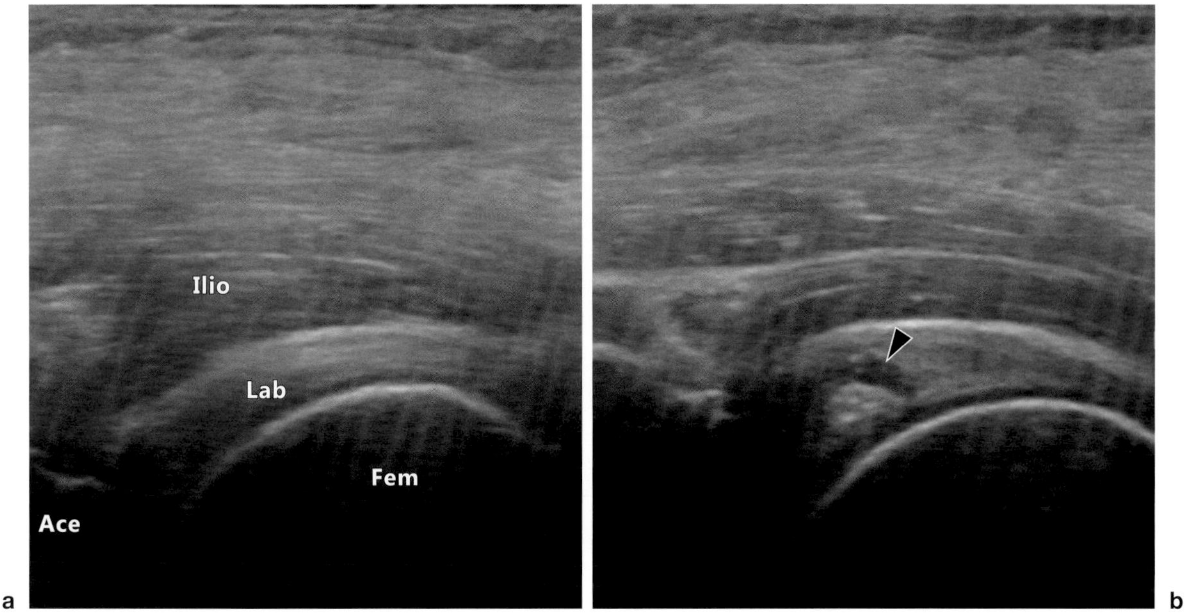

When compared with the normal side (**a**), longitudinal US image shows edematous labrum (**Lab**) with a partial defect (*arrowhead*) (**b**).

Ace acetabulum
Fem femur
Ilio iliopsoas

Expert note

Acetabular labral tears usually ensue due to repetitive trauma; likewise, they might occur as a result of traction from the iliopsoas or rectus femoris insertions as well [4].

7.10 Acetabular paralabral cyst in a 30-year-old professional football player with persistent hip pain

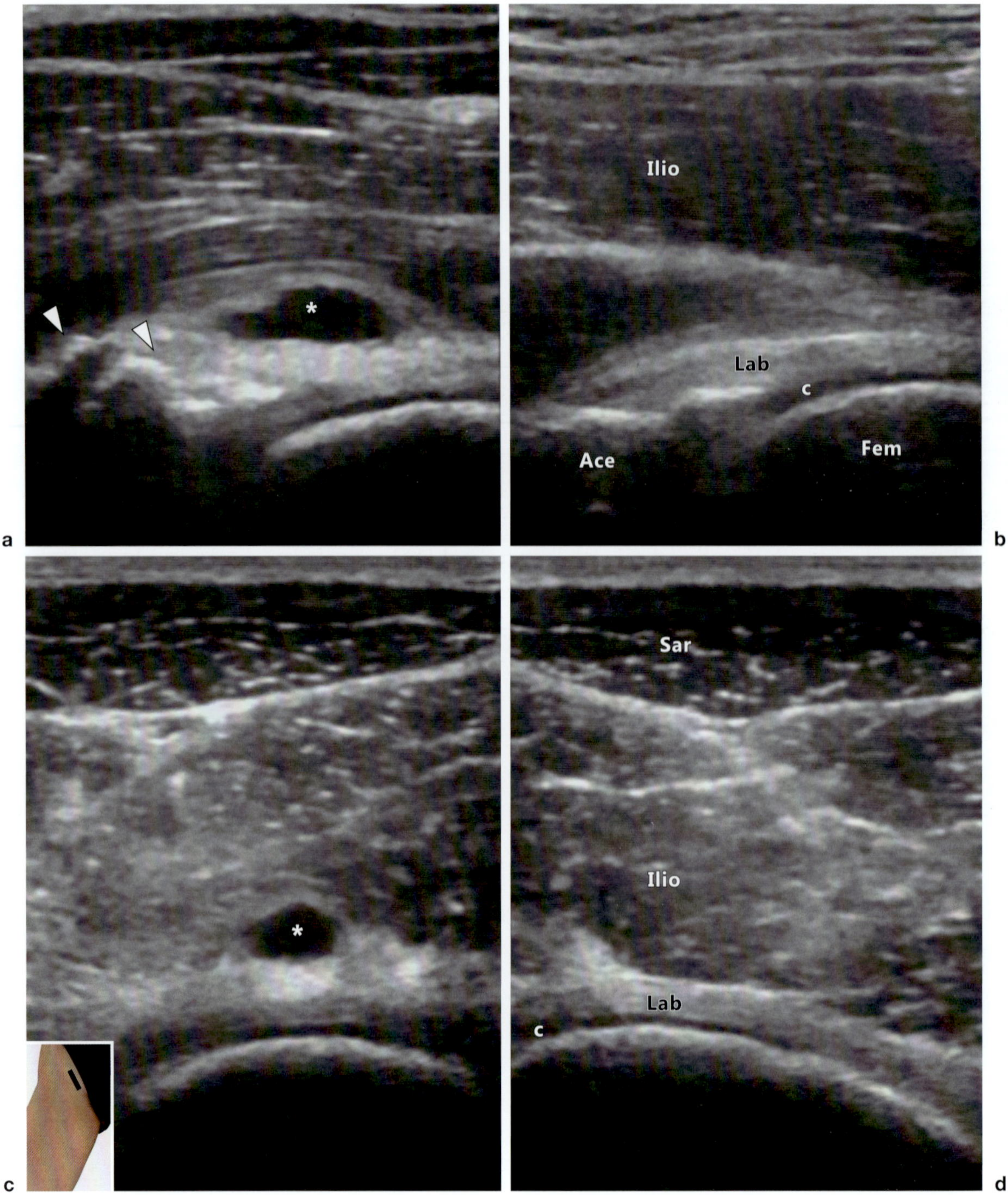

Anterior longitudinal imaging shows the paralabral cyst (*asterisk*) and cortical irregularities on the acetabulum (**Ace**) (*arrowheads*) (**a**). Normal side (**b**). Short-axis imaging also confirms the cyst (**c**). Normal side (**d**).

c	cartilage	**Lab**	labrum
Fem	femur	**Sar**	sartorius
Ilio	iliopsoas		

Expert note

By sono-palpation, US imaging can be used to confirm whether or not the observed lesion is actually the real cause of the patient's painful complaints. For sure, this would also be important as regards the treatment plan.

7.11 Healing process of the iliopsoas muscle strain in a 24-year-old professional athlete

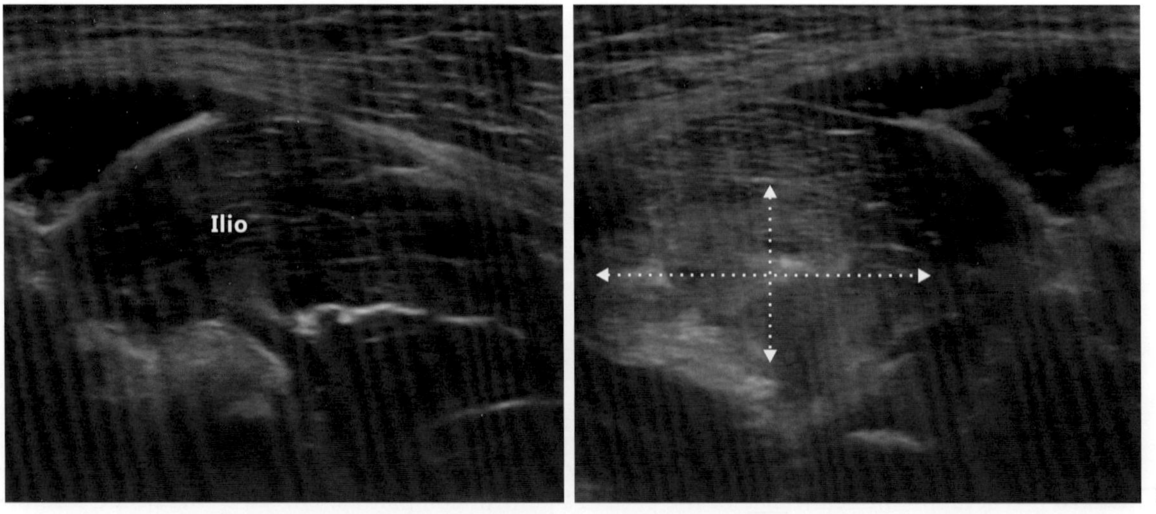

a b

He had painful snapping sensation during hip motions or walking.

When compared with the normal side (**a**), axial US image obtained over the anterior hip region shows an intramuscular, relatively well-marginated hyperechoic zone (*dashed arrows*) representing fibrous healing within the iliopsoas muscle (**b**).

Ilio iliopsoas

Expert note

Especially in subjects who are prone to overuse injuries (e.g. athletes), it is not uncommon to disclose otherwise subtle pathologies during thorough imaging. For instance, this patient was actually referred for snapping hip and accordingly dynamic assessment for the intra- and extra- articular causes had initially been performed. Meanwhile, as the US examination was extended in light of the simultaneous questioning for antecedent injuries; the above described lesion could have then been unmasked. In this sense, we strongly believe that 'dynamic imaging' does also pertain to 'interactive imaging' metaphorically.

Tensor fascia lata strain in a 41-year-old man with chronic pain on the lateral hip and thigh

7.12

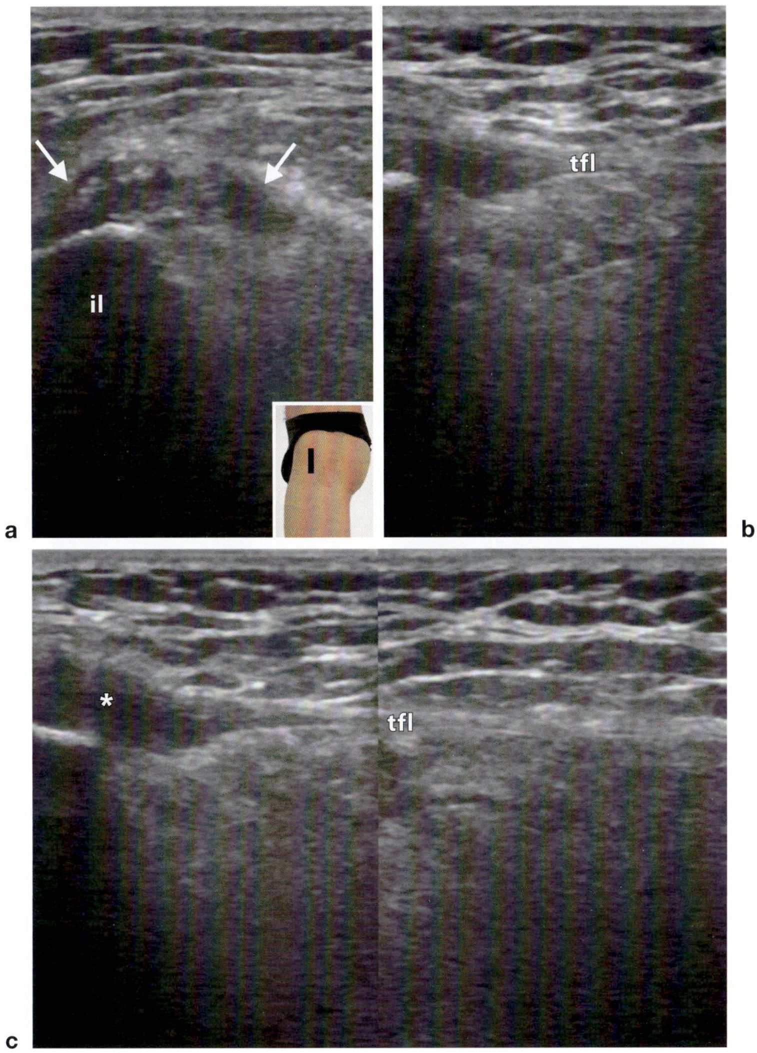

Ober test was positive in physical examination.

Axial imaging over the lateral side of the iliac crest (**il**) shows thickened tensor fascia lata (**tfl**) with heterogenous echogenicity (*arrows*) (**a**). When compared with the normal side (**b**), split-screen longitudinal imaging also depicted the swollen muscle at its origin (*asterisk*) (**c**).

Expert note

Dynamic US imaging can also be coupled with physical examination using specific maneuvers (as mentioned above). This is also an area of interest after the harvesting of bone grafts when similar abnormalities can be found as well.

7.13 Bilateral trochanteric bursitis in a 63-year-old woman with lateral hip pain and tenderness

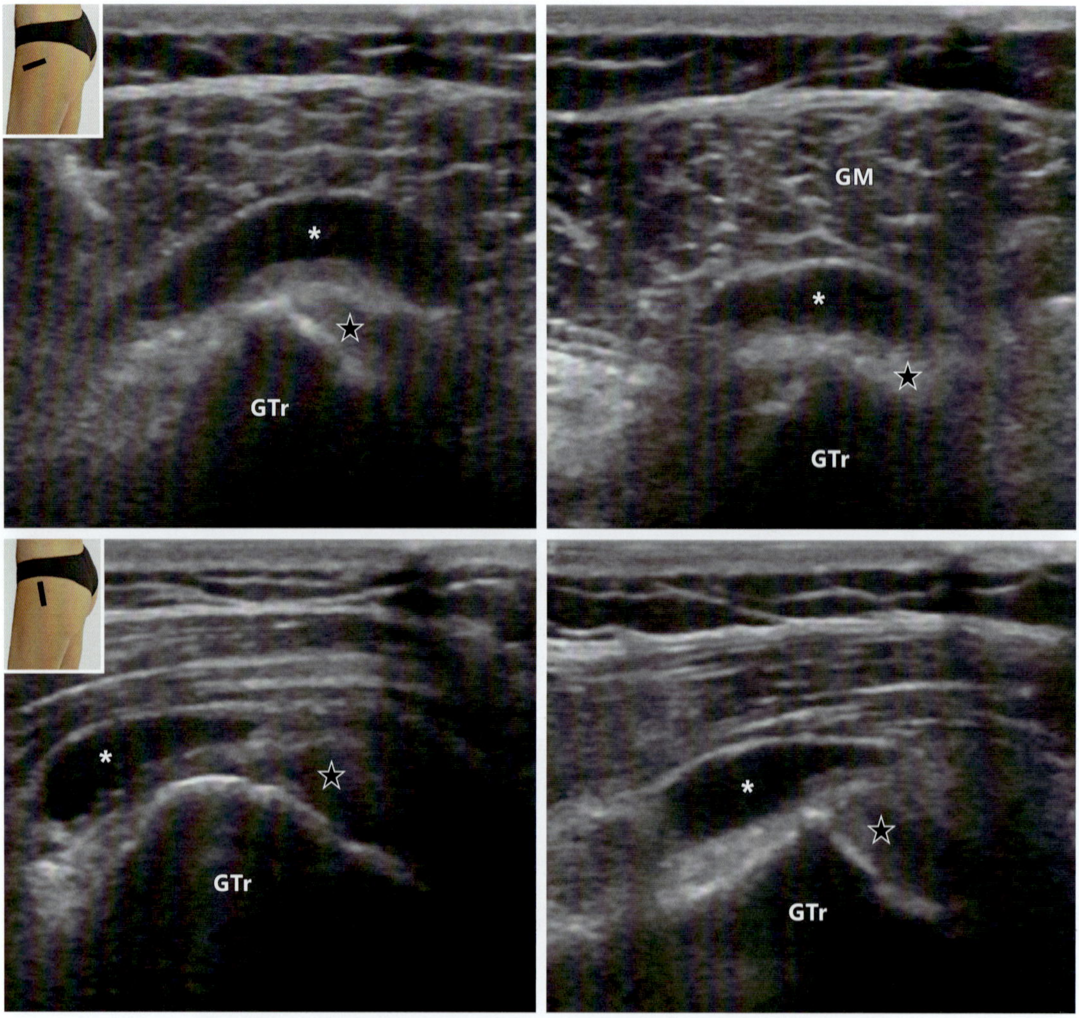

Lateral axial (**a**, **b**) and longitudinal (**c**, **d**) images demonstrate well-defined anechoic fluid collections (*asterisks*) located between the deep fibers of the gluteus maximus (**GM**) muscle, gluteus medius tendon (*stars*) and posterosuperior aspect of the greater trochanter (**GTr**).

Expert note

The sonographer should again balance between the need for optimum compression (to scan deep tissues) and the attention to keep fluid undisplaced. In the trochanteric region, bursae can be found at different layers i.e. between the hip rotator cuff tendons and overlying gluteus maximus muscle, between the gluteal tendons, and between the tendons and greater trochanter [5].

Of note, in patients referred for "trochanteritis", bursitis is much more seldom than tendinopathies.

A 27-year-old woman who complained for lateral hip pain

7.14

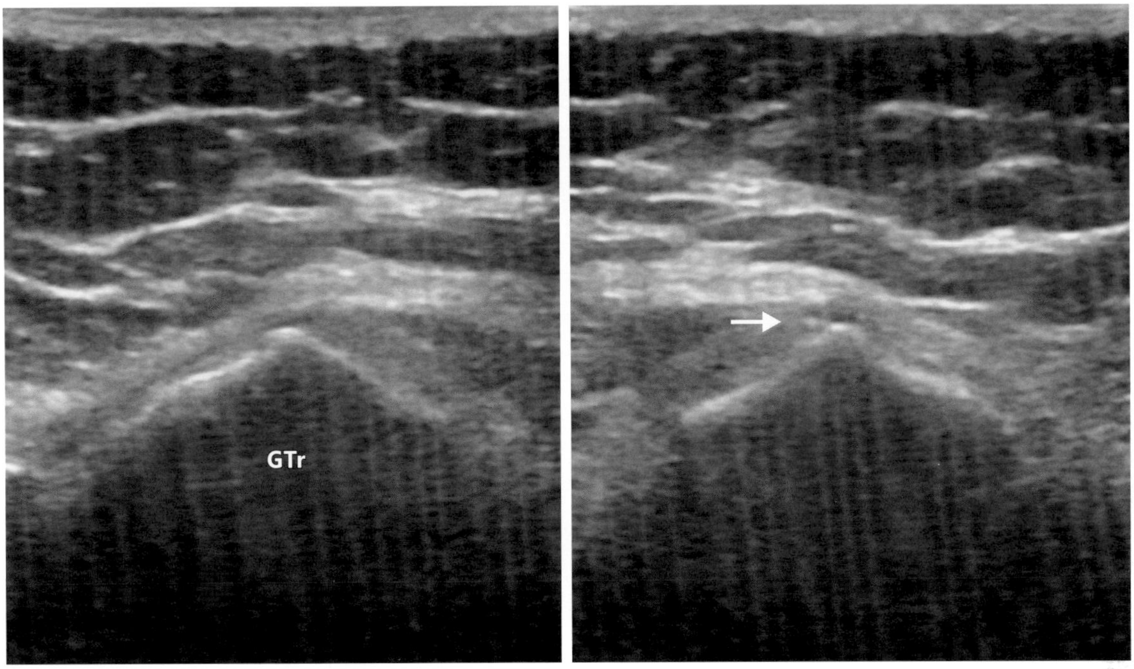

a b

When compared with the less symptomatic side (**a**), axial US image over the greater trochanter (**GTr**) demonstrates a small bony spur (*arrow*), painful with sono-palpation (**b**).

Expert note

Especially in obese subjects, sono-palpation is again quite helpful to attribute the "vague lateral hip pain" to trochanteric pathologies.

Although examination protocols usually suggest to scan the patient while lying on one side [6], this makes it difficult to compare the two sides and can also flatten small fluid collections. Therefore, having the patient lie in supine position during imaging and -if necessary- on one side during the injection would be easier.

7.15 Calcific gluteus medius tendinopathy in an obese 67-year-old woman with lateral hip pain

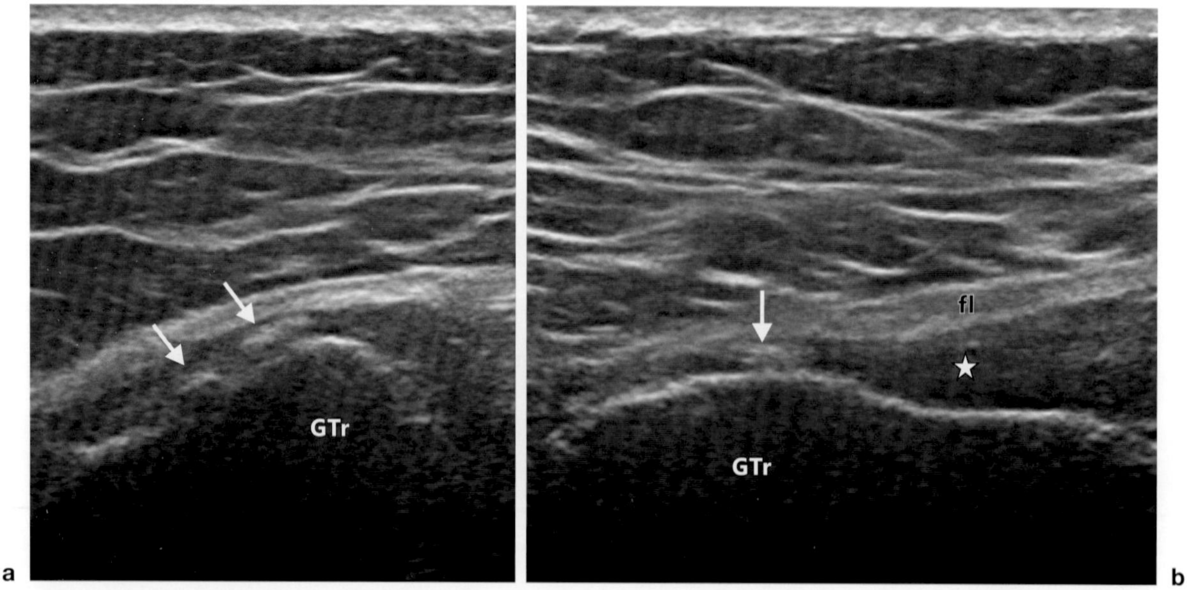

Lateral axial (**a**) and longitudinal (**b**) images obtained over the greater trochanter (**GTr**) illustrate irregular calcifications (*arrows*) within the gluteus medius tendon (*star*) insertion.

fl fascia lata

Osteitis pubis in a young professional football player with chronic groin pain

7.16

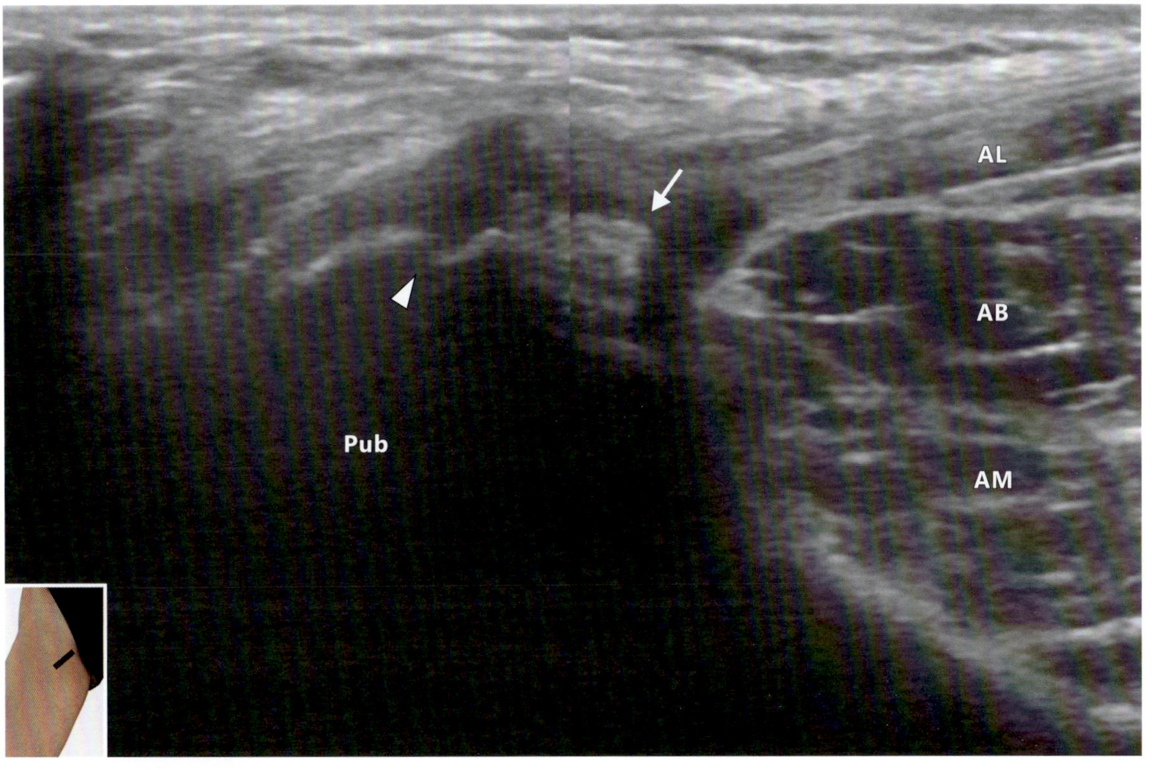

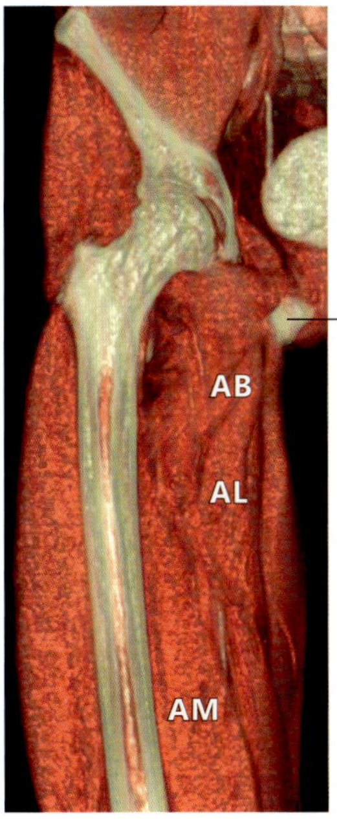

Pubic region was tender to palpation and painful on resisted adduction.

Split-screen longitudinal US imaging shows cortical irregularity (*arrowhead*) and calcification (*arrow*) at the attachment site of the hip adductor muscles.

AB	adductor brevis
AL	adductor longus
AM	adductor magnus
Pub	pubis

7.17 Osteitis pubis in a young football player who suffered from pubalgia only during sports play

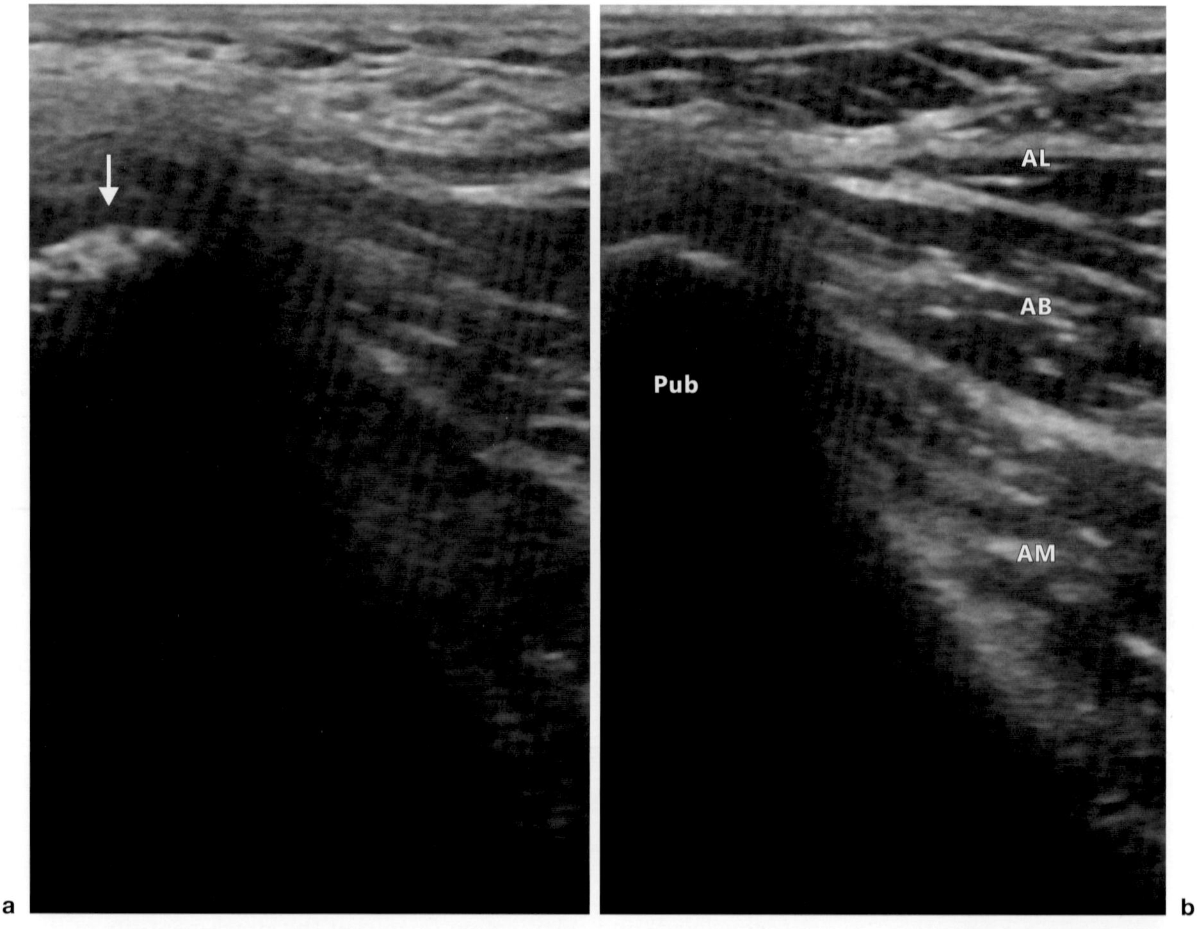

Longitudinal US imaging shows cortical irregularity (*arrow*) in the pubis (**a**). Normal side (**b**).

AB adductor brevis
AL adductor longus
AM adductor magnus
Pub pubis

Bilateral osteitis pubis in a professional athlete with chronic pelvic pain **7.18**

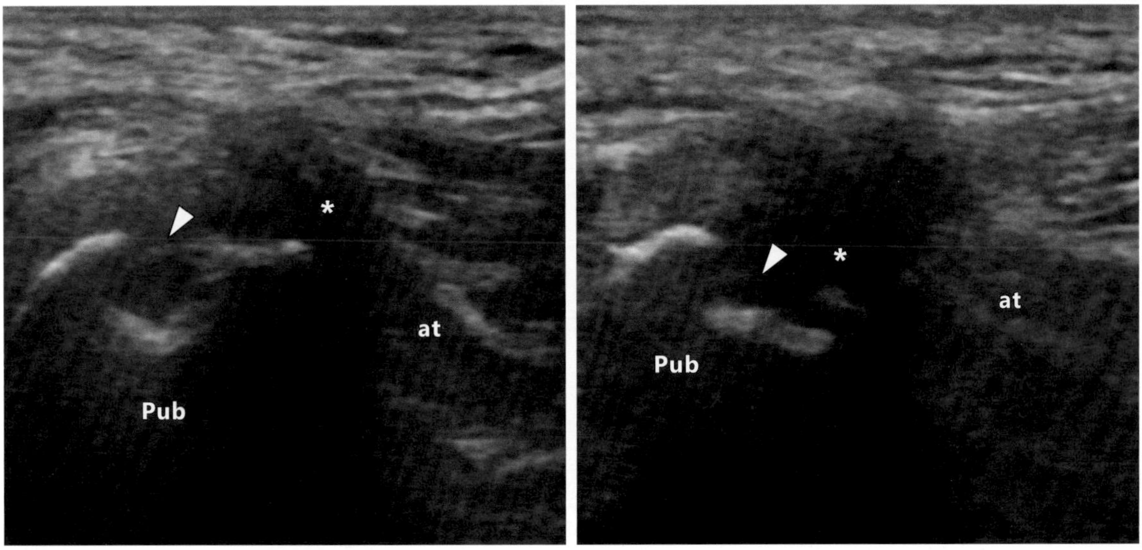

a b

Longitudinal images demonstrate cortical erosions and irregularities (*arrowheads*) on the pubis (**Pub**) with an/hypoechoic and swollen adductor tendons (**at**) at their origin (*asterisks*).

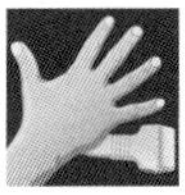

Expert note

Although the adductor longus tendon is the most commonly affected tendon among adductors pathologies, its significant rupture may also involve the superficial fibers of the adductor brevis tendon [7].

7.19 Normal view of the symphysis pubis

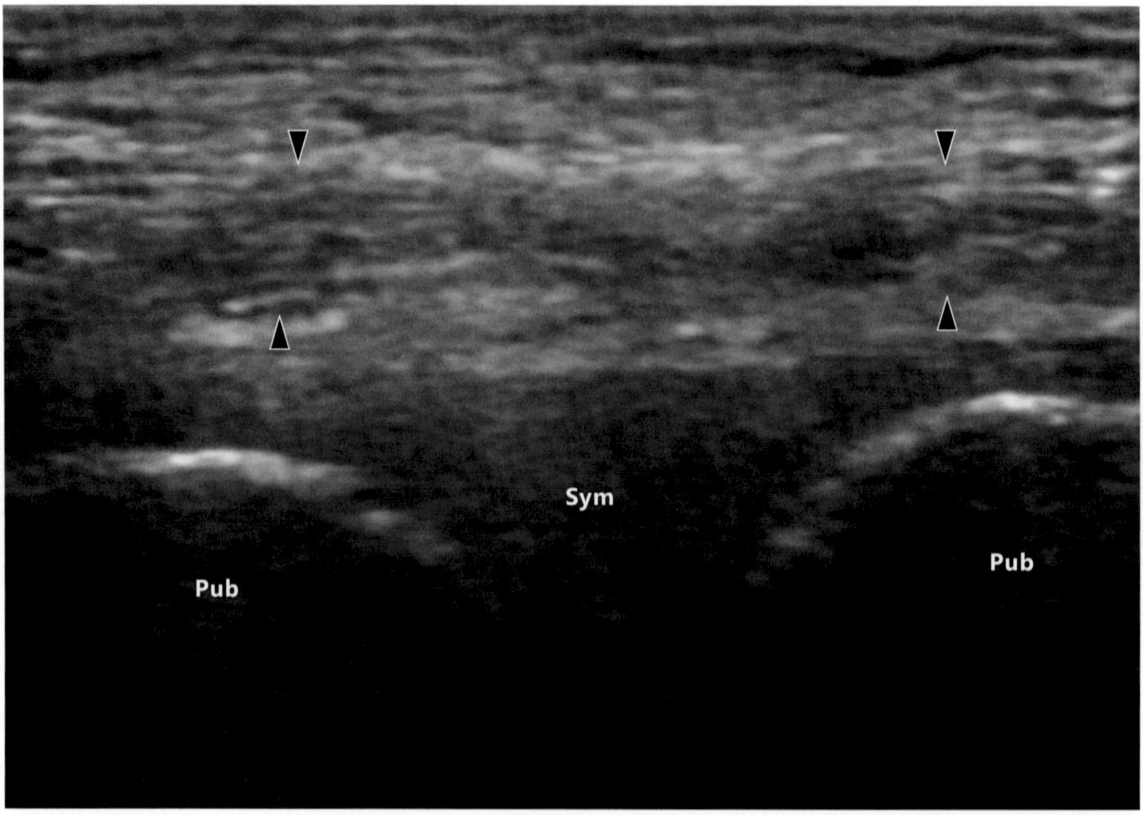

Axial US image demonstrates the normal appearance of distal rectus abdominis muscle (*arrowheads*) in relation with symphysis pubis (**Sym**).

Pub pubis

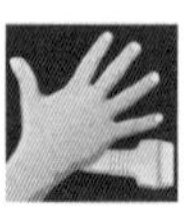

Expert note

Given the close proximity of the attachment sites of adductor and abdominal muscles, scanning from the rectus site should not be overlooked in pubalgia [8]. Pubic hair can make the examination of this area technically difficult whereby shaving may be necessary.

REFERENCES

1. Schmidt WA, Schmidt H, Schicke B, Gromnica-Ihle E. Standard reference values for musculoskeletal ultrasonography. Ann Rheum Dis. 2004; 63: 988-94.
2. Lerch S, Kasperczyk A, Warnecke J, Berndt T, Rühmann O. Evaluation of Cam-type femoroacetabular impingement by ultrasound. Int Orthop. 2013; 37: 783-8.
3. Dasgupta B, Cimmino MA, Kremers HM et al. 2012 Provisional classification criteria for polymyalgia rheumatica: a European League Against Rheumatism/American College of Rheumatology collaborative initiative. Arthritis Rheum. 2012; 64: 943-54.
4. Serner A, Tol JL, Jomaah N, Weir A, Whiteley R, Thorborg K, et al. Diagnosis of acute groin injuries: a prospective study of 110 athletes. Am J Sports Med. 2015; 43: 1857-64.
5. Steyaert A. Ultrasound evaluation of the hip. In: Özçakar L, De Muynck M, editors. Musculoskeletal ultrasound in physical and rehabilitation medicine. Milan: Edi.Ermes; 2014. p. 87-97.
6. Özçakar L, Kara M, Chang KV, Akkaya N, Hung CY, Tok F, et al. EURO-MUSCULUS/USPRM basic scanning protocols for hip. Eur J Phys Rehabil Med. 2015; 51: 635-40.
7. Steyaert A. Ultrasound evaluation of the hip. In: Özçakar L, De Muynck M, editors. Musculoskeletal ultrasound in physical and rehabilitation medicine. Milan: Edi.Ermes; 2014. p. 87-97.
8. Özçakar L, Utku B. Ultrasound images of groin pain in the athlete: a pictorial essay. PM R. 2014; 6: 753-6.

Thigh 8

- **Rectus femoris tendon -** Proximal
- **Quadriceps femoris muscle**
- **Sartorius muscle**
- **Hamstring muscles**
- **Adductor muscles**
- **Subcutaneous tissue**

8.1 Rectus femoris tendinopathy in a 32-year-old elite athlete with hip pain after long-distance running

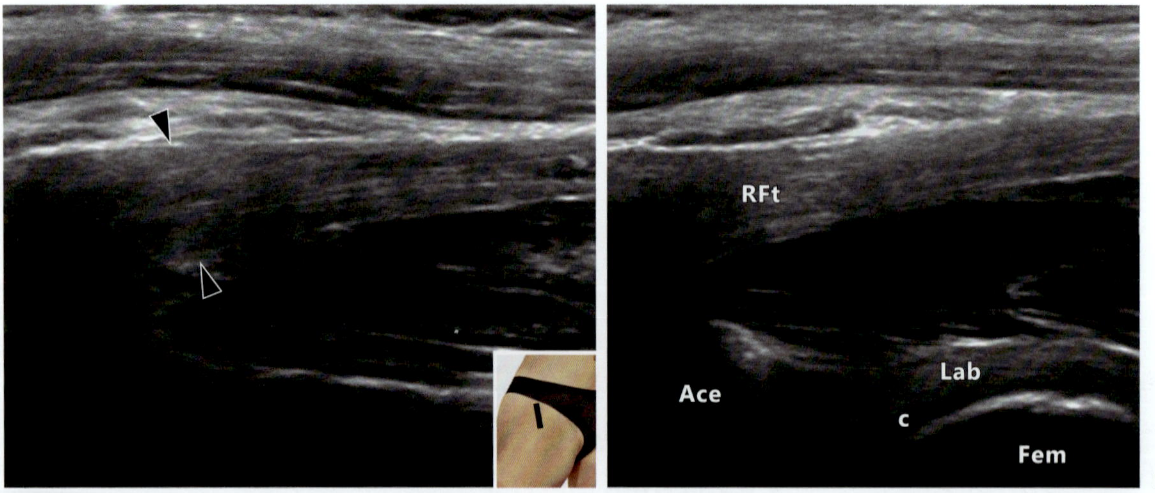

a b

Longitudinal US imaging shows thickened and a little more hypoechoic rectus femoris tendon (**RFt**) (*arrowheads*) at its origin (**a**). Normal side (**b**).

Ace acetabulum
c cartilage
Fem femur
Lab labrum

Expert note

For sure, when measuring the thickness of a tendon (an oval structure), axial view would be used to ensure its thickest point.

Type 1 strain of rectus femoris muscle in a young man after jumping

8.2

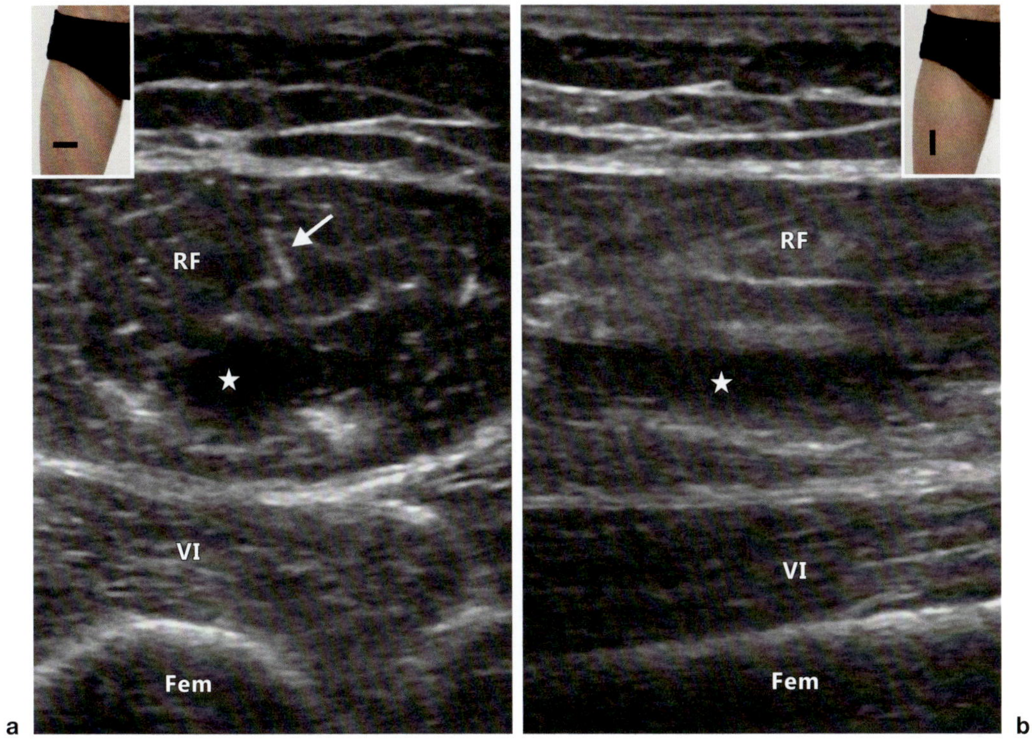

Anterior axial (**a**) and longitudinal (**b**) US images over the mid-thigh reveal hypoechoic hematoma (*stars*) in the rectus femoris muscle (**RF**). *Arrow* indicates the central aponeurosis.

Fem femur
VI vastus intermedius

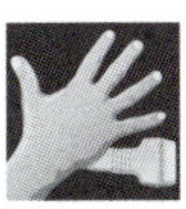

Expert note

The characteristic appearance of muscle tissue is hyperechoic dots on an anechoic background ('starry sky') in the axial view and parallel hyperechoic lines in the longitudinal view. While the hyperechoic parts correspond to the (water-poor) fibroadipose septa, anechoic parts correspond to the contractile (water-rich) muscle fibers. In case of muscle injuries, the typical findings would simply pertain to disruption of these two patterns.
In case of ruptures due to sudden contraction/elongation, one should look near central (proximal) and deep (distal) aponeurosis of the rectus femoris muscle.
Based on the severity of trauma, proximal tears affecting the central aponeurosis are divided in three stages: Type 1, small size of the tear with an ill-defined hyperechoic area surrounding the central aponeurosis; Type 2, swollen rectus femoris with an irregular focal hypoechoic area related to the hematoma surrounding the central aponeurosis; Type 3, complete disruption of the inner muscle with a large fluid collection between the retracted belly and the outer muscle [1].

8.3 Type 2 tear of the rectus femoris muscle in a young athlete after repetitive unbalanced contractions during sports play

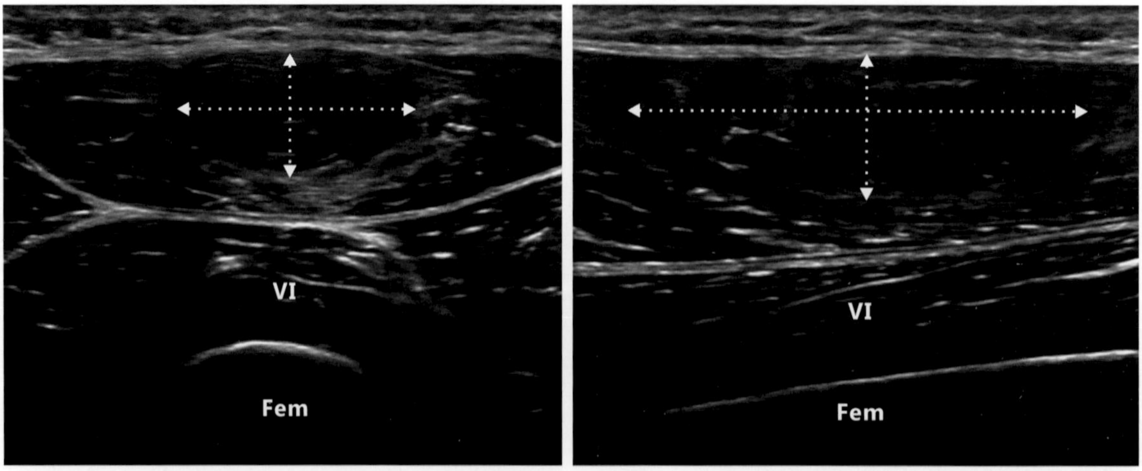

Axial (**a**) and longitudinal (**b**) US images over the anterior mid-thigh demonstrate an irregular (but relatively well-marginated) focal hypoechoic area related to organizing hematoma (*dashed arrows*) in the inner part of the rectus femoris muscle.

Fem femur
VI vastus intermedius

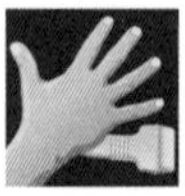

Expert note

The hyperechoic zone (gradually replacing the lesion) represents the fibrous tissue and the irregularly aligned muscle fibers in the healing process. Actually/eventually, both need to be appropriately aligned for a better restoration of the pennate structure and regain of the muscle strength. This image can probably serve as the main argument to perform stretching exercises during the follow up of strain lesions.

Vastus intermedius strain in a patient with anterior thigh pain after a forceful contraction **8.4**

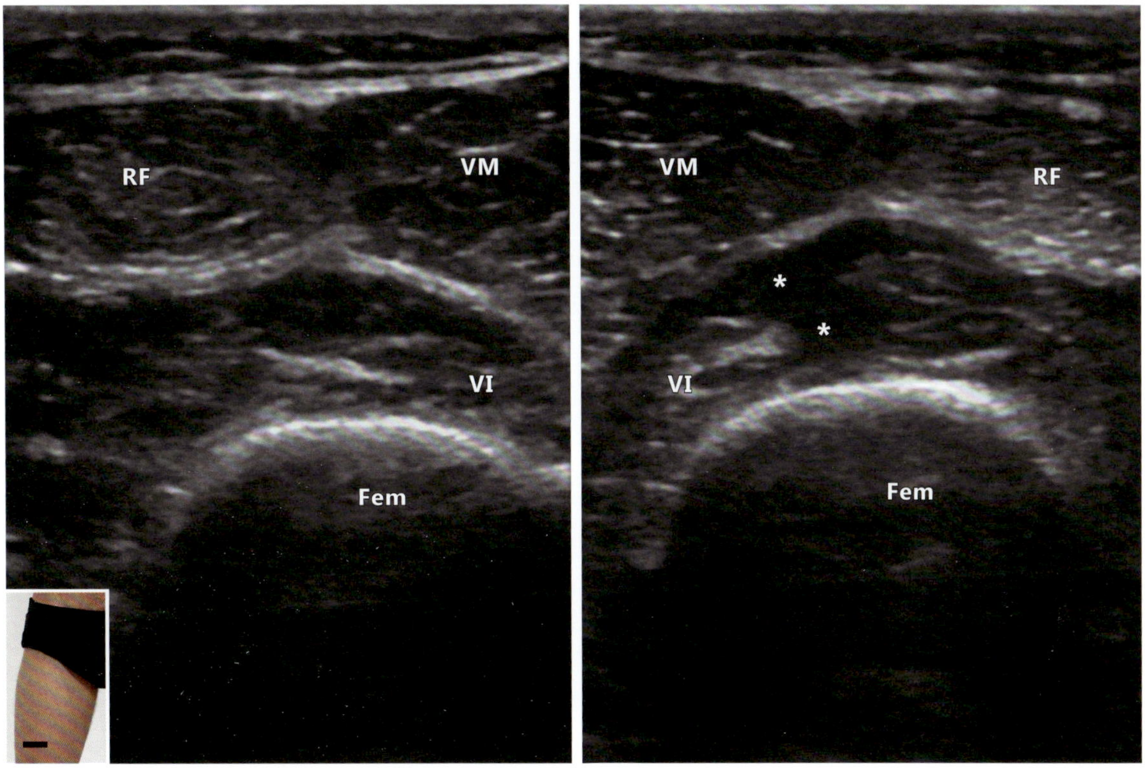

a b

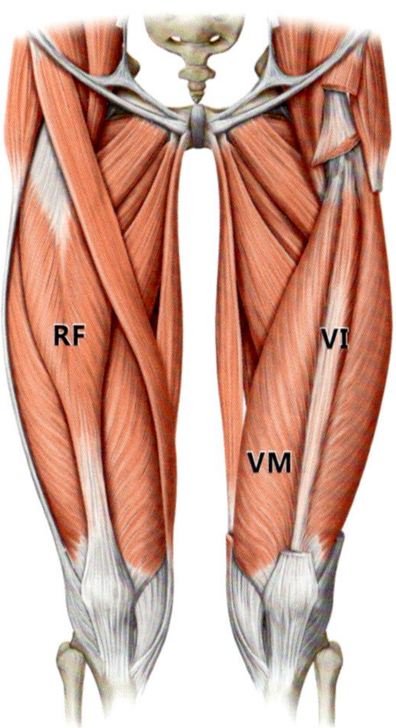

When compared with the normal side (**a**), anterior axial US image over the anterior thigh reflects anechoic hematoma (*asterisks*) of the vastus intermedius muscle (**VI**) (**b**).

Fem femur
RF rectus femoris
VM vastus medialis

Expert note

As regards strain lesions, the terms 'hematoma' and 'rupture' can usually be used interchangeably. Yet, if there is hematoma, there needs to be a preceding rupture; or if there is a rupture, hematoma is usually inevitable. Herewith, in mild injuries, the formation of a hematoma might be incomplete before 24-48 hours. As such, US examination is generally suggested to be undertaken thereafter [2].

8.5 Vastus medialis strain in a 35-year-old man with a history of blunt trauma to the anterior distal thigh

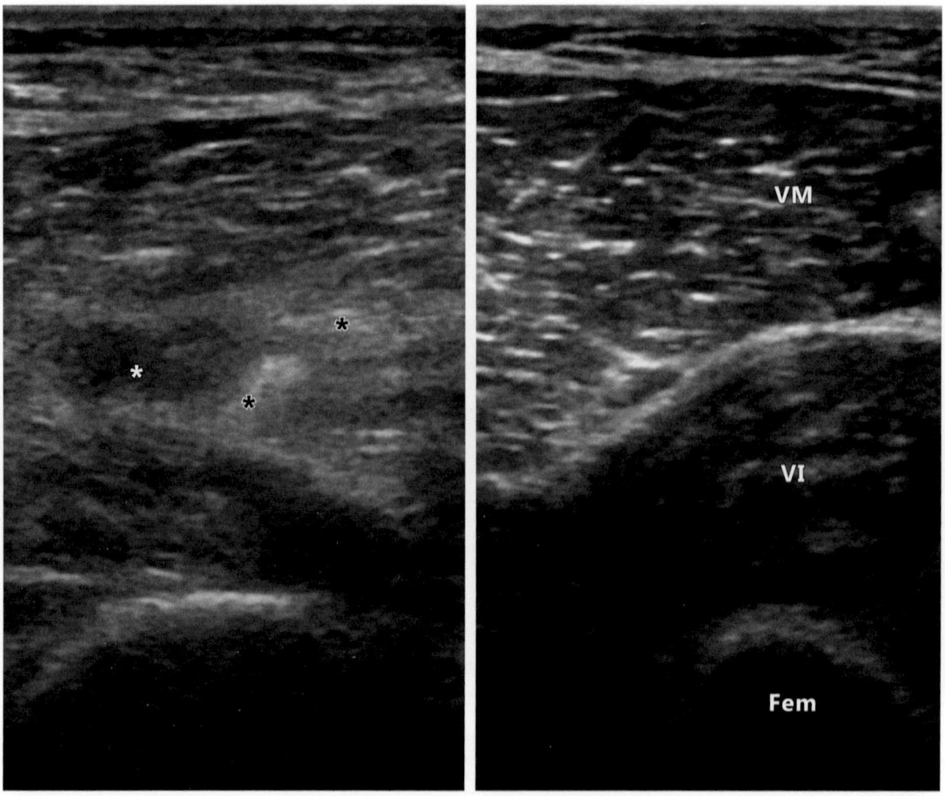

a b

Axial US image reveals hyperechoic fibrous tissue (*black asterisks*) and detachment (*white asterisk*) of the vastus medialis muscle (**VM**) fascicles (**a**). Normal side (**b**).

Fem femur
VI vastus intermedius

Expert note

In early phase of ectopic ossification, "zone phenomenon" can be seen i.e. a sequence of hypo/hyper/hypoechoic zones without shadows. At that time, x rays will still be negative. After 2-3 weeks with progressive maturation, peripheral hypoechoic zone may become hyperechoic in sheet-like or egg-shell-like calcified rim view which is considered in favor of myositis ossificans. The centre of the lesion and the underlying bony cortex cannot be seen due to posterior acoustic shadowing of the peripheral calcifications. At the peripheral zone, there is usually a marked Doppler activity [2, 3].

Although the characteristics of calcifications are specific, it is essential to obtain a standard radiograph in order to confirm the diagnosis and to exclude other calcified lesions, including paraosteal and soft-tissue sarcomas.

Myositis ossificans in a 35-year-old man with anterior thigh pain and prior contusion history **8.6**

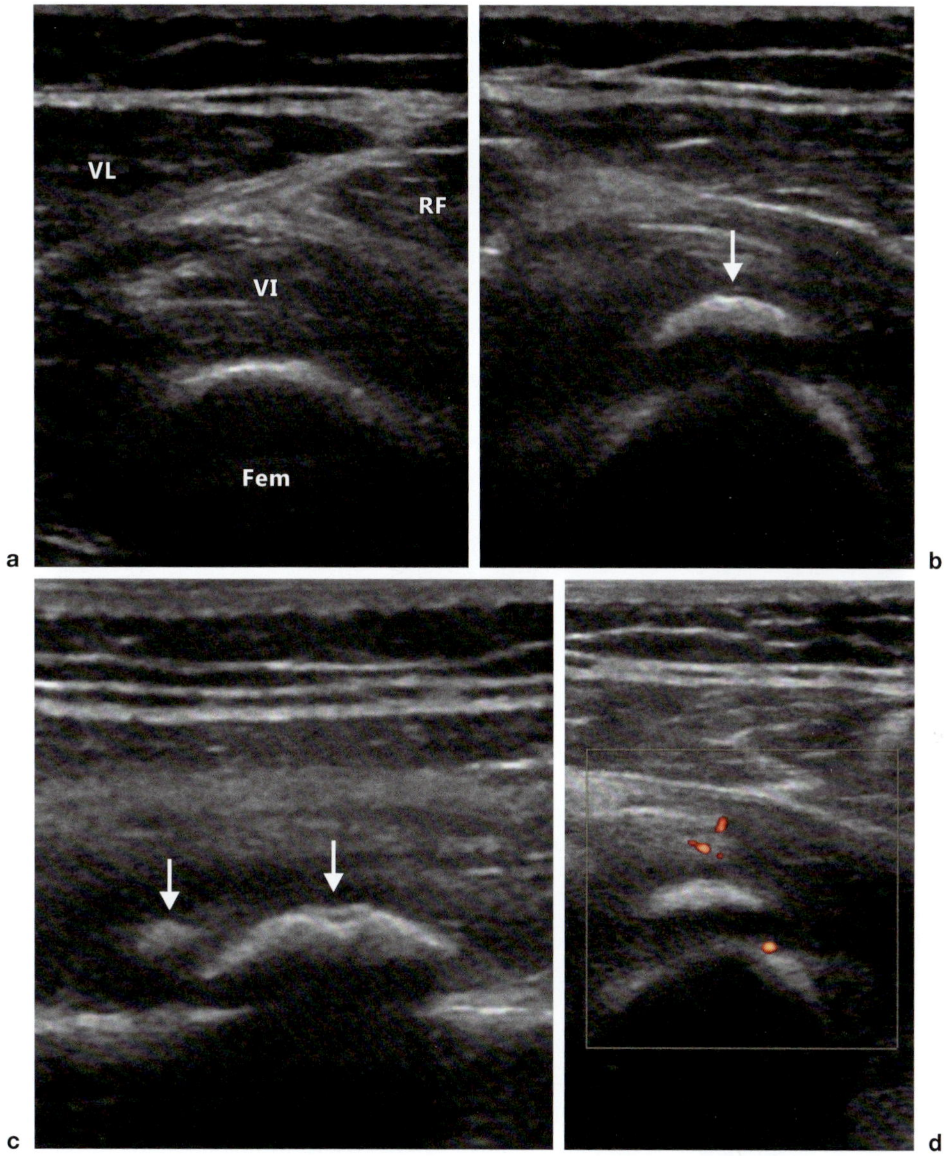

When compared with the normal side (**a**), axial (**b**) and longitudinal (**c**) US images over the quadriceps femoris muscle reveal hyperechoic calcifications (*arrows*) in the vastus intermedius (**VI**) reflecting myositis ossificans. Power Doppler image detects perilesional low flow states in the axial view (**d**).

Fem femur
RF rectus femoris
VL vastus lateralis

8.7 Myositis ossificans in a 23-year-old rugby player 6 weeks after the initial strain

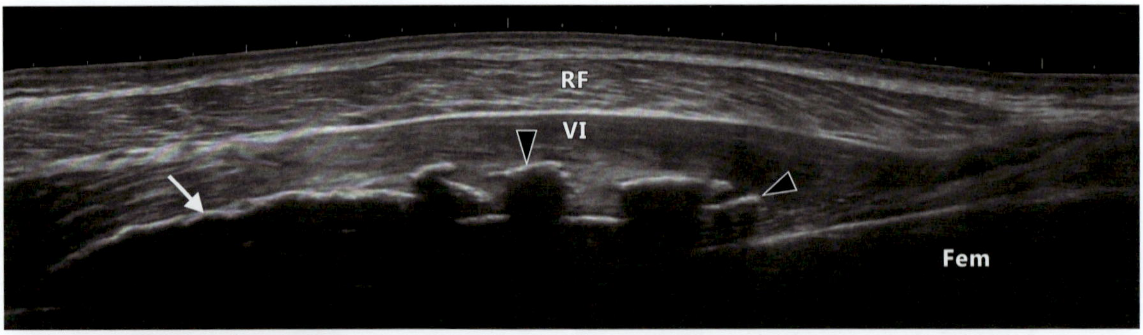

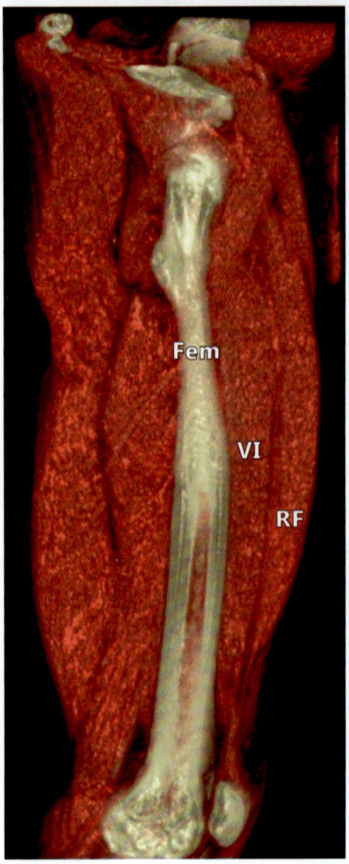

Longitudinal panoramic US image identifies a linear, huge ossification (*arrow*), and multiple irregular hyperechoic foci (*arrowheads*) adjacent and parallel to the femur (**Fem**) with posterior acoustic shadowing inside the vastus intermedius muscle (**VI**).

RF rectus femoris

Expert note

Aside from its role in the very early diagnosis of ossifications, repeat US imaging is definitely very convenient for the long term follow-up of these sports injuries. Especially ruptures in close proximity to bones (as here in vastus intermedius not rectus femoris) should be carefully watched in this regard.

Quadriceps femoris muscle atrophy after a contusion trauma to the femoral nerve in a 25-year-old man with a 6-week history of thigh pain **8.8**

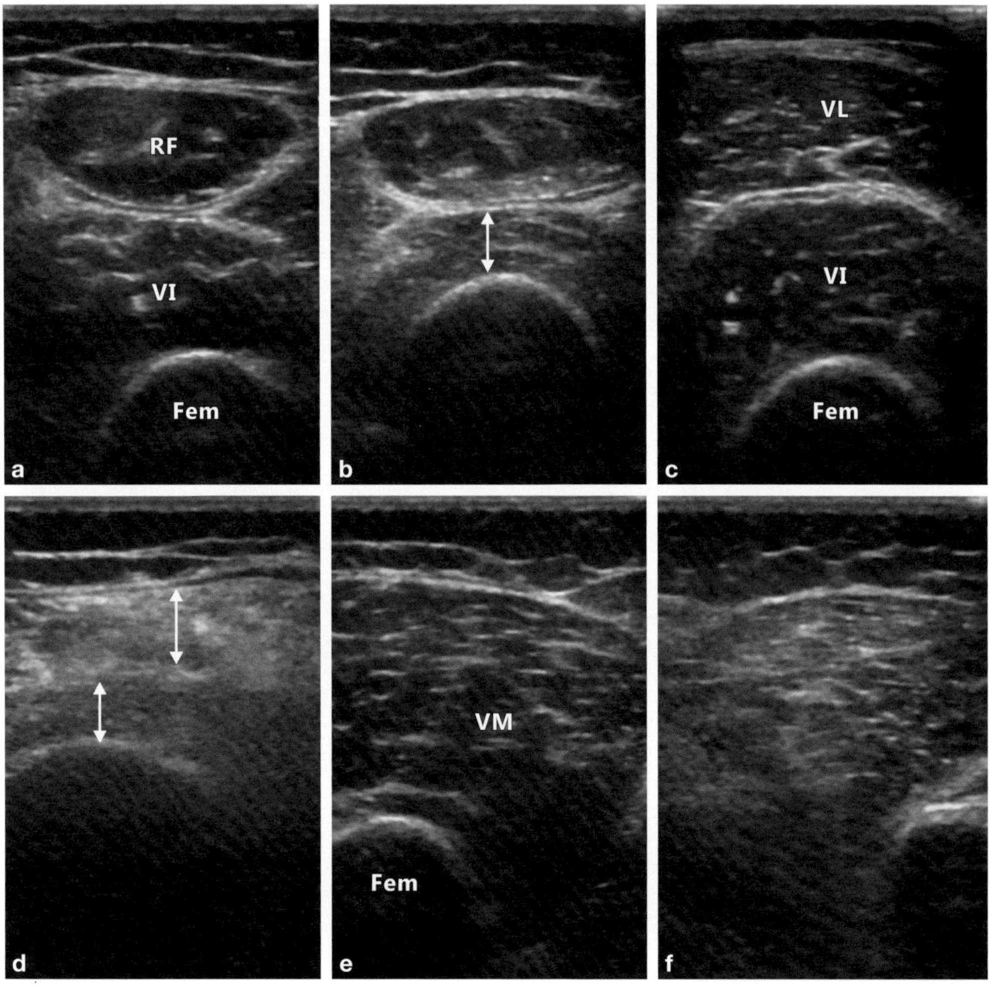

When compared with the normal side (**a**), axial US image obtained over the anterior mid-thigh reveals marked atrophy with increased echogenicity (*double arrow*) in the vastus intermedius muscle (**VI**) (**b**). Axial images over the lateral side at the same level show normal views for the vastus lateralis (**VL**) and VI muscles (**c**), whereas significant atrophy with hyperechogenicity (*double arrows*) again on the affected side (**d**). Comparison for vastus medialis (**VM**) on the distal third of the anteromedial thigh illustrates similar changes but less atrophy, consecutively (**e**, **f**).

Fem femur

RF rectus femoris

Expert note

While the US finding of atrophy is self-explanatory, concomitant hyperechogenicity is usually attributed to fibroadipose replacement of the muscle tissue.

Thigh

8.9 Quadriceps femoris muscle atrophy due to femoral nerve palsy in a 35-year-old woman

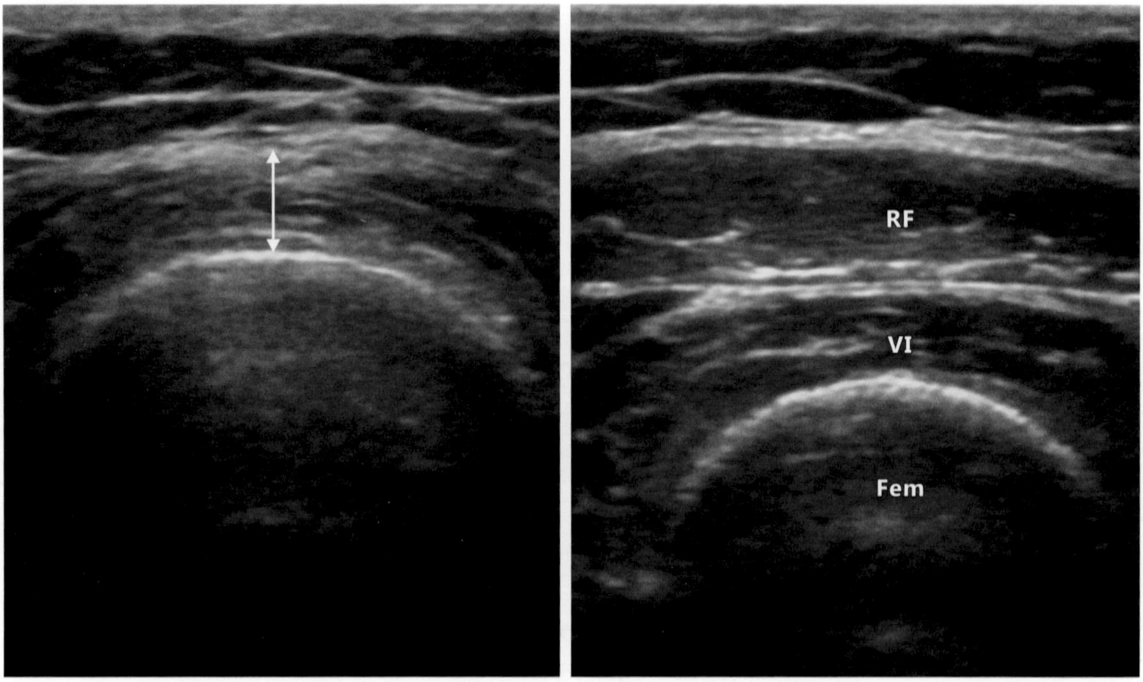

Axial US image over the anterior mid-thigh demonstrates signs of denervation atrophy (decreased thickness and increased echogenicity) more in the rectus femoris (**RF**) and less in the vastus intermedius (**VI**) muscles (*double arrow*) (**a**). Normal side (**b**).

Fem femur

A 43-year-old man was admitted with a swelling just above the knee joint **8.10**

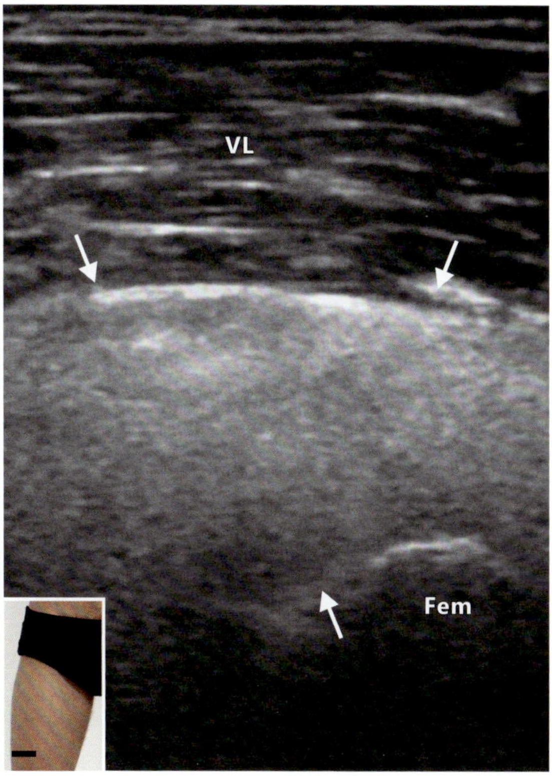

Axial US imaging reveals a large diffuse hyperechoic lesion in the vastus intermedius muscle reminiscent of a malignant mass lesion (*arrows*).

Fem femur
VL vastus lateralis

Expert note

US imaging has a pivotal role in the initial assessment of mass lesions. Small size (<5 cm), no/less vascularity and clear-cut margins suggest that the lesion is more likely to be benign. In this patient, contrast-enhanced magnetic resonance imaging confirmed the diagnosis as liposarcoma.

8.11 Healing sartorius strain in a young woman with neuropathic pain in the medial lower leg for the last six months

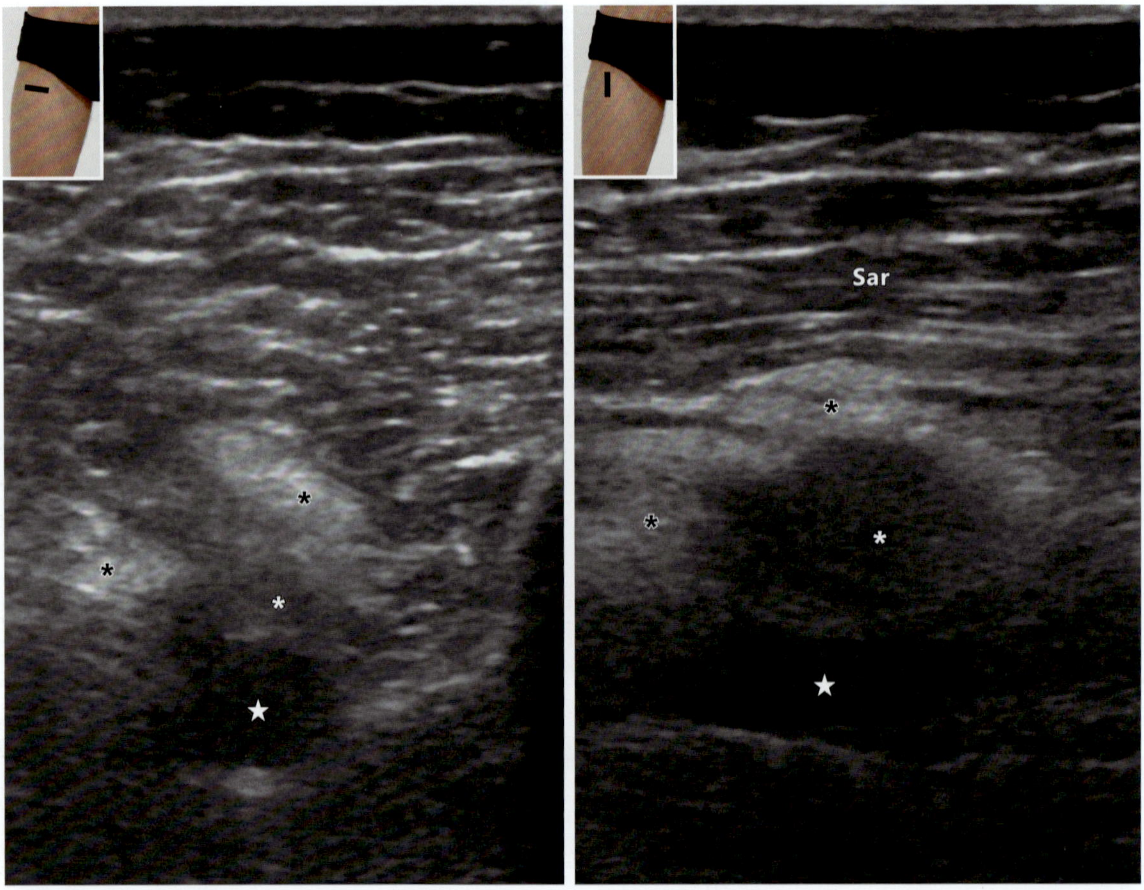

a b

Axial (**a**) and longitudinal (**b**) US images reveal healing process of the sartorius (**Sar**) strain with perilesional fibrosis (*black asterisks*) and edema (*white asterisks*). Please note the close relationship between the lesion and the superior edge of the adductor hiatus (Hunter canal). *Stars* indicates femoral artery.

Expert note

Since neurovascular structures course through muscle compartments (beneath the sartorius muscle), their possible entrapment due to a nearby muscle lesion would not sound unexpected. In this sense, there is no need to mention that US imaging can 'see both'.

Another important remark would be to distinguish these hyperechoic zones from early ossifications as well. Close follow up (repeat imaging) or the search for typical findings of ectopic ossification (i.e. cloudy appearance or zone phenomenon) would help in this regard.

Semitendinosus-biceps myotendinous strain in a young swimmer who presented with posterior thigh pain 8.12

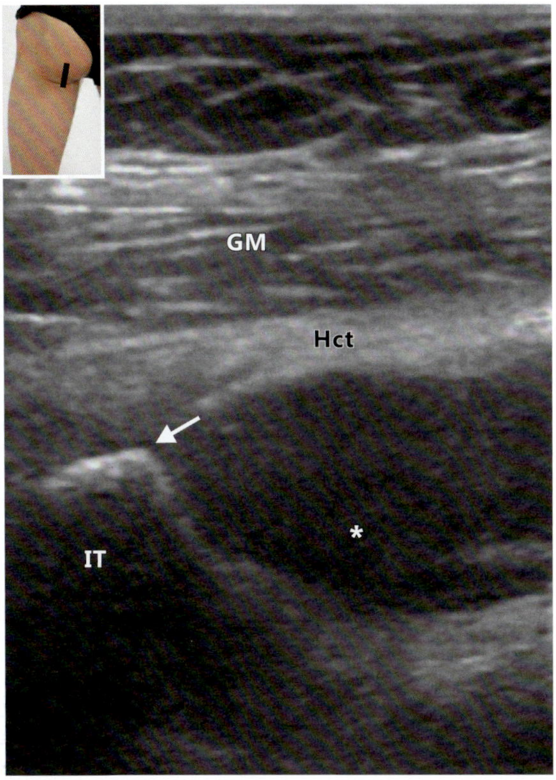

Posterior longitudinal US image illustrates a large, hypoechoic hematoma (*asterisk*) in the hamstrings muscles possibly due to exostosis (*arrow*) near to ischial tuberosity (**IT**).

GM gluteus maximus
Hct conjoined tendon of hamstring

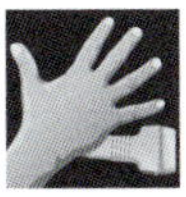

Expert note

Interestingly, while scanning for a strain lesion in the hamstrings; a possible underlying cause was also uncovered with the help of sono-palpation. This case exemplifies the practical role of US imaging for muscle injuries in the acute setting and also how an unexpected finding might tailor the rest of the imaging algorithm. Likewise, in this patient, the exostosis was later on confirmed with the radiographs as well.

8.13 Hamstrings strain and edematous sciatic nerve in a 17-year-old football player who had pain and mild sciatica in the posterior thigh

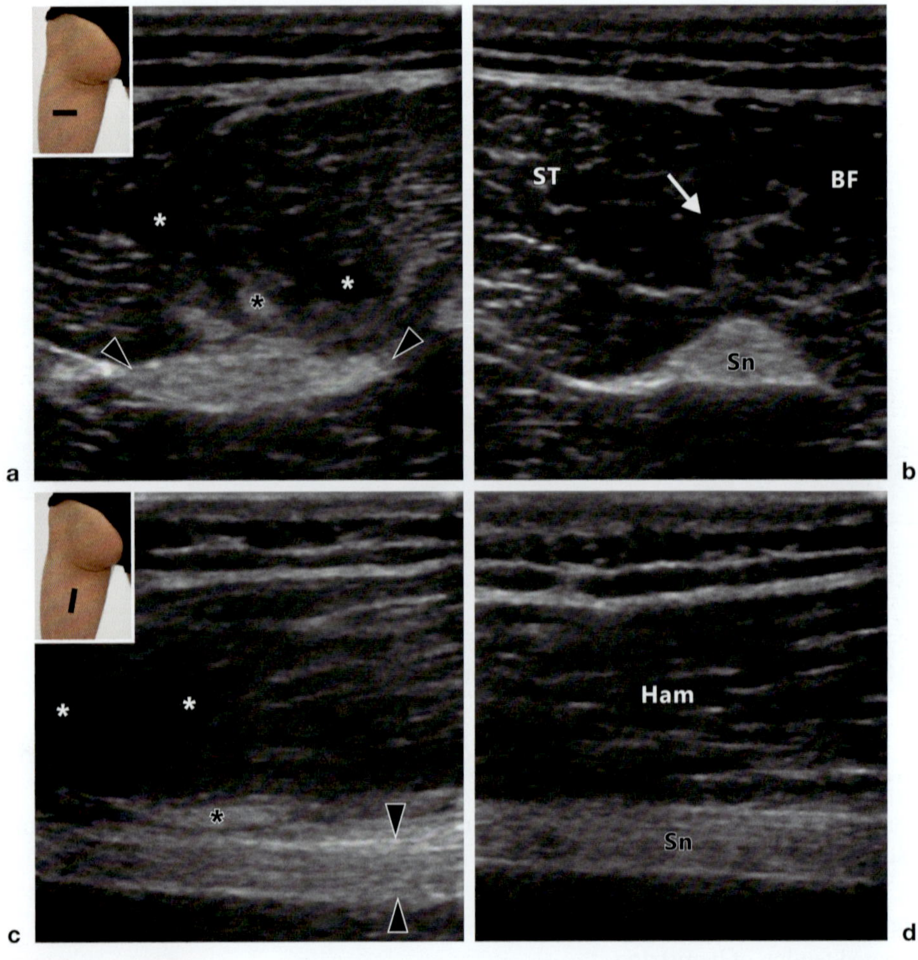

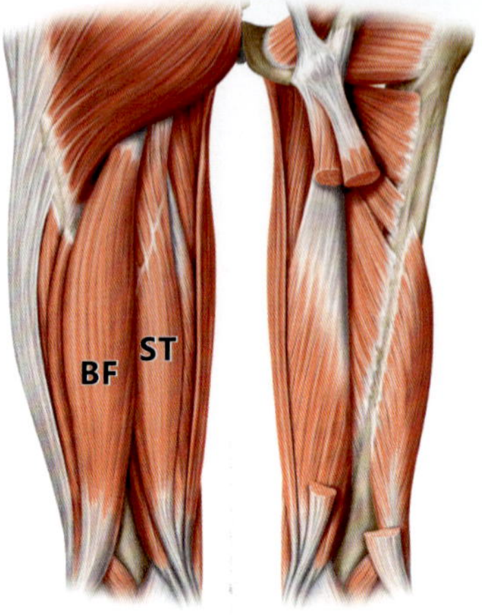

Axial (**a**) and longitudinal (**c**) US images over the posterior thigh demonstrate injured conjoined tendon (*arrow*) of the semitendinosus (**ST**) and biceps femoris (**BF**) muscles with disruption (*white asterisks*) and healing process (*black asterisks*) of the fascicles. Note that the immediately underlying sciatic nerve (**Sn**) is widened and edematous (*arrowheads*) (**a**). Normal side (**b**, **d**).

Ham hamstring

Expert note

The most commonly involved muscles are the biceps femoris (2/3) and the semitendinosus (1/3) muscles in acute hamstring injuries [4].

Semitendinosus muscle tear in a 40-year-old patient after jumping down from a higher place **8.14**

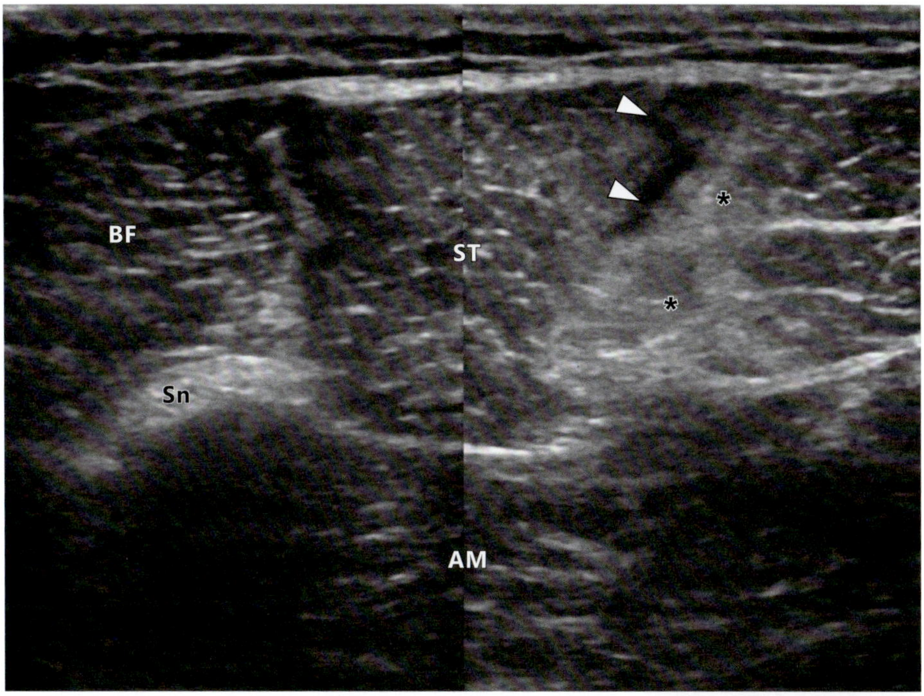

Posterior split-screen axial US image over the proximal thigh demonstrates a hyperechoic zone of healing process (*asterisks*) next to a superficial/vertical tear (*arrowheads*) of semitendinosus muscle (**ST**).

AM adductor magnus
BF biceps femoris
Sn sciatic nerve

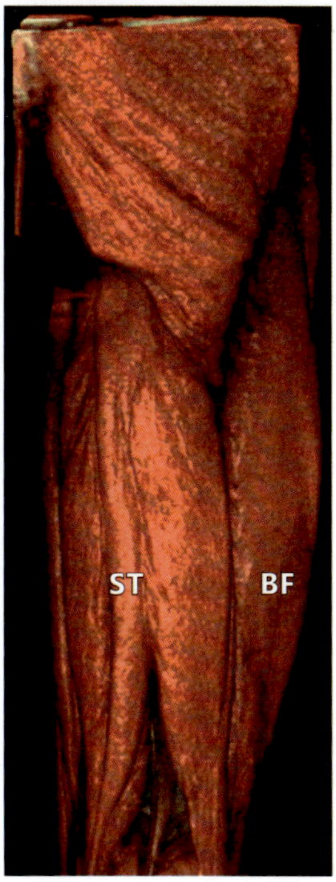

8.15 Biceps femoris muscle strain in a patient with posterior thigh pain after heavy lifting

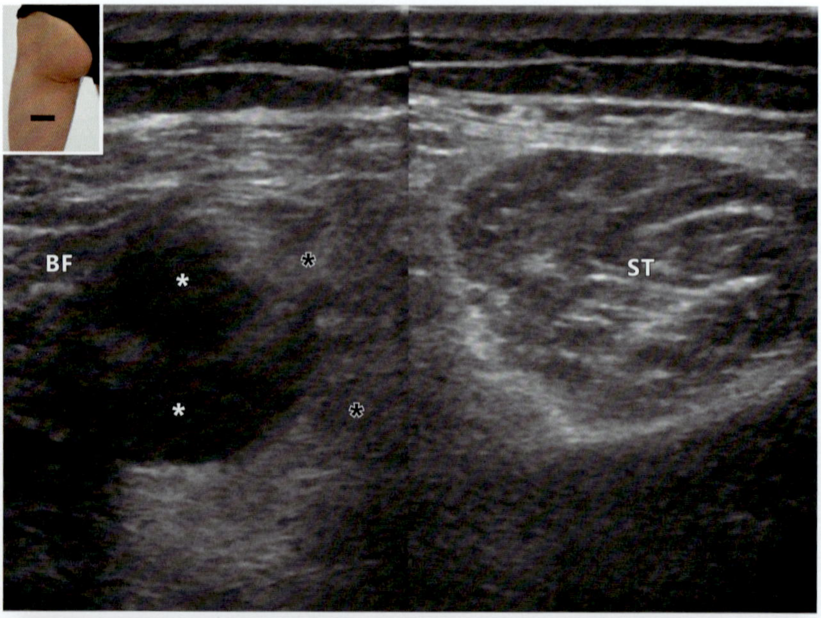

a

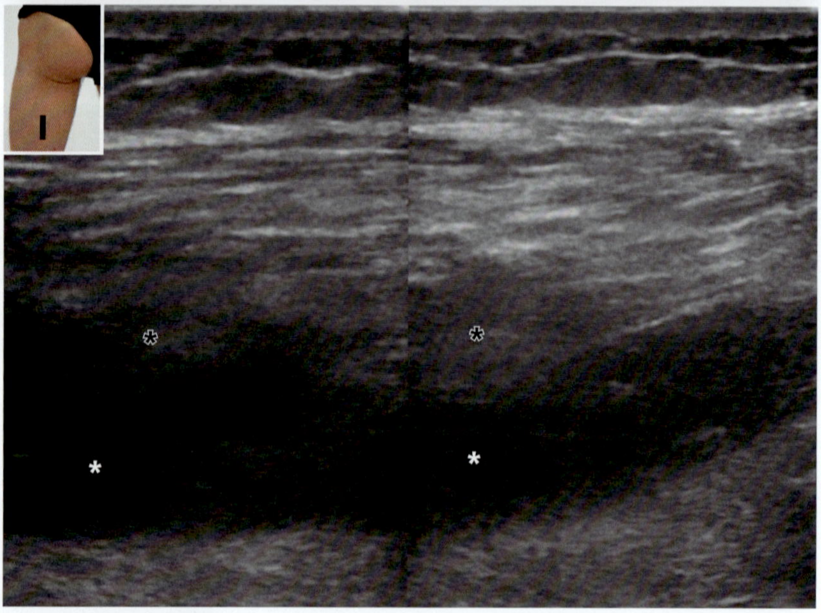

b

Split-screen axial (**a**) and longitudinal (**b**) US images over the posterior distal thigh show a large irregular hypoechoic area reflecting hematoma and focal discontinuity of the biceps femoris muscle (**BF**) fascicles (*white asterisks*) with interstitial edema (*black asterisks*).

ST semitendinosus

Semitendinosus strain in a young dancer with posterior distal thigh pain 8.16

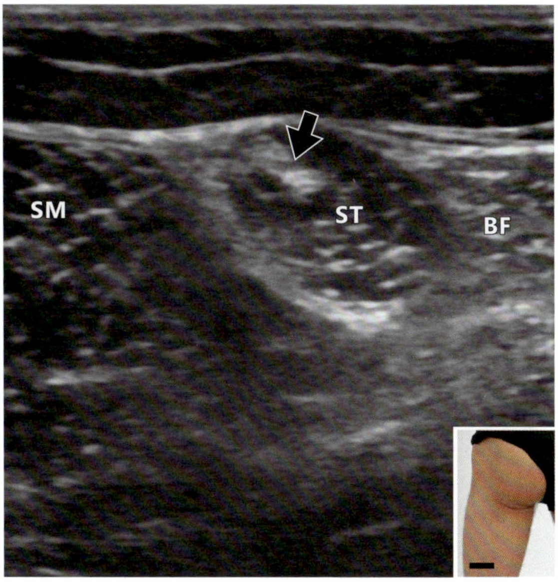

The pain started during rehearsals three weeks ago.

Axial US imaging shows a small area of fibrosis (*arrow*) in the semitendinosus muscle (**ST**) which seems to reflect an already/partially healed strain lesion.

BF biceps femoris
SM semimembranosus

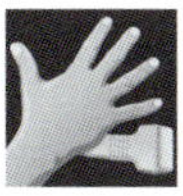

Expert note

Again, localizing these small lesions would definitely be easier with sono-palpation. Additionally, as persistent (even small) intramuscular fibrosis lessens the overall muscle strength, it may also predispose to future tears. For sure, this should always be kept in mind especially in professional athletes.
During imaging, slight isometric contraction can also be performed to better evaluate if the muscle belly widens in a harmonic or non-harmonic manner.

8.17 Biceps femoris muscle injury due to recurrent bleeding episodes in a 43-year-old patient who has been under dialysis for a long period

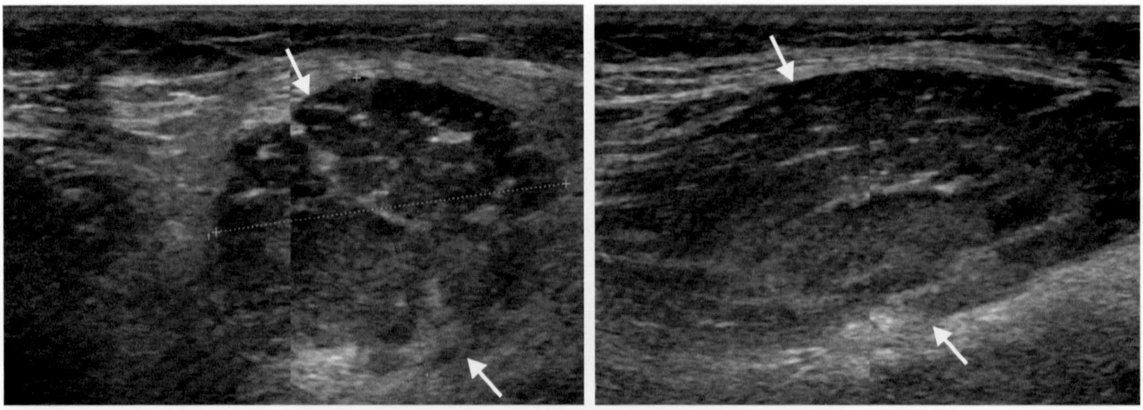

a b

Split-screen axial (**a**) and longitudinal (**b**) US images over the posterior thigh show a significant enlargement of biceps femoris muscle (*arrows*) with a heterogenous hypo/hyperechoic appearance.

Expert note

Once again, considering its convenience (i.e. patient friendly, bed-side application, etc.), US imaging is incomparable as regards the follow up of various muscle injuries in chronic illnesses.

US-guided injection in an adult patient with semitendinosus strain after jumping down from a higher place

8.18

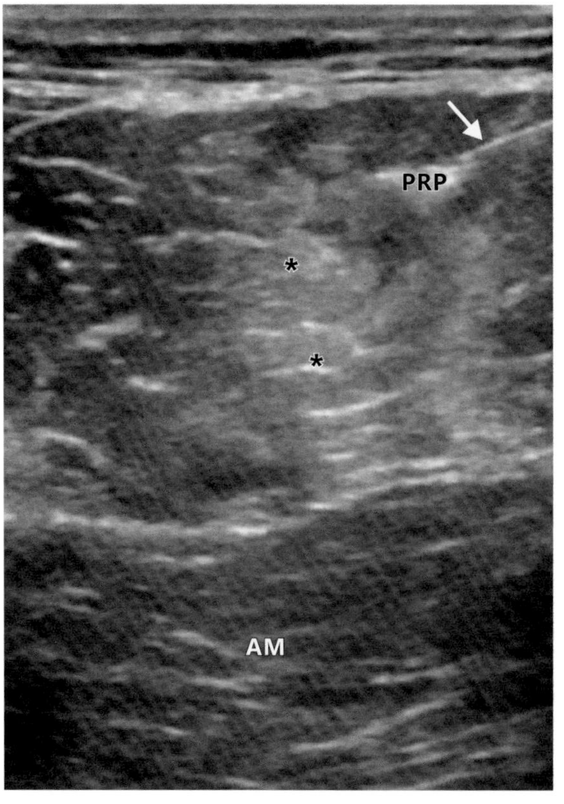

Axial US image over the posterior midthigh shows the needle (*arrow*) during the platelet-rich plasma (**PRP**) injection (direct in-plane technique) for semitendinosus muscle. Note the hyperechoic tissue due to healing process (*asterisks*) next to the injection area.

AM adductor magnus

8.19 Adductor longus tear in a basketball player who suffered groin pain after a match

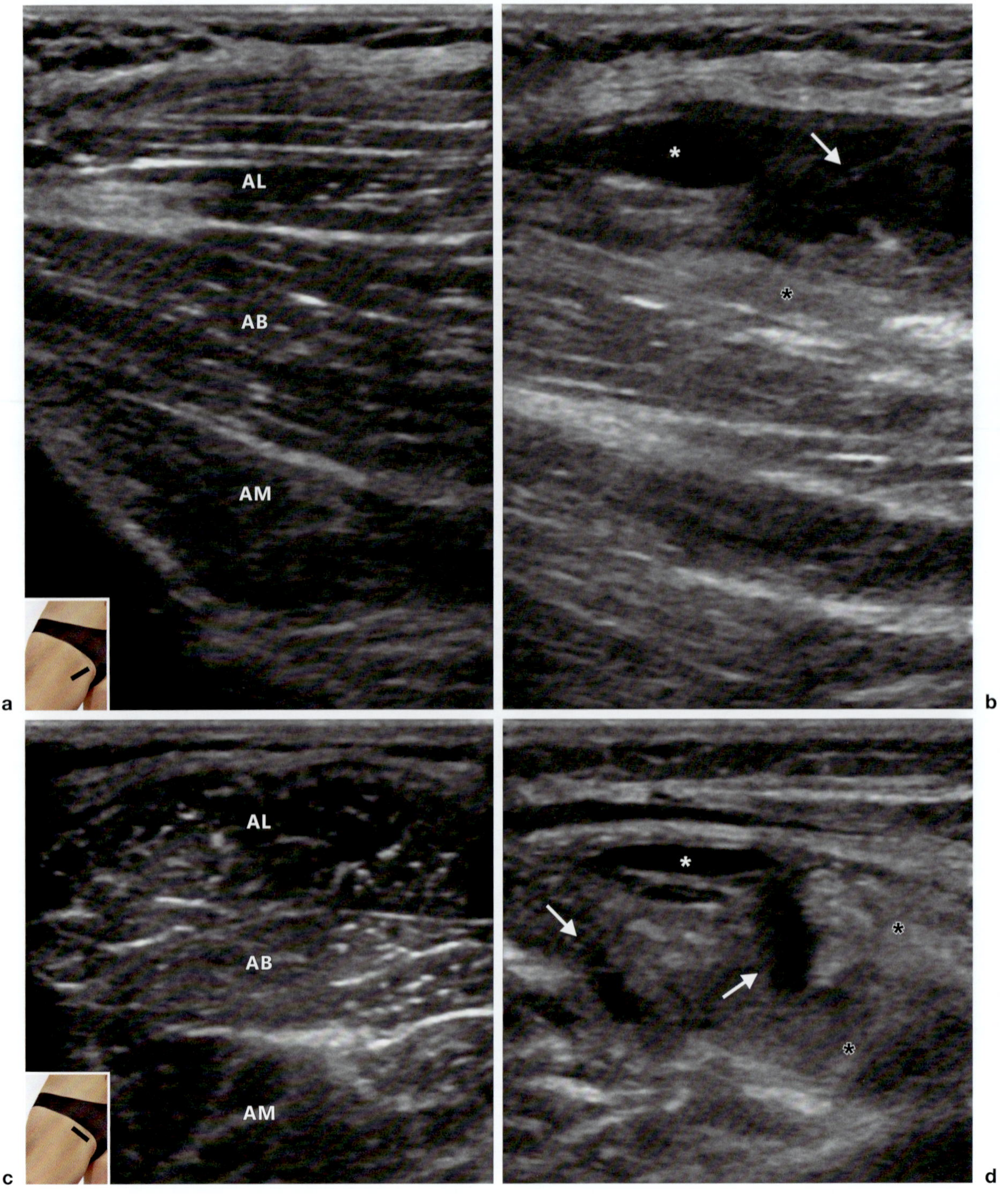

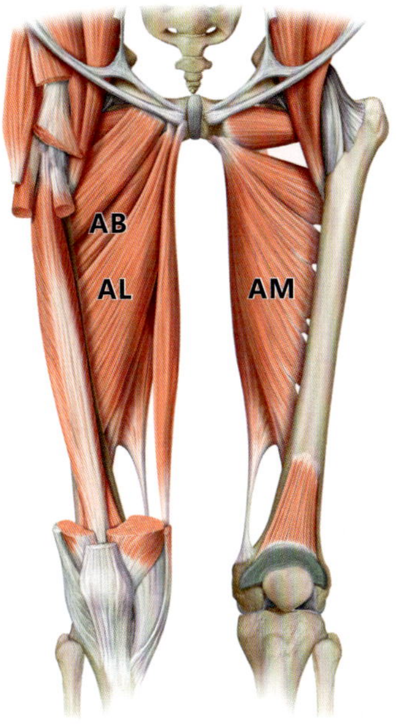

When compared with the normal side (**a**, **c**), longitudinal (**b**) and axial (**d**) US images over the adductor muscles demonstrate anechoic hematoma (*white asterisk*) and hyperechoic healing process of the muscle fascicles (*black asterisks*) reflecting the myotendinous strain. Please note the hypoechoic appearance of the resorbed/organizing hematoma (*arrows*).

AB adductor brevis
AL adductor longus
AM adductor magnus

Expert note

The majority of acute groin injuries encompasses the adductor injuries with a ratio of 2/3 (especially the adductor longus). Iliopsoas and proximal rectus femoris injuries are also commonly encountered for approximately 2/5 of all injuries [5].

8.20 Adductor longus strain in a 57-year-old woman with groin pain for the last one month

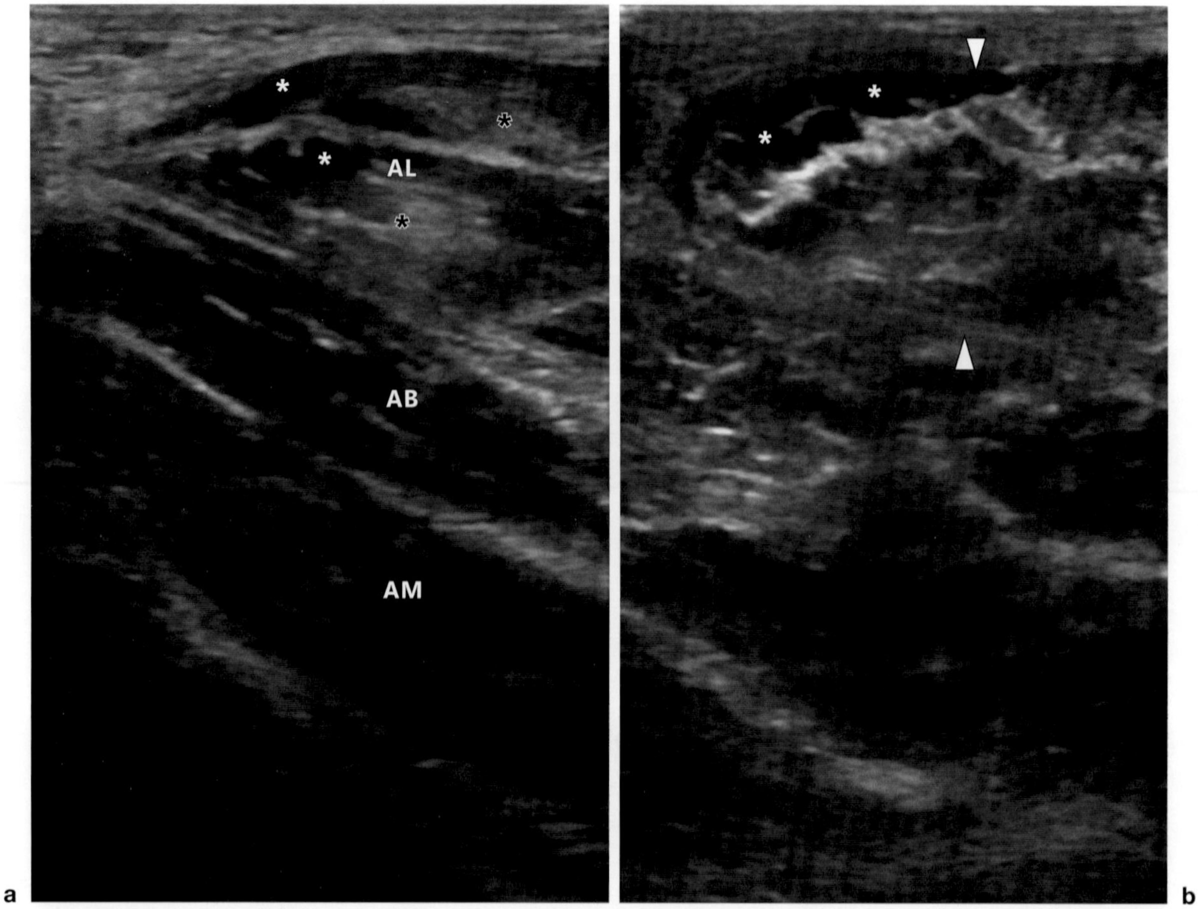

Longitudinal (**a**) and axial (**b**) US images show an anechoic area of hemorrhage and separated fascicles (*white asterisks*) as well as fibrosis (*black asterisks*) within the proximal portion of adductor longus muscle (**AL**) (*arrowheads*).

AB adductor brevis
AM adductor magnus

Healing adductor longus strain in a 32-year-old football player with inner thigh pain and tenderness 8.21

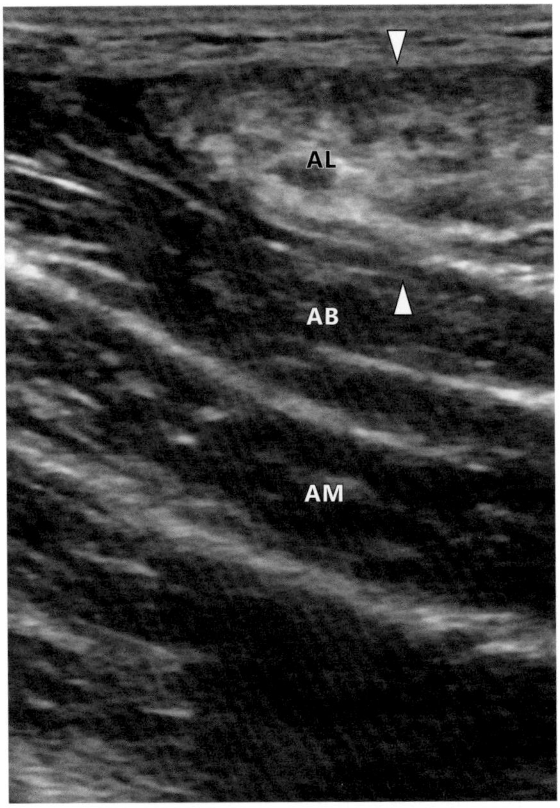

Pain developed after a strong shoot six weeks ago.

Longitudinal US imaging over the adductor muscles reveals a heterogenous area representing a residual scar tissue (*arrowheads*) in the adductor longus muscle (**AL**).

AB adductor brevis
AM adductor magnus

8.22 Healing phase of an adductor longus tear in a veteran footballer with proximal thigh pain

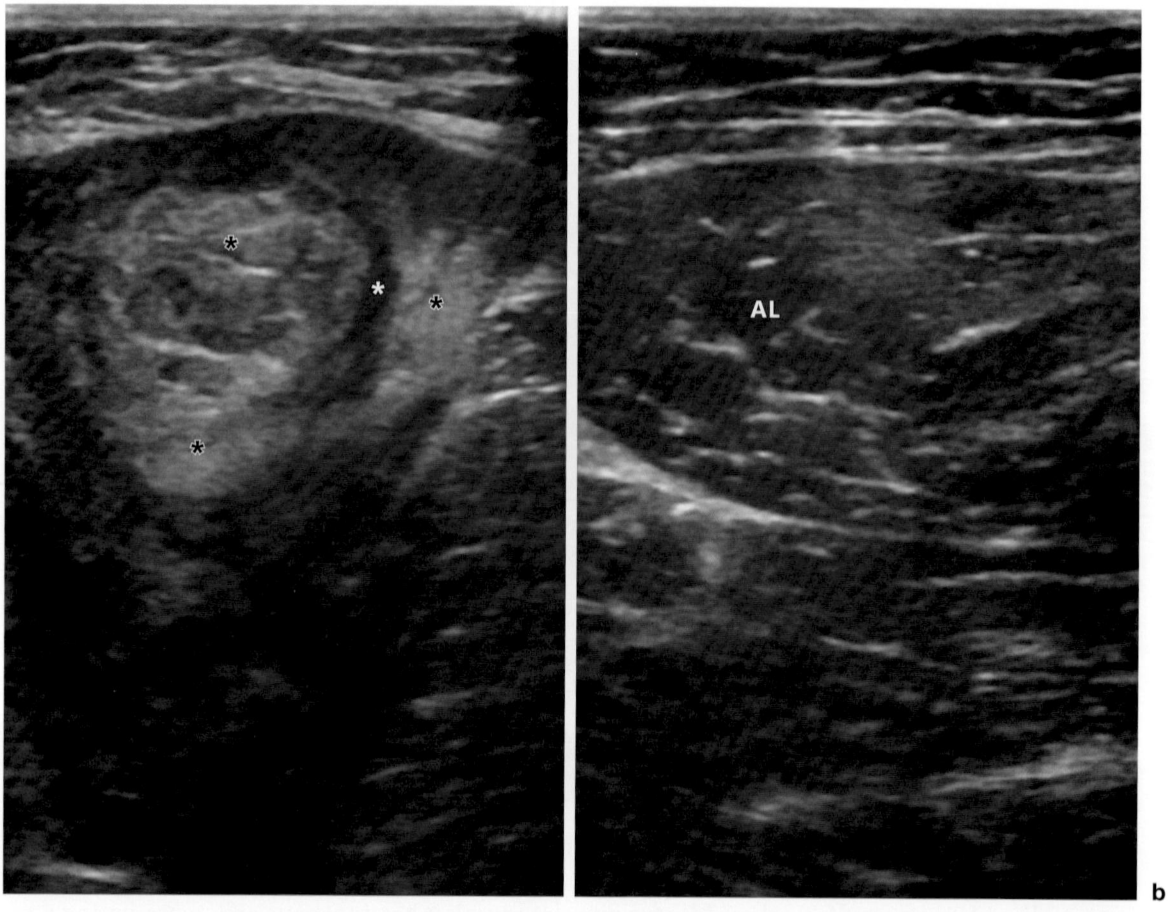

Axial US image of the adductor longus muscle (**AL**) depicts areas of hyperechoic healing fibrotic tissue (*black asterisks*) embracing the remnants of ruptured fascicles (*white asterisk*) (**a**). Normal contralateral side (**b**).

Hip adductor strain and myositis ossificans in a 32-year-old woman who had contusion trauma two months ago

8.23

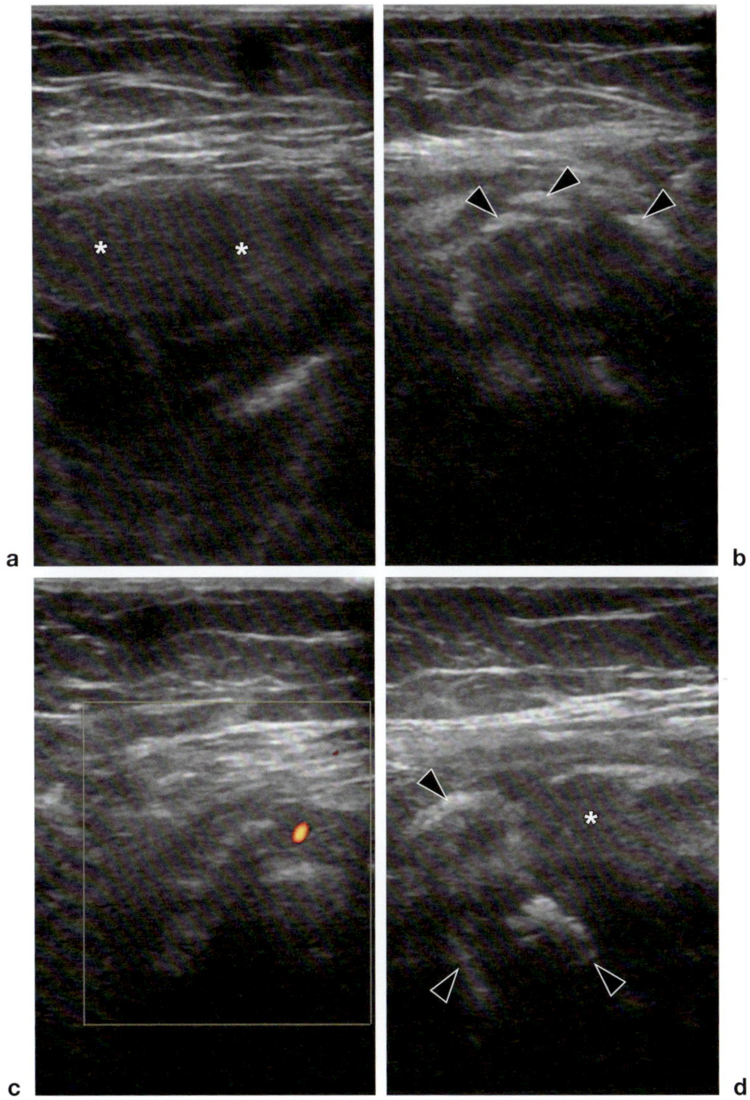

Axial (**a**-**c**) and longitudinal (**d**) US images obtained over the medial thigh demonstrate disrupted adductor muscles in hypoechoic appearance related to hemorrhagic changes (*asterisks*) (**a**), and irregularly shaped calcifications (*arrowheads*) in the muscle (**b**, **d**) with increased power Doppler signal (**c**).

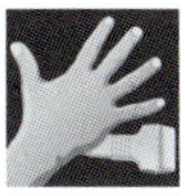

Expert note

Osteosarcoma or metastasis with cortical break-through could also give a similar image. If there is no clear history of muscle trauma, additional X-rays and/or magnetic resonance imaging should be considered.

8.24 Adductor longus abscess in a 55-year-old man with proximal thigh pain

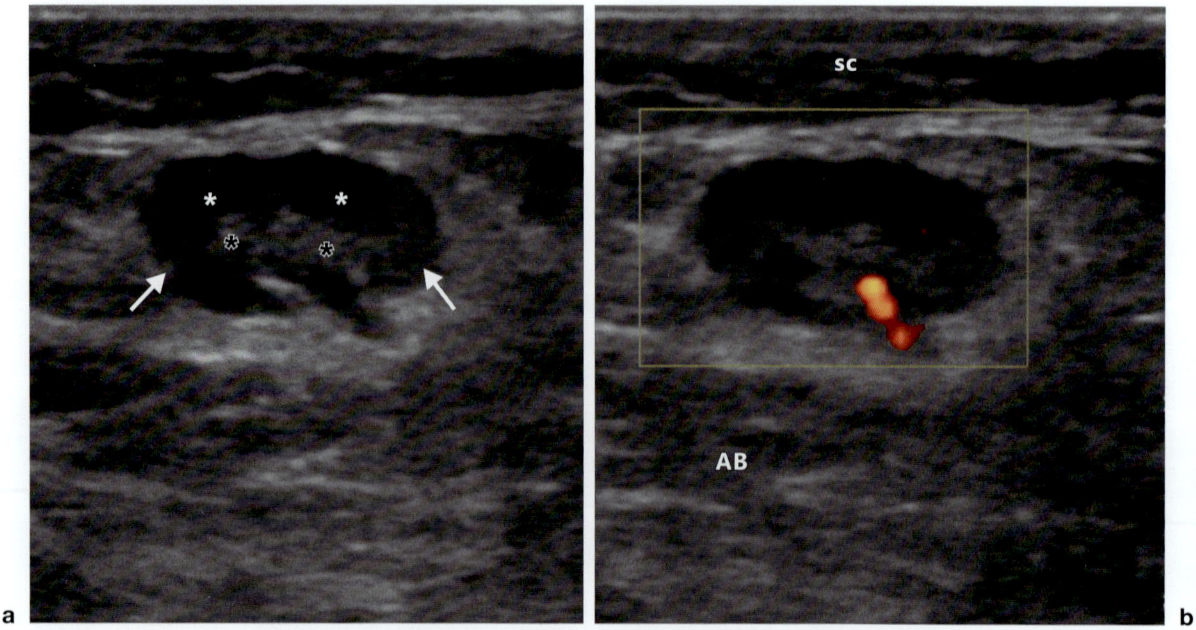

Axial US image shows internal fluid-filled areas (*white asterisks*) and debris (*black asterisks*) consistent with a local abscess formation (*arrows*) in the adductor longus muscle (**a**). Power Doppler imaging exhibits peripheral hyperemia as well (**b**).

AB adductor brevis
sc subcutaneous tissue

Intrafascial lipoma in a 47-year-old woman with a painful lump in the anterior thigh for three months

8.25

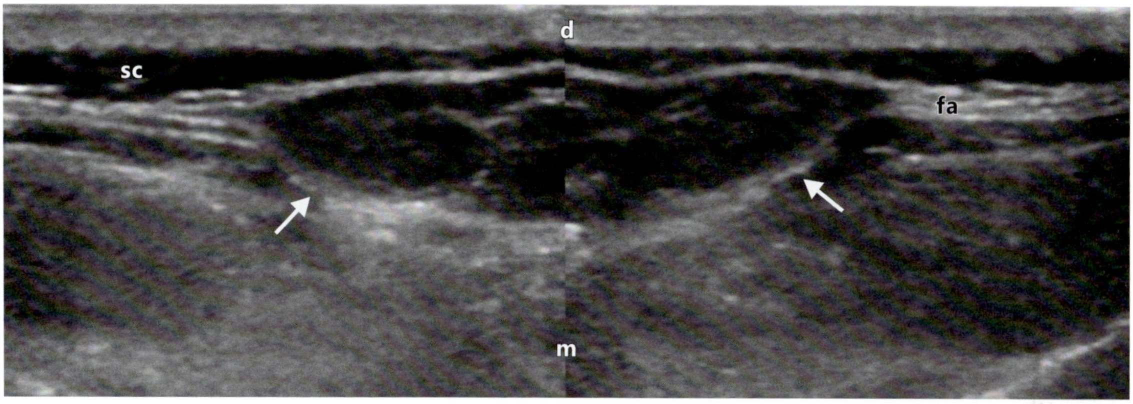

Split-screen longitudinal US image demonstrates an elongated, hypoechoic mass (*arrows*) inside the fascia, in similar echogenicity with the subcutaneous tissue (**sc**).

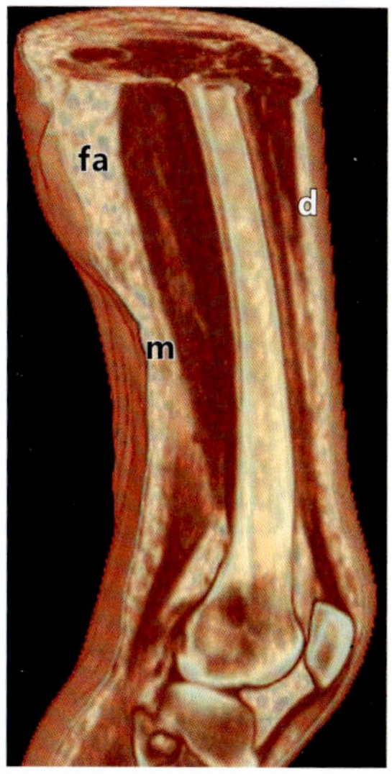

d dermis
fa fascia
m muscle

8.26 Lipoma in a 40-year-old woman with a swelling on the extensor surface of the thigh

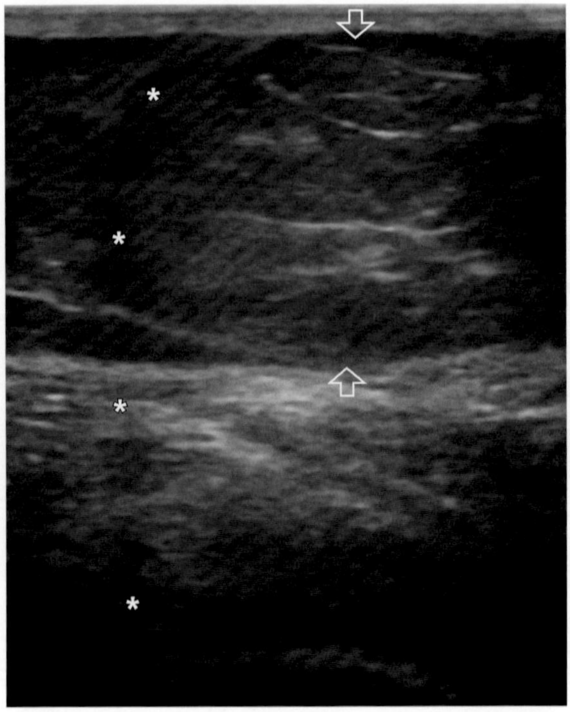

Longitudinal US image shows a non-uniformly bounded, hypoechoic mass (*arrows*) with its lateral shadowing artifact (*asterisks*).

Expert note

Although lipomas are usually well-defined masses, they may sometimes lack clear margins. In that case, the shadowing artifacts might be helpful for delineating their shape. Indisputably, vascularity of the mass should also be evaluated in order not to overlook a possibly malignant etiology.
Certainly, for intra- or intermuscular lipomas/masses, one should be further careful and possibly consult for additional magnetic resonance imaging.

Chronic unexplained medial thigh pain in a 50-year-old man

8.27

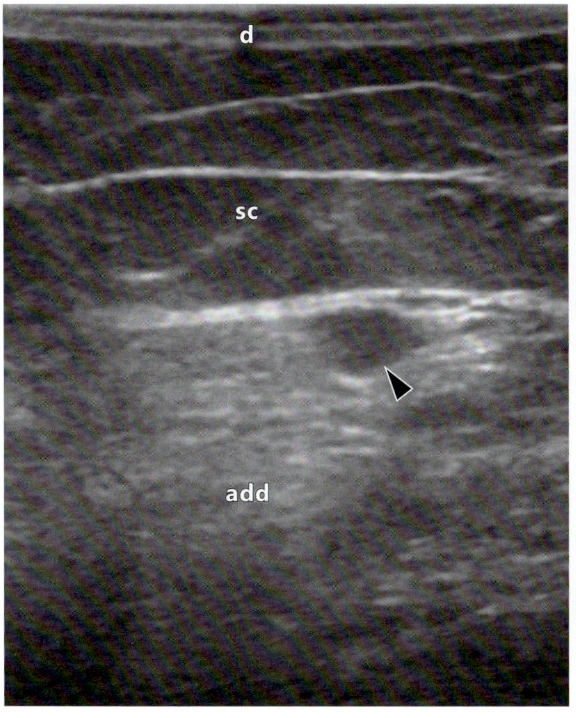

a

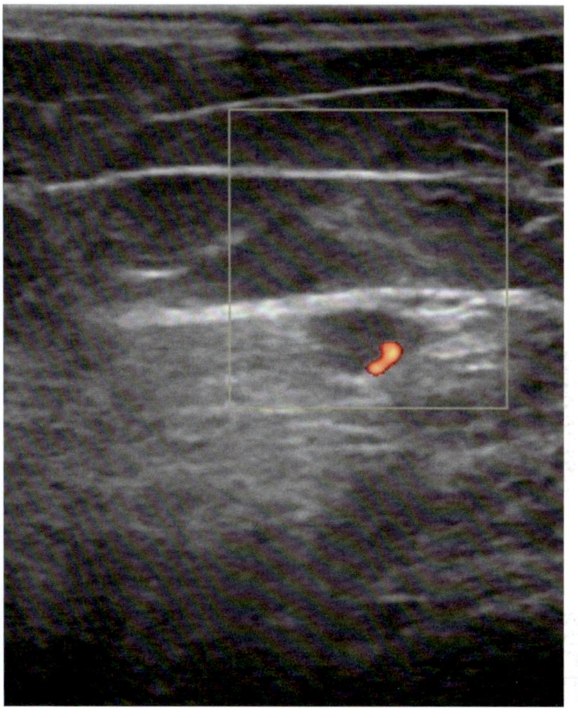

b

Axial images show an intramuscular, well-defined, hypoechoic lesion (*arrowhead*) close to the superficial fascia (**a**). Peripheral vascular flow signal is present on power Doppler imaging (**b**).

add adductors
d dermis
sc subcutaneous tissue

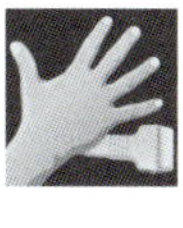

Expert note

This patient had been scanned at different centers using various imaging techniques all of which had been inconclusive. Herewith, sono-palpation easily localized the lesion during US evaluation.

REFERENCES

1. Bianchi S, Martinoli C. Thigh. In: Bianchi S, Martinoli C, editors. Ultrasound of the musculoskeletal system. Berlin: Springer; 2007. p. 611-36.
2. Tok F. Ultrasound imaging in Sports Medicine. In: Özçakar L, De Muynck M, editors. Musculoskeletal ultrasound in physical and rehabilitation medicine. Milan: Edi.Ermes; 2014. p. 125-39.
3. Valle M, Zamorani MP. Muscle and tendon. In: Bianchi S, Martinoli C, editors. Ultrasound of the musculoskeletal system. Berlin: Springer; 2007. p. 45-96.
4. Petersen J, Thorborg K, Nielsen MB, Skjødt T, Bolvig L, Bang N, et al. The diagnostic and prognostic value of ultrasonography in soccer players with acute hamstring injuries. Am J Sports Med. 2014; 42: 399-404.
5. Serner A, Tol JL, Jomaah N, Weir A, Whiteley R, Thorborg K, et al. Diagnosis of acute groin injuries: a prospective study of 110 athletes. Am J Sports Med. 2015; 43: 1857-64.

Knee 9

- **Suprapatellar recess**
- **Quadriceps femoris tendon** - Distal
- **Tibial tuberosity**
- **Patellar tendon**
- **Infrapatellar bursae**
- **Patella**
- **Medial collateral ligament**
- **Medial meniscus**
- **Pes anserinus**
- **Iliotibial band**
- **Lateral collateral ligament**
- **Biceps femoris tendon**
- **Femoral cartilage** - Distal
- **Semimembranosus-gastrocnemius bursa**

9.1 Suprapatellar effusion in a 60-year-old man with anterior knee pain and swelling

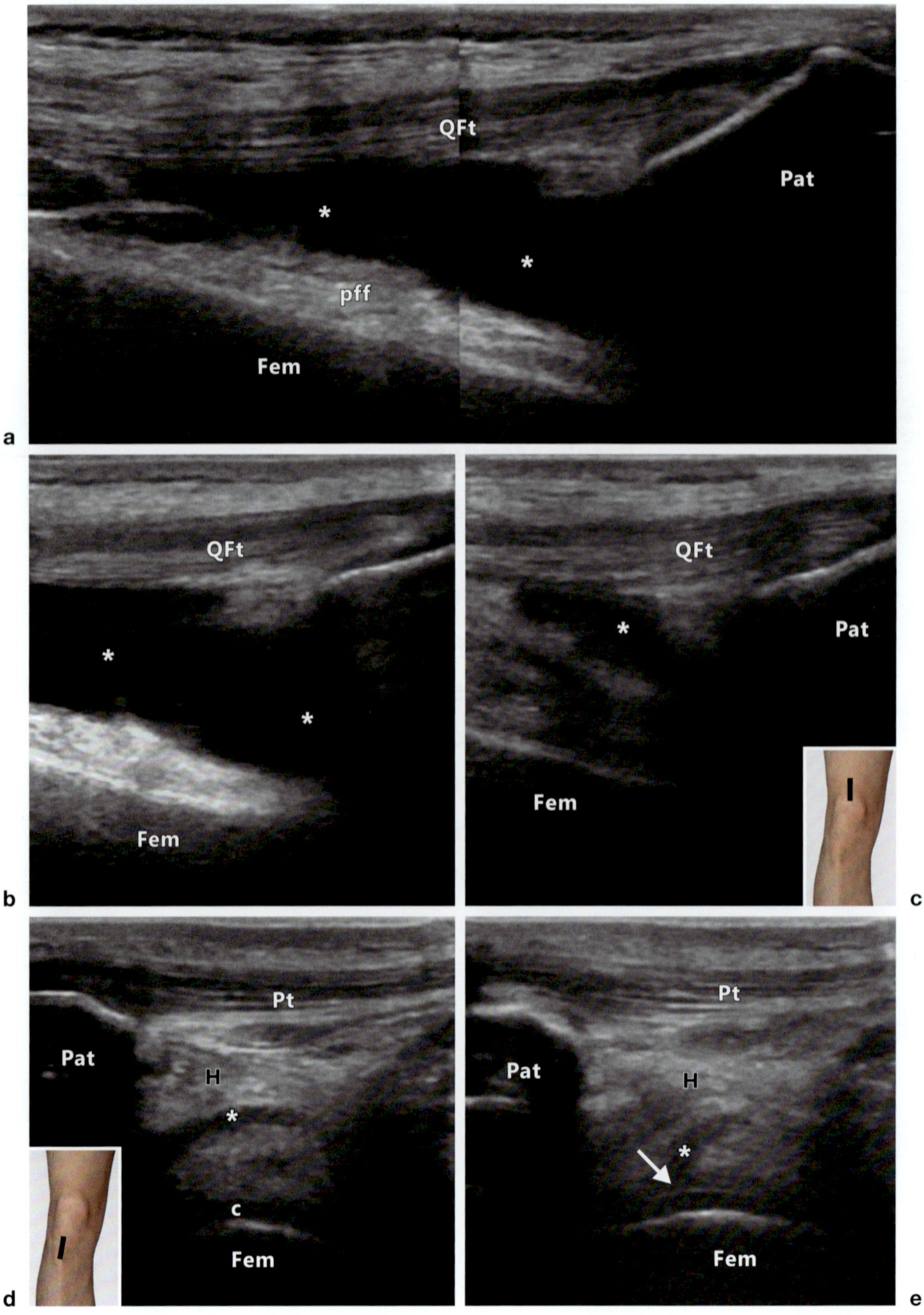

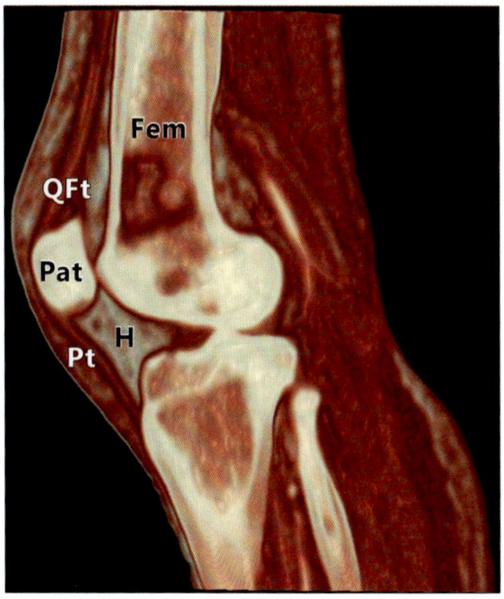

Split-screen (**a**) and longitudinal (**b**, **c**) US images over the suprapatellar region reveal effusion in the suprapatellar bursae (*asterisks*), more prominent on the symptomatic side (**a**, **b**). Longitudinal views over the infrapatellar region (**d**, **e**) also reveal joint fluid (*asterisks*) extending into the Hoffa's fat pad (**H**). Please note the cartilage interface sign (*arrow*) due to the overlying effusion.

c	hyaline cartilage of the femoral trochlea
Fem	femur
Pat	patella
pff	prefemoral fat pad
Pt	patellar tendon
QFt	quadriceps femoris tendon

Expert note

Although joint effusion is more commonly evaluated/found in the suprapatellar recess, fluid might also be found to extend in the infrapatellar recess i.e. commonly inside the Hoffa's fat pad.

9.2 Suprapatellar effusion and Baker cysts in a 66-year-old man with knee osteoarthritis

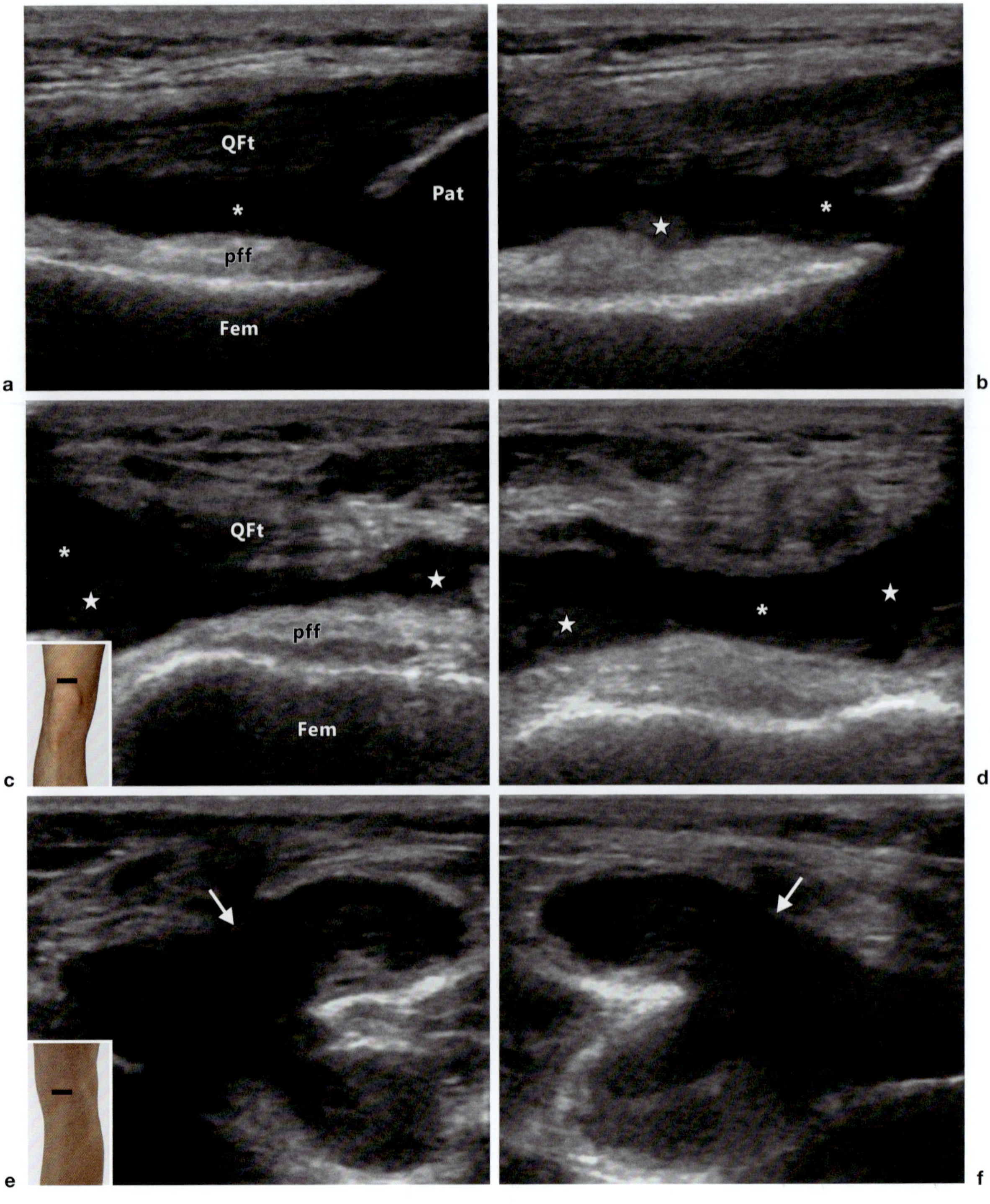

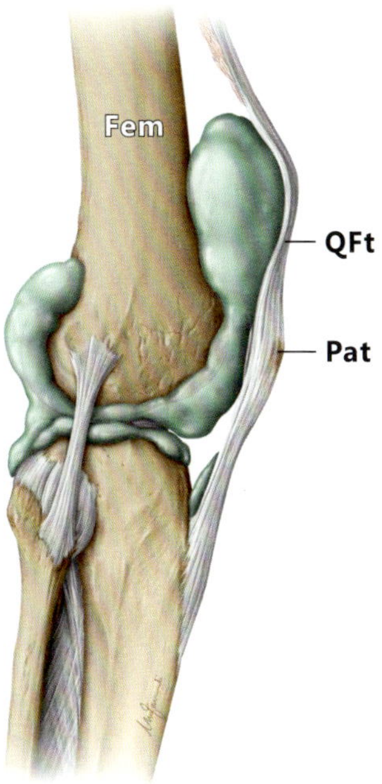

Anterior longitudinal (**a**, **b**) and axial (**c**, **d**) US images show suprapatellar effusion (*asterisks*) and synovial folds (*stars*). Posterior axial images (**e**, **f**) also demonstrate large boomerang-shaped Baker cysts bilaterally (*arrows*).

Fem femur
Pat patella
QFt quadriceps femoris tendon

Expert note

The presence of fluid in the anterior compartment(s) might necessitate the search for Baker cysts on the posterior sides in relevant clinical scenarios.
Herewith, one should also keep in mind that a Baker cyst is sometimes referred as a 'symptom' (of an underlying degeneration) not a diagnosis. Presence of joint effusion and/or Baker cyst has been reported to correlate with worse pain or poorer function [1].

9.3 Bilateral suprapatellar effusion in a 48-year-old woman with anterior knee pain and intermittent swelling

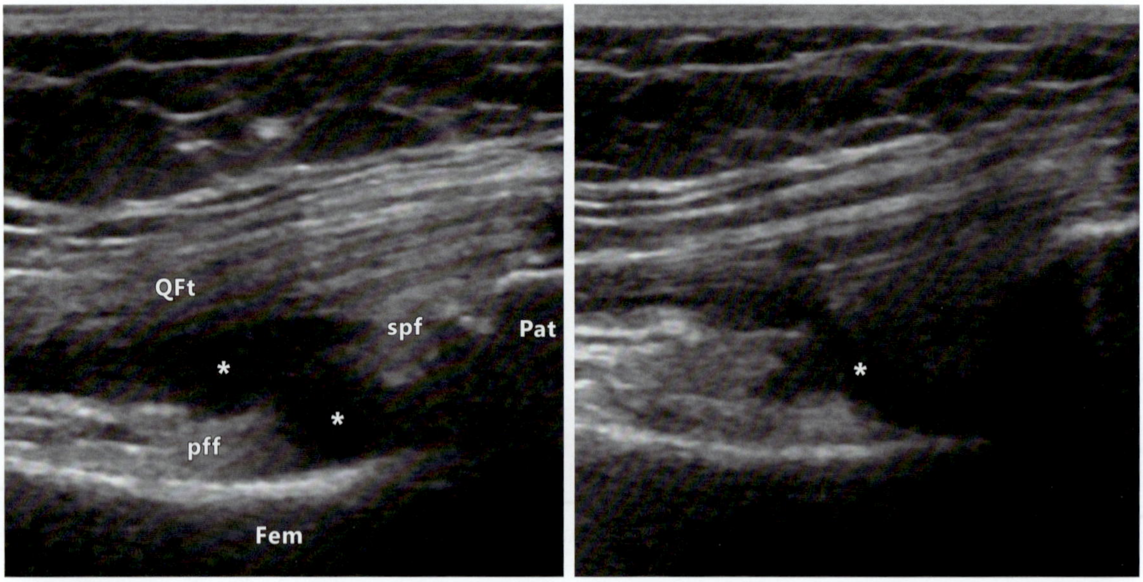

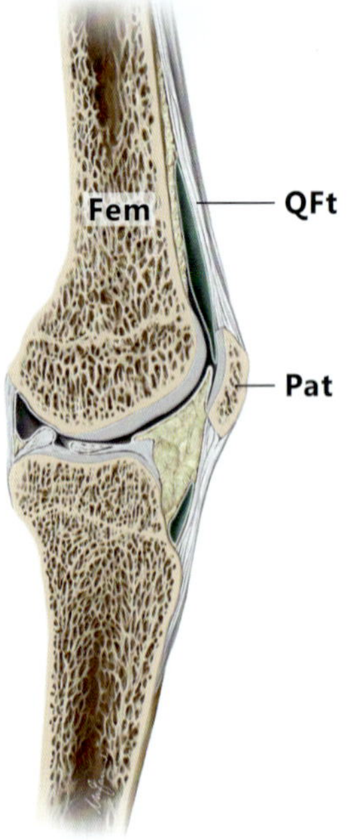

Longitudinal US scans reveal effusion in the suprapatellar recesses (*asterisks*) on both sides (**a**, **b**).

Fem	femur
Pat	patella
pff	prefemoral fat pad
QFt	quadriceps femoris tendon
spf	suprapatellar fat pad

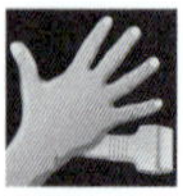

Expert note

Mild flexion of the knee joint during imaging for fluid in the anterior compartment(s) also helps better visualize the quadriceps femoris tendon which is aligned more parallel to the US probe.

Chronic knee effusion in a 67-year-old woman with tenderness and swelling at the suprapatellar region

9.4

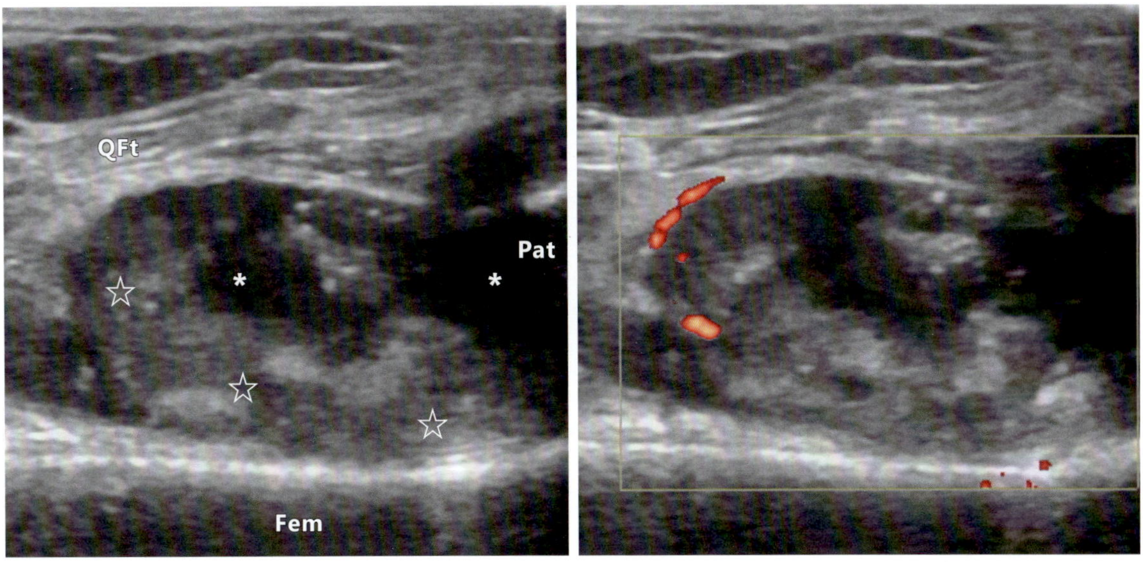

Longitudinal US image (**a**) shows a distended lateral pouch of the suprapatellar bursa filled with fluid (*asterisks*) and synovial thickenings (*stars*). Power Doppler image reveals mild hyperemia (**b**).

Fem femur
Pat patella
QFt quadriceps femoris tendon

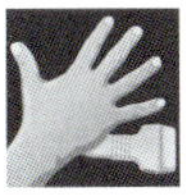

Expert note

Knee OA can demonstrate synovial hypertrophy or effusion in almost half of the patients. While synovial hypertrophy is defined as synovial thickening of ≥4 mm, the presence of effusion is based on the size of fluid being less or more than 4 mm in the suprapatellar recess [2].

9.5 Suprapatellar hematoma in a patient with painful knee swelling after a direct trauma to the joint

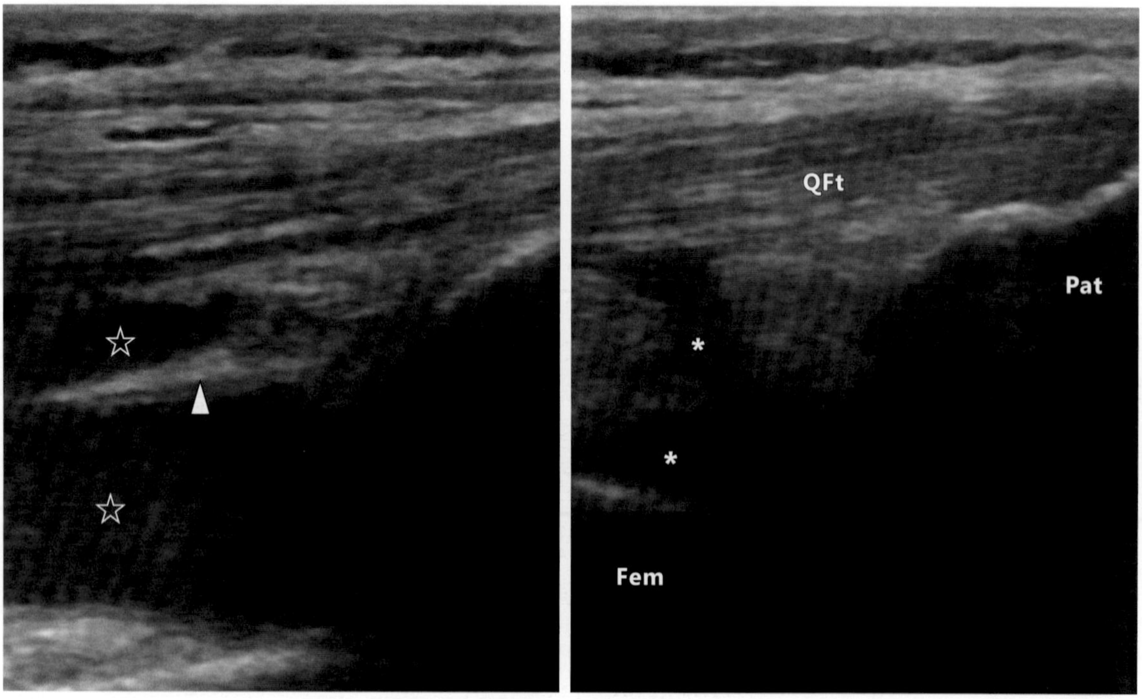

a b

Longitudinal US image (**a**) shows hypoechoic hematoma (*stars*) filling the suprapatellar recess and an incomplete suprapatellar septum/plica (*arrowhead*). Normal side with mild effusion (*asterisks*) (**b**).

Fem femur
Pat patella
QFt quadriceps femoris tendon

Expert note

While imaging for fluid in the suprapatellar bursa, positioning of the knee joint is noteworthy and yet to be taken into account. While mild knee flexion would facilitate the detection of fluid in the midline (separating the layers of the bursa), full extension usually displaces the fluid to the medial and lateral pouches [3]. Further, when the patient is lying on the back, legs will often fall in external rotation and because of gravity, the fluid will tend to accumulate more laterally.

Suprapatellar effusion and synovial calcification in an elderly woman with chronic painful knee swelling **9.6**

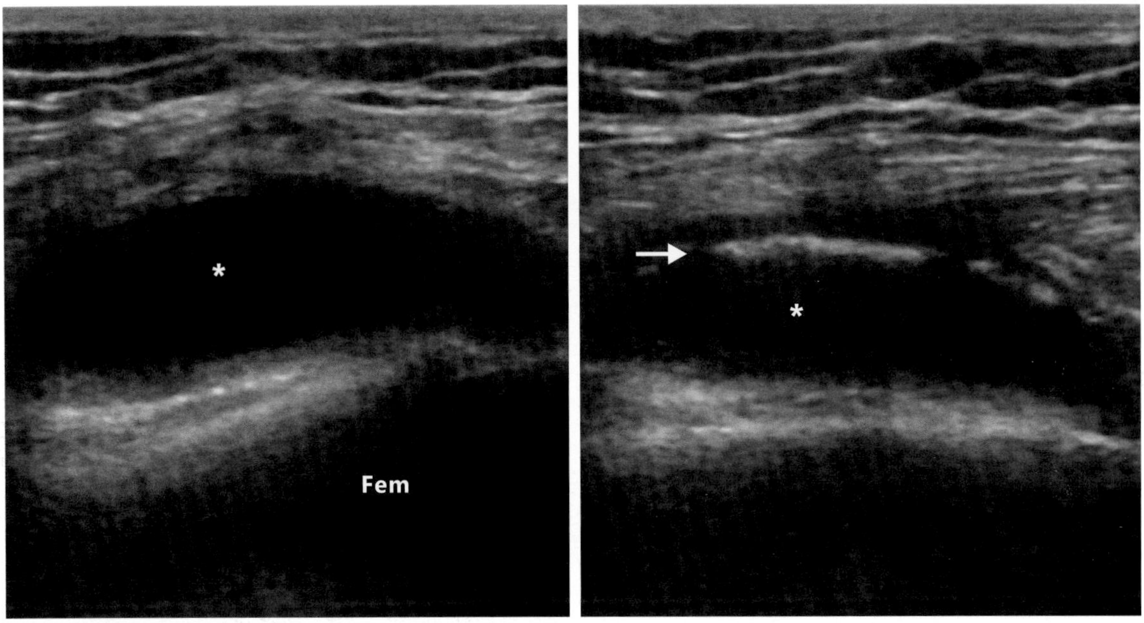

Axial US images over the suprapatellar region demonstrate hypo/anechoic effusion (*asterisks*) on both sides (**a**, **b**). Also note the large/marginal linear calcification (*arrow*) without posterior acoustic shadowing artifact (**b**).

Fem femur

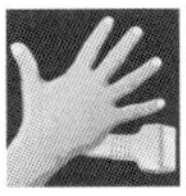

Expert note

While synovial calcifications are generally observed in chronic cases, crystal deposition diseases should also be kept in mind in the differential diagnosis [4].

9.7 Suprapatellar effusion in a 67-year-old man with painful swelling and limited knee flexion

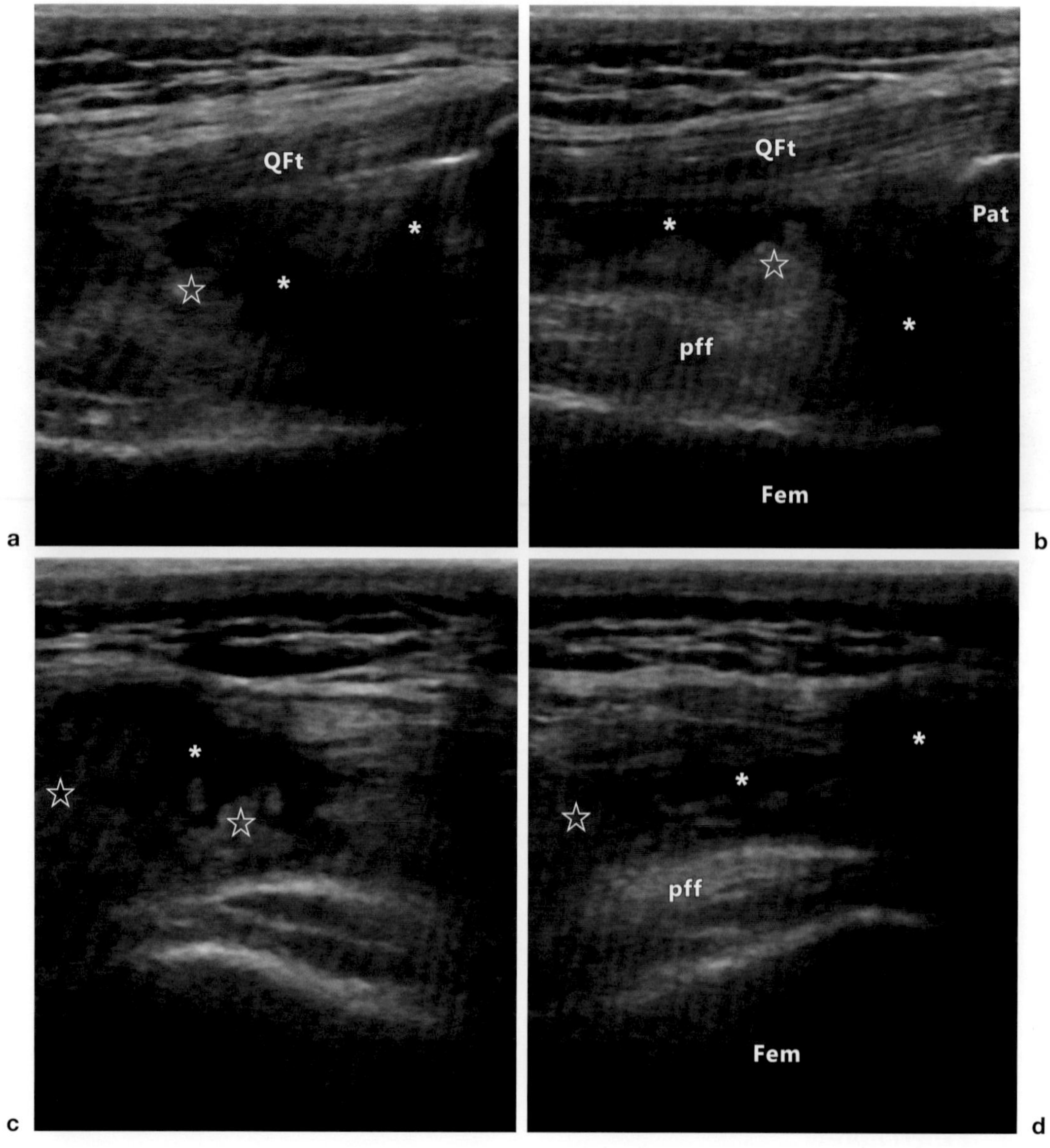

Longitudinal (**a**, **b**) and axial (**c**, **d**) US images over the suprapatellar region reveal anechoic effusion (*asterisks*) and hypoechoic synovial hypertrophy (*stars*) in the suprapatellar bursa.

Fem femur
Pat patella
pff prefemoral fat pad
QFt quadriceps femoris tendon

Synovitis in a 46-year-old woman with rheumatoid arthritis for 12 years **9.8**

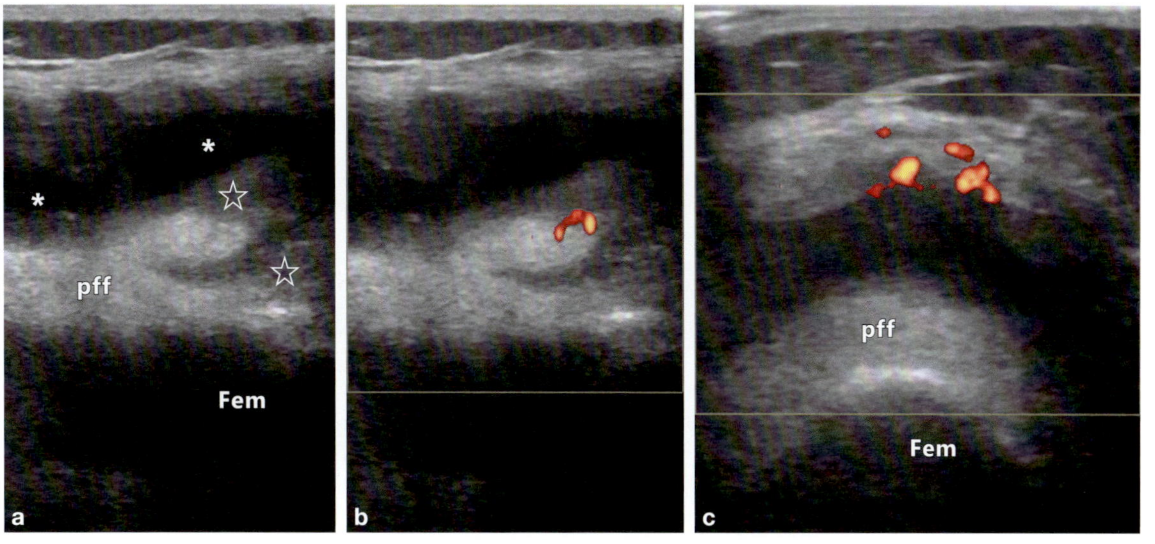

She had painful knee swelling with a positive patellar ballottement test.

Longitudinal US image over the suprapatellar region shows anechoic effusion (*asterisks*) and hypoechoic synovial hypertrophy (*stars*) in the suprapatellar bursa (**a**). Power Doppler images on both longitudinal (**b**) and axial (**c**) scans demonstrate synovial inflammation.

Fem femur
pff prefemoral fat pad

9.9 US-guided drainage of the suprapatellar effusion in a 60-year-old man with knee osteoarthritis

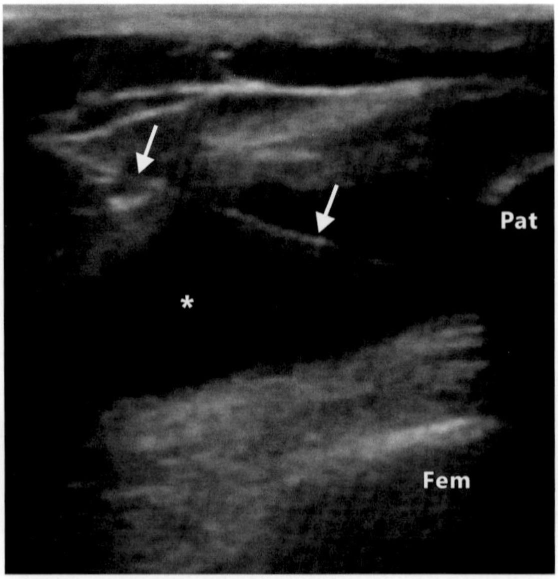

Longitudinal US image demonstrates the hyperechoic needle (*arrows*) within the fluid collection (*asterisk*) during aspiration (direct in-plane technique).

Fem femur
Pat patella

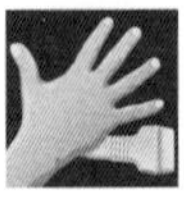

Expert note

US imaging is definitely paramount for precise guidance as regards the onward intervention i.e. not only during the procedure itself but also for better clinical decision making in advance [5]. Sonographers can easily understand what the exact diagnosis is, where exactly they should intervene and what exactly they need to do (e.g. aspiration, injection with different alternatives).

Suprapatellar hemorrhage in a 50-year-old man with painful knee swelling **9.10**

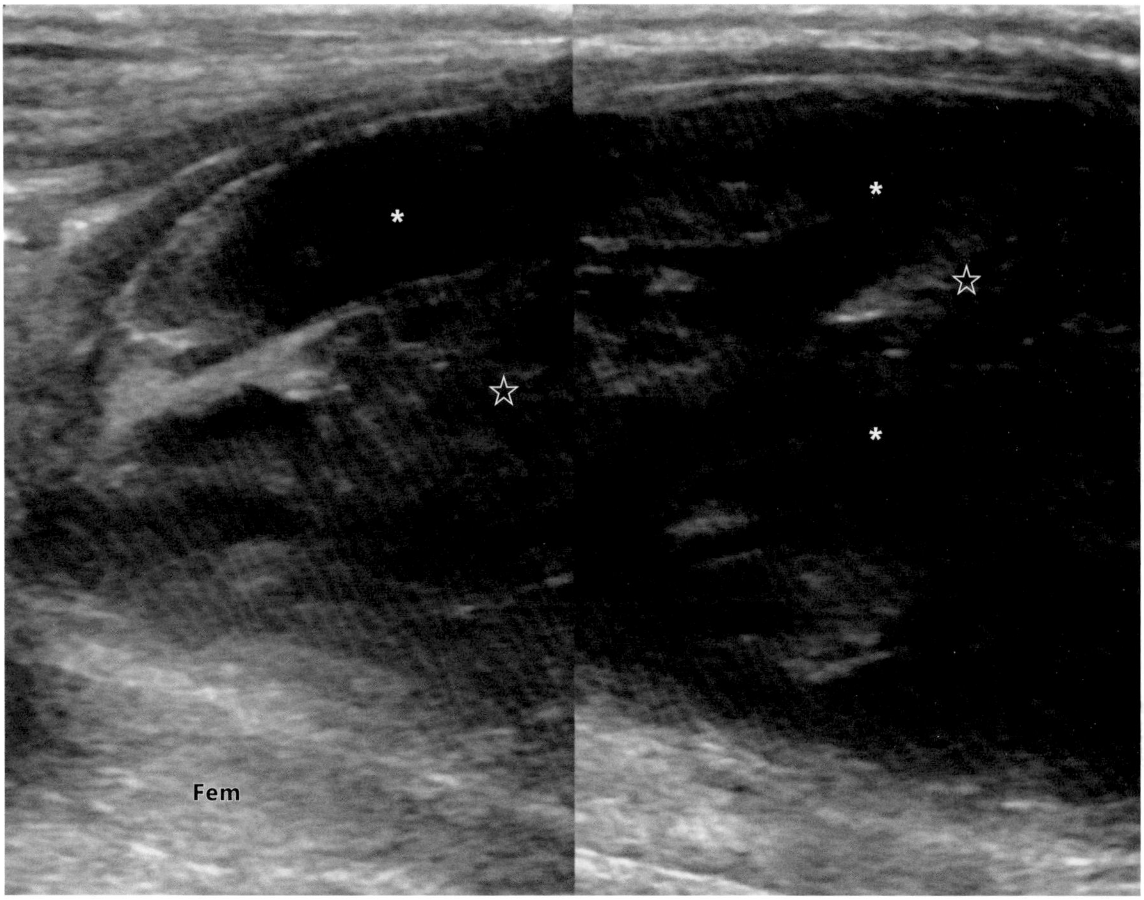

He was receiving hemodialysis for chronic renal disease.

Split-screen US image shows a large, irregular, hypo/anechoic content (*asterisks*) filling the suprapatellar recess. Irregular fibrous stranding within the collection reflects hypoechoic fibrin organization (*stars*).

Fem femur

Expert note

Owing to its several advantages (e.g. patient friendly, portable, convenient, does not contain radiation), US imaging provides great feasibility in patients with chronic morbidities. Intrabursal/articular hemorrhage may be encountered particularly in patients who have bleeding disorders or are using anticoagulant drugs.

9.11 Patellar degeneration in a 50-year-old woman with anterior knee pain and a history of knee surgery 25 years ago

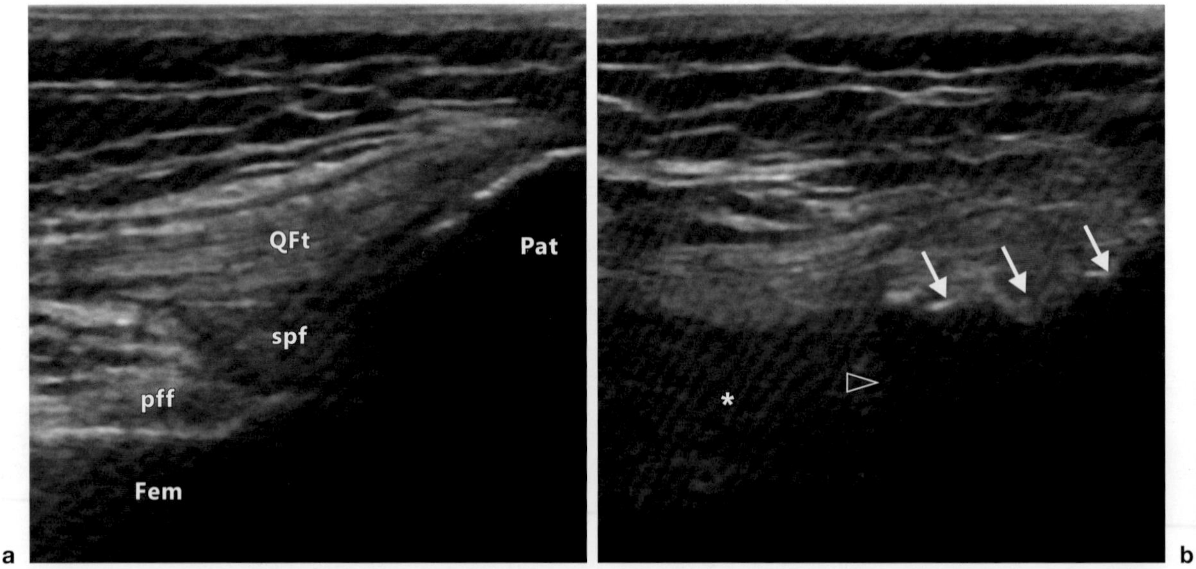

When compared with the normal side (**a**), longitudinal US image over the suprapatellar region (**b**) shows effusion (*asterisk*) at the suprapatellar recess and cortical irregularities (*arrows*) on the superior pole of patella (**Pat**). Please also note the sharp and well-defined posterior acoustic shadowing (*arrowhead*) due to the changed contour of the patella.

Fem femur
pff prefemoral fat pad
QFt quadriceps femoris tendon
spf suprapatellar fat pad

Repaired quadriceps tendon in a 57-year-old man after a traumatic knee injury **9.12**

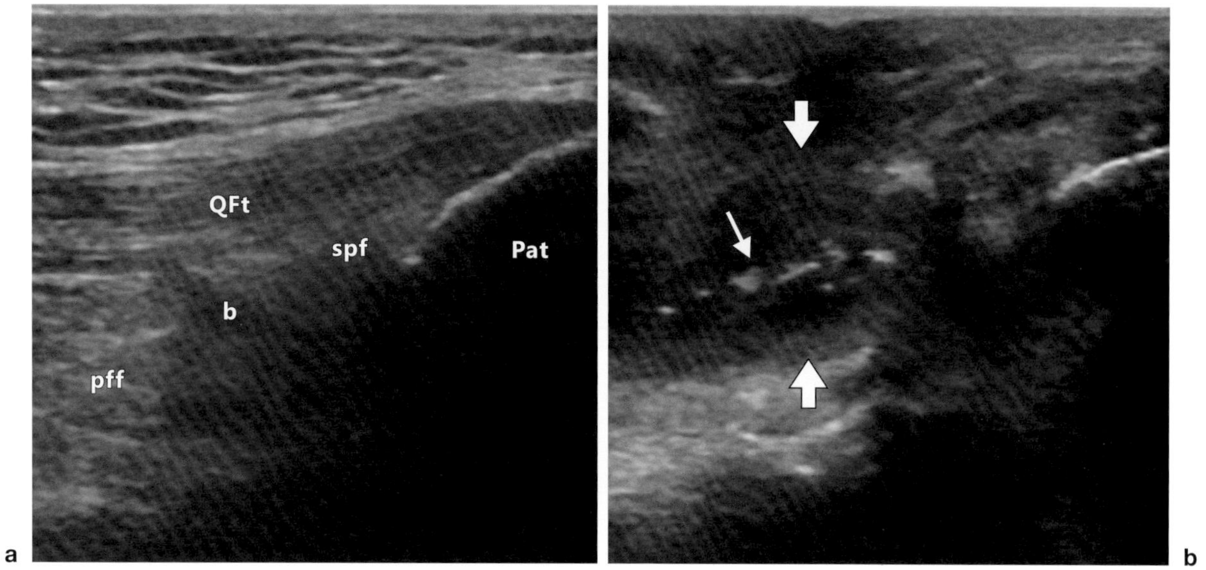

When compared with the normal side (**a**), longitudinal US view shows the repaired full-thickness tear (*thick arrows*) with swollen and hypoechoic irregular margins and bright linear echoes corresponding to intratendinous suture materials (*thin arrow*) (**b**).

b suprapatellar bursa
Pat patella
pff prefemoral fat pad
QFt quadriceps femoris tendon
spf suprapatellar fat pad

Expert note

While close follow-up is very convenient with US imaging, in early post-operative cases, the scanning could be challenging due to excessive edema. As such, it is usually suggested that US imaging would better be used if the follow-up shows unexpected signs, not when it is uneventful.

9.13 A 51-year-old man with bone-tendon-bone reconstruction for the anterior cruciate ligament

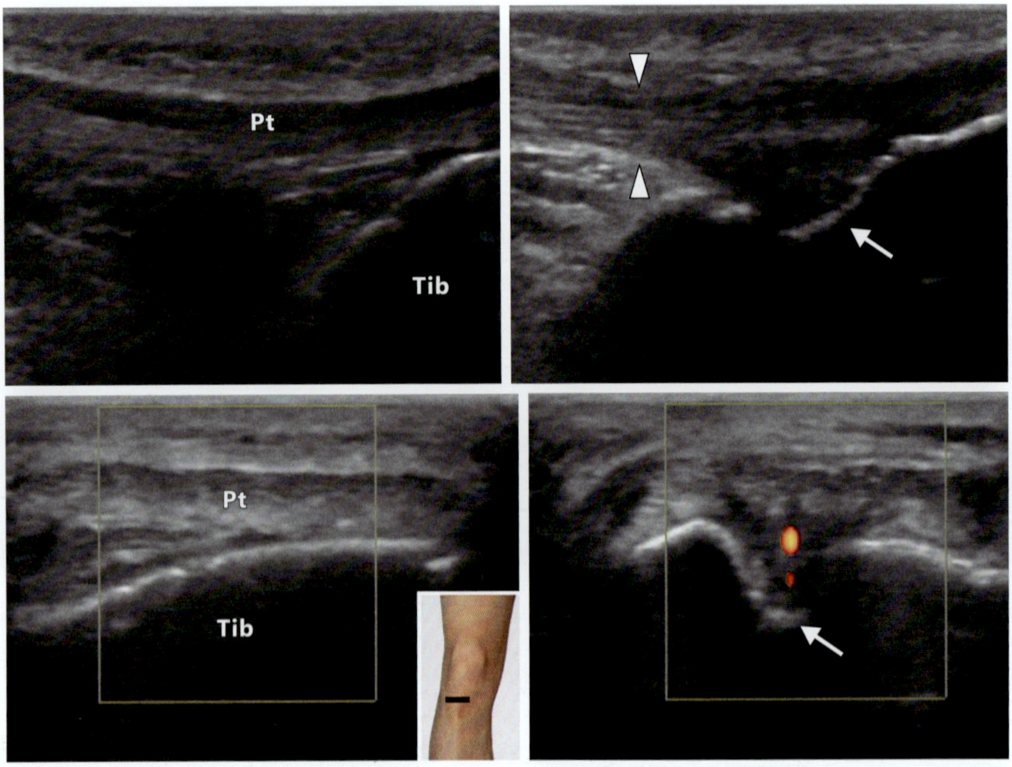

When compared with the normal side (**a**, **c**), longitudinal (**b**) and axial (**d**) US images demonstrate swelling (*arrowheads*) on the distal part of the patellar tendon (**Pt**) and a cortical defect of the tibial groove (*arrows*) at the level of the healing graft area with low power Doppler signal.

Tib tibia

Expert note

Owing to its convenience, US imaging can be used for the prompt follow-up of postoperative musculoskeletal conditions. The wide spectrum would encompass certain bony lesions as well as soft tissue injuries. Similar to fracture follow-up (callus healing); in this patient, US imaging was performed due to persistent local/painful findings after surgery. Aside from the edematous patellar tendon, healing bony cortex (still displaying Doppler flow) was clearly seen. Herein, in contrast to a similar finding of an inflammatory enthesopathy, it would be noteworthy that this Doppler finding is more perceived as "healing". However, it should be interpreted in light of the clinical findings, for sure.

Bilateral Osgood-Schlatter disease in a 14-year-old boy **9.14**

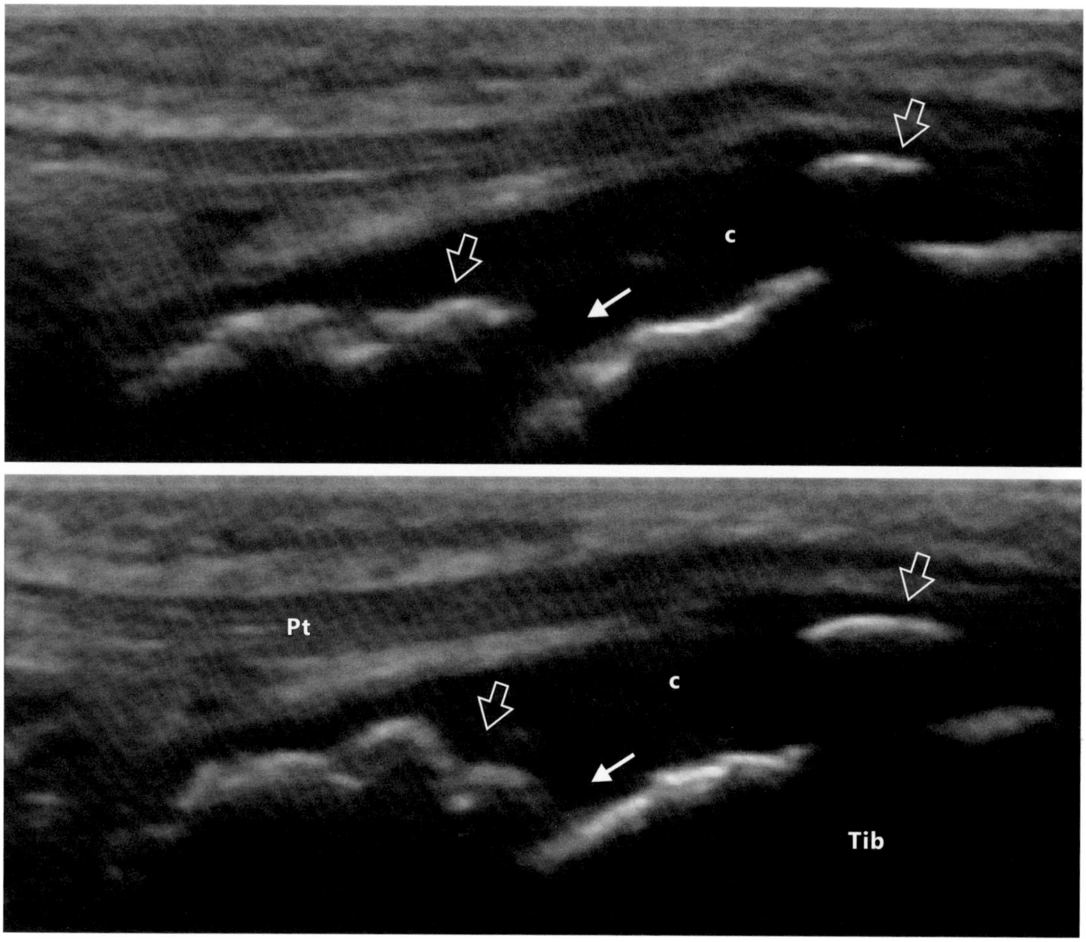

a

b

He presented with focal tenderness and chronic pain on the tibial tuberosity (**Tib**).

Longitudinal US images of the anterior tibial surface reveal significant bony irregularities and small avulsions from the apophyseal cartilage (*void arrows*). Please note the plenty amount of anechoic hyaline cartilage (**c**) and the zone of epiphyseal plates (*thin arrows*) on both sides.

Pt patellar tendon

Expert note

The amount of articular cartilage in children can really be overwhelming and should therefore be cautiously evaluated in order not to misinterprete as fluid. This is also the case for epiphyseal plates whereby erroneous diagnosis of a fracture could otherwise be inevitable. Swelling of the distal patellar tendon insertion and the bursa can also be present in case of Osgood-Schlatter disease.

9.15 Osgood-Schlatter disease in a 35-year-old man

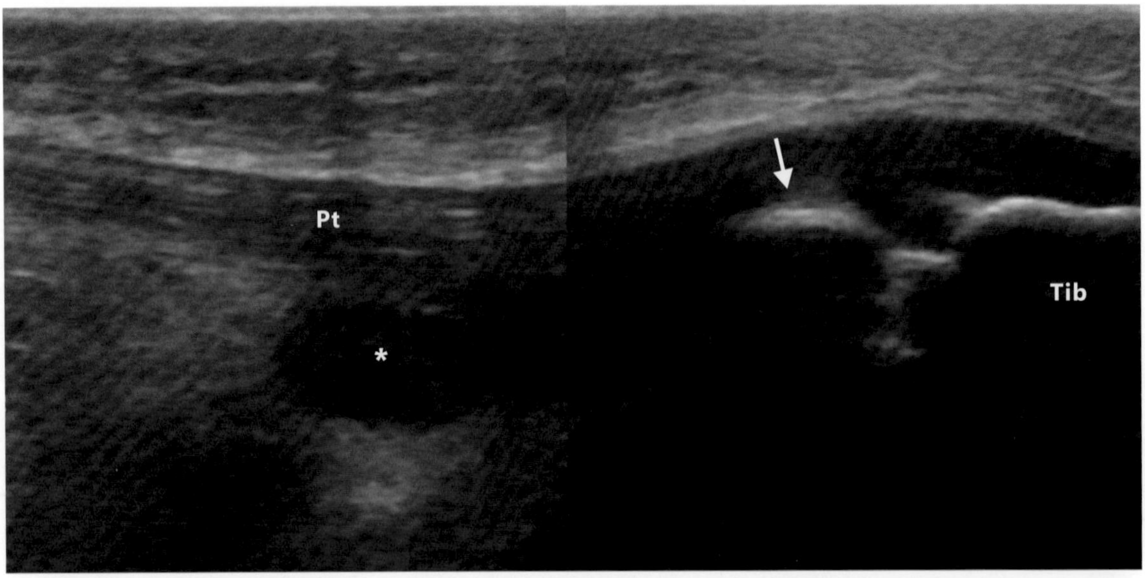

The scenario was complicated by acute and painful infrapatellar bursitis.

Split-screen longitudinal US image shows a fragmented apophysis (*arrow*) of the anterior tibial surface and fluid in the deep infrapatellar bursa (*asterisk*).

Pt patellar tendon
Tib tibial tuberosity

Expert note

Although this disease is chronic, it is usually an accompanying problem which might make the clinical findings overt. On the other hand, it is also not uncommon to diagnose the underlying (otherwise asymptomatic) Osgood-Schlatter disaase when examining for a painful knee for bursitis/tendinitis.

Bilateral Osgood-Schlatter disease in a 15-year-old gymnast **9.16**

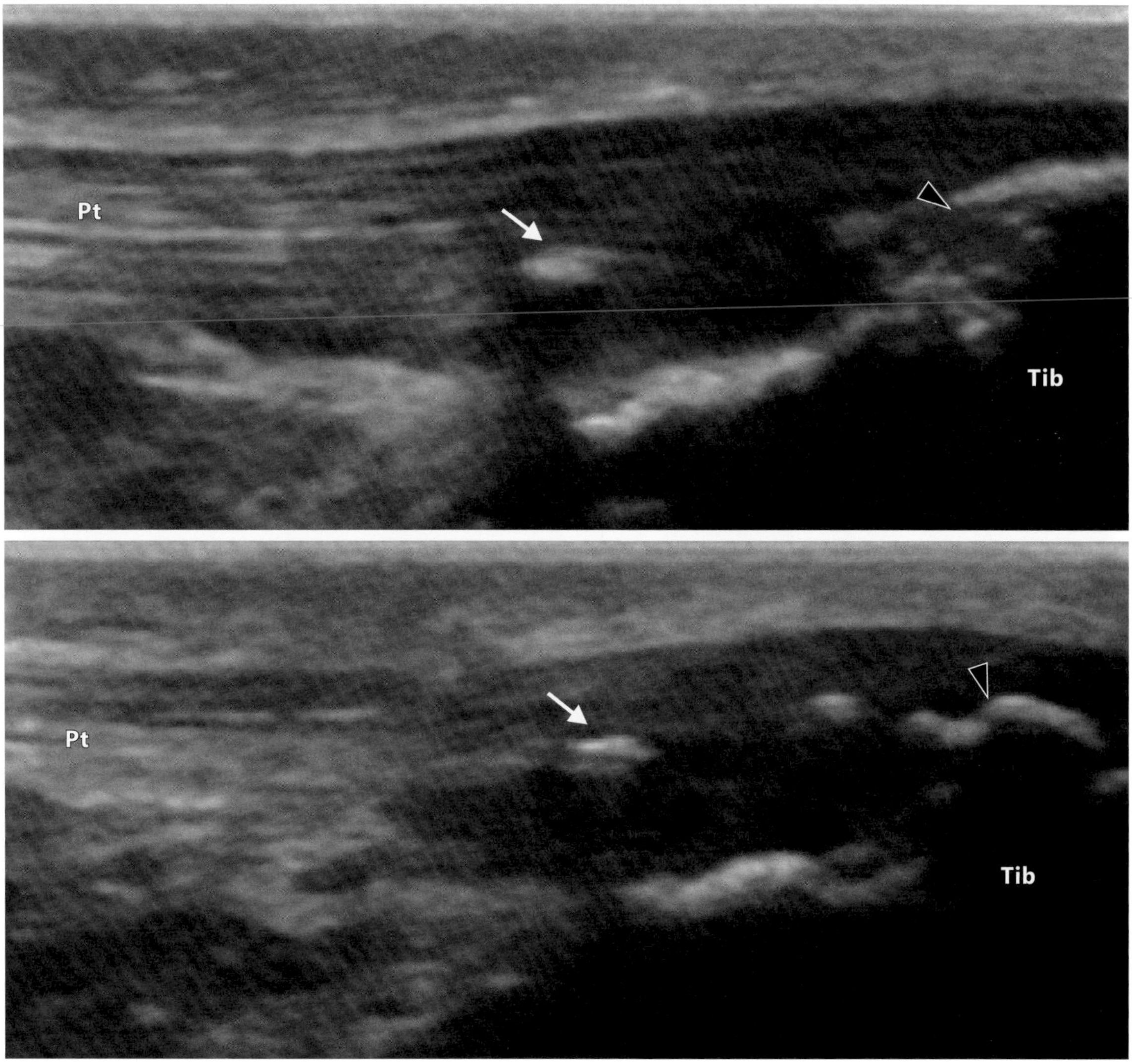

She presented with left sided anterior knee pain during and after training.

Longitudinal US images reveal bilateral cortical irregularities (*arrowheads*) of the tibial tuberosity (**Tib**) and small hyperechoic calcific foci (*arrows*) within the patellar tendons (**Pt**).

Expert note

Since comparison is not only an advantage but also a prerequisite in US imaging, physicians can easily inform their patients in advance as regards their bilateral disease involvement and the relevant precautions when necessary.

9.17 Bilateral Osgood-Schlatter disease in a 19-year-old basketball player

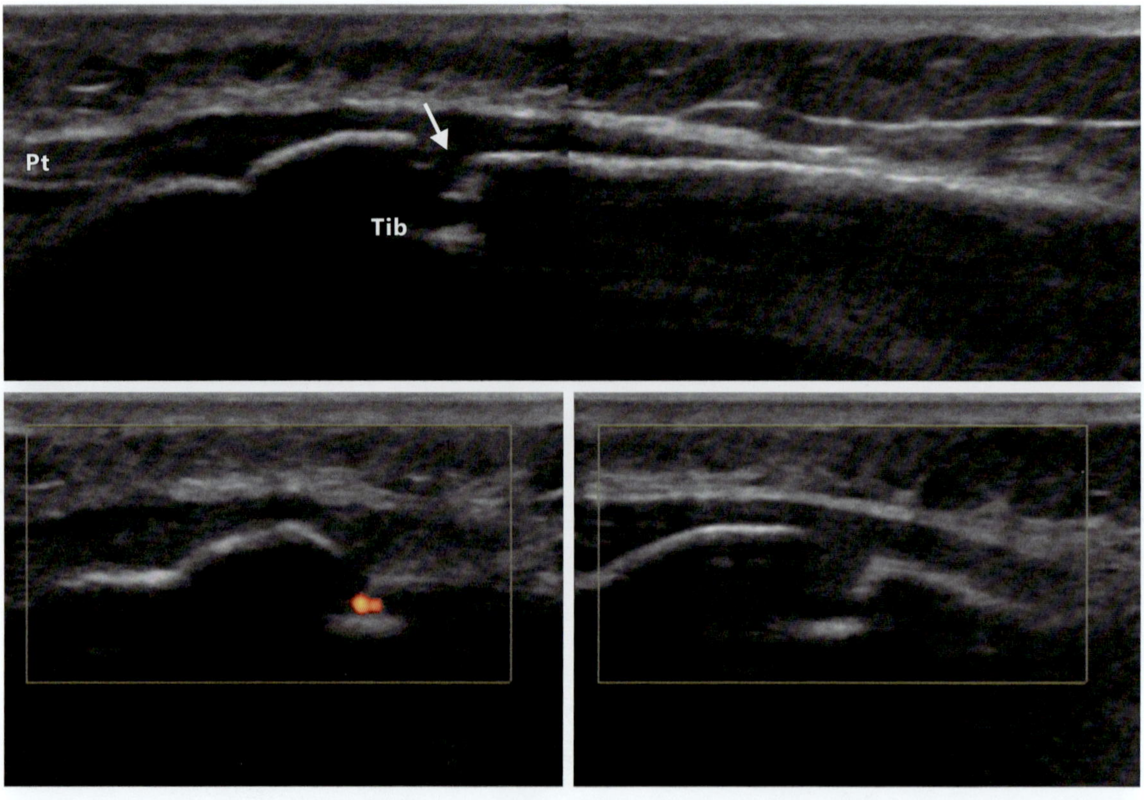

a b c

He had knee pain for about two months and was unable to adequately complete jumping activities.

Split-screen longitudinal US view (**a**) shows a cortical irregularity (*arrow*) on the tibial tuberosity (**Tib**). Power Doppler image reveals hyperemia on the symptomatic side (**b**) but not on the asymptomatic side (**c**).

Pt patellar tendon

Patellar tendinitis in a 23-year-old amateur volleyball player **9.18**

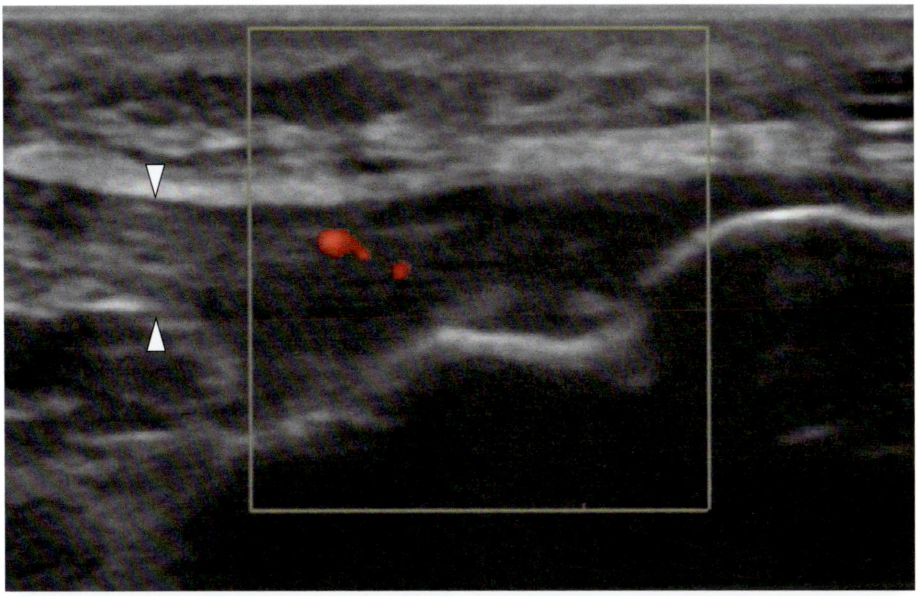

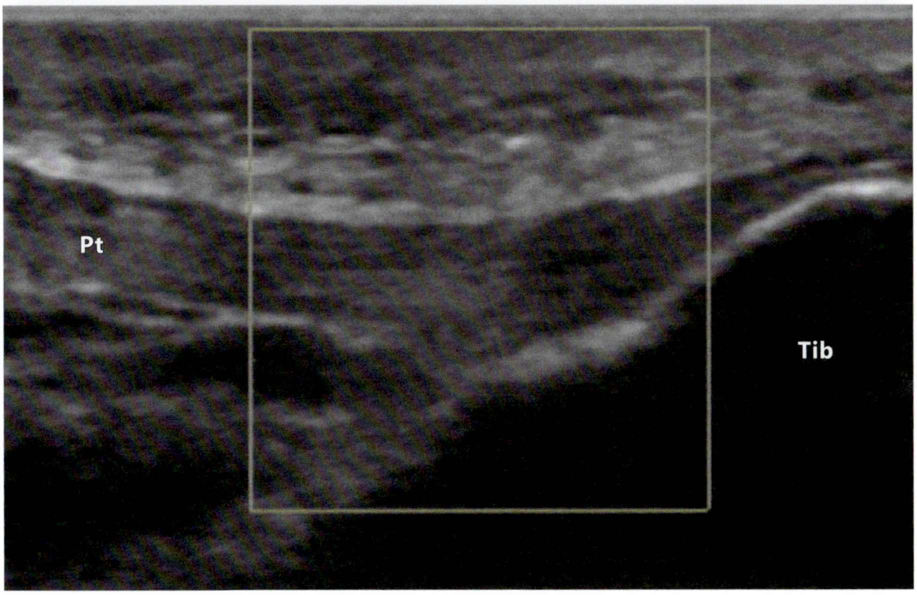

He suffered anterior knee pain especially on descend from jumping.

Longitudinal US image shows a markedly thickened and hypoechoic patellar tendon (**Pt**) (*arrowheads*) which reveals mild hyperemia on power Doppler imaging (**a**). Normal side (**b**).

Tib tibial tuberosity

9.19 Patellar tendon abnormality in a 30-year-old athlete

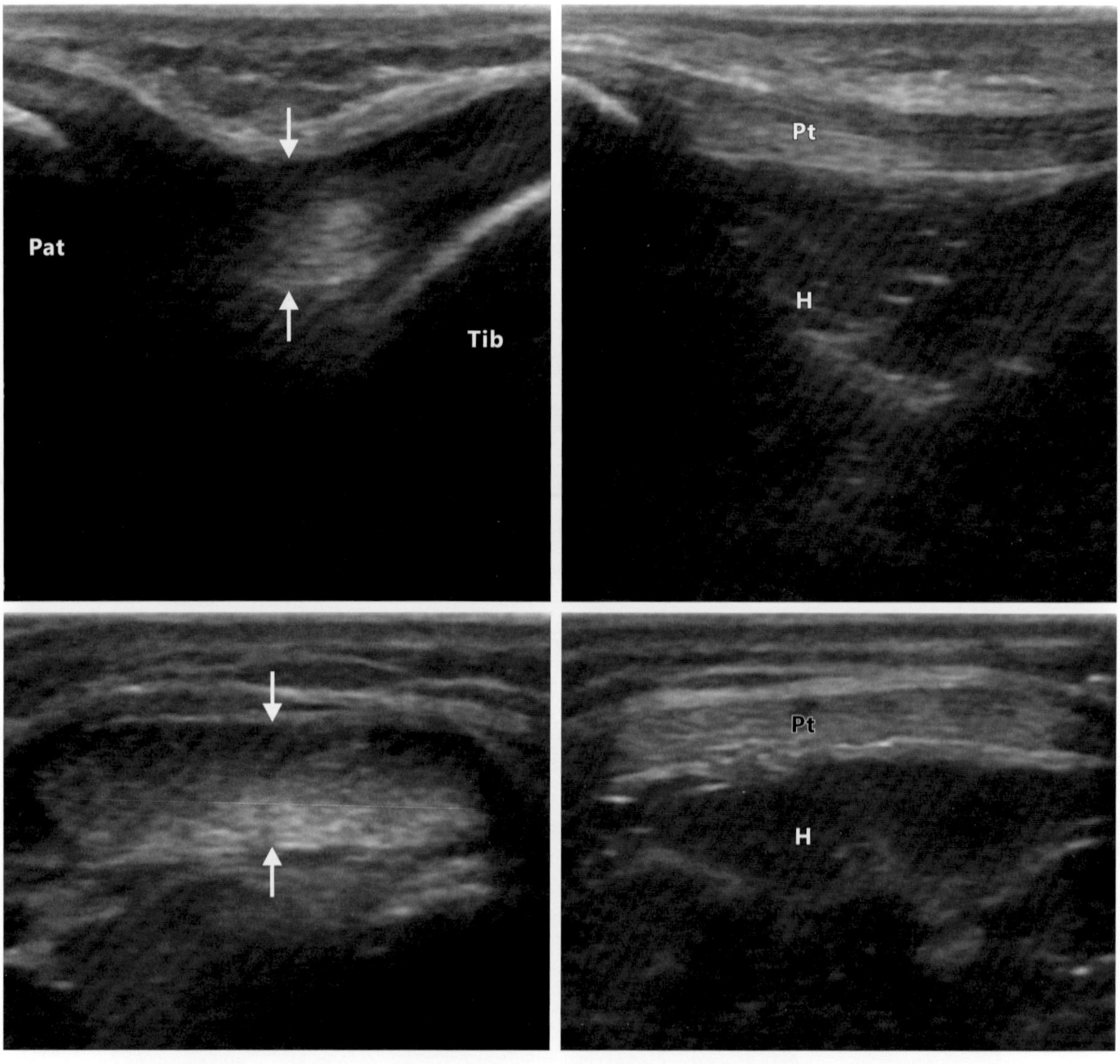

a b c d

He had femoral nerve palsy with anterior thigh atrophy and knee pain.

Longitudinal (**a**) and axial (**c**) US images over the anterior aspect of the knee obtained during mild knee flexion show an enlarged and bowing patellar tendon (*arrows*). Corresponding normal views (**b**, **d**).

H	Hoffa's fat pad	**Pt**	patellar tendon
Pat	patella	**Tib**	tibia

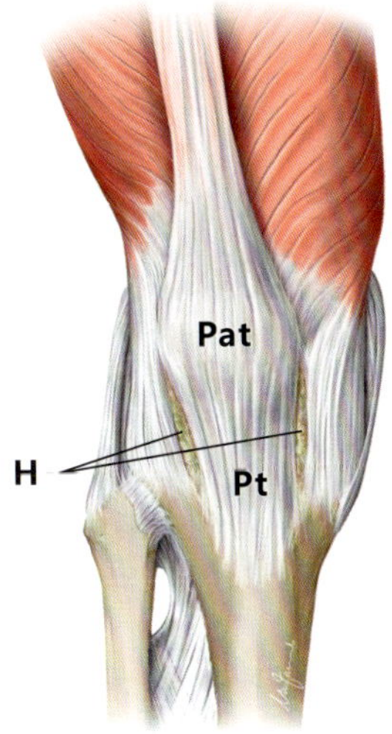

Expert note

Normally, mild knee flexion is usually performed to make the patellar and quadriceps tendons more straight and better visualized [6]. However, in this patient, probably due to weakened quadriceps strength and a consequent patellar malalignment; the tendon could only be imaged as bowing. Of additional note, using different/reference measurements, US imaging can well be used to assess and quantify joint subluxations.
A practical remark would be that the patella and tibia can not be visualized at the same time on the asymptomatic side. However, on the symptomatic side they can be easily seen simultaneously; this is indicative of patella baja.

9.20 Superficial infrapatellar and prepatellar bursitis in a 44-year-old woman after a fall on the flexed knee

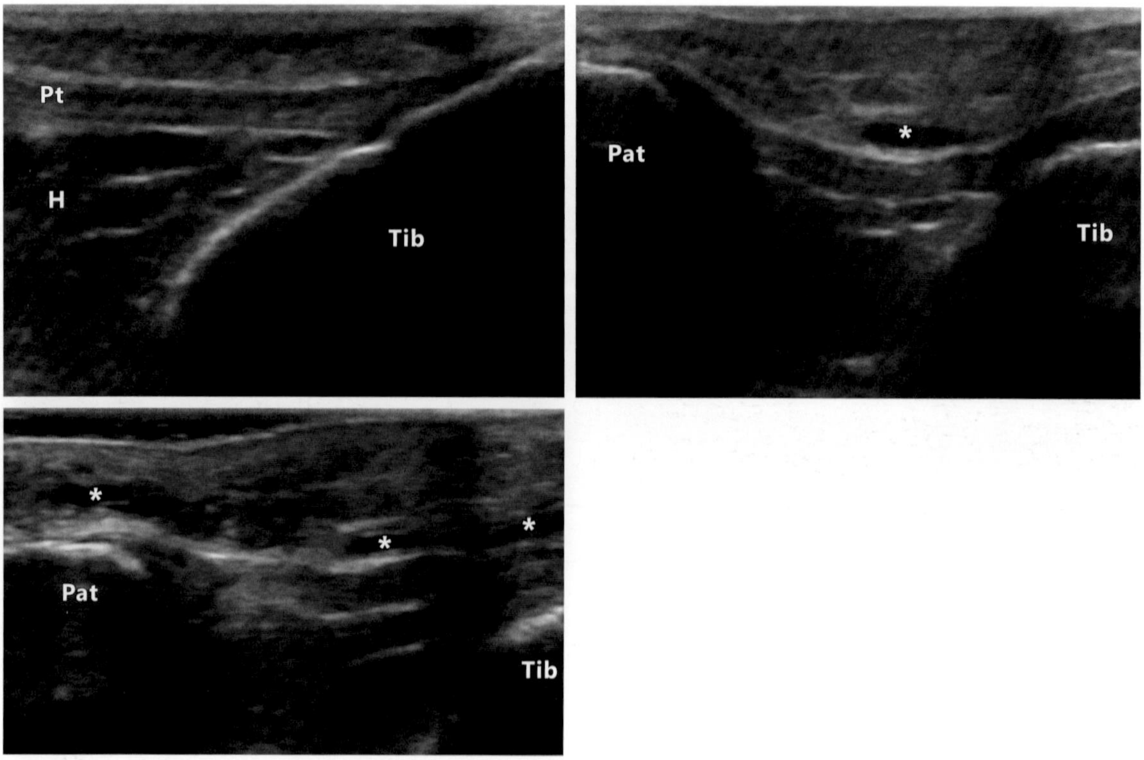

When compared with the normal side (**a**), longitudinal US images obtained over the anterior aspect of the knee during extension (**b**) and flexion (**c**) reveal small fluid collections (*asterisks*) superficial to the distal patellar tendon (**Pt**) and patella (**Pat**) (*star*).

H Hoffa's fat pad
Tib tibia

Expert note

Once again, while dynamic imaging is easily performed in these conditions; the sonographer should be careful (i.e. applying mild compression) in searching for small and quite superficial areas of fluid accumulation.

Hoffa's disease (Hoffitis) in a middle-aged man **9.21**

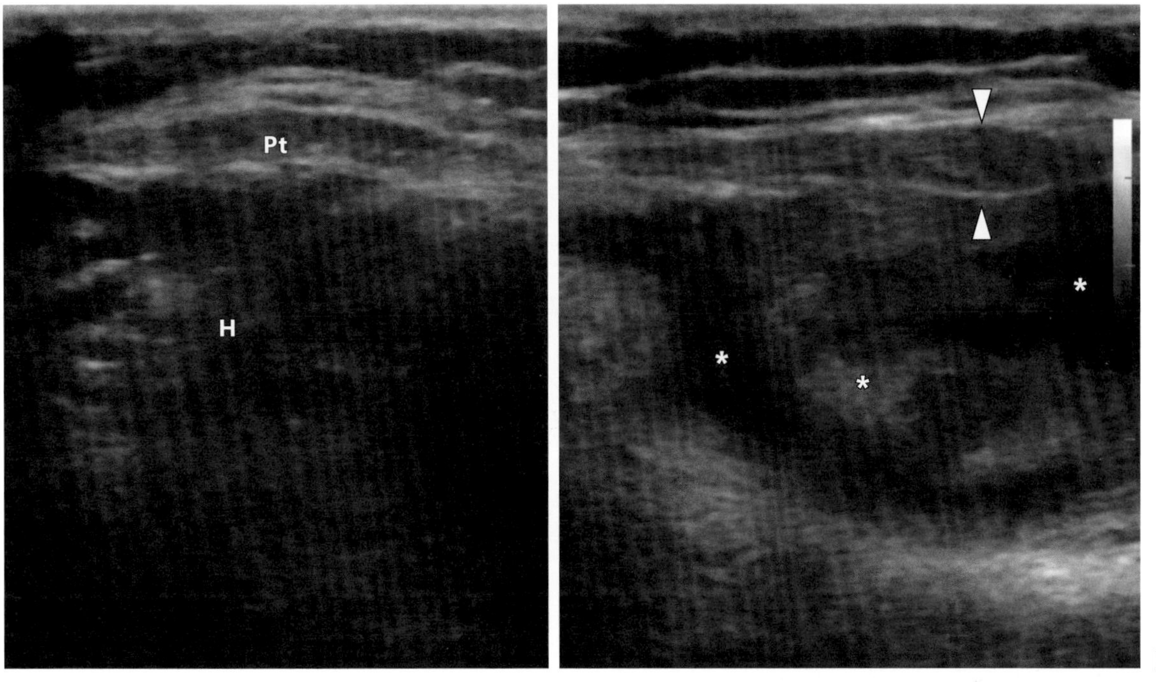

a b

He had anterior knee pain and tenderness at the inferior pole of the patella.

When compared with the normal side (**a**), axial US image shows focal thickening (*arrowheads*) of the patellar tendon (**Pt**) and swollen and edematous (*asterisks*) Hoffa's fat pad (**H**) with heterogenous appearance (**b**).

9.22 Superficial infrapatellar bursitis in a patient with 10-year history of systemic lupus erythematosus

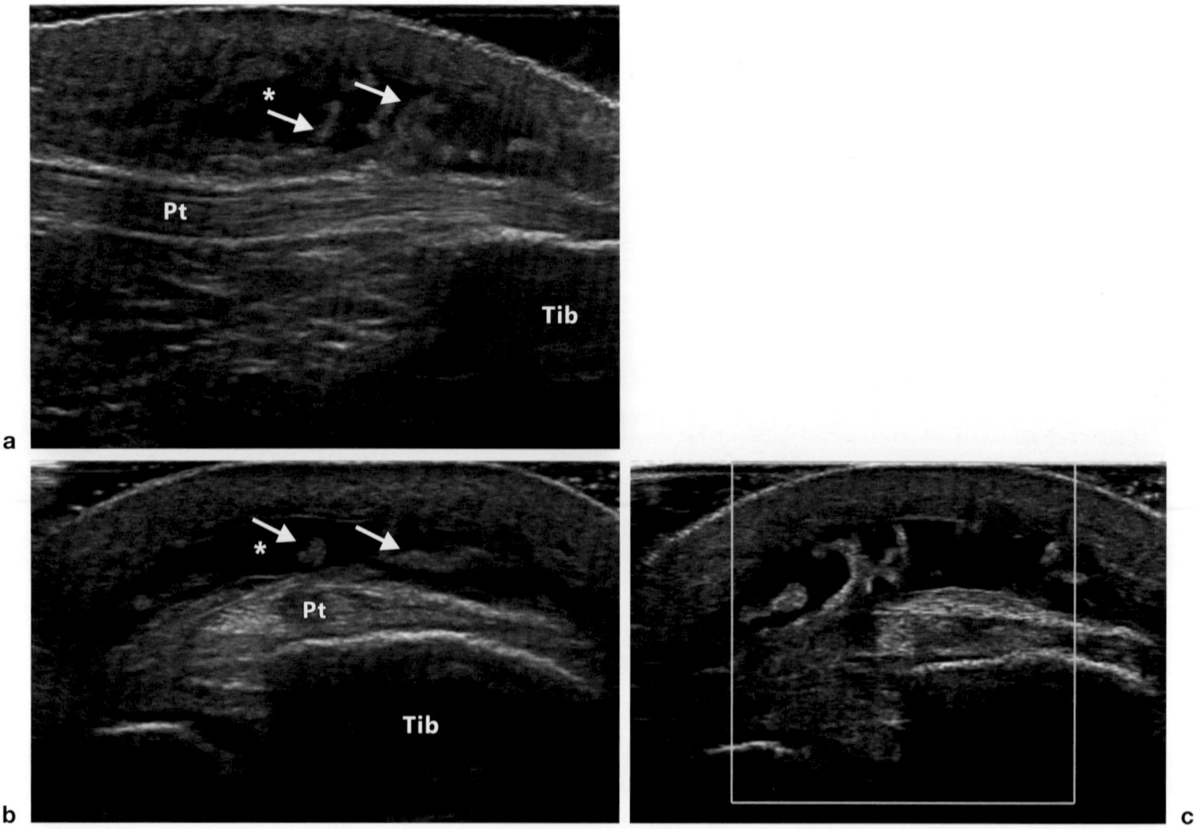

Longitudinal (**a**) and axial (**b**, **c**) US images over the anterior aspect of the knee demonstrate thickened and heterogeneous superficial infrapatellar bursa filled with fluid collection (*asterisks*) and internal septations of the hypertrophied synovium (*arrows*). Power Doppler imaging is unremarkable (**c**).

Pt patellar tendon
Tib tibial tuberosity

Expert note

Owing to the very superficial localization of the pathology, the images were acquired with the use of extra gel and very gentle probe compression. Despite the overlying chronic bursitis, patellar tendon seems to be quite normal and perhaps with relatively increased echogenicity due to the enhanced through transmission artifact.

Superficial infrapatellar bursitis in a 50-year-old woman after a local blunt trauma

9.23

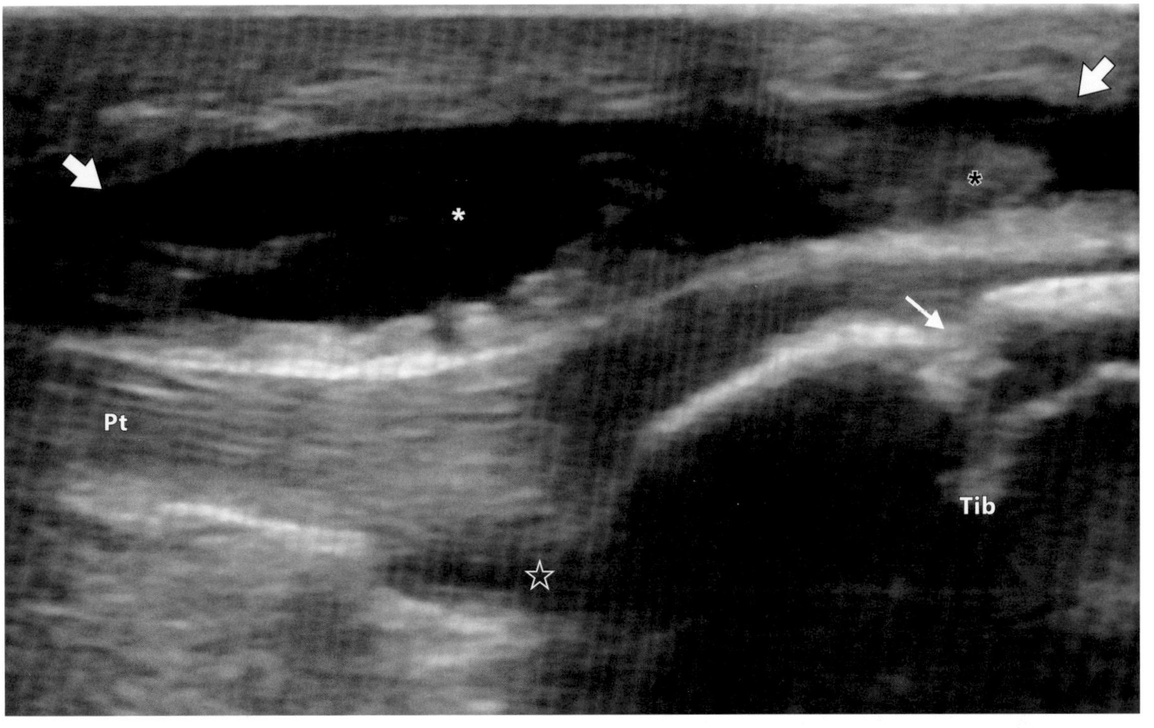

Longitudinal US image over the infrapatellar region shows marked distension (*thick arrows*) of the superficial infrapatellar bursa with effusion (*white asterisk*) and synovial hypertrophy (*black asterisk*) as well as bony irregularity (*thin arrow*) on the anterior tibial surface.
Please also note the small effusion (*star*) in the deep infrapatellar bursa between the deep tendon margin and the tibia (**Tib**).

Pt patellar tendon

Knee

9.24 Distal patellar tendinopathy and deep infrapatellar bursitis in a middle-aged man

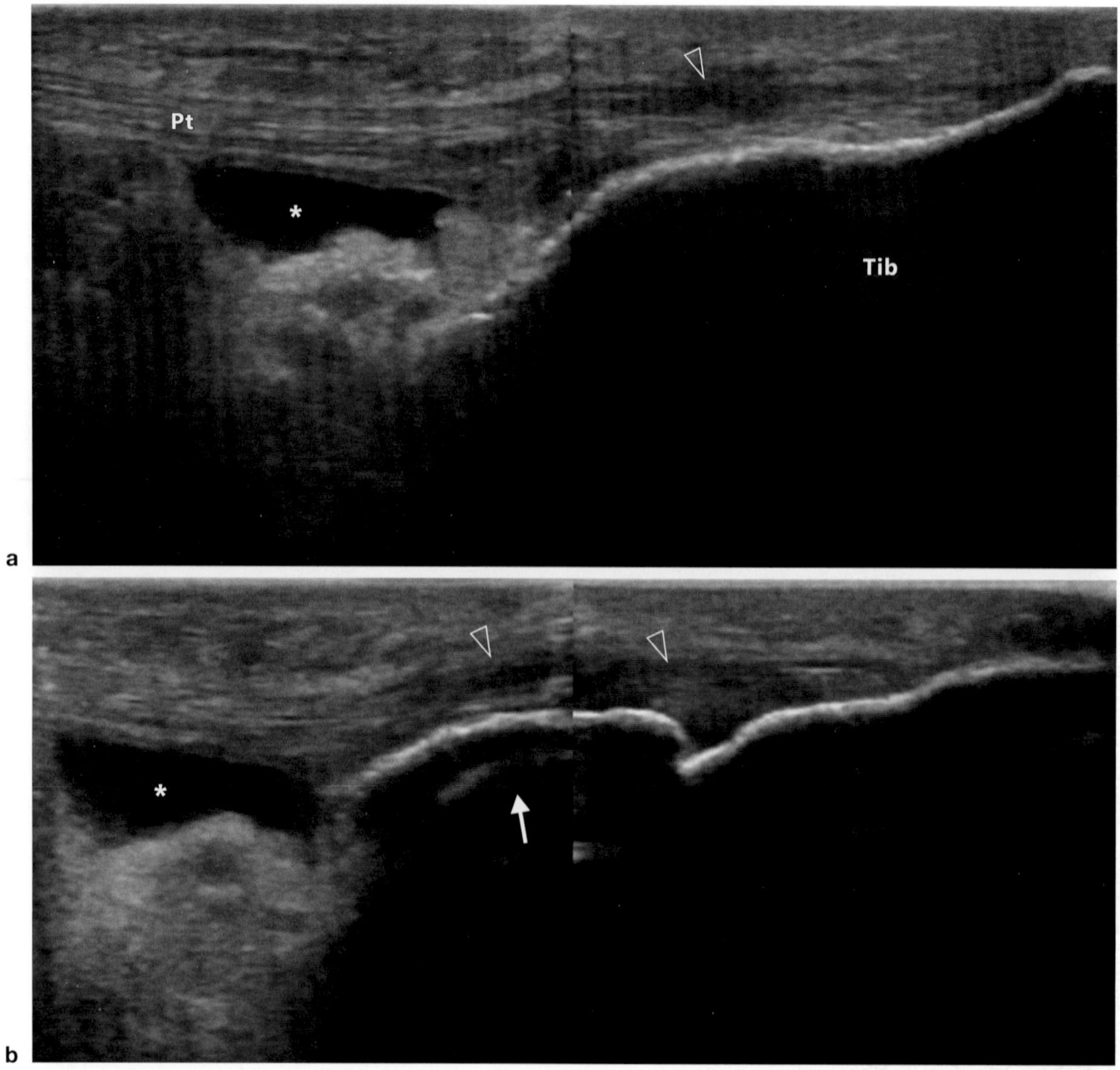

Longitudinal split-screen US images of the infrapatellar region (**a**, **b**) reveal effusion in the deep infrapatellar bursa (*asterisks*) associated with edematous (*arrowheads*) distal patellar tendon (**Pt**). A large cortical sequela (*arrow*) of a likely Osgood-Schlatter disease is also seen (**b**).

Tib tibial tuberosity

Chronic prepatellar bursitis in a 42-year-old woman with painful knee swelling **9.25**

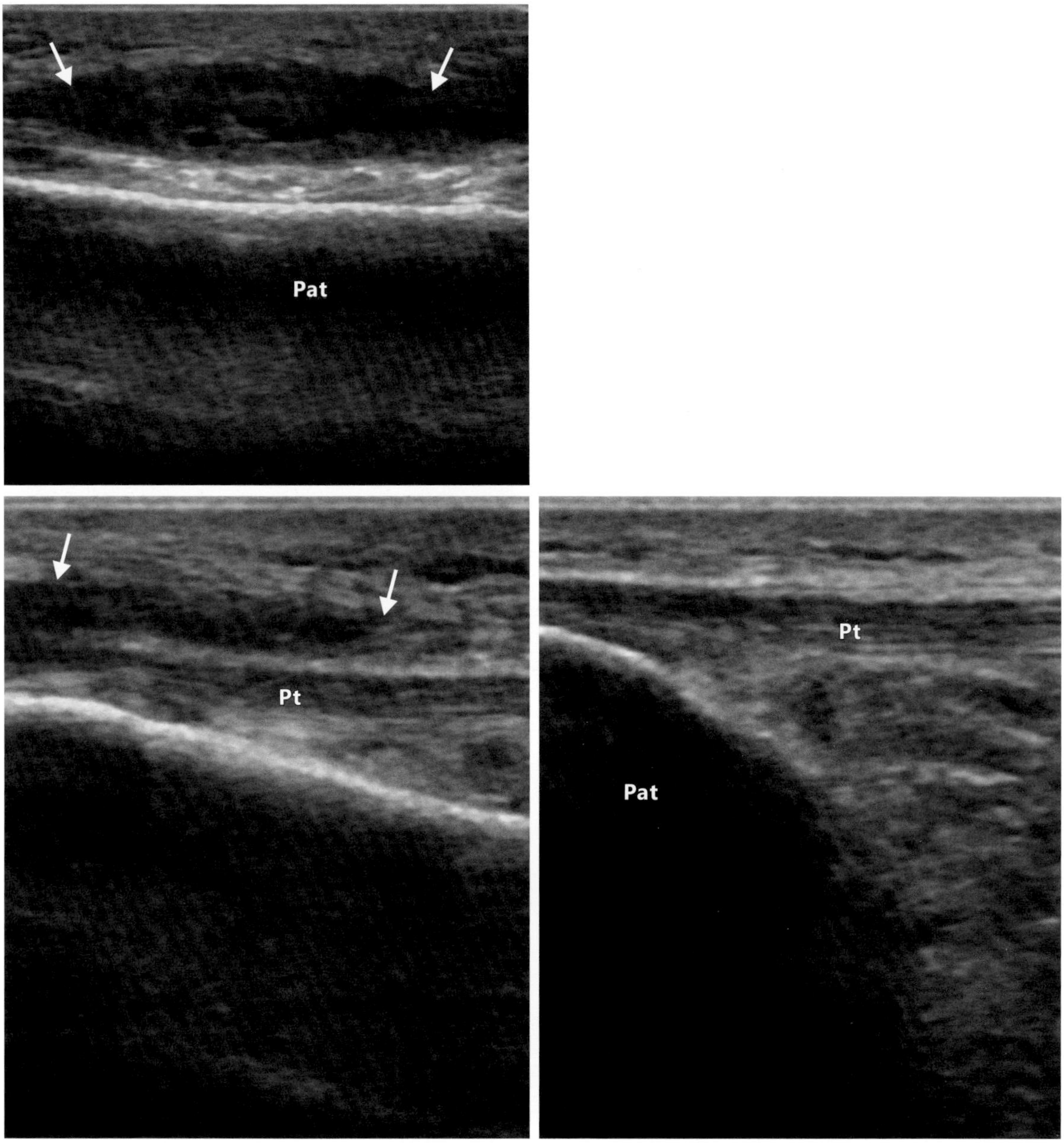

a b c

Axial US imaging over the patella (**Pat**) demonstrates marked thickening of the prepatellar bursa (*arrows*) with internal hypoechoic appearance (**a**). Longitudinal US imaging (**b**) shows the distal extension of the bursa over the patellar tendon (**Pt**). Longitudinal view of the normal side (**c**).

9.26 Intraarticular loose body in a 55-year-old man with a 5-year history of knee pain and recurrent swelling

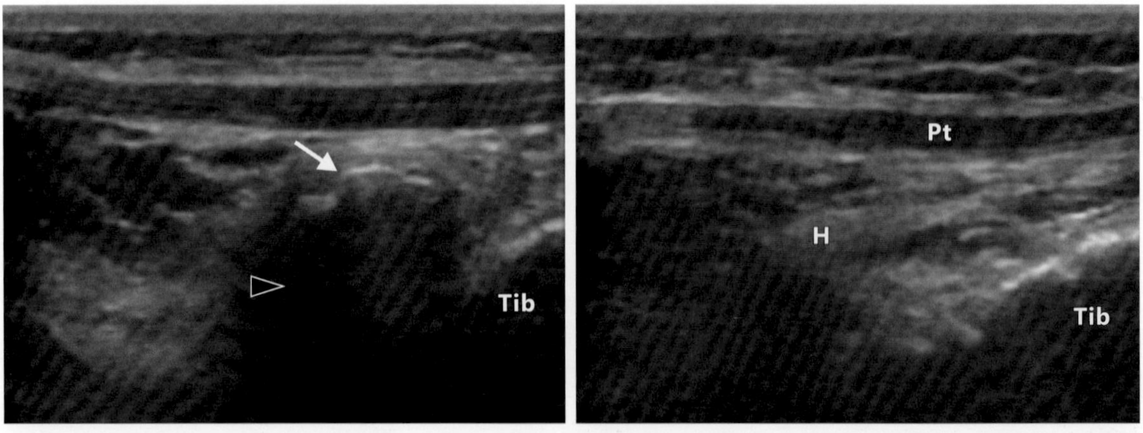

a b

Longitudinal US image (**a**) demonstrates a calcified loose body (*arrow*) within the deep infrapatellar recess close to tibia (**Tib**). Note also its posterior acoustic shadowing artifact (*arrowhead*). Normal side (**b**).

H Hoffa's fat pad
Pt patellar tendon

Expert note

In some patients who describe symptoms of joint locking, different loose bodies can be observed. Herein, the advantage of US would be the availability of imaging at any angle of the joint either statically or dynamically. Yet, it is possible to move next to the patient (while lying, sitting or standing) and perform the scanning at any position he/she describes to be symptomatic.

Patellar hypoplasia in a 3-year-old boy with the complaint of limping 9.27

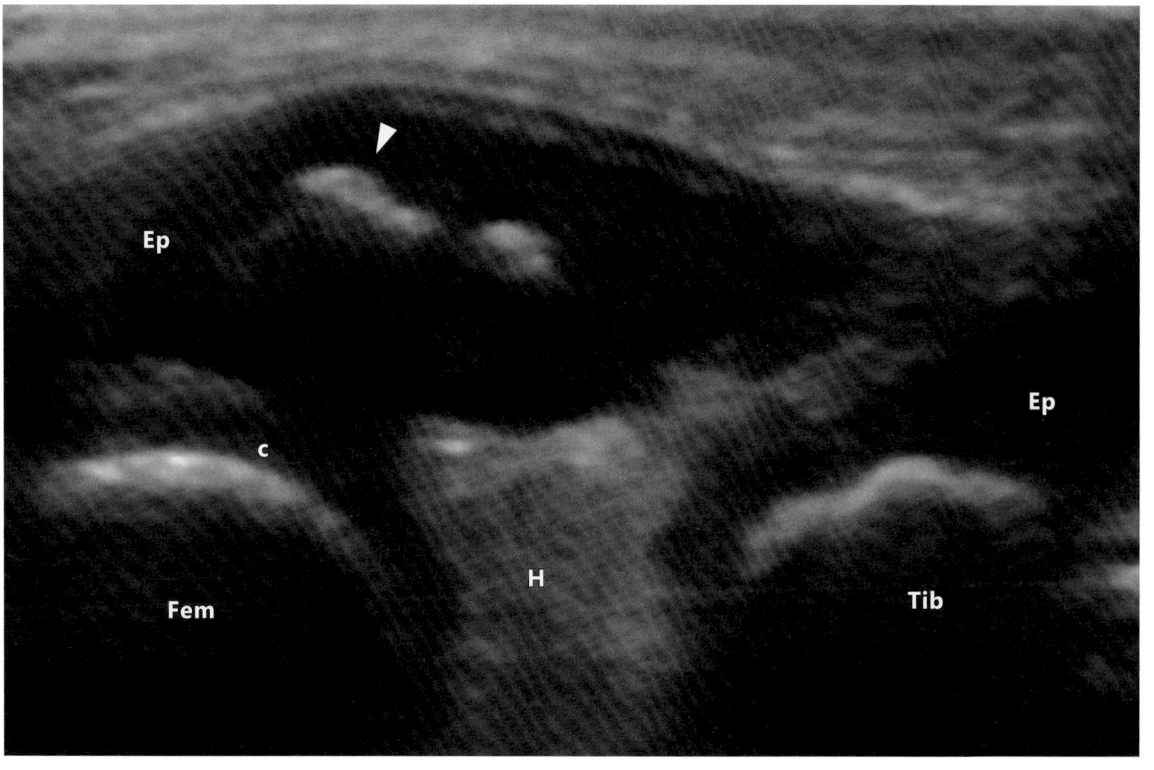

Longitudinal US imaging over the anterior knee shows the large amount of unossified epiphyseal cartilage (**Ep**) in the patella and tibia (**Tib**). Articular cartilage (**c**) over the distal femoral condyle and ossification zone of the patella (*arrowhead*) are also observed.

Fem femur
H Hoffa's fad pad

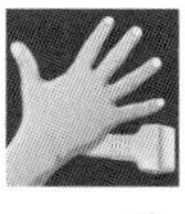

Expert note

Again, the amount of cartilage in small children can be overwhelming [7]. While this would pose challenges during the examination (e.g. misdiagnosis for effusion), it could sometimes provide ease as well. For instance, although the probe is positioned over the patella in this case, the joint can readily be scanned, even with better visibility for the Hoffa's fat pad. This is for sure owing to the anechoic property of the hyaline cartilage.

9.28 Medial collateral ligament injury in a 45-year-old patient with medial knee pain after a fall on the ground

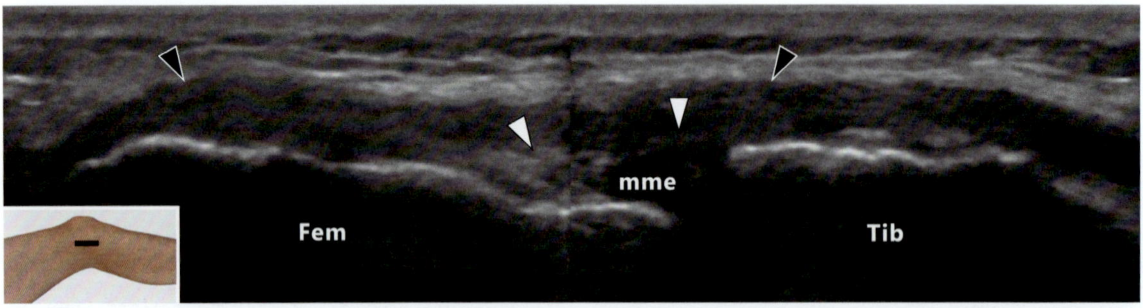

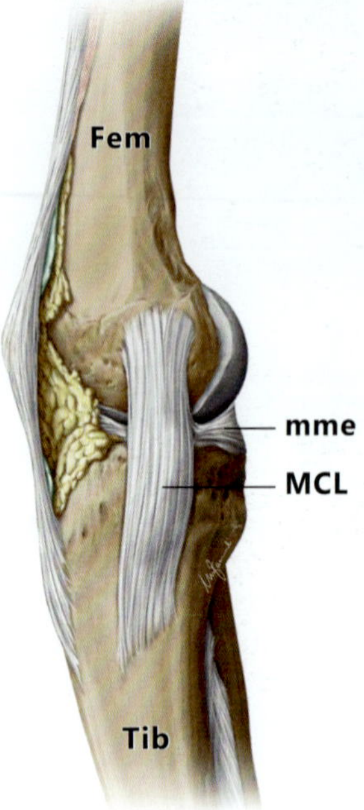

Longitudinal split-screen US image over the medial knee joint demonstrates hypoechoic appearance of the thickened but intact superficial layer of the medial collateral ligament (*black arrowheads*).
Please note the intact deep layer of the ligament (*white arrowheads*).

Fem femur
MCL medial collateral ligament
mme medial meniscus
Tib tibia

Follow-up for medial collateral ligament injury in an amateur soccer player **9.29**

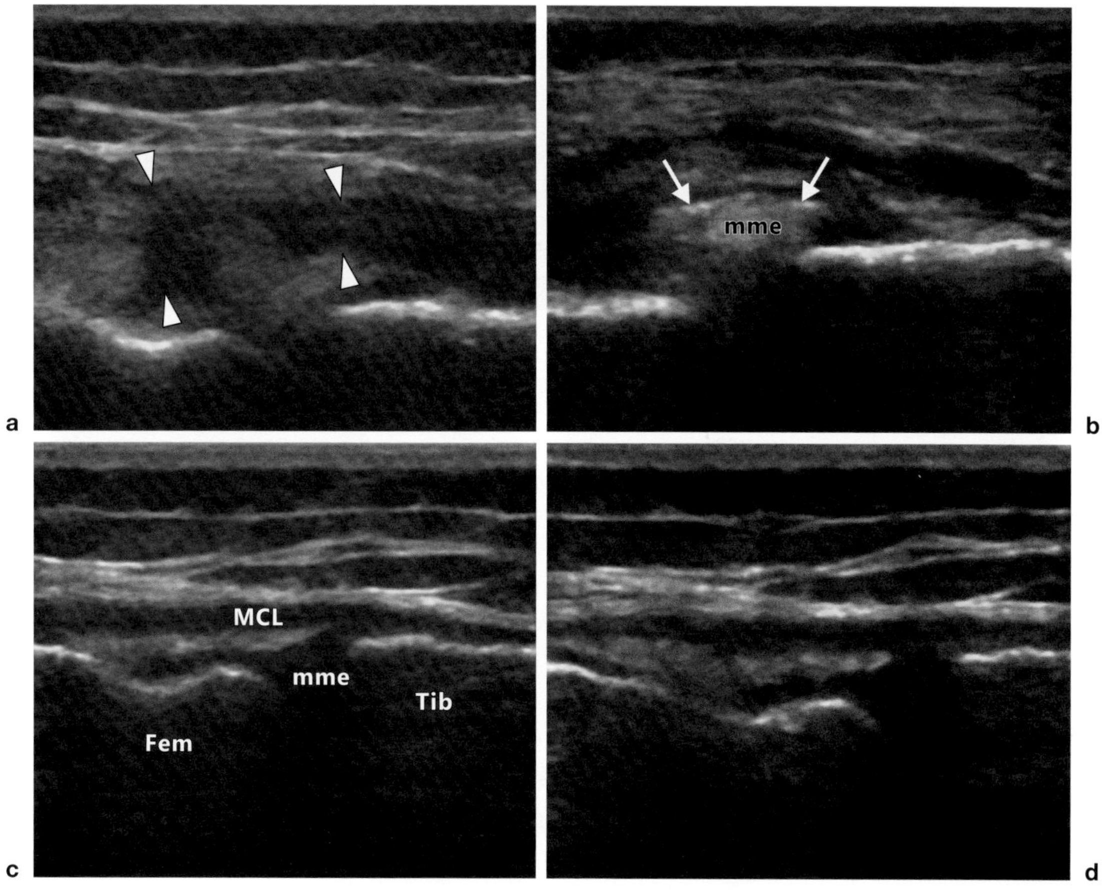

Longitudinal US image over the medial joint line reveals irregular, thickened, inhomogeneously hypoechoic medial collateral ligament (**MCL**) (*arrowheads*) due to edema (**a**). Repeat examination after treatment shows less edema and irregularity in the ligament with mild extrusion (*arrows*) of the medial meniscus (**mme**) (**b**). Corresponding views on the contralateral side at two examinations (**c**, **d**).

Fem femur
Tib tibia

Expert note

Normally, the proximal (meniscofemoral) portion of the MCL is thicker than the distal (meniscotibial) portion. Likewise, in this case, the edematous thicknening of the ligament seems to be more predominant in the proximal portion as well. Herewith, the presence of an additional partial rupture can be confirmed either with compression of the US probe or application of the valgus stress test. Concerning the meniscal extrusion, imaging can also be performed while the patient is standing which might make it further salient.

9.30 Pellegrini-Stieda lesion in a 45-year-old ex-football player with pain and tenderness on the medial aspect of the knee

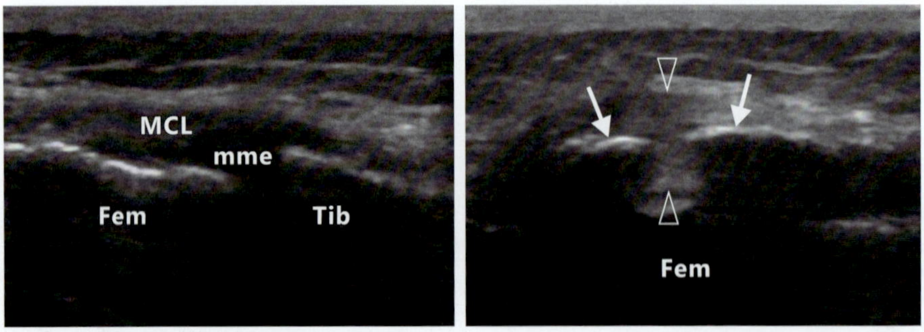

When compared with the normal medial collateral ligament (**MCL**) (**a**), longitudinal US image over the medial aspect of the knee shows irregular areas of calcifications (*arrows*) at the proximal side of the thickened ligament (*arrowheads*) (**b**).

Fem femur
Tib tibia
mme medial meniscus

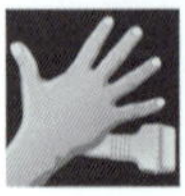

Expert note

As in other cases of calcifications, US needs to be considered as the best imaging modality for early diagnosis, even during the period when X-ray or computed tomography might be negative.

9.31 Pellegrini-Stieda lesion in a 50-year-old woman with chronic pain on the medial aspect of the knee

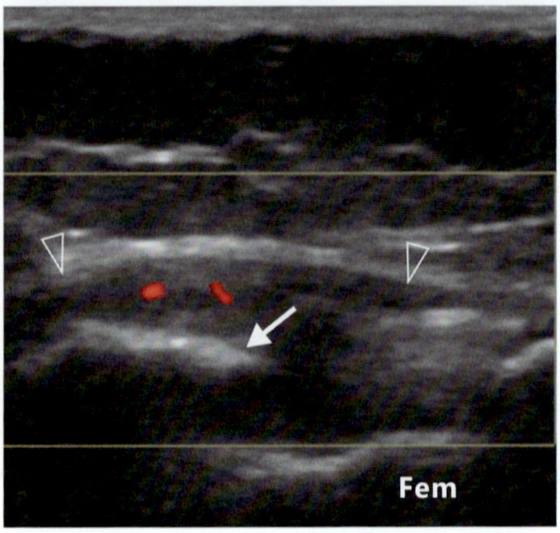

Longitudinal US (power Doppler) image over the medial knee shows calcification (*arrow*) within the medial collateral ligament (*arrowheads*) and vascular flow signals.

Meniscal extrusion in a young-aged woman who had medial knee pain after a fall from the stairs **9.32**

a
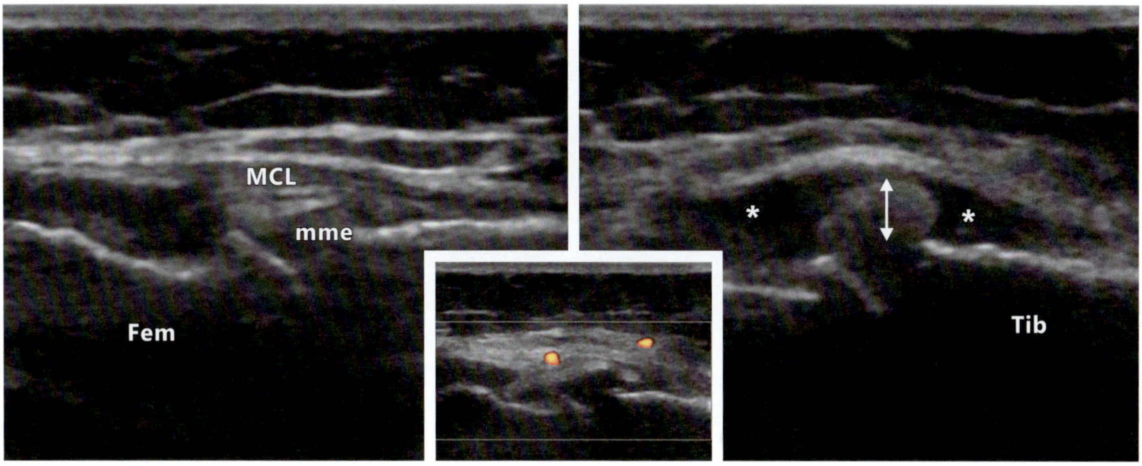

b

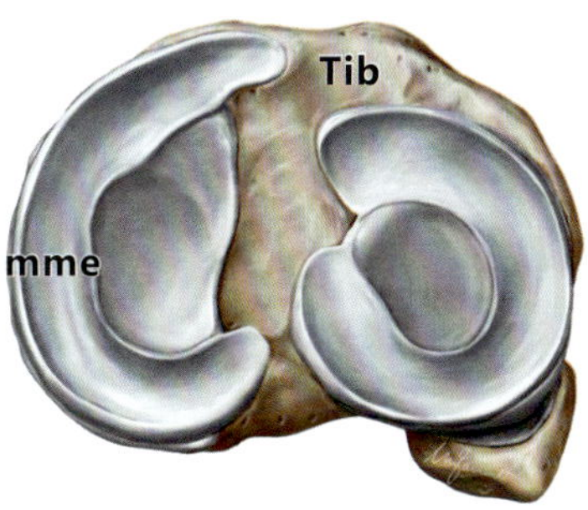

When compared with the normal side (**a**), longitudinal US image on the medial knee joint (**b**) shows extrusion (*double arrow*) in the medial meniscus (**mme**) stretching the overlying edematous (*asterisks*) medial collateral ligament (**MCL**). Local vascularity is also seen in power Doppler imaging (*small figure*).

Fem femur
Tib tibia

Expert note

Protrusion of the medial menisci has been defined as the distance between the peripheral border of the meniscus and the outline of the tibial plateau being >2 mm [8, 9].

9.33 Meniscal extrusion in a patient with intermittent catching sensation and knee pain

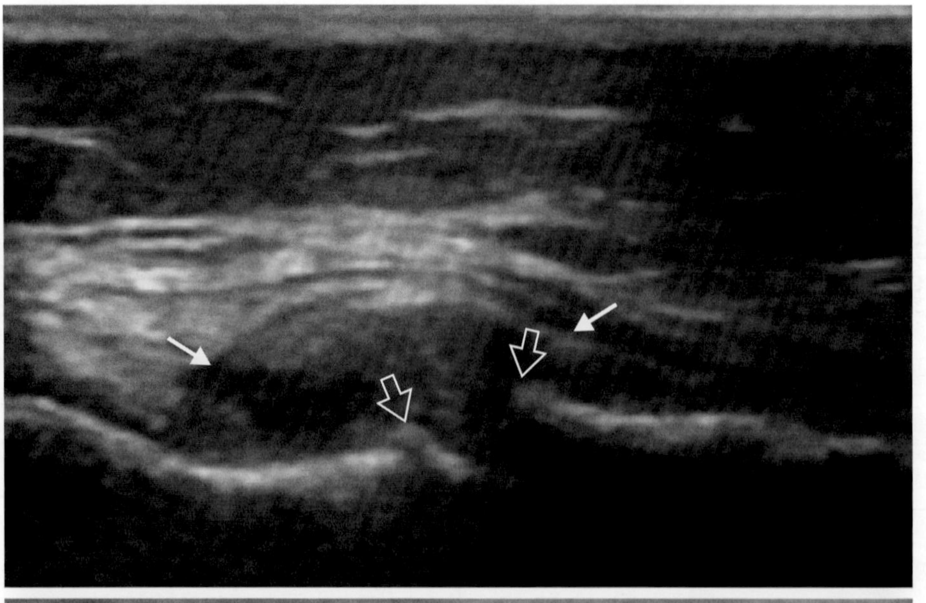

a

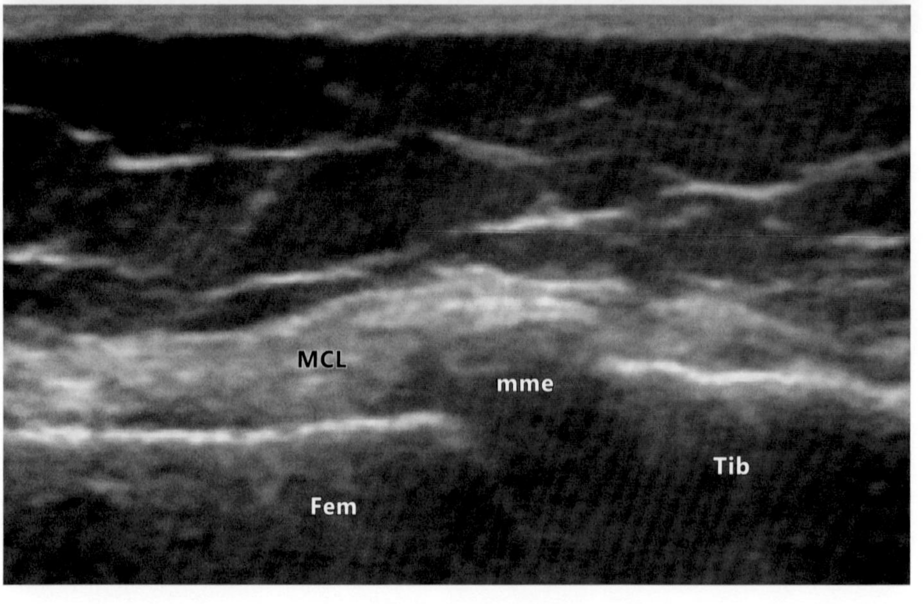

b

Longitudinal US image over the medial knee joint demonstrates joint space narrowing, small osteophytes (*void arrows*) and extrusion (*thin arrows*) of the medial meniscus (**mme**) (**a**). Normal contralateral side (**b**).

Fem femur
MCL medial collateral ligament
Tib tibia

Bilateral meniscal extrusion in a 54-year-old woman with medial knee osteoarthritis 9.34

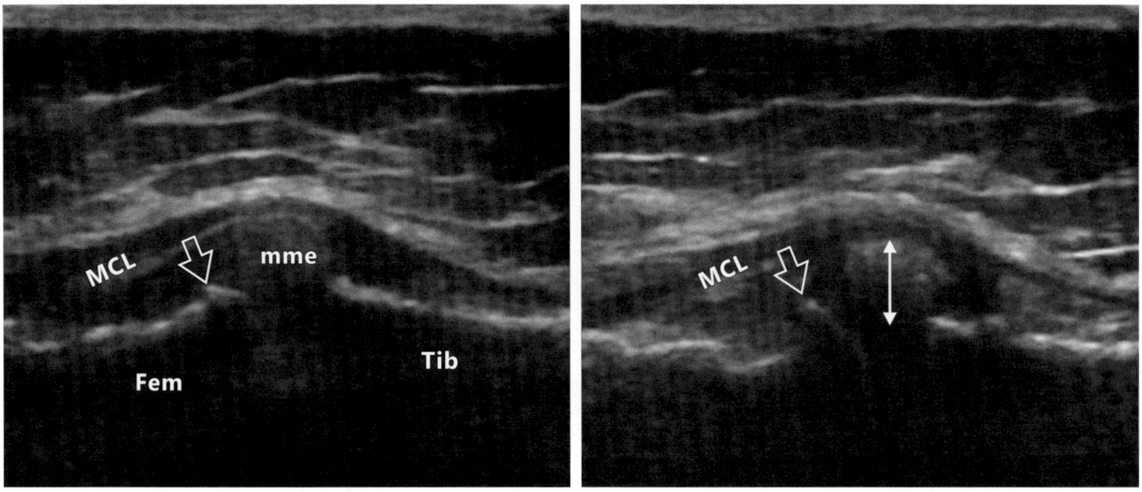

a b

Longitudinal US images over the medial joint line show extrusion of the medial menisci (**mme**) that stretch the overlying medial collateral ligaments (**MCL**), and small (**a**) and medium (**b**) sized osteophytes (*void arrows*). Measurement for the meniscal extrusion can also be performed as shown (*double arrow*) (**b**).

Fem femur
Tib tibia

9.35 Medial knee osteoarthritis with meniscus degeneration in an elderly woman

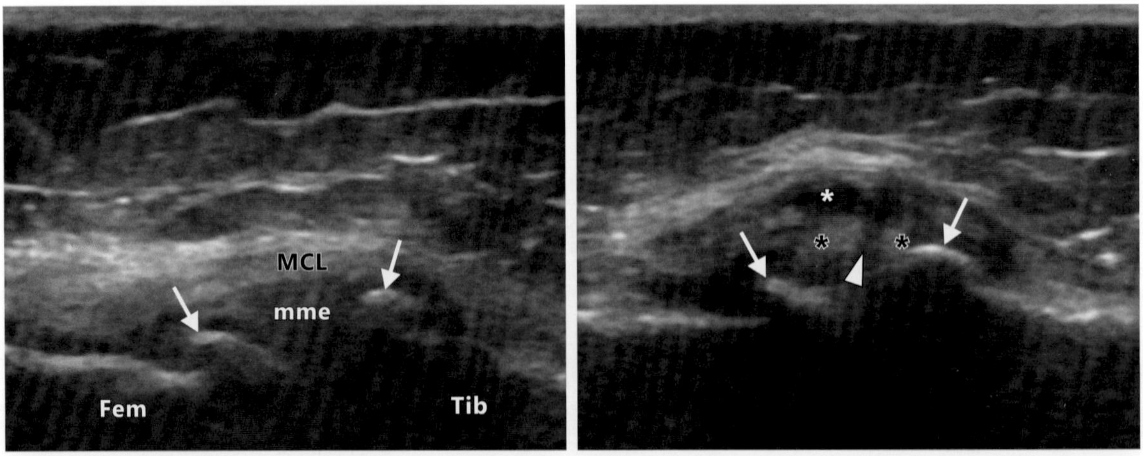

The patient had pain radiating along the internal aspect of the knee.

When compared with the asymptomatic side (**a**), medial longitudinal US image shows narrowing of the joint space, ruptured (*arrowhead*) and degenerated (*black asterisks*) medial meniscus (**mme**) (**b**). A small meniscal cyst (*white asterisk*) can also be seen immediately deep to the bulging medial collateral ligament (**MCL**) (**b**). Please note that the marginal medium sized osteophytes (*arrows*) are present bilaterally.

Fem femur
Tib tibia

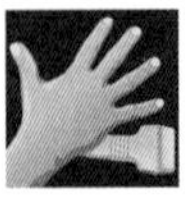

Expert note

US is more sensitive to detect knee osteophytes than radiography, and the presence/size of osteophytes evaluated with US is a significant predictor for arthroscopic degenerative changes in the articular cartilage of the medial compartment [10].

Knee osteoarthritis in a 50-year-old woman with bilateral knee pain during walking and going up/down the stairs

9.36

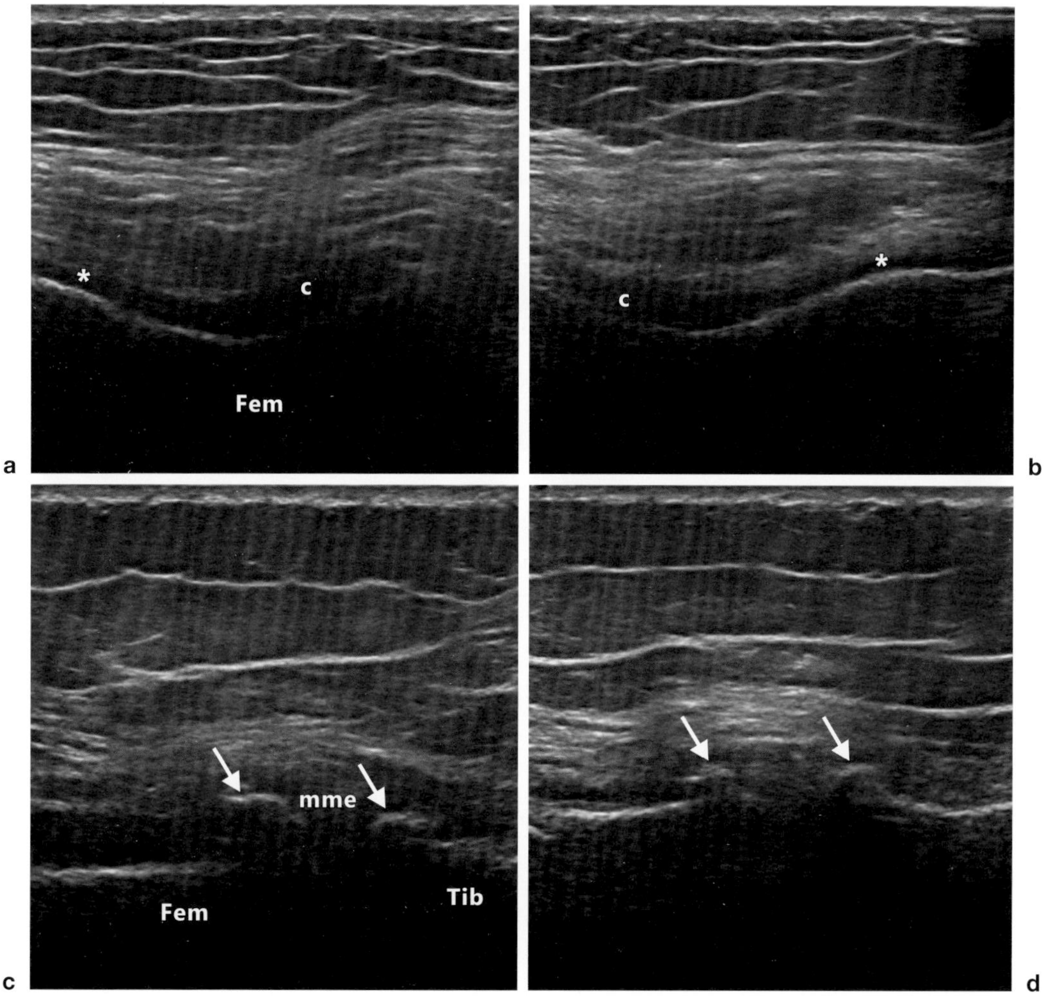

Axial US images obtained over the femoral trochlea show narrowing (*asterisks*) of the hyaline cartilage (**c**) on the lateral sides (**a**, **b**). Longitudinal images over the medial knee joint demonstrate bony irregularities at the joint surfaces related to medium (**c**) and small (**d**) sized osteophytes (*arrows*).

Fem femur
mme medial meniscus
Tib tibia

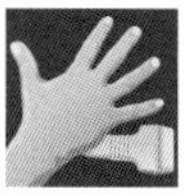

Expert note

According to their size, these osteophytes are generally classified as small, medium and large [10].

9.37 Knee osteoarthritis in a 45-year-old man who had medial knee pain below the joint

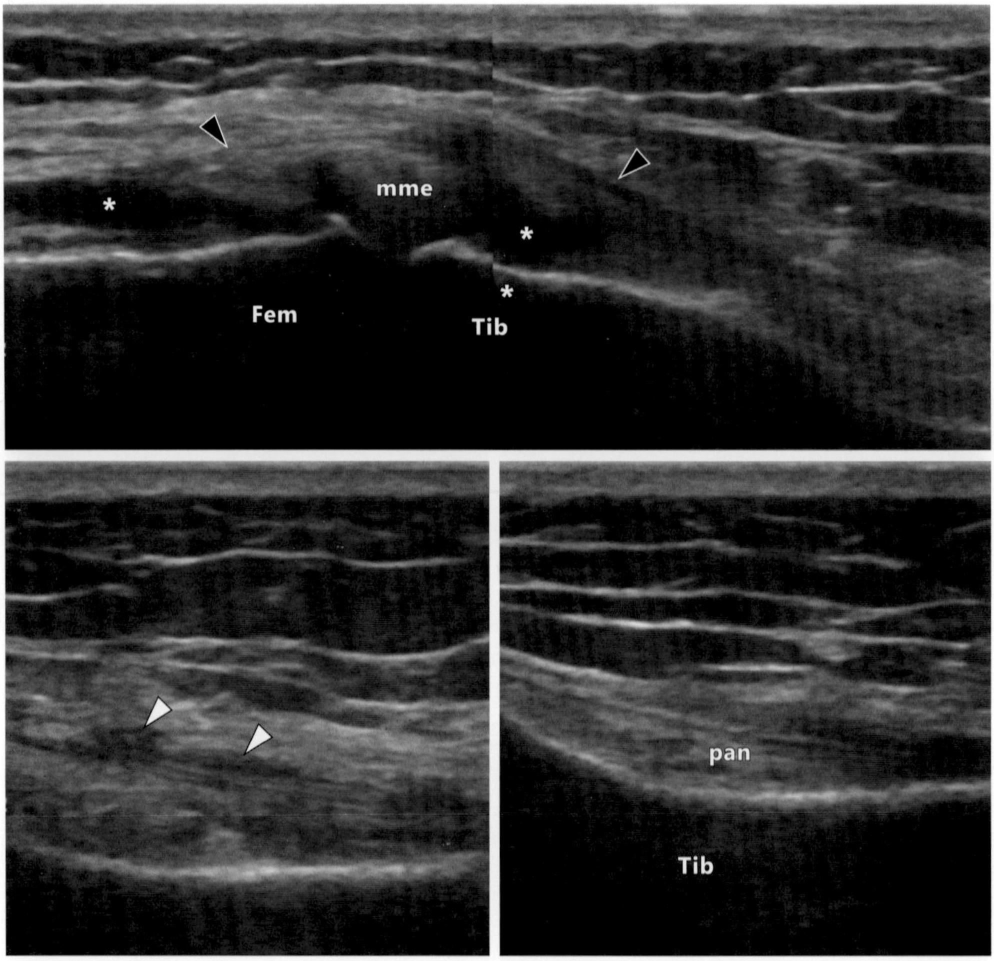

a b c

Longitudinal split-screen US image over the medial knee reveals joint effusion (*asterisks*) and extrusion of the medial meniscus (**mme**) that stretches the overlying medial collateral ligament (*black arrowheads*) (**a**). Longitudinal oblique US image over the tibial insertion of the pes anserine complex (**pan**) demonstrates mild effusion in the bursa (*white arrowheads*) (**b**). Normal side (**c**).

Fem femur **Tib** tibia

Expert note

Although pes anserine region is not the initial place for exploring knee joint effusion, overflowing fluid can for sure be detected in relevant cases. On the contrary, if the patient is found to have such a fluid, suprapatellar scanning for knee joint effusion should never be skipped.

Pes anserine tendinopathy in a 50-year-old woman with pain and tenderness over the inner knee **9.38**

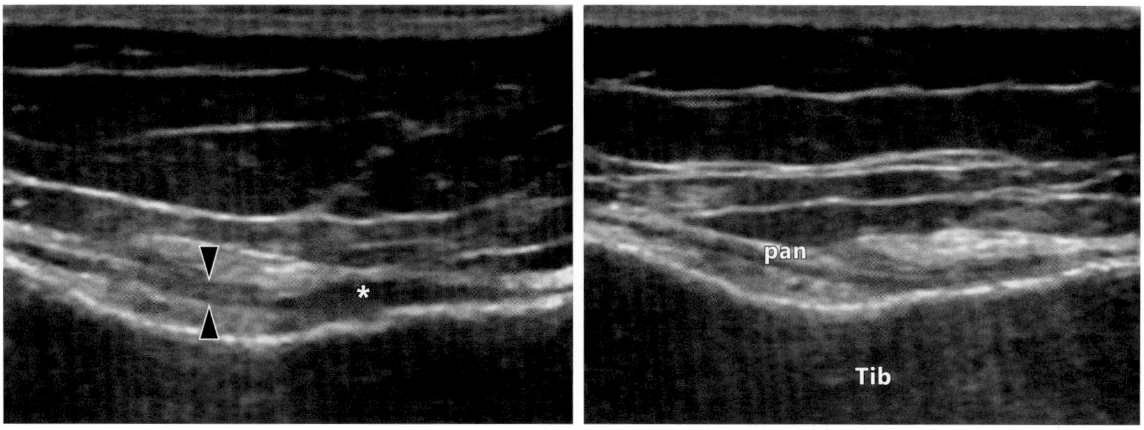

a b

Longitudinal oblique US image over the pes anserine complex (**pan**) demonstrates mild edema (*asterisk*) and overall thickening of the tendons (*arrowheads*) attaching on the anteromedial aspect of the proximal tibial metaphysis (**a**). Normal contralateral side (**b**).

Tib tibia

Expert note

Pes anserine region is another typical painful area in patients with knee problems (osteoarthritis). Again, delicate sono-palpation definitely prompts the treatment (including interventions) of such patients.

9.39 Pes anserine bursitis in a middle-aged man

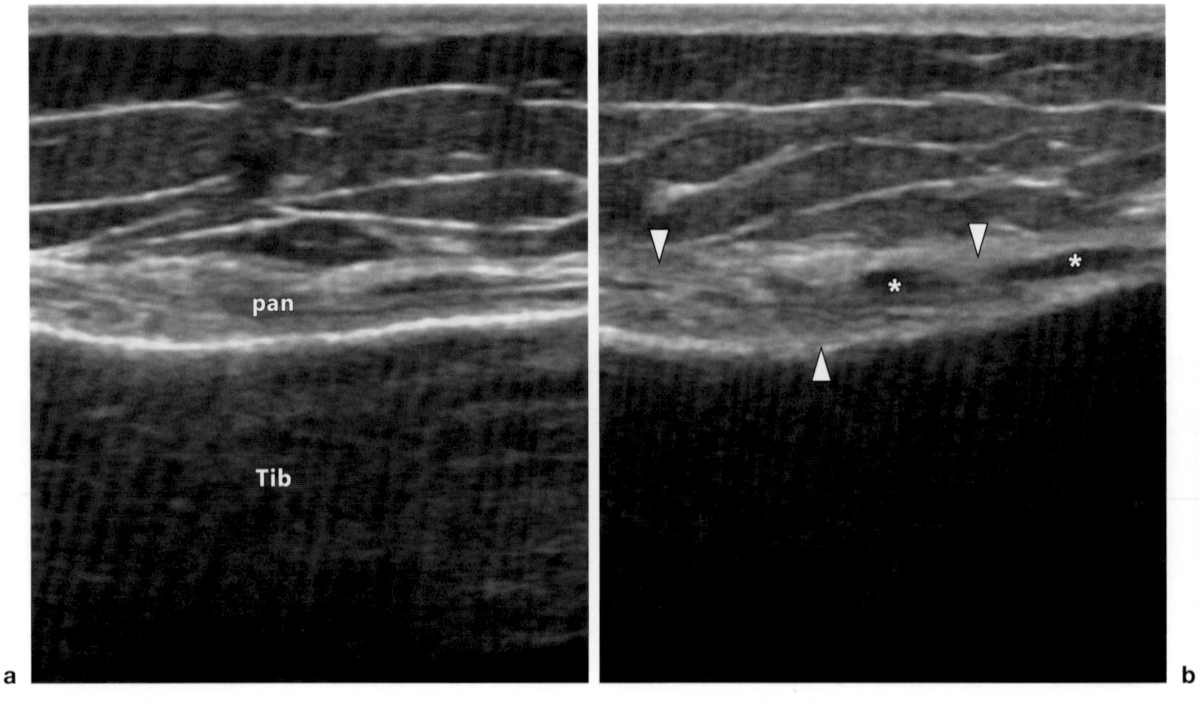

The patient had medial knee pain particularly on palpation or during resisted internal rotation/flexion of the knee.

When compared with the normal pes anserine complex (**pan**) (**a**), longitudinal oblique US image (**b**) shows fluid (*asterisks*) in the bursa and thickened pes anserine tendons (*arrowheads*).

Tib tibia

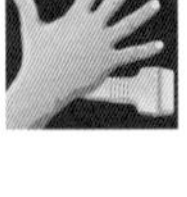

Expert note

Despite the local/overlying fat tissue in obese subjects, pes anserine complex is localized quite superficially. Also considering the fact that the amount of fluid in the bursa is usually not overwhelming, the sonographer should be cautious while scanning for bursitis.

Bilateral pes anserine bursitis in a 46-year-old obese woman with knee pain during walking or climbing 9.40

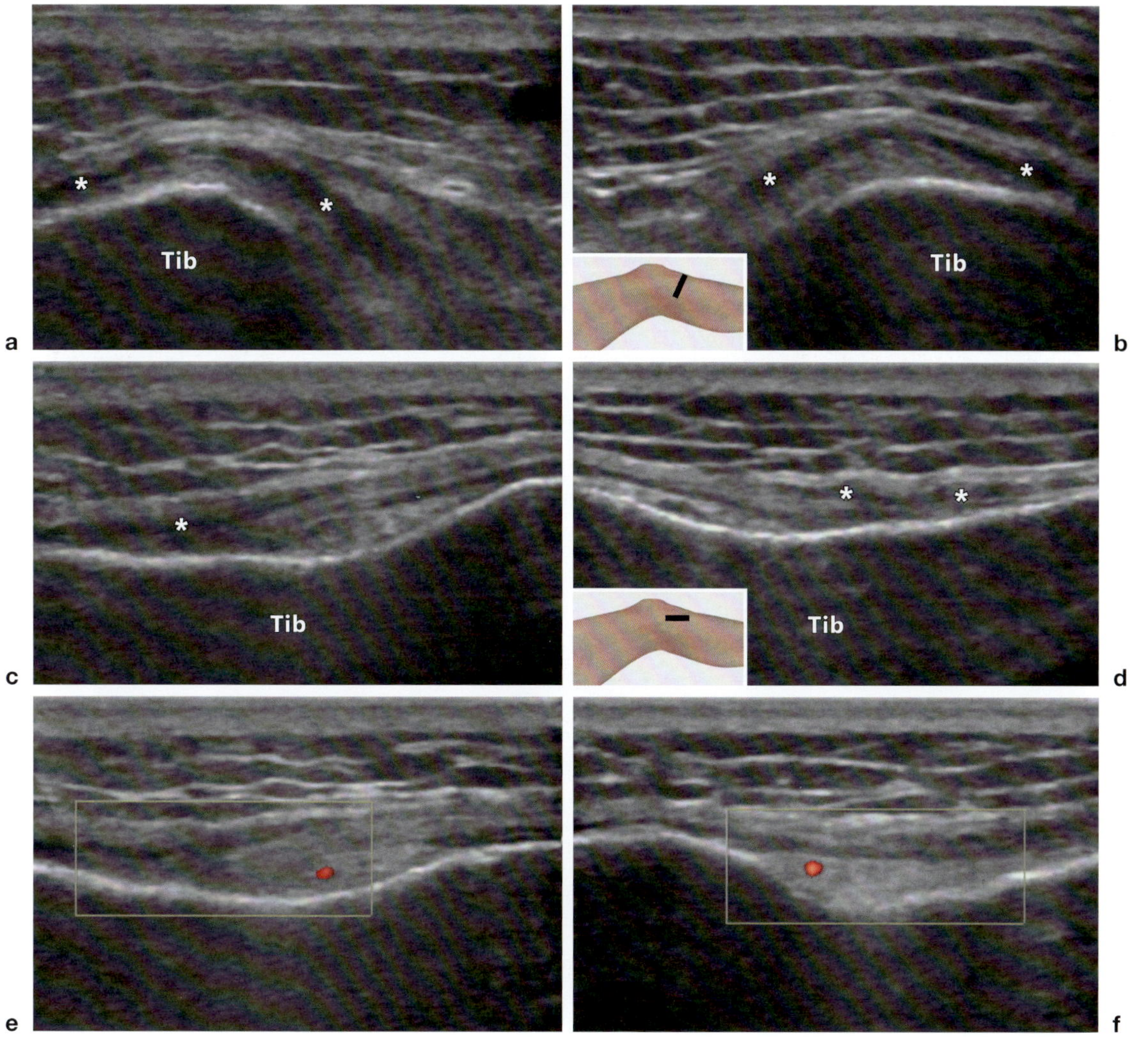

Axial (**a**, **b**) and longitudinal (**c**, **d**) US images of the pes anserine complex show fluid (*asterisks*) at the tendon insertions. Power Doppler images demonstrate only flow signals pertaining to the inferior medial genicular arteries (**e**, **f**).

Tib tibia

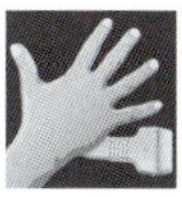

Expert note

Although not a strict rule, the fluid accumulation in the pes anserine bursa is usually localized superficial to the tendons. Herewith, the genicular arteries (deep to the tendons) can also/sometimes be misinterpreted as fluid. In this regard, power Doppler imaging can definitely be confirmatory [6].

9.41 Distal iliotibial band tendinopathy in a middle-aged woman with lateral knee pain

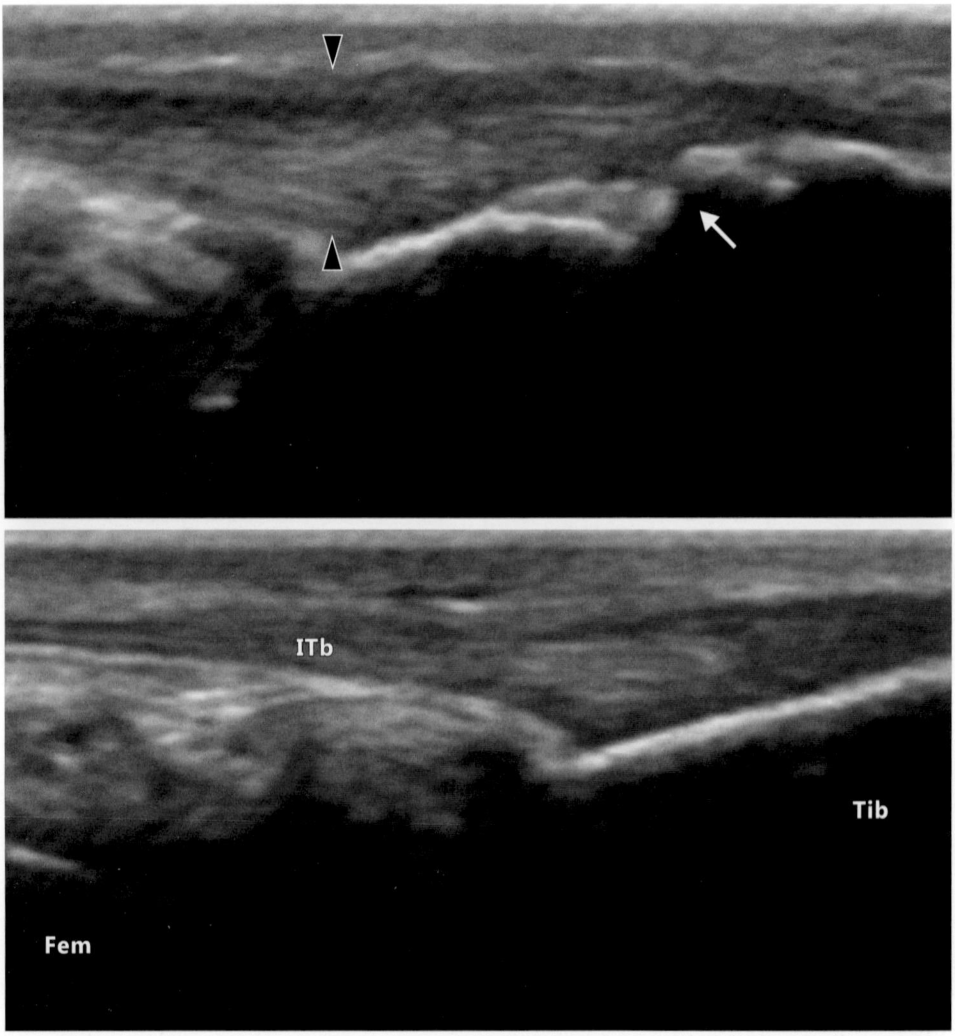

Longitudinal US image over the lateral knee demonstrates a swollen and hypoechoic insertional portion (*arrowheads*) of the distal iliotibial band (**ITb**) with blurred margins (**a**). Also note the irregularity of the ipsilateral Gerdy's tubercle (*arrow*). Contralateral normal side (**b**).

Fem femur
Tib tibia

Expert note

Bony abnormalities are usually indicative of more chronic problems.

Iliotibial band friction syndrome in a 45-year-old woman

9.42

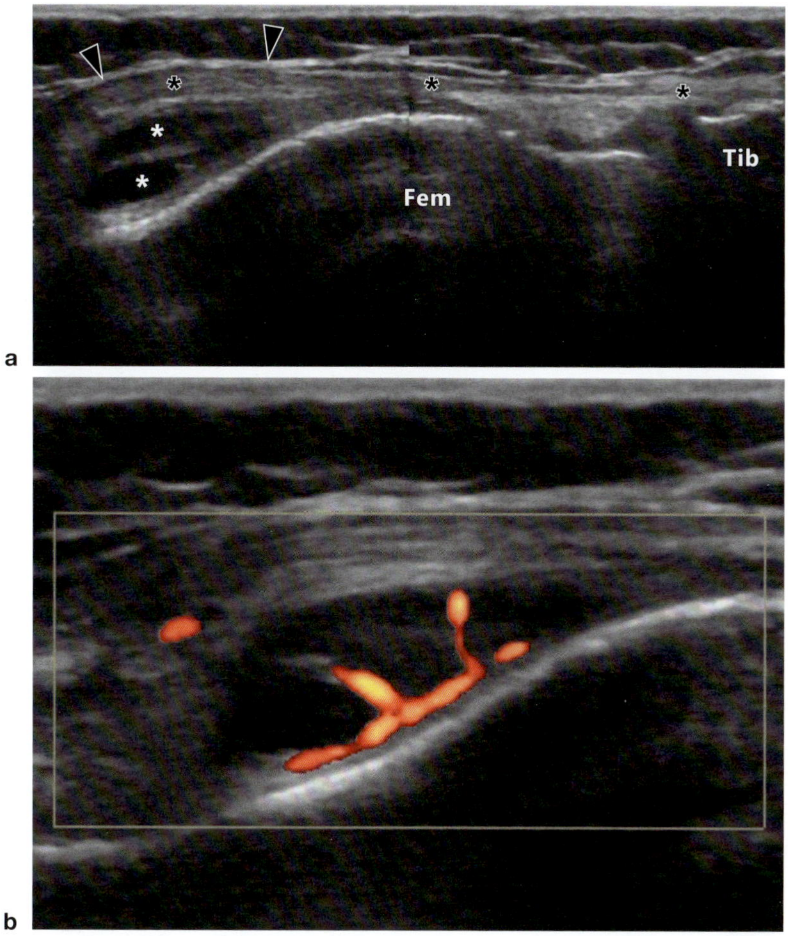

She had pain and tenderness on the lateral part of the knee joint with walking or running.

Longitudinal split-screen US image reveals thickening (*arrowheads*) of the iliotibial band (*black asterisks*) proximally, and hypo/anechoic enlargement of the bursa (*white asterisks*) (**a**). Power Doppler imaging demonstrates signs of hyperemia reflecting inflammation (**b**).

Fem femur
Tib tibia

Expert note

On the lateral side of the knee, the iliotibial band passes very close to the lateral femoral condyle and this is exactly the place where the friction ensues. Typically, in patients with iliotibial band friction syndrome, the US findings are local thickening of the band and fluid accumulation in the bursa between the band and the condyle.

9.43 Iliotibial band friction syndrome in a 35-year-old man with pain and tenderness at the lateral knee region

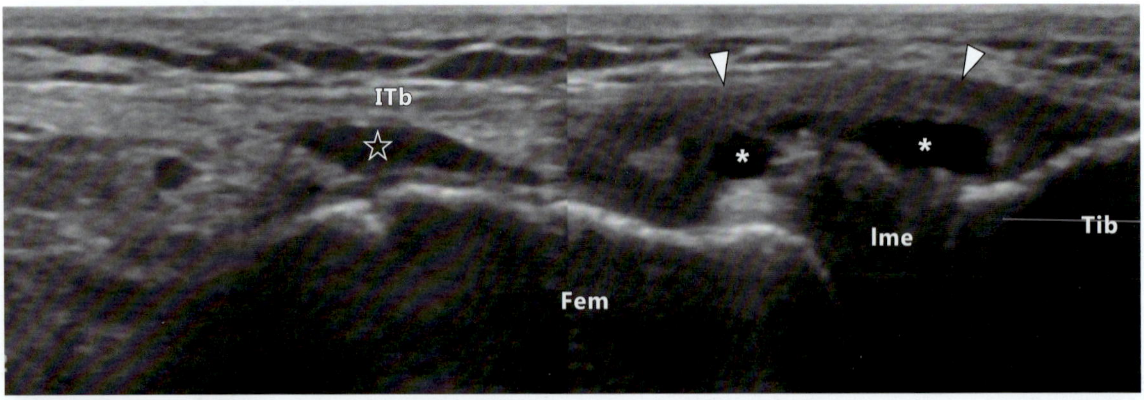

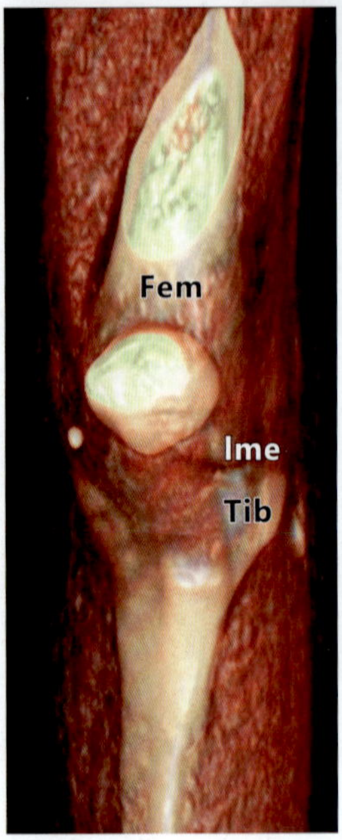

Longitudinal split-screen US image over the lateral knee demonstrates hypoechoic swelling (*arrowheads*) of the distal iliotibial band (**ITb**), fluid collection within the joint space (*asterisks*) and synovial bursa (*star*).

Fem femur
Ime lateral meniscus
Tib Gerdy's tubercle of the tibia

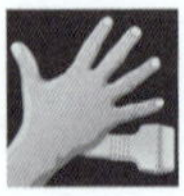

Expert note

In this patient, the involvement of the iliotibial band is actually not much typical but more distal. Anechoic appearance next to a meniscus can well be due to a meniscal cyst, dynamic imaging with probe compression or scanning for accompanying meniscal problems can be performed for clarification.

Iliotibial band friction syndrome in a 27-year-old woman with lateral knee pain **9.44**

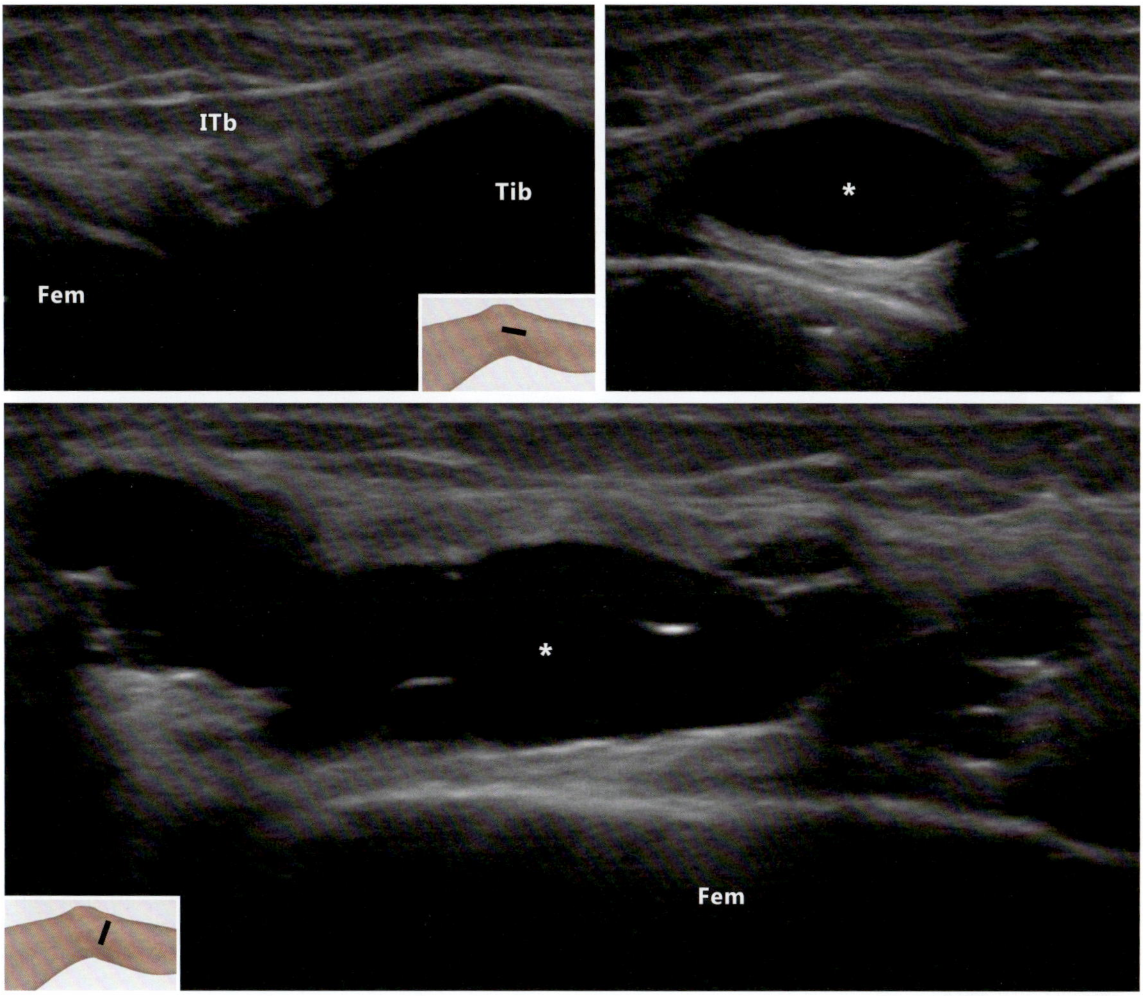

a b c

When compared with the normal side (**a**), longitudinal (**b**) and axial (**c**) US images over the lateral knee joint demonstrate a well-defined ganglion cyst (*asterisks*) which seems to stretch the overlying distal iliotibial band (**ITb**).

Fem femur
Tib tibia

9.45 Lateral collateral ligament injury in a 34-year-old man with knee pain and mild focal tenderness

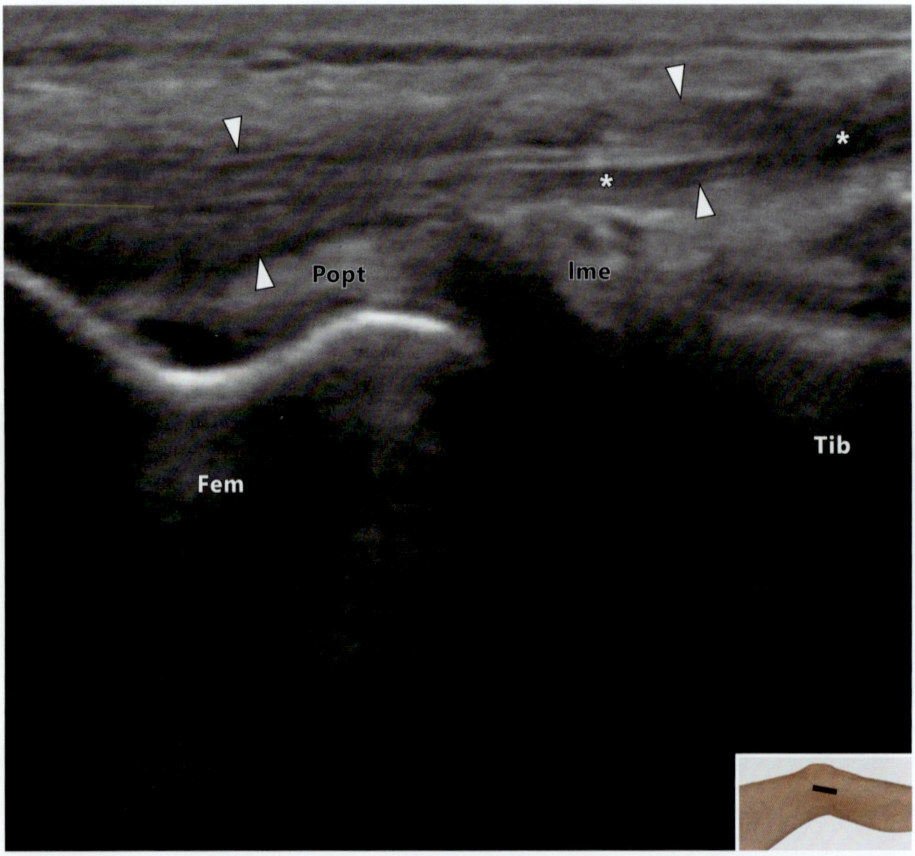

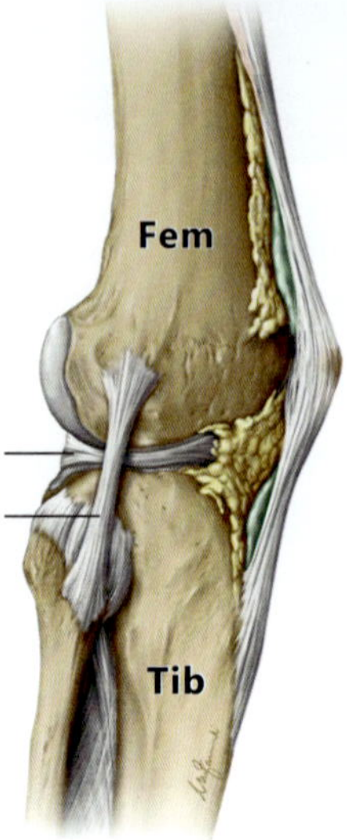

Video 10

Longitudinal US image obtained over the lateral knee joint illustrates partial detachment (*asterisks*) of the fibrillary structure of the lateral collateral ligament (*arrowheads*).

Fem	femur	**Popt**	popliteus tendon
lcl	lateral collateral ligament	**Tib**	tibia
lme	lateral meniscus		

Expert note

Due to its steep alignment, scanning for the lateral collateral ligament is quite difficult. However, if the notch where the popliteus tendon takes off is taken as the landmark and the probe is positioned as much parallel as possible to the ligament, the ligament can be imaged. Fine probe adjustment is again necessary while scanning is directed distally. Similar to the medial collateral ligament, dynamic assessment under stress manuevers might also be contributory [3].

Biceps femoris tendinitis in a 43-year-old man with a 2-month history of posterolateral knee pain after starting karate

9.46

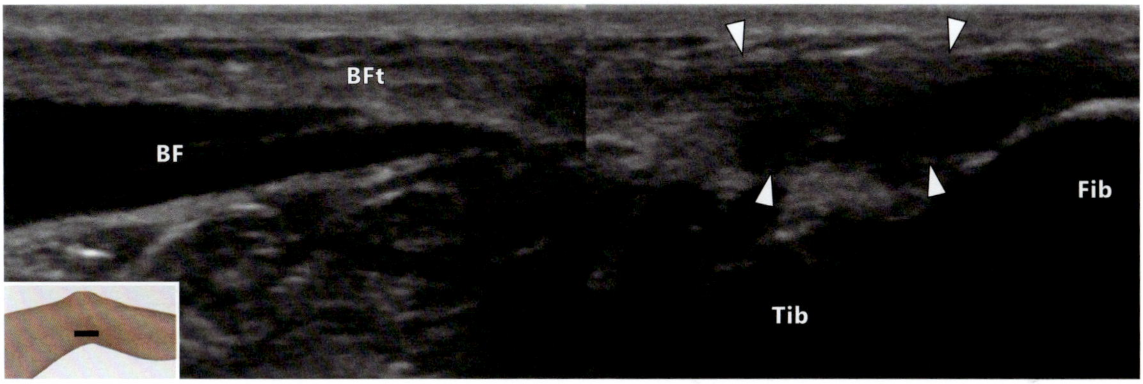

Longitudinal split-screen US image over the distal biceps femoris tendon (**BFt**) reveals an irregular, swollen and hypoechoic tendon (*arrowheads*).

BF biceps femoris
Fib fibula
Tib tibia

9.47 Knee osteoarthritis in a 57-year-old woman with bilateral chronic and progressive knee pain

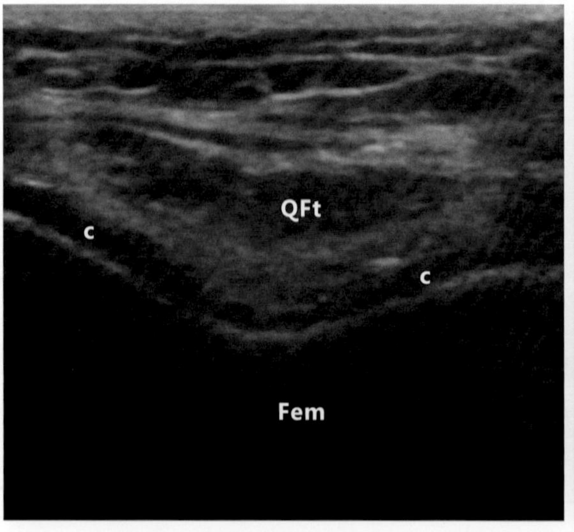

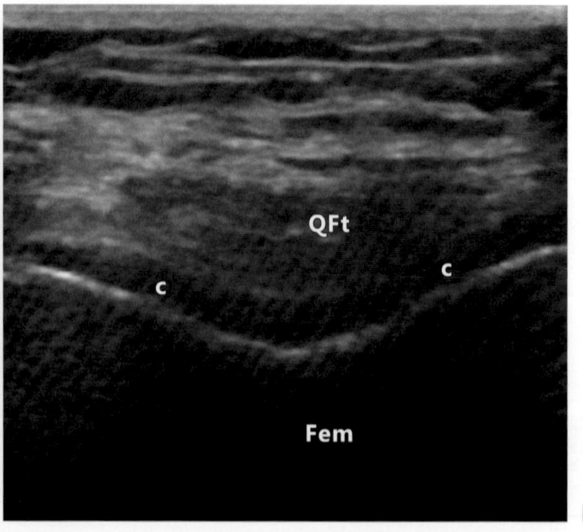

Axial US images obtained over the trochlear cartilage (**c**) illustrate diffusely irregular and thin cartilage with blurred margins on both sides.

Fem femur
QFt quadriceps femoris tendon

Expert note

While the distal femoral articular cartilage can not be visible in the neutral position (due to the overlying patella), axial imaging on the suprapatellar view with maximum knee flexion can make it be nicely seen. Cartilage thickness is usually measured on the mid-points of the condyles and the intercondylar notch. As such, either quantitative (thickness measurement) or semi-quantitative (grading from 0 to 6) assessment has been shown to be reliable and valid in relevant subjects [11].

Chondrocalcinosis in a 49-year-old hypothyroid woman with chronic pain and tenderness in the knee joint **9.48**

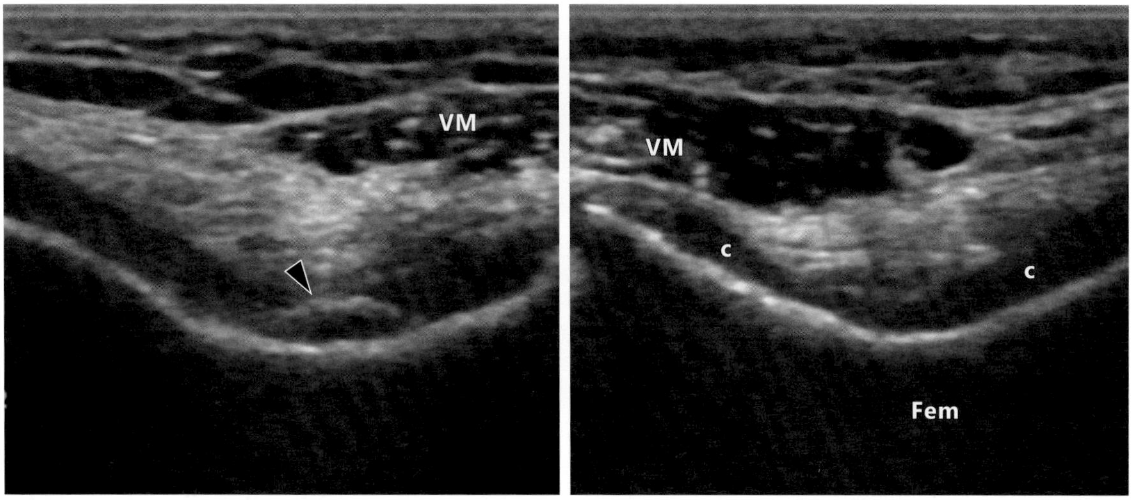

a b

Axial US image (**a**) over the anterior suprapatellar region (obtained with maximum knee flexion) reveals a linear calcification (*arrowhead*) inside the femoral trochlear cartilage (**c**) consistent with calcium pyrophosphate deposition disease (CPPD). Normal side (**b**).

Fem femur
VM vastus medialis

Expert note

In case of pseudogout, the deposits typically reside within the hyaline cartilage (as a thin hyperechoic band) in contrast to gout where they are found as perfectly overlying [12]. CPPD calcifications in cartilage and periarticular tissues are defined in Table 9.1 [13].

Table 9.1 CPPD calcifications

Pattern	
I	Thin hyperechoic bands, parallel to the surface of the hyaline cartilage (frequently observed in the knee)
II	A "punctate" pattern, composed of several thin hyperechoic spots, more common in fibrous cartilage and tendons
III	Homogeneous hyperechoic nodular or oval deposits localized in bursae and articular recesses

9.49 Baker cyst in a 58-year-old man with posteromedial knee pain and swelling

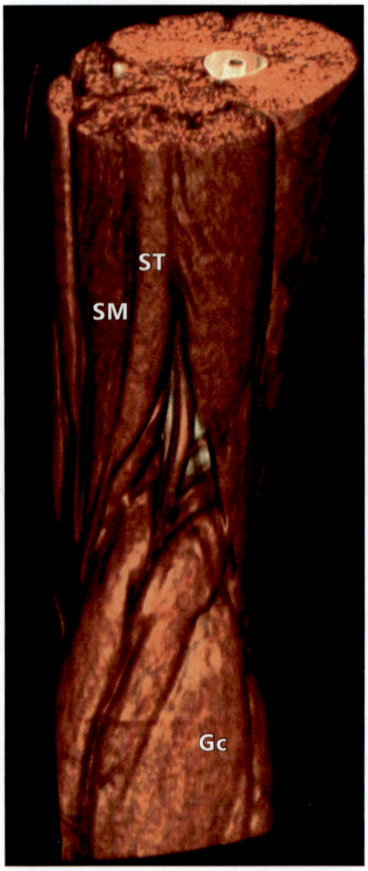

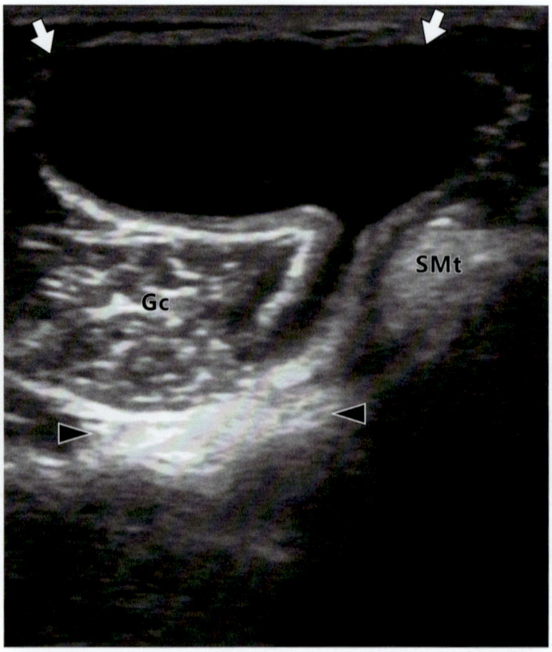

Axial US imaging reveals a Baker cyst (*arrows*) filling the upper part of the semimembranosus-gastrocnemius bursa with a characteristic "talk bubble" appearance. Please note the enhanced through-transmission artifact on the medial head of the gastrocnemius muscle (**Gc**), semimembranosus tendon (**SMt**) and deeper (*arrowheads*).

ST semitendinosus

Expert note

The most common disorders associated with Baker cysts are underlying meniscal pathology (particularly posterior horn of the medial meniscus), anterior cruciate ligament and chondral tears. As such, the US examination might be tailored to also encompass meniscal and ligament imaging in pertinent cases [14, 15].

Baker's cyst in a 60-year-old man with knee pain and tension posteriorly **9.50**

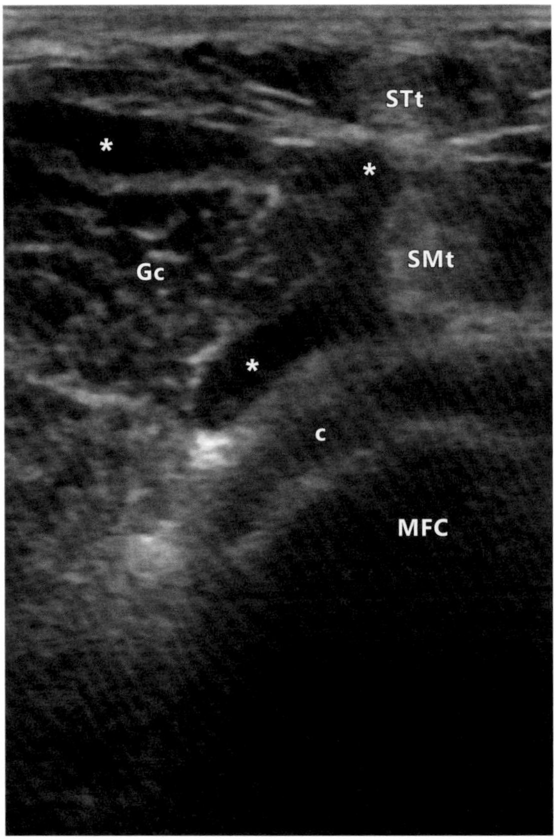

Posterior axial US imaging shows mild enlargement of the semimembranosus-gastrocnemius bursa (*asterisks*).

c	cartilage
Gc	medial head of gastrocnemius muscle
MFC	medial femoral condyle
SMt	semimembranosus tendon
STt	semitendinosus tendon

Knee

Expert note

Baker cyst is known to originate from the "v-shaped" or "boomerang shaped" semimembranosus-gastrocnemius bursa. Accordingly, this bursa is the exact place to scan for Baker cysts. Herewith, although some fluid can be observed in relevant subjects, it is not always possible/appropriate to call it a cyst and "dilatation of the bursa" would preferrably be a better terminology.

Although it is quite simple to scan a simple cyst; oft-times, the assessment might become really challenging. Yet, the anisotropy pertaining to the two hamstring tendons might easily be misinterpreted as fluid. Further dangerous would be a possible attempt to drain it or to inject it otherwise with steroids.

The medial localization of this bursa and the prompt recognition of the relevant anatomy (gastrocnemius muscle, semimembranosus and semitendinosus tendons) can also avoid erroneously diagnosing the popliteal vessels (with a more lateral localization) as Baker cysts.

9.51 Baker cyst in a 9-year-old girl with knee pain and a palpable lump at the posteromedial knee

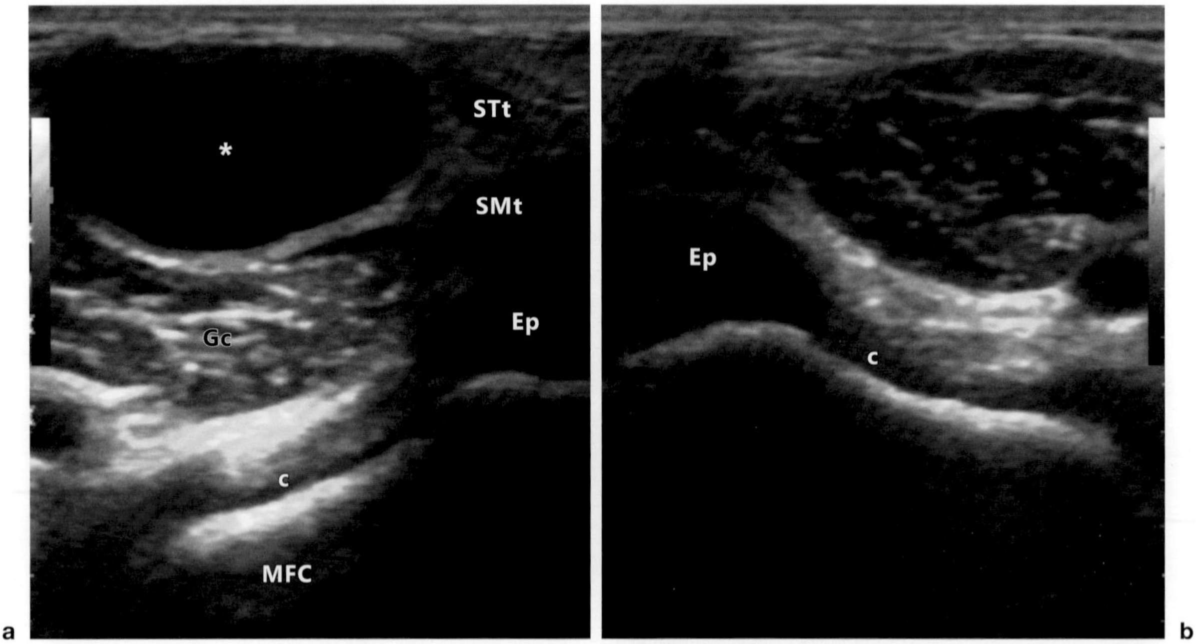

Posterior axial US image illustrates an anechoic Baker cyst (*asterisk*) (**a**). Normal contralateral side (**b**). Please note the articular cartilage (**c**) and the epiphyseal plate (**Ep**).

Gc medial head of gastrocnemius muscle
MFC medial femoral condyle
SMt semimembranosus tendon
STt semitendinosus tendon

Expert note

In children, the challenge/necessity to not misinterprete a nearby anechoic structure as Baker cyst is even mounted. Yet, depending on the age of the child the presence/amount of epiphyseal cartilage would be noteworthy.

Intrabursal calcified loose body in a 55-year-old woman with posteromedial knee pain and lump **9.52**

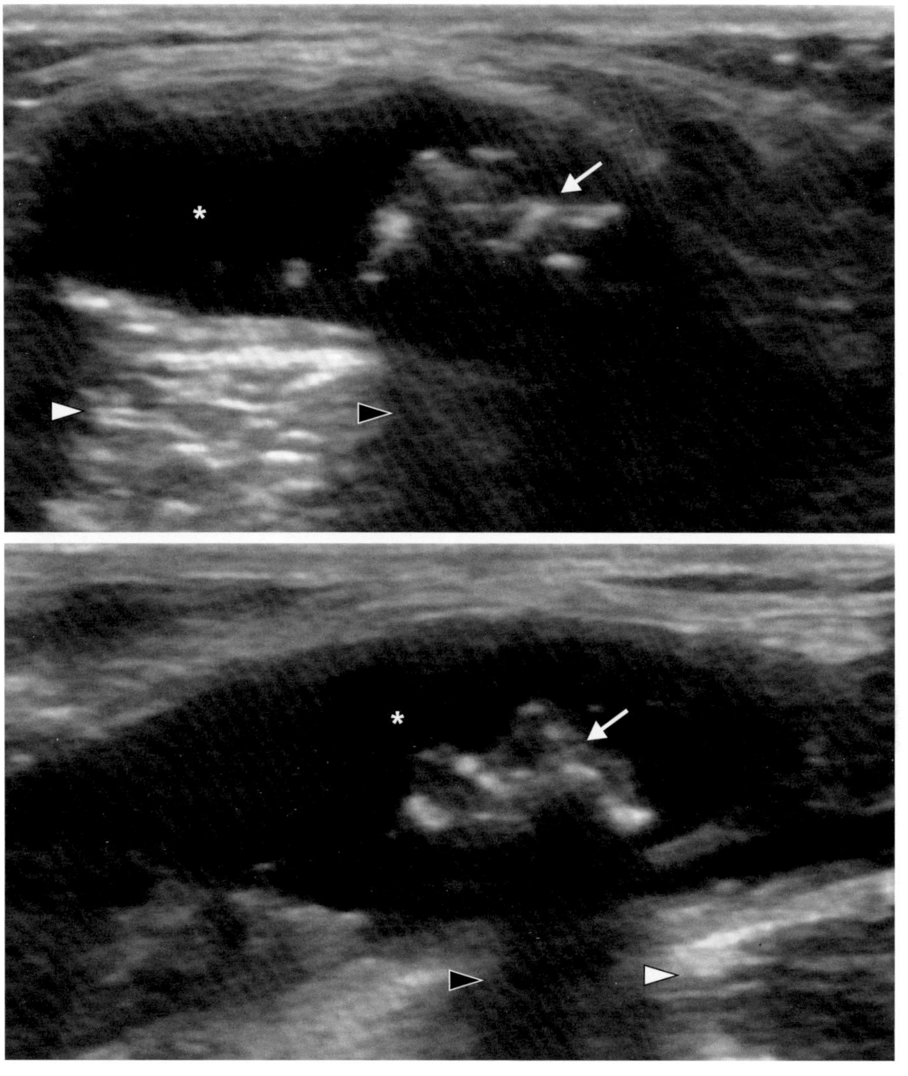

a

b

Axial (**a**) and longitudinal (**b**) US images of the popliteal fossa show fluid collection (*asterisks*) with a large irregular calcification (*arrows*). Please note the contrast between the echogenicities of fluid and calcification, and also between their pertinent artifacts i.e. enhanced through-transmission (*white arrowheads*) and acoustic shadowing (*black arrowheads*).

Expert note

Calcified or (osteo)chondral fragments may be kept in the cyst by the valve mechanism and may complete its lumen with time. In case of doubt, changing the patient's position might help better localize the intracystic fragments (loose bodies) [14].

9.53 Intrabursal calcified loose body in a 63-year-old woman with posteromedial knee pain and lump

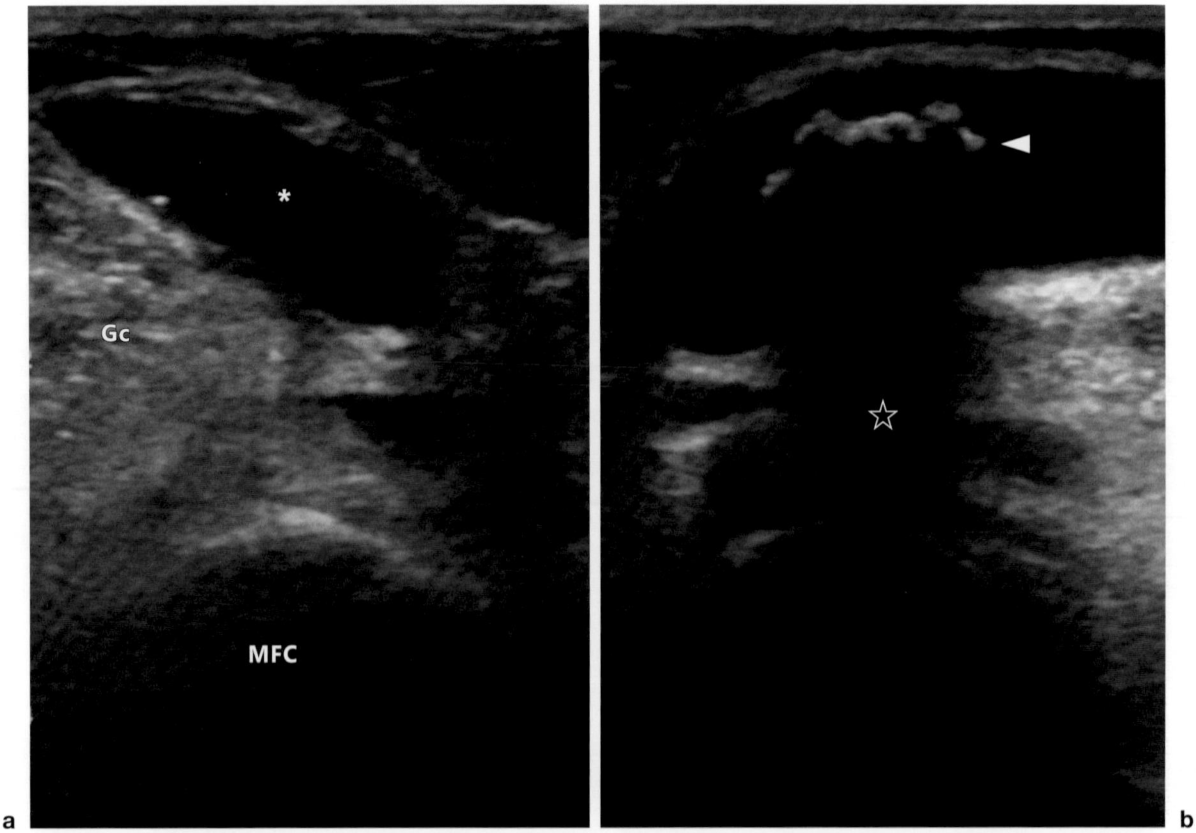

Axial (**a**) and longitudinal (**b**) US images over the posteromedial aspect of the popliteal fossa demonstrate a large Baker cyst (*asterisk*) that contains a linear calcification (*arrowhead*) giving a sharp posterior acoustic shadowing artifact (*star*).

Gc medial head of gastrocnemius muscle
MFC medial femoral condyle

Baker cyst rupture in a 57-year-old man with a non-painful mass in the posteromedial knee **9.54**

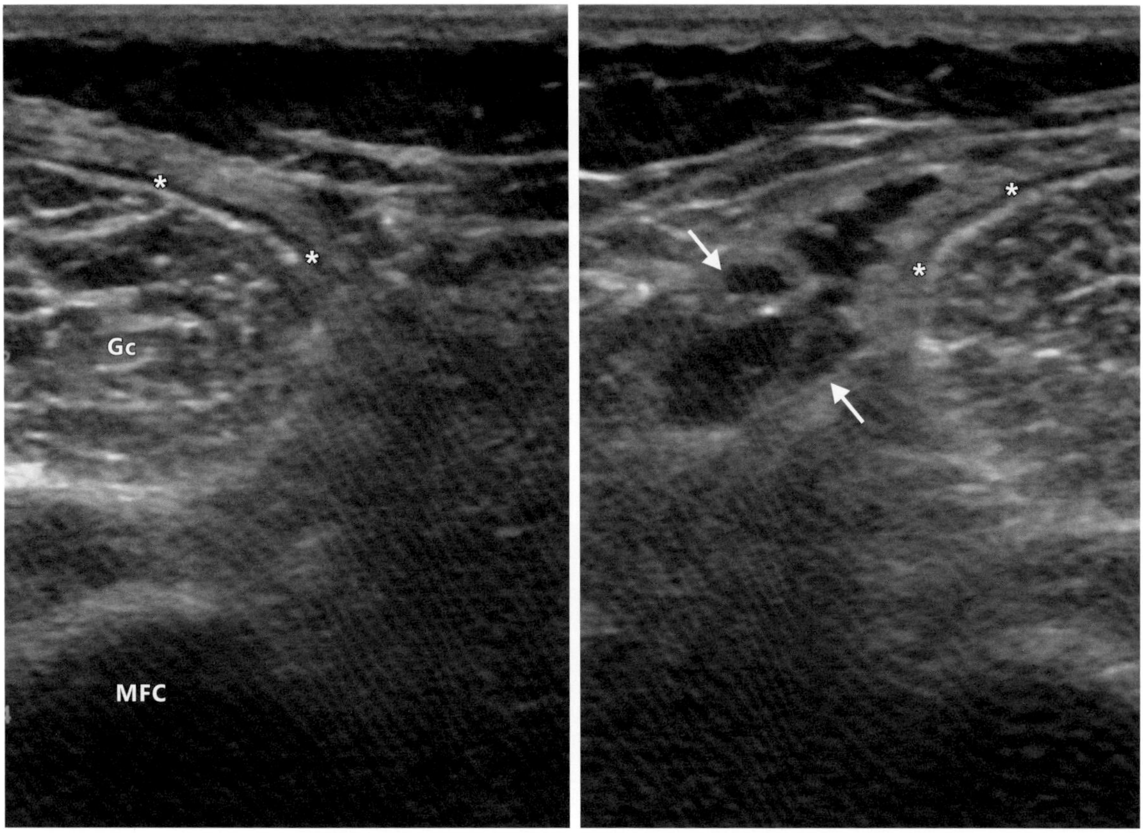

a b

When compared with the normal side (**a**), posterior axial US imaging shows ruptured and organized Baker cyst (*arrows*) spreading into the subcutaneous fatty tissue (**b**). Please note that the bursa seems to be otherwise quite normal (*asterisks*).

Gc medial head of gastrocnemius muscle
MFC medial femoral condyle

Expert note

Substantial (proximal to distal) imaging would definitely be necessary to understand whether this collection has any connection with the bursa or it is a remnant from a previous rupture.

9.55 Ruptured Baker cyst in a 10-year-old girl with juvenile idiopathic arthritis

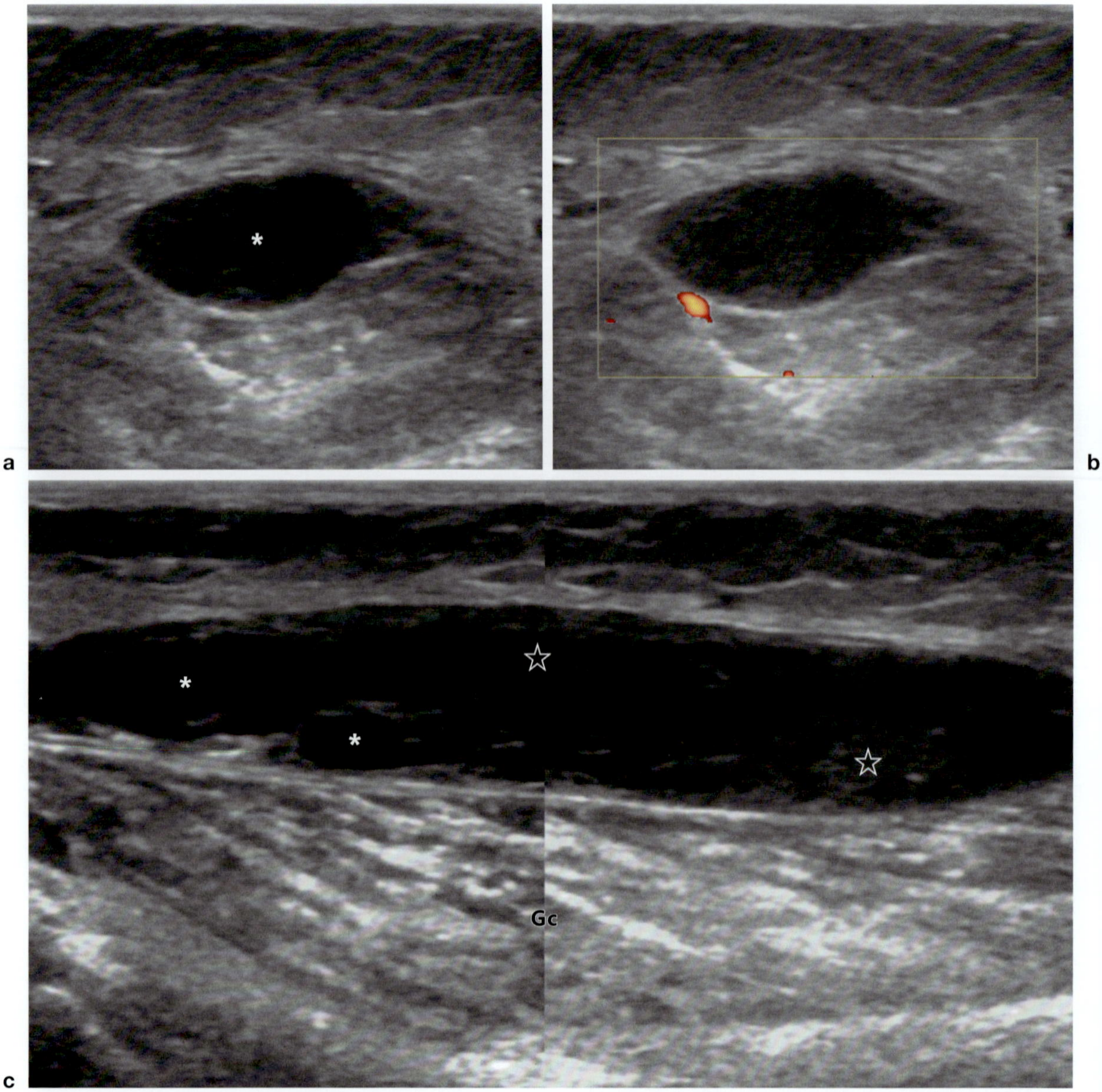

Axial (**a**) and split-screen longitudinal (**c**) US images depict hypoechoic fluid (*asterisks*) and organized synovial hypertrophy (*stars*) within the gastrocnemius-semimembranosus bursa spreading throughout the muscle superficially. Power Doppler image shows mild peripheral hyperemia (**b**).

Gc gastrocnemius

Complicated Baker cyst rupture in an elderly woman with pain and difficulty during knee bending

9.56

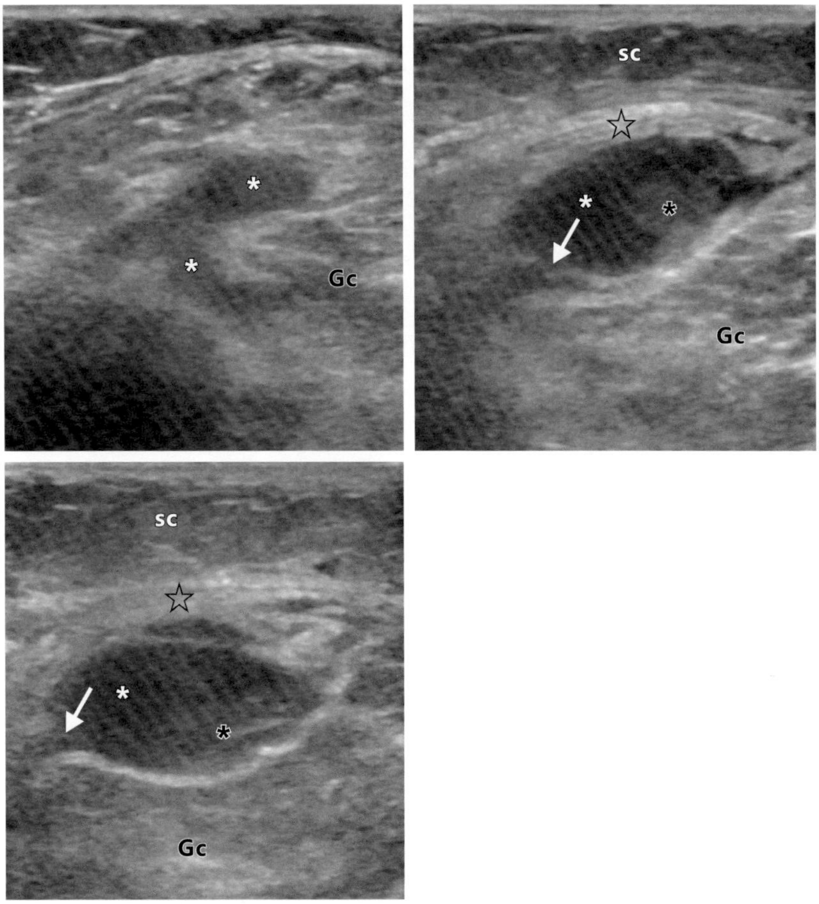

a b c

Axial US images at different levels (from proximal to distal) show enlarged bursa filled with hypoechoic fluid (*white asterisks*) (**a**) and encapsulated (*stars*) fluid accumulation within the medial head of the gastrocnemius muscle (**Gc**) (**b**, **c**). Synovial thickenings (*black asterisks*) and the possible area of the rupture (*arrows*) can also be seen. Note that the subcutaneous tissues (**sc**) are also edematous distally (**b**, **c**).

Expert note

Rupture of the Baker cyst (usually inside the gastrocnemius muscle) can ensue and usually/clinically masquerades as thrombophlebitis in clinical practice. While the scenario is named as "pseudothrombophlebitis", its (differential) diagnosis might pose great challenges to the clinician. As such, in relevant patients (especially with a known diagnosis of Baker cyst), US can readily be used for prompt diagnosis if they describe acute complaints in the calf or sudden disappearance of their otherwise palpable cysts.
While the rupture will often occur at the distal tip of the cyst (causing an arrow-like image), as shown in this case, the exuberant involvement may also affect the subcutaneous tissues.

9.57 Primary hydatid cyst (echinococcosis) in a 62-year-old woman with a painful and progressively enlarged popliteal mass

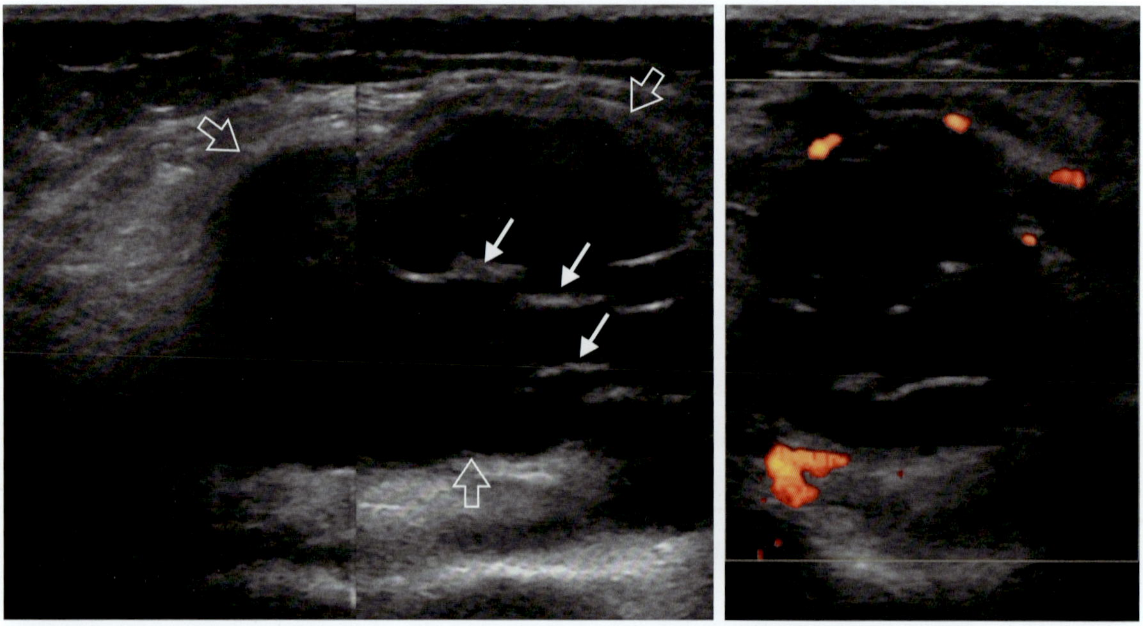

a b

Initially the mass was diagnosed as Baker cyst.

Axial split-screen US image shows a large cystic lesion with a round, well-defined capsule (*void arrows*) including septations (*thin arrows*) within the gastrocnemius muscle (**a**).
Power Doppler imaging reveals increased peripheral vascular signals within the cyst wall and surrounding tissue (**b**).

Expert note

While scanning for a suspicious Baker cyst after physical examination can be unremarkable (especially in obese subjects); at other times, the "palpated" mass can turn out to be not a simple cyst as well.

REFERENCES

1. Malas FÜ, Kara M, Kaymak B, Akinci A, Özçakar L. Ultrasonographic evaluation in symptomatic knee osteoarthritis: clinical and radiological correlation. Int J Rheum Dis. 2014; 17: 536-40.
2. D'Agostino MA, Conaghan P, Le Bars M, Baron G, Grassi W, Martin-Mola E, et al. EULAR report on the use of ultrasonography in painful knee osteoarthritis. Part 1: prevalence of inflammation in osteoarthritis. Ann Rheum Dis. 2005; 64: 1703-9.
3. Özçakar L, Kara M, Chang KV, Tok F, Hung CY, Akkaya N, et al. EURO-MUSCULUS/USPRM. Basic scanning protocols for knee. Eur J Phys Rehabil Med. 2015; 51: 641-6.
4. McCarthy G. Basic calcium phosphate crystal deposition disease. In: Hochberg MC, Silma AJ, Smolen JS, Weinblatt ME, Weisman MH, editors. Philadelphia: Elsevier; 2011. p. 1889-98.
5. De Muynck M, Parlevliet T, De Cock K, Vanden Bossche L, Vanderstraeten G, Özçakar L. Musculoskeletal ultrasound for interventional physiatry. Eur J Phys Rehabil Med. 2012; 48: 675-87.
6. Batmaz İ, Malas FÜ, Özçakar L. Ultrasound evaluation of the knee. In: Özçakar L, De Muynck M, editors. Musculoskeletal ultrasound in physical and rehabilitation medicine. Milan: Edi.Ermes; 2014. p. 99-110.
7. Chang KV, Şahin Onat Ş, Lee CW, Kara M, Hung CY, Özçakar L. EURO-MUSCULUS/USPRM basic scanning protocols revisited in children. Eur J Phys Rehabil Med. 2016; 52: 887-901.
8. Van Holsbeeck M, Introcaso JH. Musculoskeletal ultra-sonography. Radiol Clin North Am. 1992; 30: 907e25.
9. Friedman L, Finlay K, Jurriaans E. Ultrasound of the knee. Skeletal Radiol 2001; 30: 361e77.
10. Koski JM, Kamel A, Waris P, Waris V, Tarkiainen I, Karvanen E et al. Atlas-based knee osteophyte assessment with ultrasonography and radiography: relationship to arthroscopic degeneration of articular cartilage. Scand J Rheumatol. 2016; 45: 158-64.
11. Lee CL, Huang MH, Chai CY, Chen CH, Su JY, Tien YC. The validity of in vivo ultrasonographic grading of osteoarthritic femoral condylar cartilage: a comparison with in vitro ultrasonographic and histologic gradings. Osteoarthritis Cartilage. 2008; 16: 352-8.
12. Kılıç E, Akgül Ö, Kılıç G, Özgöçmen S. Ultrasound imaging in rheumatic diseases. In: Özçakar L, De Muynck M, editors. Musculoskeletal ultrasound in physical and rehabilitation medicine. Milan: Edi.Ermes; 2014. p. 161-83.
13. Frediani B, Filippou G, Falsetti P, Lorenzini S, Baldi F, Acciai C, et al. Diagnosis of calcium pyrophosphate dihydrate crystal deposition disease: ultrasonographic criteria proposed. Ann Rheum Dis. 2005; 64: 638-40.
14. Martinoli C, Bianchi S. Knee. In: Bianchi S, Martinoli C, editors. Ultrasound of the musculoskeletal system. Berlin: Springer; 2007. p. 637-745.
15. Artul S, Jabaly-Habib H, Artoul F, Habib G. The association between Baker's cyst and medial meniscal tear in patients with symptomatic knee using ultrasonography. Clin Imaging. 2015; 39: 659-61.

Calf 10

- Subcutaneous tissue
- Periosteum
- Gastrocnemius

10.1 Variceal dilatation in a 65-year-old woman who had calf pain during walking

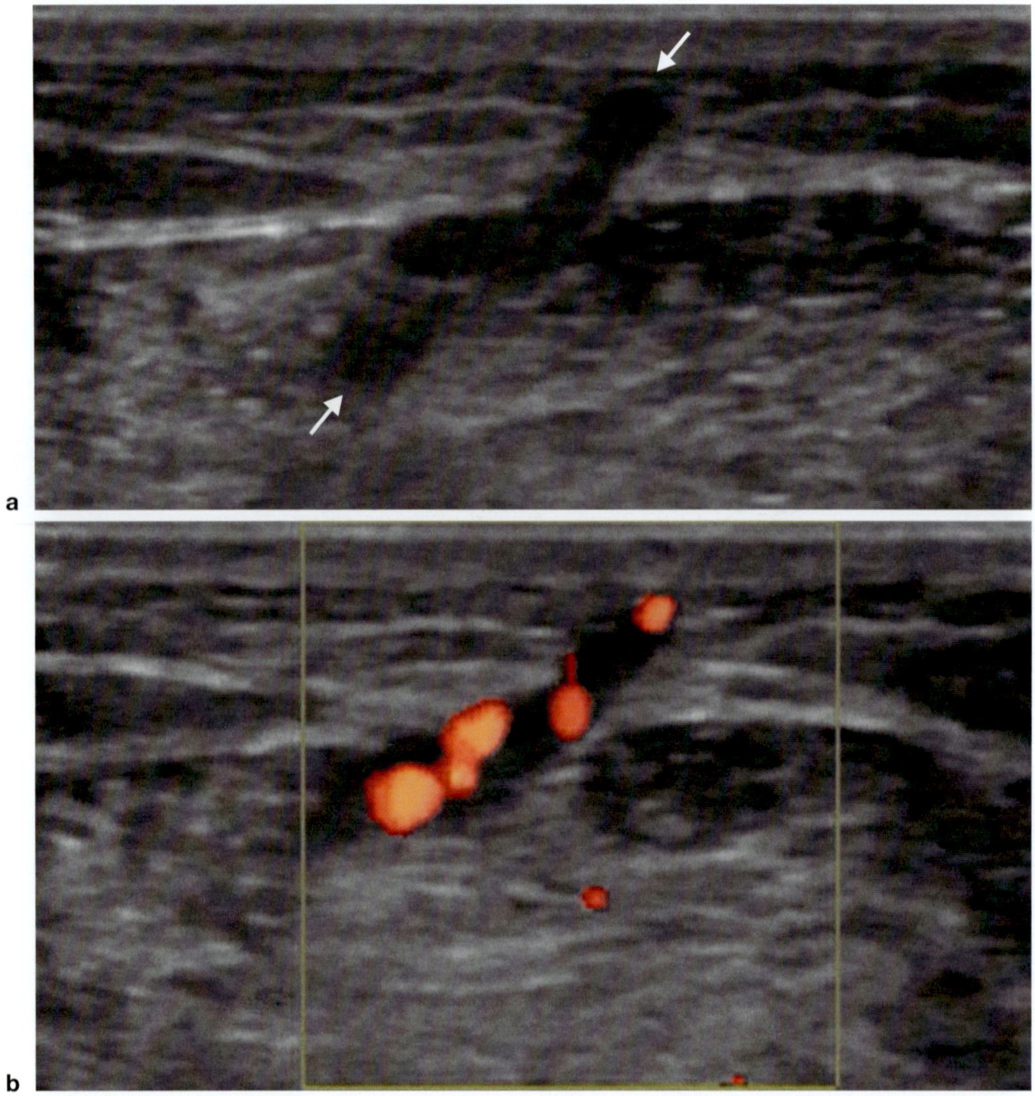

Longitudinal US images (with gentle probe positioning) demonstrates an abnormally dilated hypoechoic superficial vein (*arrows*) in the subcutaneous tissue (**a**) and low-flow signal on power Doppler imaging (**b**).

Expert note

Compression of the probe a little more might induce collapse of such a superficial vein; therefore the sonographer should be cautious especially while exploring venous pathologies of this kind.

Foreign body in a 40-year-old carpenter who had a previous gunshot injury **10.2**

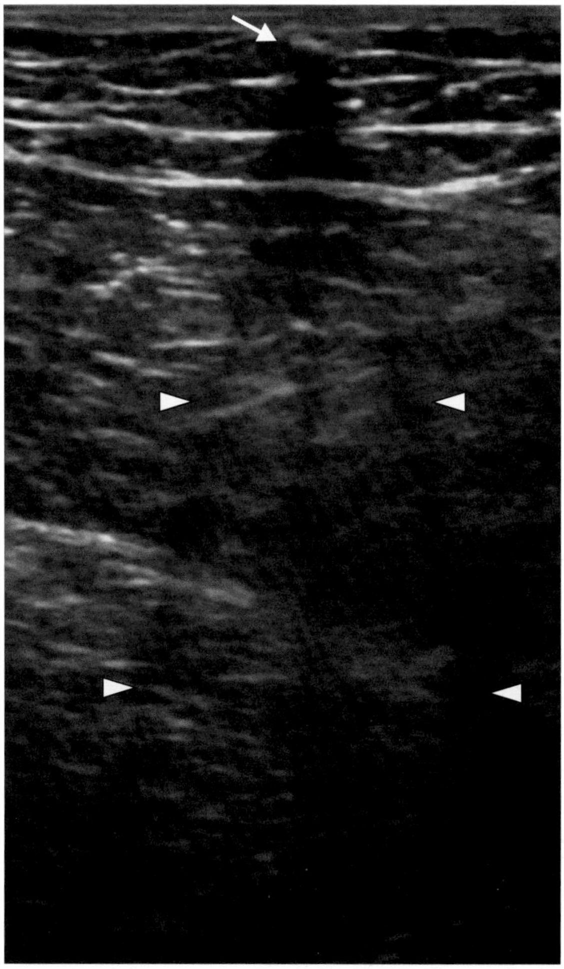

Longitudinal US image shows a small hyperechoic piece of bullet (*arrow*), which is very superficial in the subcutaneous tissue of the calf, giving a huge comet-tail artifact (*arrowheads*).

Expert note

While the foreign objects cannot always be recognized at the initial glance, particular/relevant artifacts make them almost impossible to be overlooked. Herewith, it is noteworthy that even during surgery, very small objects might not be easily detected despite microscopy. In this sense, US imaging can also be used to precisely navigate an onward surgery.

10.3 Lipedema in a 50-year-old woman with a 3-year history of diffuse swelling in distal lower limbs proximal to the ankle joints

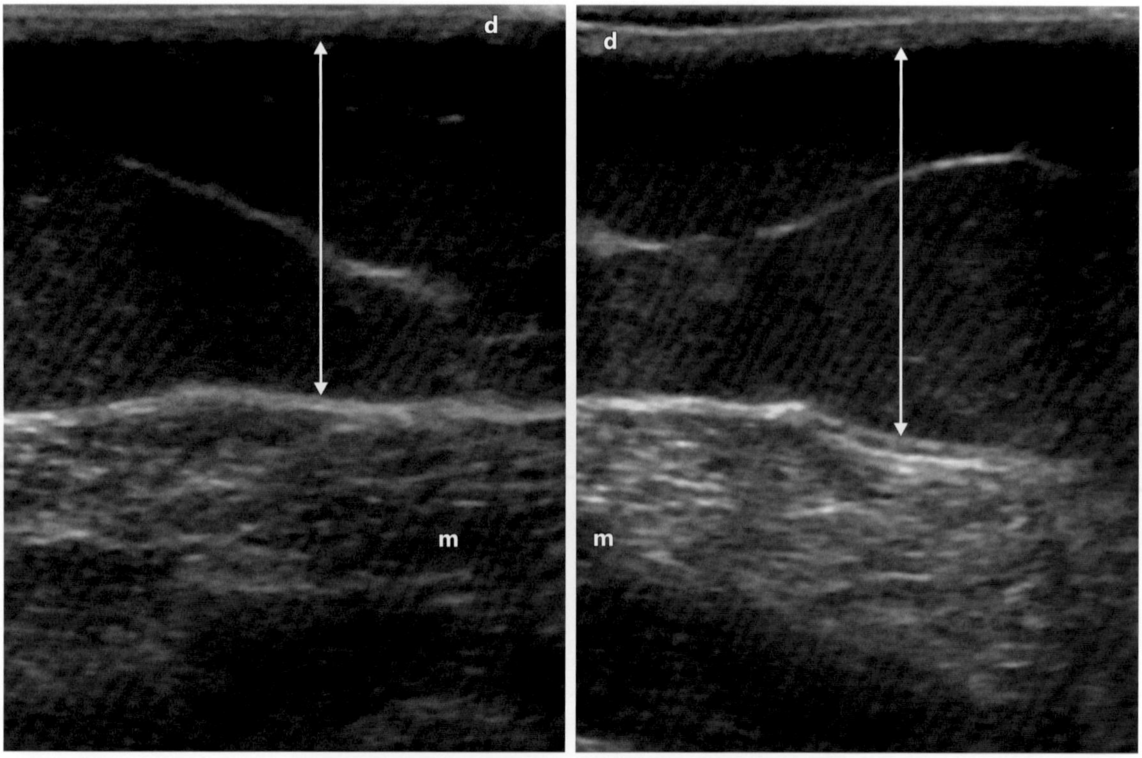

a b

Axial US images over the anteromedial leg show significant and diffuse thickening of the subcutaneous fat tissue (*double arrows*) bilaterally.

d dermis
m muscle

Expert note

In lymphedema, there is an image of hyperechoic "islands" surrounded by hypoechoic "streams". In edema, the borders of the fascia and underlying tissues are often blurred. On the other hand, in this figure, the septae in the subcutis and the fasciae are rather sharp.

Lymphedema in a 44-year-old woman with calf swelling **10.4**

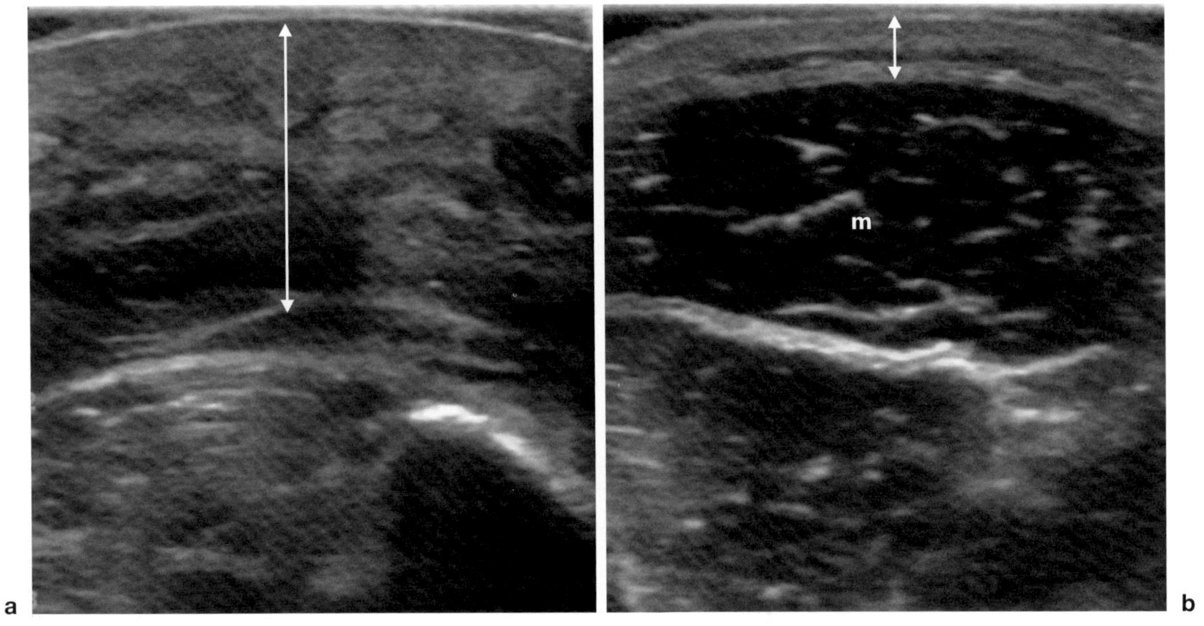

Axial US image over the calf demonstrates blurred, heterogenous and thickened dermis and subcutaneous fat layers (*double arrow*) due to lymphedema (**a**). Normal side (**b**).

m muscle

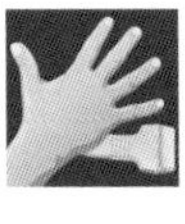

Expert note

It is quite obvious that the edema pertains to both the dermis and subcutaneous fat layers in between which the stratification can no more be distinguished. Due to the heterogenous character of the edema, the underlying muscle tissue is not well visualized either.

10.5 Lymphedema in the lower extremity of a 57-year-old woman with a history of pelvic malignancy

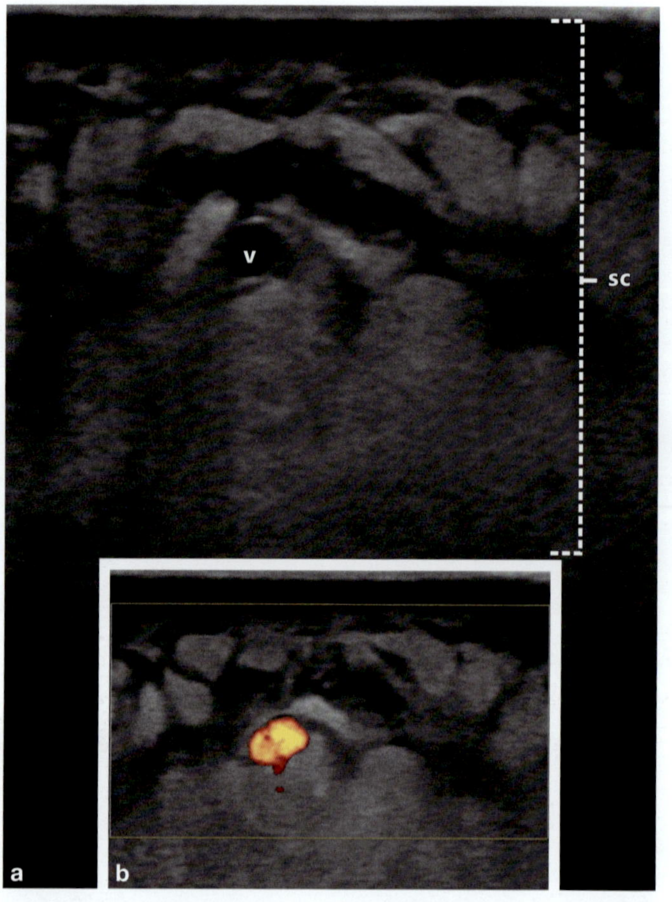

B-mode (**a**) and power Doppler US (**b**) images show irregular thicknening of the subcutaneous tissue (**sc**) with dilated veins (**v**).

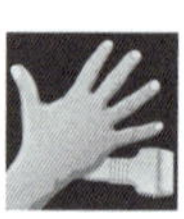

Expert note

For sure, the use of power Doppler imaging can help better demonstrate accompanying complications like cellulitis.

Localized neurofibroma in a 35-year-old woman with extreme pain over the medial knee **10.6**

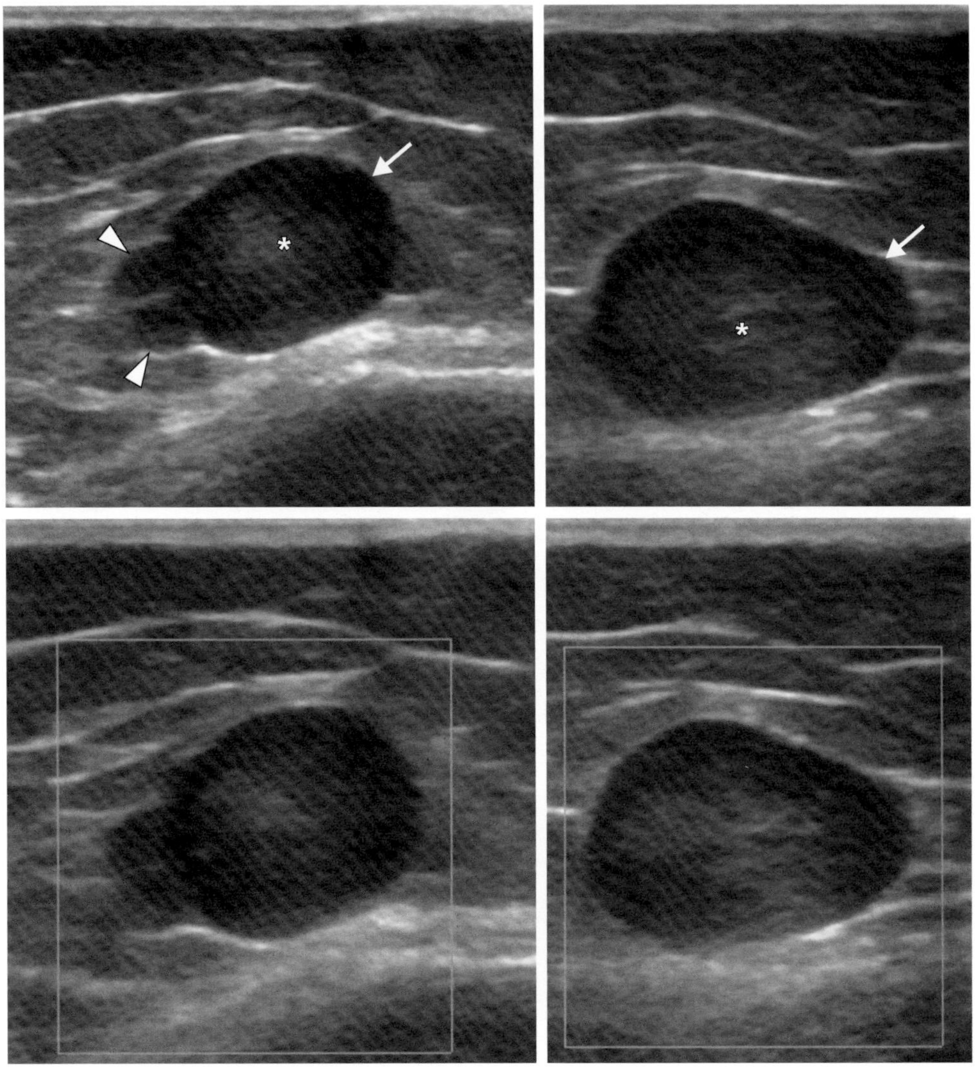

a b c d

Axial (**a**) and longitudinal (**b**) US images over the medial knee show a well-demarcated oval mass (*arrows*) with two small satellite nodules (*arrowheads*) in the subcutaneous tissue. It appears peripherally hypoechoic and centrally hyperechoic representing the target sign (*asterisks*). Power Doppler images reveal no flow signal (**c**, **d**).

Expert note

Neurofibromas (in contrast to schwannomas) typically display no vascular flow [1]. While their locations (or anatomical origin) can usually be delineated, it might sometimes be impossible when they reside in the subcutaneous tissue and only be detected as scattered "bubble-like" structures.

10.7 Thrombophlebitis in the saphenous vein of an elderly man with leg pain and discomfort

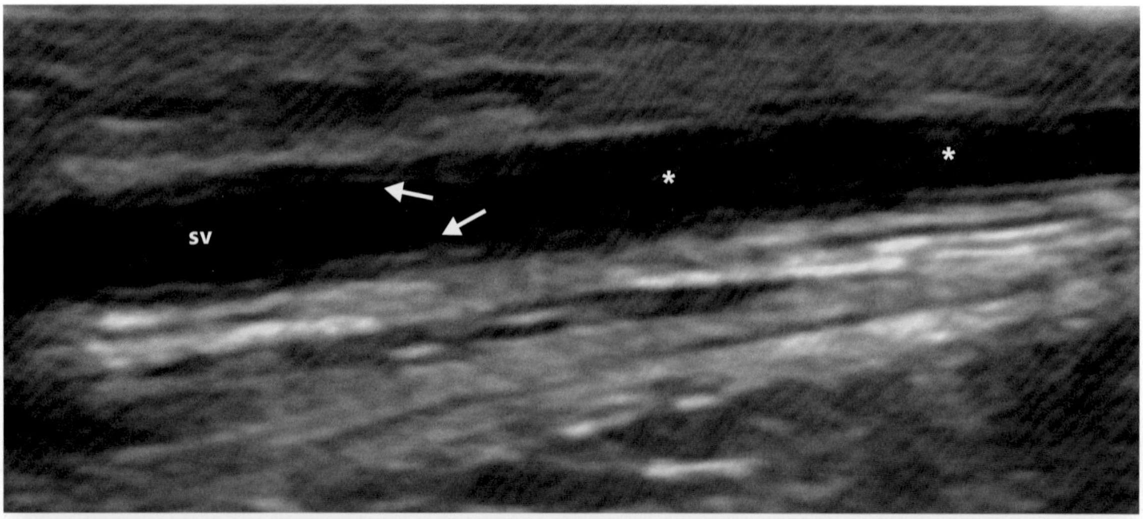

a

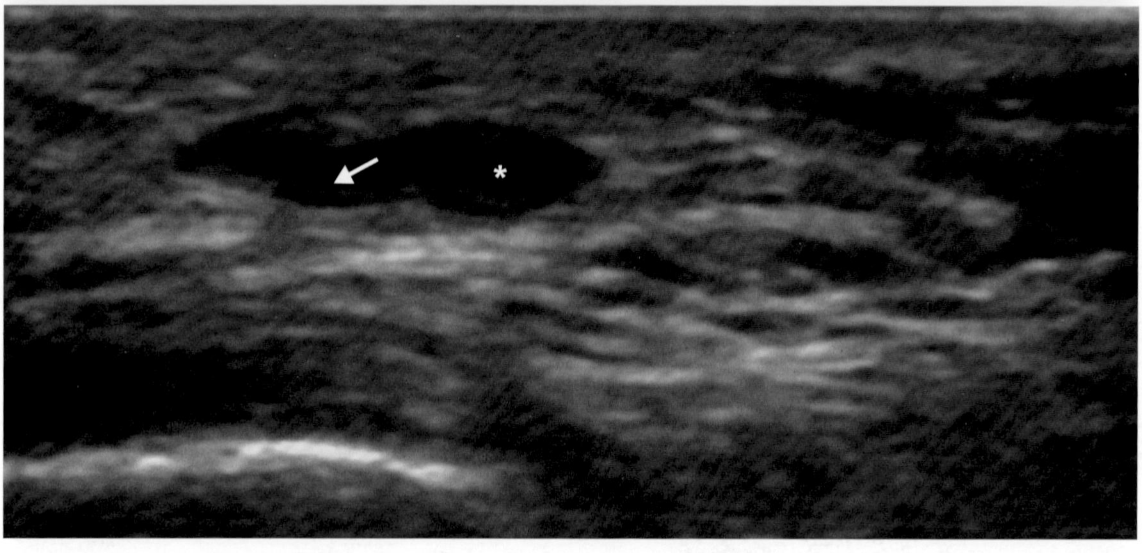

b

Longitudinal (**a**) and axial (**b**) B-mode US images of the leg show the thickening of the wall (*arrows*) and the hypoechoic thrombus in the lumen (*asterisks*).

sv saphenous vein

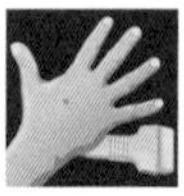

Expert note

Indisputably, further evaluations as regards the flow parameters can be done using Doppler imaging.

Shin splint over the tibia in a young-aged runner after heavy training before the season **10.8**

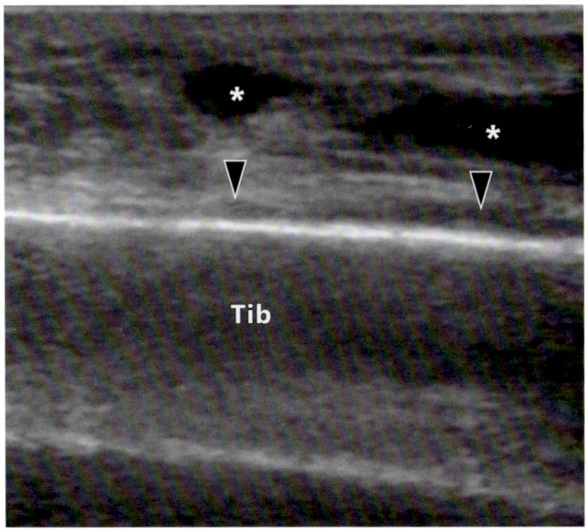

Longitudinal US image of the anterior aspect of tibia (**Tib**) shows hypo/anechoic fluid collection (*asterisks*) and periosteal reaction (*arrowheads*) overlying the bony cortex.

Hematoma in a 28-year-old football player with pain on the anterior tibia after a match trauma **10.9**

a 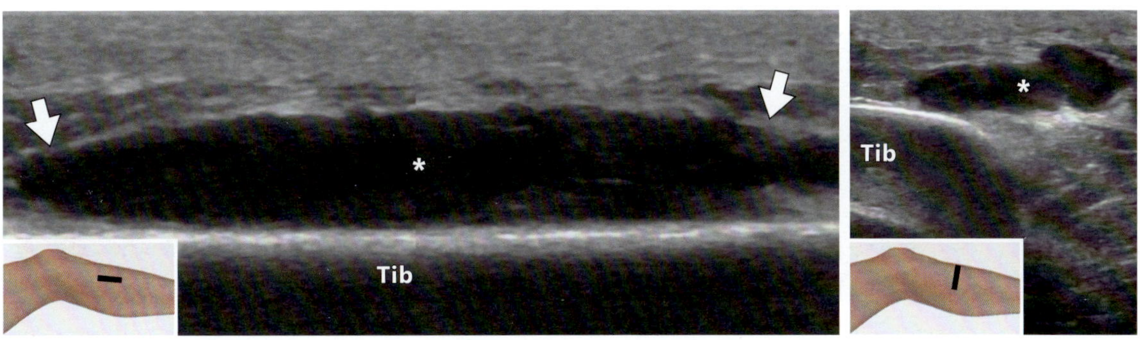 b

Longitudinal split-screen (**a**) and axial (**b**) US images demonstrate a large hypo/anechoic collection (*asterisks*) resembling a peri/subperiosteal hematoma (*arrows*).

Expert note

Aside from its user-dependency, the most important disadvantage of US imaging is the inability to assess intraosseous pathologies. Nonetheless, lesions involving the cortex or the periosteum are undoubtedly in sight and can easily be located with sono-palpation.

10.10 Tennis leg in a 34-year-old player with a painful and swollen calf

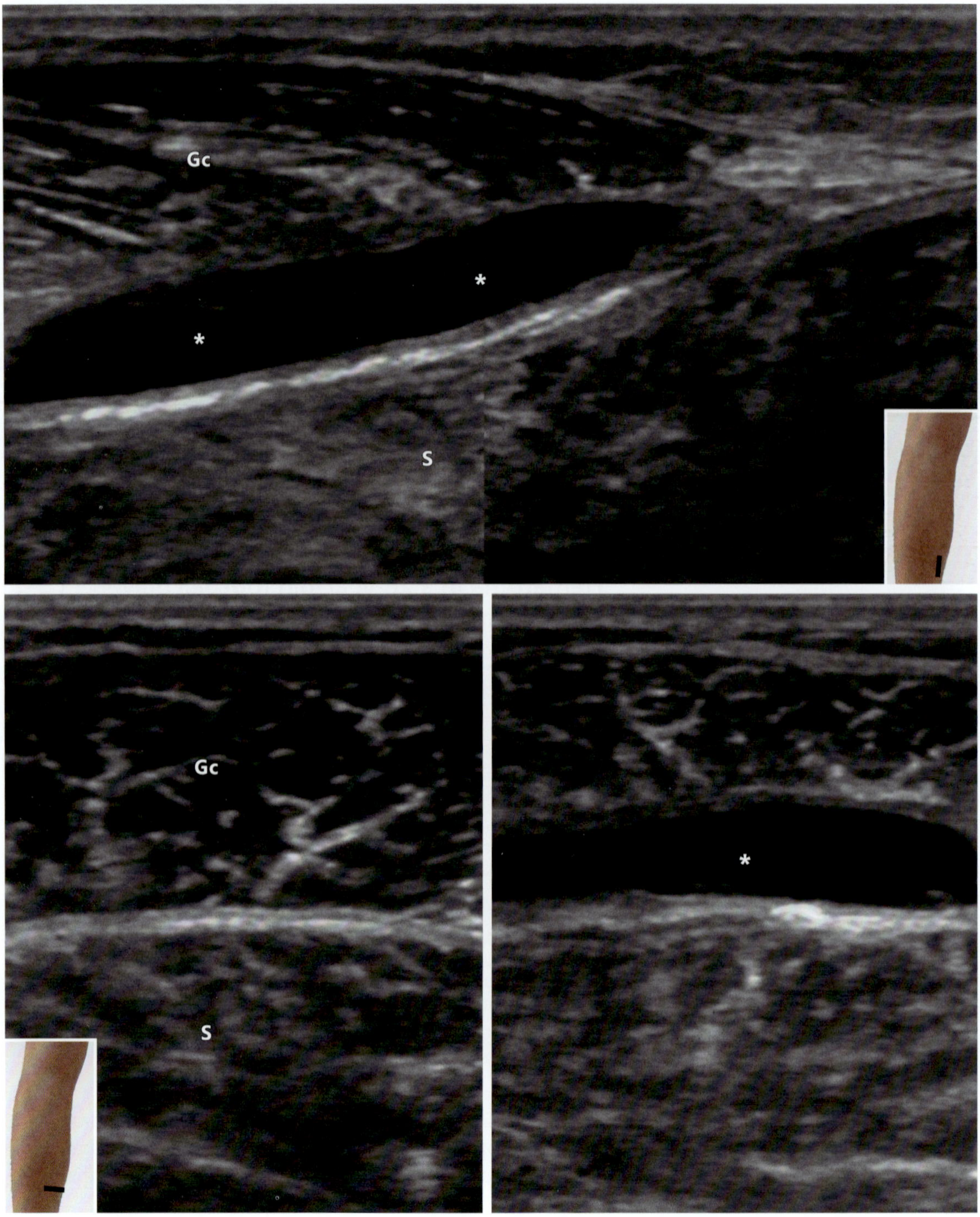

a

b

c

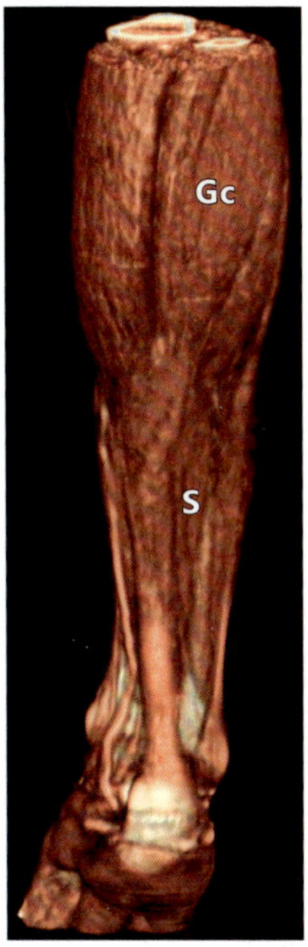

The athlete had to leave the match after a snap sensation in his midcalf.

Longitudinal split-screen (**a**) and axial (**c**) US images show a well-defined anechoic fluid/blood collection (*asterisks*) caused by myofascial tear of the gastrocnemius muscle (**Gc**). Normal axial view on the contralateral (**b**).

S soleus

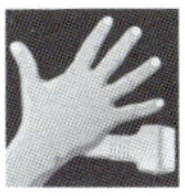

Expert note

By and large, tennis leg is one of the most commonly encountered myotendinous injuries in sports traumatology. Medial head of the gastrocnemius muscle is affected, usually during lateral sports. While local hematoma may be present exactly on the ruptured area, oft-times it might spread along the layers of the fascia far proximally.

10.11 Venous insufficiency in a 60-year-old woman with local sharp pain and swelling after long-standing activities

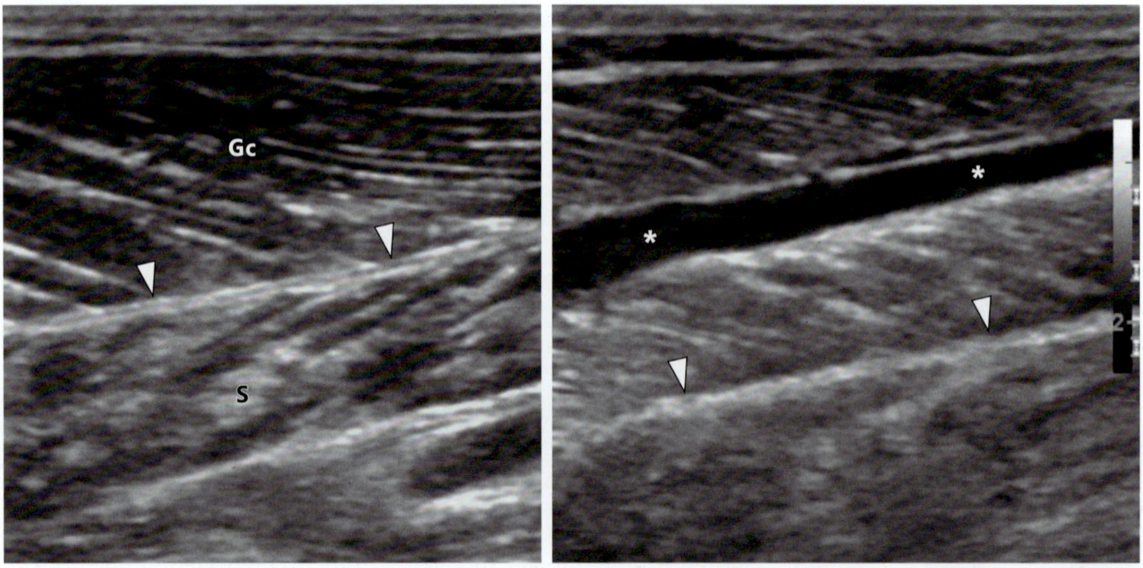

a b

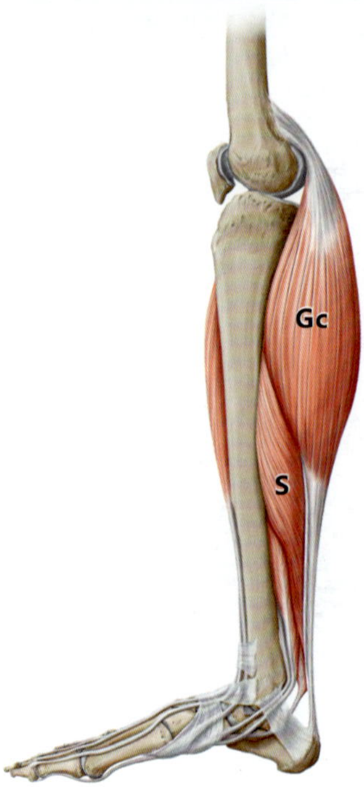

When compared with the normal side (**a**), longitudinal US imaging (**b**) reveals dilated gemellary vein (*asterisks*) crossing through the medial head of the gastrocnemius muscle (**Gc**). Intermuscular aponeurosis is shown by the *white arrowheads*.

S soleus

Expert note

Dilated deep veins with less tortuosity can masquerade as linear blood accumulations between the outer fascia layers. As such, sonographers should be cautious against an erroneous diagnosis of "tennis leg" in relevant patients.

Healing tennis leg (complete tear) in a 42-year-old patient with calf pain and swelling after a fall during skiing

10.12

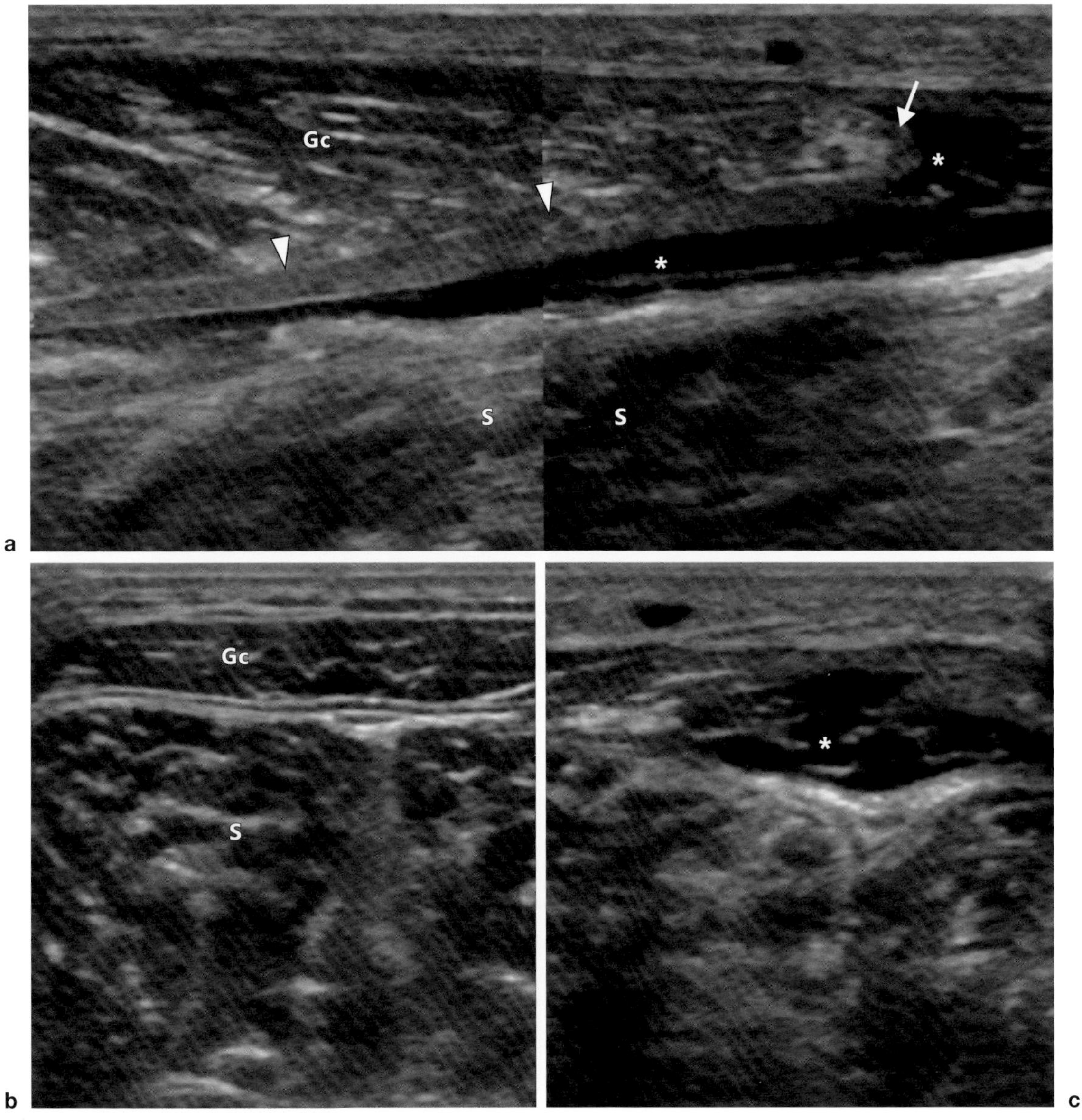

Longitudinal split-screen (**a**) and axial (**c**) US images over the distal gastrocnemius muscle (**Gc**) reveal a myotendinous tear with a slight retraction of the stump (*arrow*) surrounded by a large hematoma (*asterisks*). *Arrowheads* indicate the walls of the hematoma which become thickened and organized. Normal axial view on the contralateral side (**b**).

S soleus

10.13 Healing tennis leg (partial tear) in a sportman after four weeks of injury

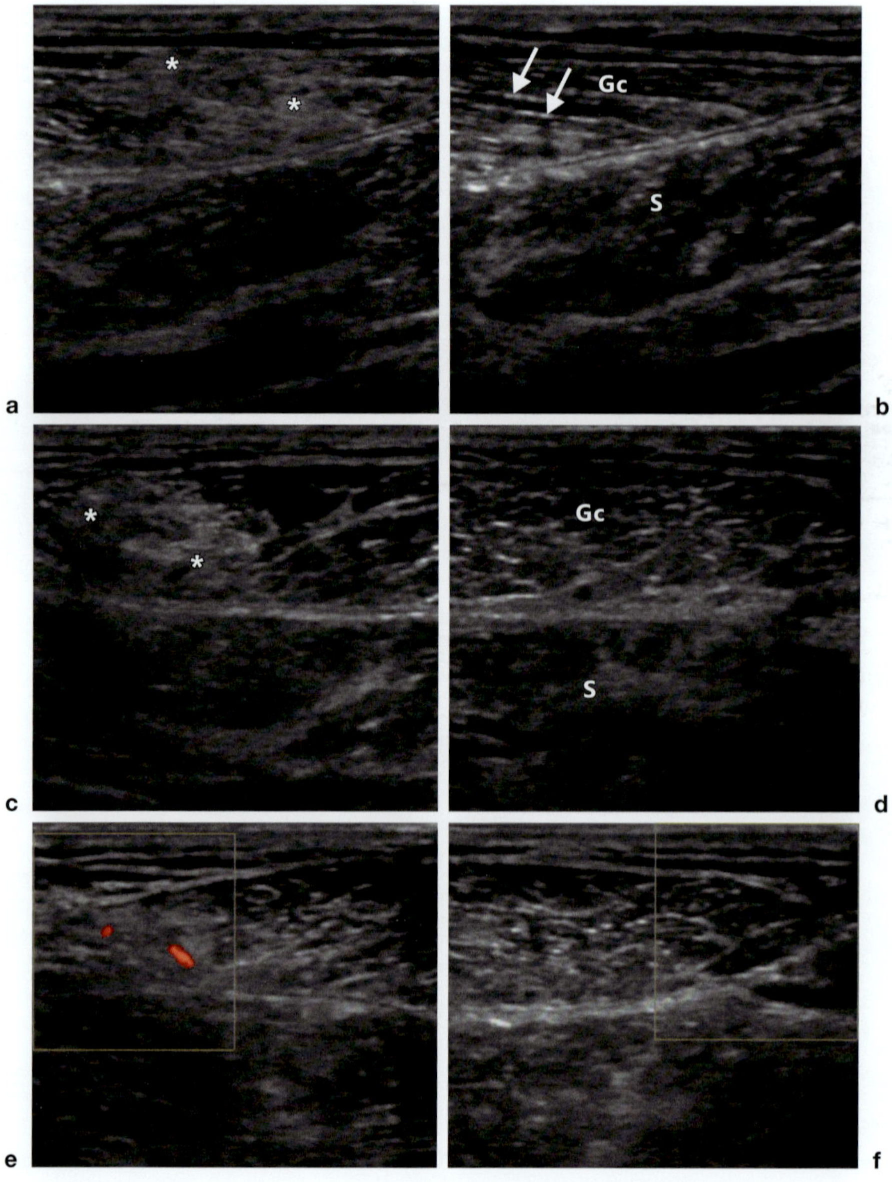

Longitudinal (**a**) and axial (**c**) US images obtained over the posteromedial aspect of the midcalf demonstrate partially disrupted and edematous gastrocnemius muscle (**Gc**) fascicles (*asterisks*). Power Doppler imaging identifies increased vasculature consistent with inflammation/repair (**e**). Contralateral side displays the normal pennation pattern (*arrows*) in longitudinal view (**b**). Normal side axial view (**d**) and Doppler imaging (**f**).

S soleus

Reparative/healing process of tennis leg in a patient after sports trauma **10.14**

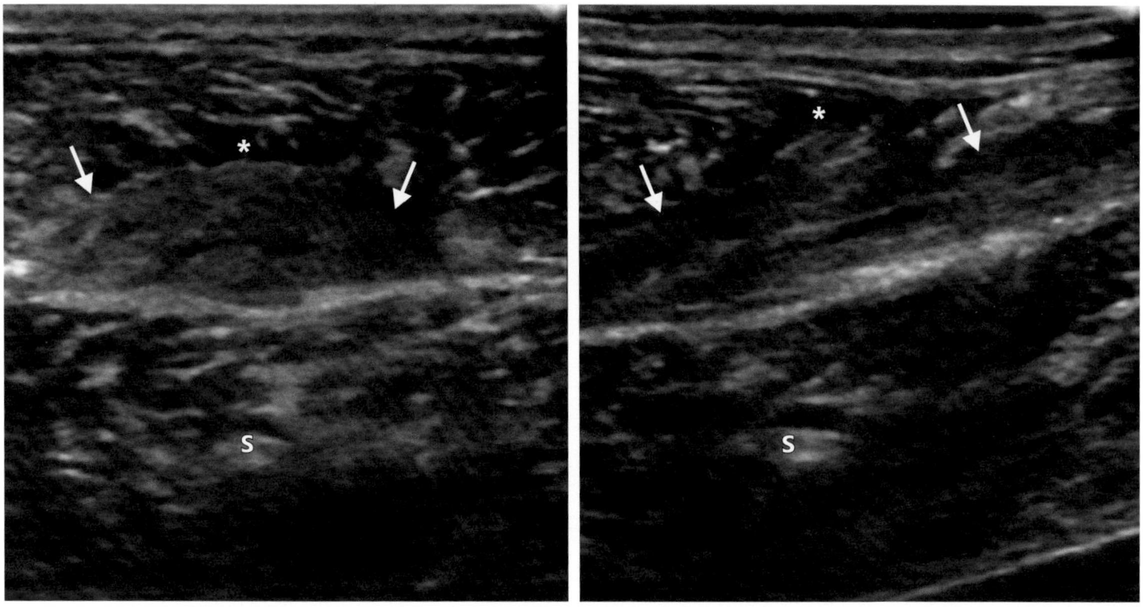

a b

Axial (**a**) and longitudinal (**b**) US images over the myotendinous junction of the gastrocnemius muscle depict healing of the tear as a hyperechoic area (fibrous tissue) (*arrows*). Note the anechoic appearance where the muscle fascicles are separated/retracted (*asterisks*).

S soleus

Calf

Expert note

Axial scans are appropriate to distinguish partial from complete tears as these images can completely reveal the medial head of the gastrocnemius. On the other hand, longitudinal US images are more reliable to show the proximal retraction. Another method to show the presence of a partial or complete rupture is dynamic examination of the foot with dorsal and plantar flexion in prone position which illustrates the intact soleus gliding under an immobile disinserted medial head [2]. Likewise, one can ask for isometric contraction to see if the area is contractile or not.

10.15 Gastrocnemius muscle tear in a 42-year-old man with calf pain and ecchymosis after blunt leg trauma

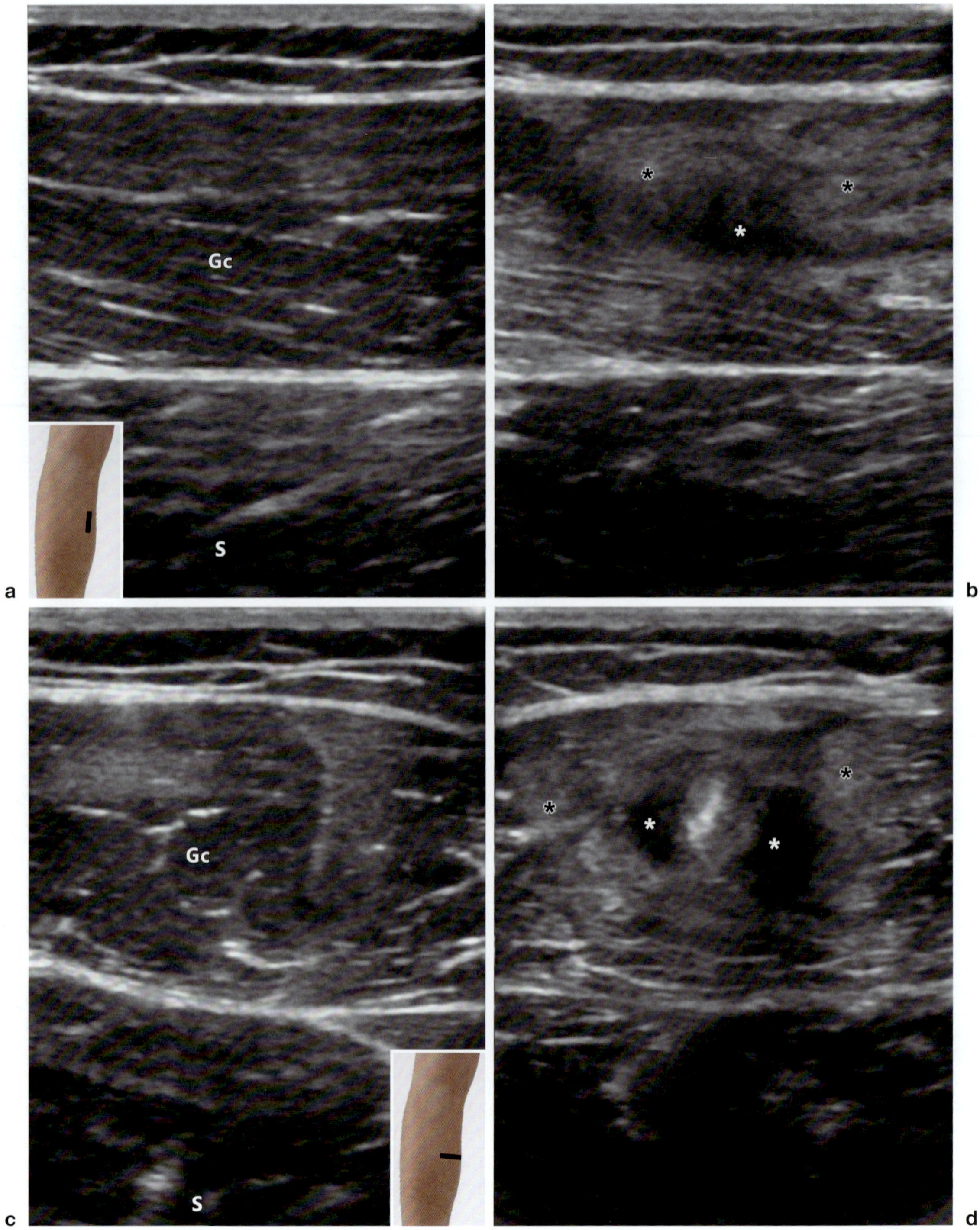

When compared with the normal side (**a**, **c**), longitudinal (**b**) and axial (**d**) US images demonstrate hemorrhagic infiltration (*black asterisks*) and partial disruption (*white asterisks*) of the medial head of the gastrocnemius muscle (**Gc**).

S soleus

Expert note

Since located more proximally, this type of an intrasubstance tear of the gastrocnemius muscle is not termed as 'tennis leg'. As mentioned before, this is an illustration of possible central location in the muscle belly due to blunt trauma.

Polymyositis in a 31-year-old woman with a 6-month duration of widespread myalgias **10.16**

a 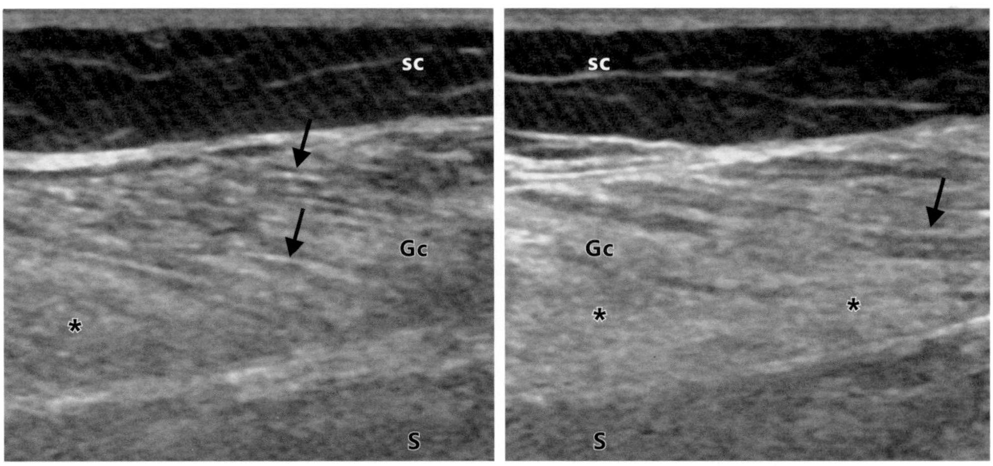 b

She had progressive difficulty in climbing the stairs or rising from a chair.

Longitudinal US images (**a**, **b**) over the medial head of the gastrocnemius muscle (**Gc**) reveal bilateral intramuscular irregular hyperechoic areas (*asterisks*) where there is partial loss of the normal (*arrows*) fibroadipose septa (pennation pattern) as well.

sc subcutaneous tissue

Expert note

Apart from traumatic/overuse injuries, US imaging can also be used for inflammatory or neurogenic muscle disorders. Changes in the muscle architecture, echogenicity or vascularity are the usual parameters that are assessed in such conditions.

In acute inflammatory myopathies, US imaging can demonstrate increased echogenicity and minor change in muscle thickness but with preserved deep bone reflection. It is different from the increased echogenicity with strong attenuation in deeper layers that is seen in muscular dystrophy or the advanced stages of myositis when muscle destruction and following fibrosis have taken place [3].

10.17 Healing process of tennis leg in a marathon athlete after a long run three weeks ago

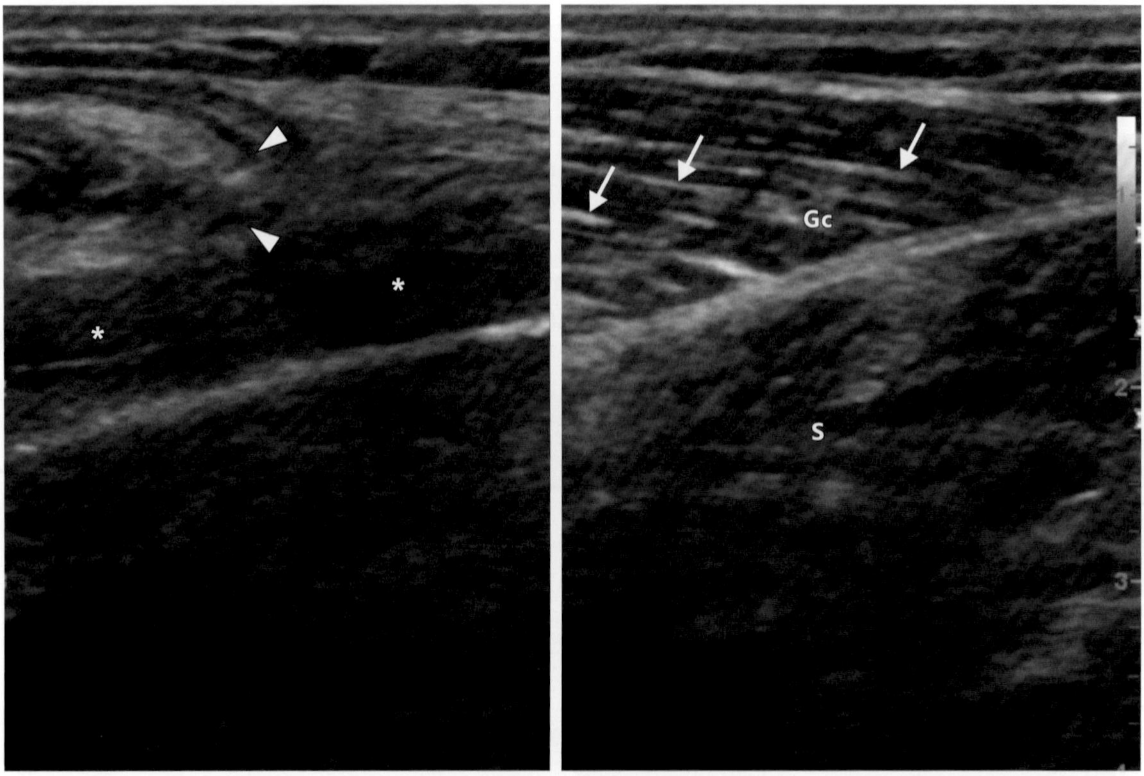

a b

Longitudinal US imaging shows hyperechoic deformed/retracted gastrocnemius muscle fascicles (*arrowheads*) and a hypoechoic zone of organizing hematoma (*asterisks*) (**a**). Normal pennation pattern (*arrows*) on the contralateral side (**b**).

Gc gastrocnemius
S soleus

Expert note

In case the muscle fibers are involved, normal pennation structure of the muscle is lost and a blunt ending separated from the distal tendon would be the typical eventuality.

Arteriovenous malformation in the calf region of an otherwise healthy 40-year-old man **10.18**

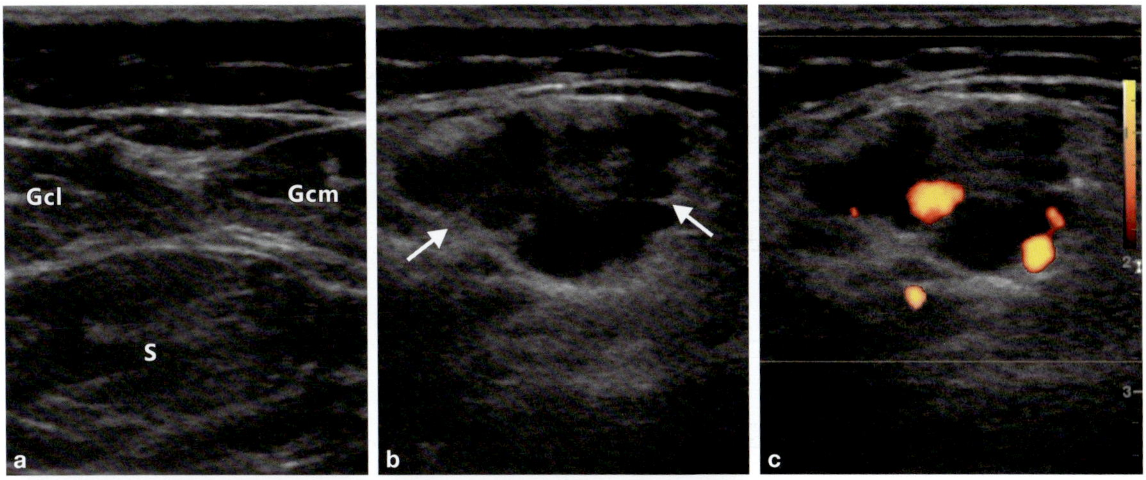

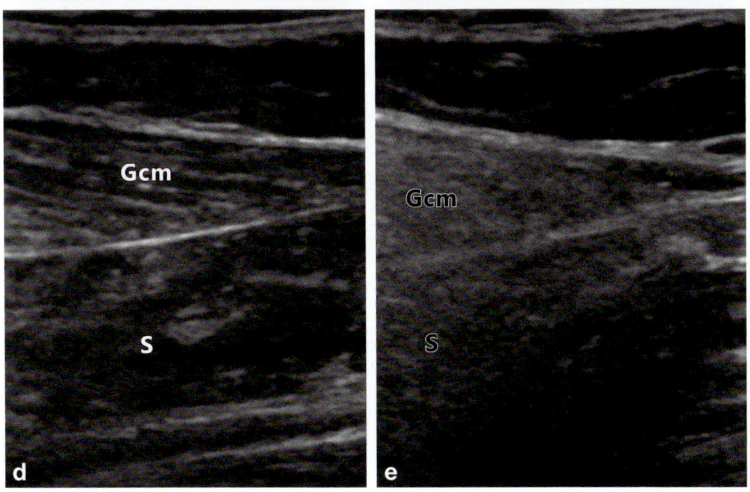

When compared with the normal side (**a**), axial US image over the posterior proximal leg reveals a focal, heterogeneous lesion with well-defined margins (*arrows*) resembling an arteriovenous malformation (**b**). Power Doppler imaging (**c**). Longitudinal US image shows the normal appearance of the medial head of the gastrocnemius muscle (**Gcm**) distally (**d**). Hyperechoic muscles -with loss of normal architecture- reflect possible damage on the affected side (**e**).

Gcl lateral head of the gastrocnemius muscle
S soleus

Expert note

Here is another case whereby substantial US imaging unmasks several associated pathologies in details. Inarguably, these findings should be interpreted with in-depth physical examination for prompt clinical decision making.

REFERENCES

1. Kara M. Ultrasound imaging for peripheral nerve problems. In: Özçakar L, De Muynck M, editors. Musculoskeletal ultrasound in physical and rehabilitation medicine. Milan: Edi.Ermes; 2014. p. 141-60.
2. Bianchi S, Martinoli C. Leg. In: Bianchi S, Martinoli C, editors. Ultrasound of the musculoskeletal system. Berlin: Springer; 2007. p. 745-72.
3. Zaidman CM, van Alfen N. Ultrasound in the assessment of myopathic disorders. J Clin Neurophysiol. 2016; 33: 103-11.

Ankle and Foot 11

- **Tibiotalar joint**
- **Talonavicular joint**
- **Tibialis anterior tendon**
- **Tibialis posterior tendon**
- **Fibularis longus tendon**
- **Subcutaneous tissue** - Ankle
- **Retrocalcaneal bursa**
- **Retroachilles bursa**
- **Calcaneal enthesis** - Superior
- **Achilles tendon**
- **Soleus tertius**
- **Plantar fascia**
- **Subcutaneous tissue** - Plantar
- **Anterior talofibular ligament**
- **Deltoid ligament**
- **Tibiofibular ligament**
- **First metatarsophalangeal joint**
- **Second metatarsophalangeal joint**
- **Tarsometatarsal joint**
- **Abductor hallucis**
- **Submetatarsal bursa**
- **Metatarsal bone**
- **Extensor hallucis longus tendon**
- **Subcutaneous tissue** - Dorsal

11.1 Tibiotalar joint effusion in a 36-year-old man with ankle pain

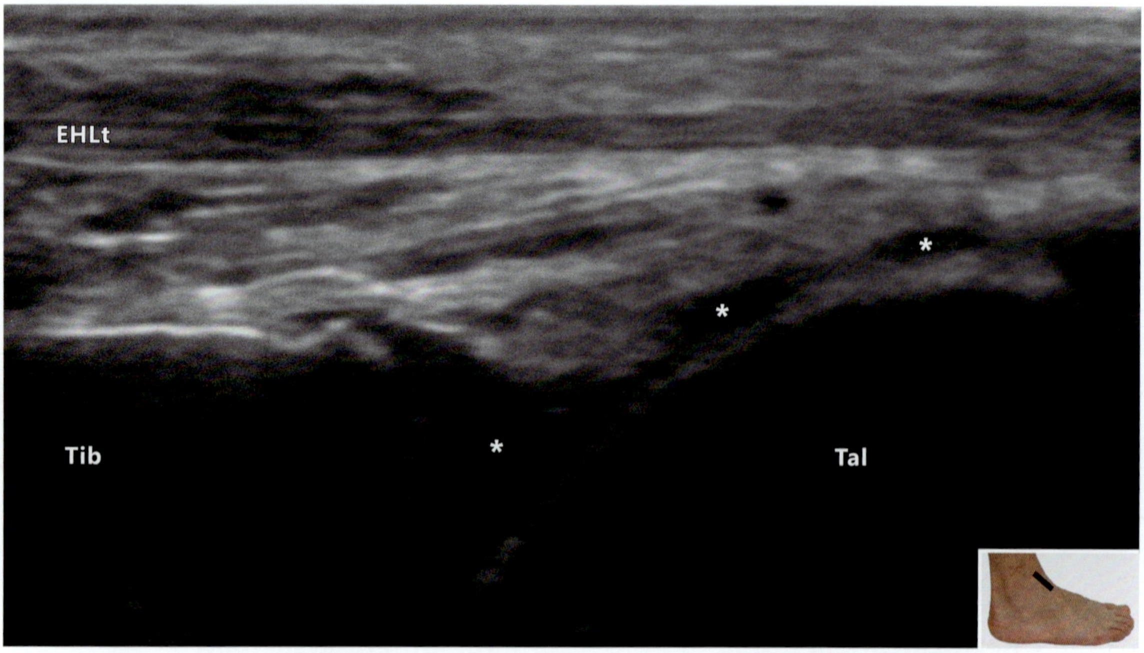

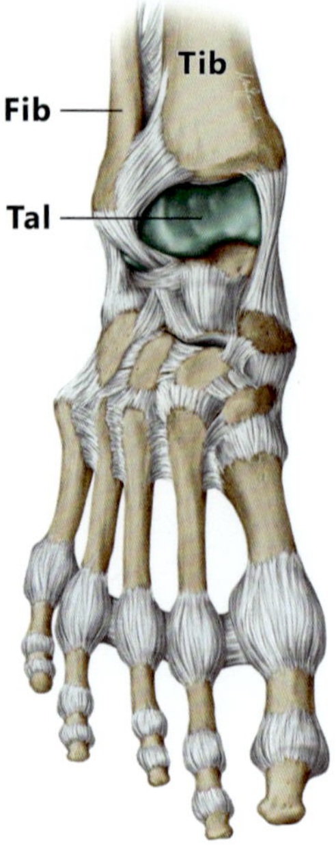

Longitudinal US imaging over the dorsal aspect of the tibiotalar joint demonstrates mild fluid (*asterisks*).

EHLt extensor hallucis longus tendon
Fib fibula
Tal talus
Tib tibia

Expert note

The most commonly scanned joint for effusion in the ankle is the tibiotalar joint. Herewith, similar to the wrist/hand, there are several joints that can be scanned and the US imaging should be tailored according to the complaints and physical examination of the patient. When the patient is lying down, the ankle will often be positioned in slight inversion/plantar flexion. Small amounts of fluid might not be visible in this way. Bringing the ankle in neutral position or dorsiflexion will "push" the fluid into the anterior recess.

Talonavicular joint effusion in a young woman with prior ankle inversion sprain 11.2

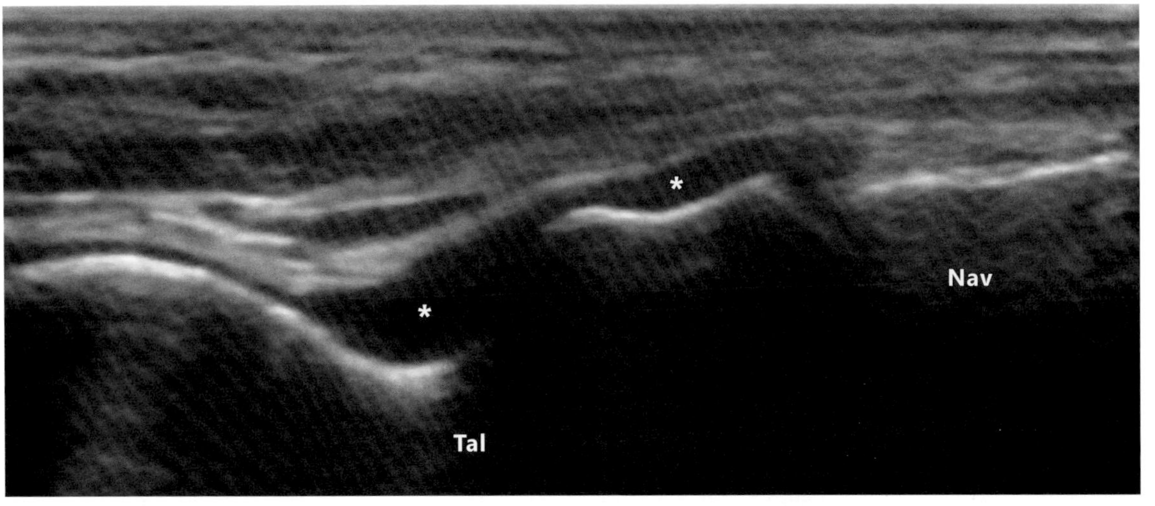

Longitudinal US imaging over the dorsal aspect of the talonavicular joint shows fluid accumulation (*asterisks*).

Nav navicular
Tal talus

11.3 Talonavicular joint effusion in an 18-year-old athlete with foot pain after an inversion sprain

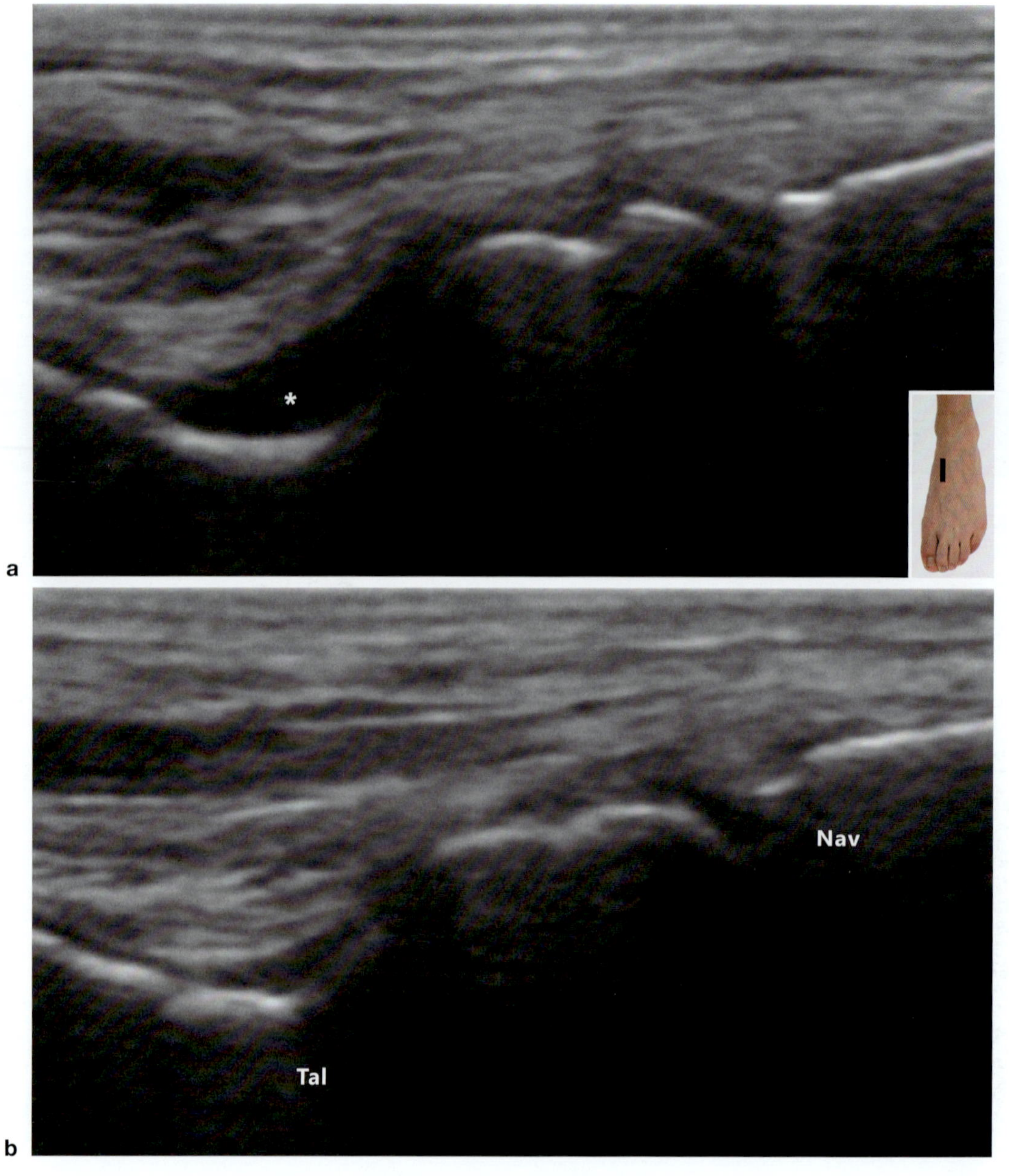

Longitudinal US image of the talonavicular joint demonstrates a small amount of anechoic fluid (*asterisk*) (**a**). Contralateral normal side for comparison (**b**).

Nav navicular
Tal talus

Joint effusion in a 35-year-old man with a history of spondyloarthritis 11.4

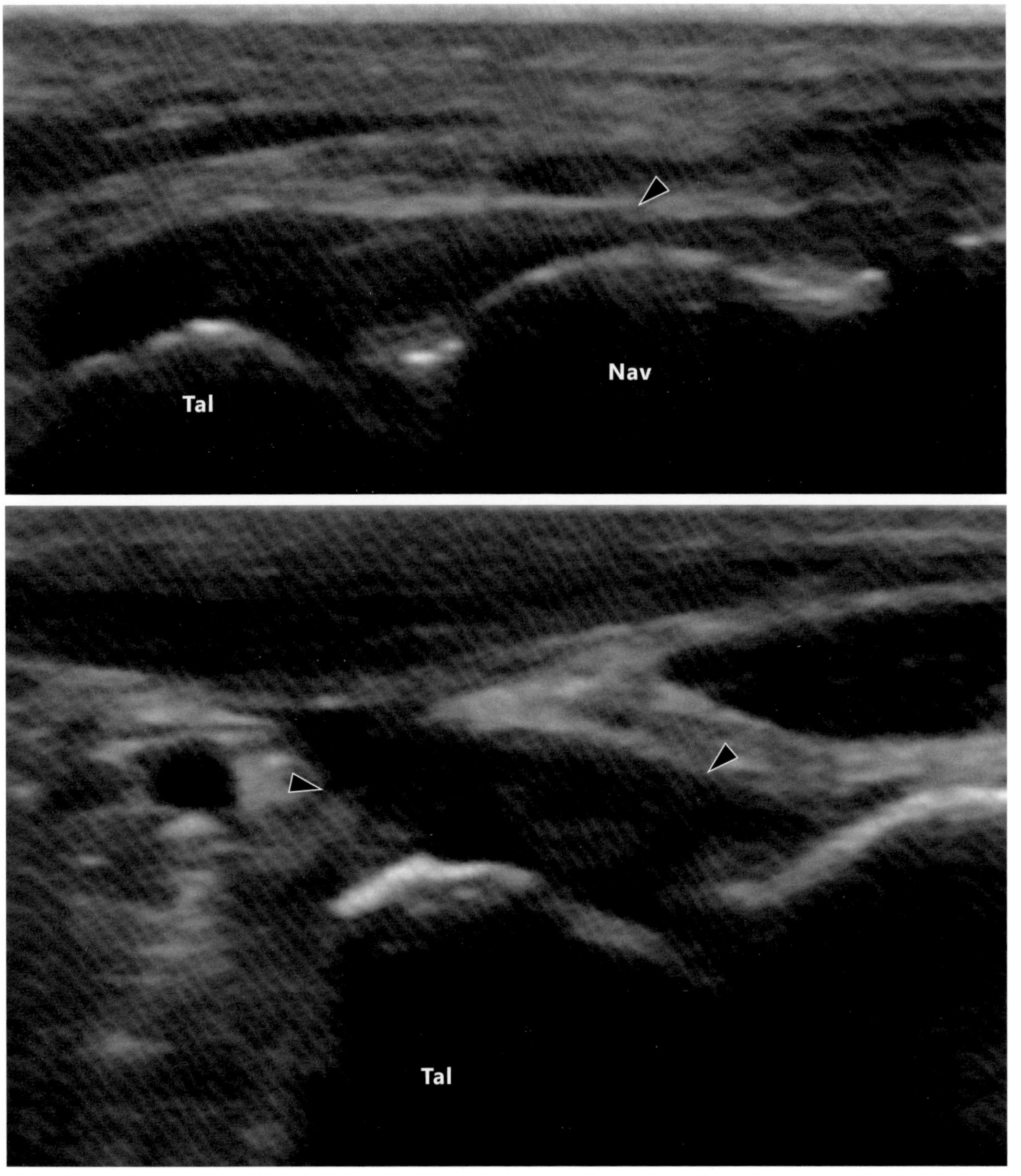

a

b

Longitudinal (**a**) and axial (**b**) US images over the dorsal aspect of the talonavicular joint show swelling (*arrowheads*) due to anechoic fluid and hypoechoic synovial hypertrophy.

Nav navicular
Tal talus

11.5 Talonavicular joint arthritis in a 60-year-old woman with longstanding rheumatoid arthritis

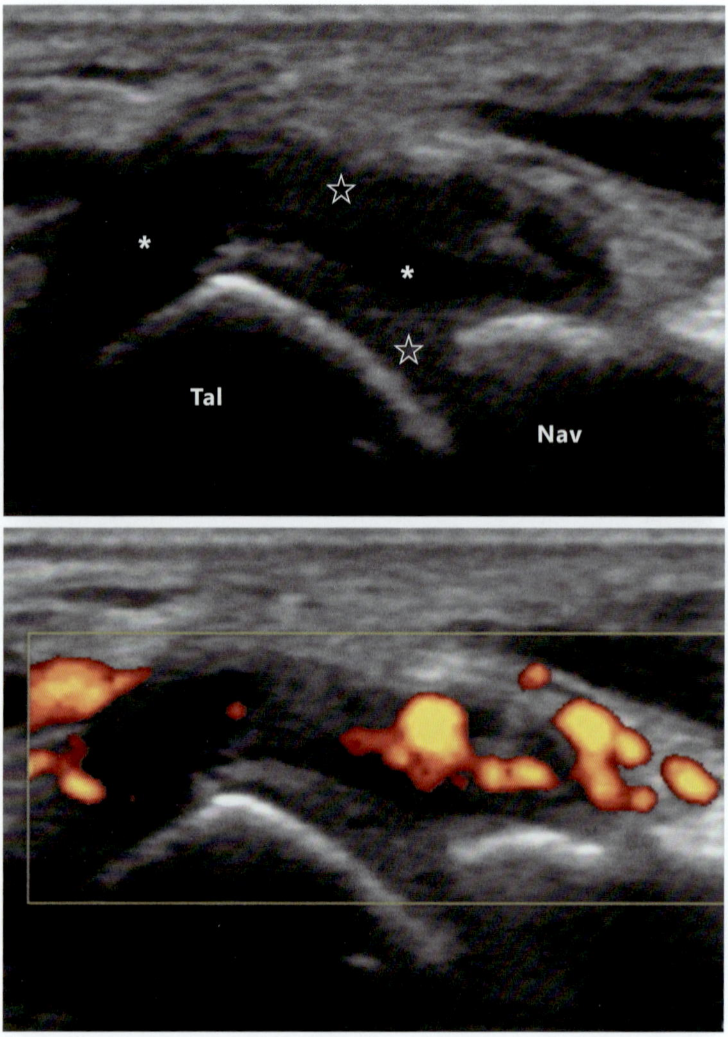

a

b

Dorsal view of the talonavicular joint illustrates effusion (*asterisks*) and synovial hypertrophy (*stars*) (**a**). Increased blood flow (active synovitis, grade II) is seen on power Doppler imaging (**b**).

Nav navicular
Tal talus

Expert note

Semi-quantitative grading (0-III) of synovitis can reliably be done using either the gray-scale or power Doppler images [1].

Tibialis anterior tendinopathy in a 45-year-old man with ankle pain

11.6

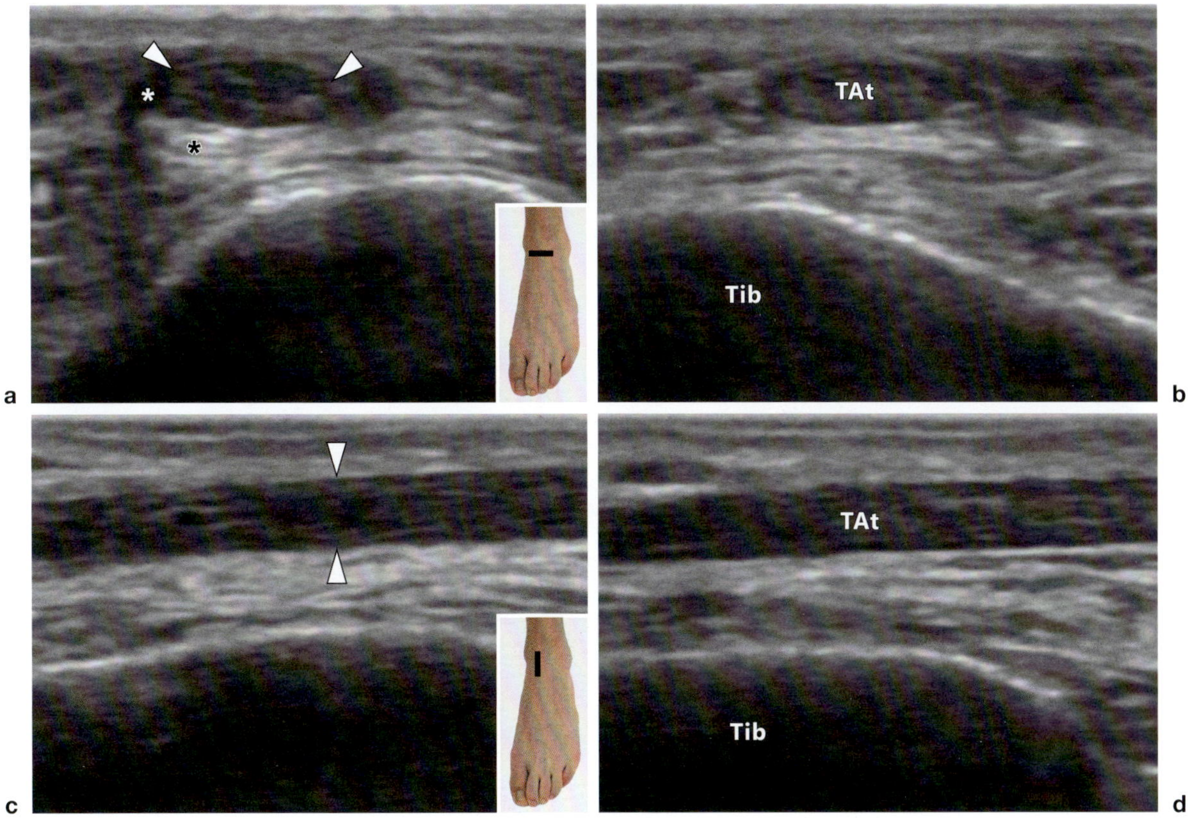

Axial (**a**) and longitudinal (**c**) US images over the anterior ankle show abnormal echotextural appearance (*arrowheads*) of the tibialis anterior tendon (**TAt**) with mild fluid around it (*white asterisk*). Normal contralateral side (**b**, **d**).
Please also note the enhanced through transmission artifact (*black asterisk*).

Tib tibia

11.7 Chronic tenosynovitis of the tibialis posterior tendon in a patient with rheumatoid arthritis

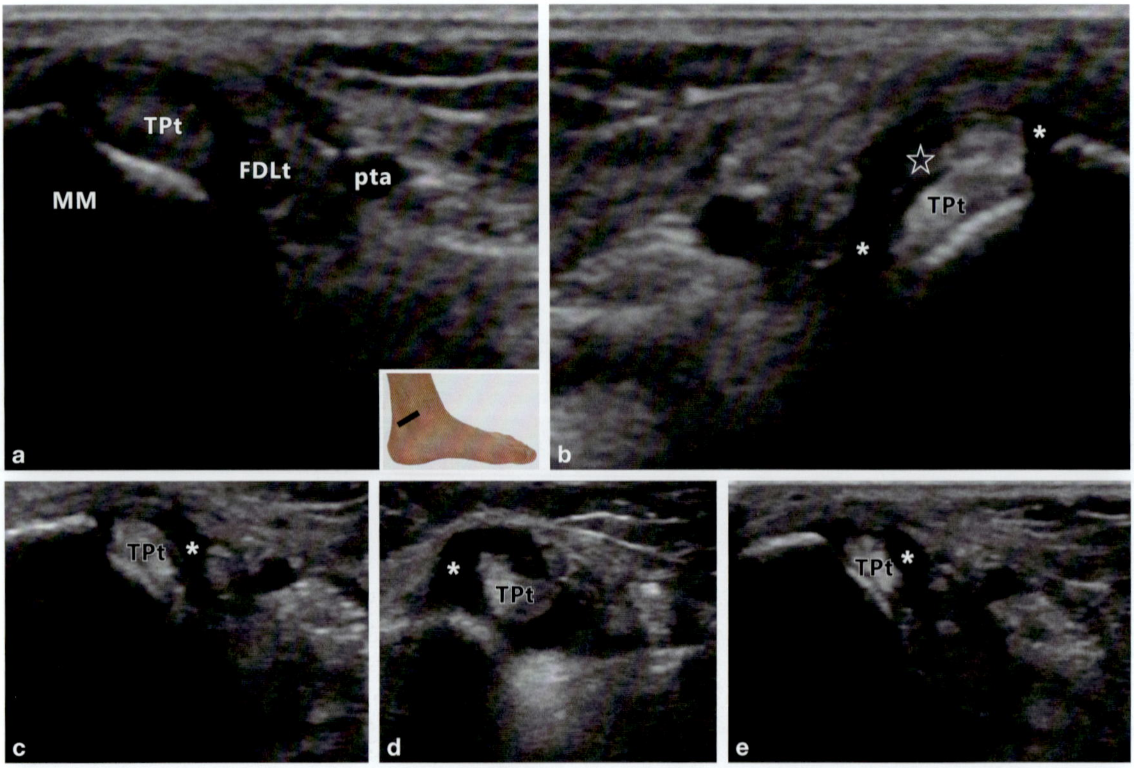

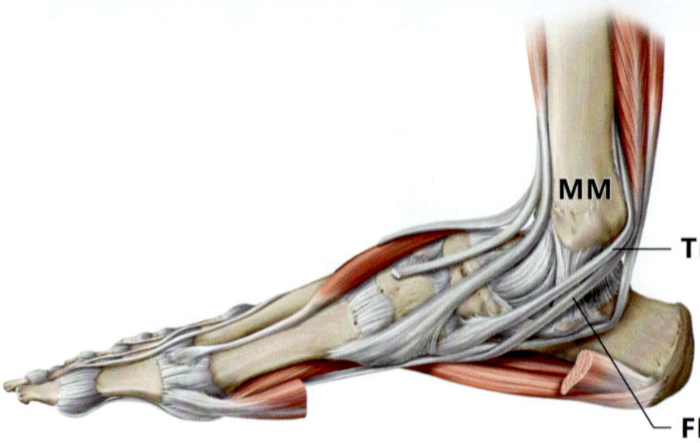

Video 11

When compared with the normal side (**a**), axial US images reveal anechoic fluid collection (*asterisks*) and synovial proliferation (*star*) within the tibialis posterior tendon (**TPt**) sheath obtained at different levels (**b**-**e**).

FDLt	flexor digitorum longus tendon
MM	medial malleolus
pta	posterior tibial artery

Expert note

Finding some fluid around tendons where they are covered with synovial sheaths or at their distal attachments could be acceptable to a certain amount (e.g. ≤4 mm for tibialis posterior) [2]. Therefore, before ascertaining that it is pathological, comparison is indisputably needed.

Tibialis posterior tendinopathy in a middle-aged obese woman with ankle pain and swelling **11.8**

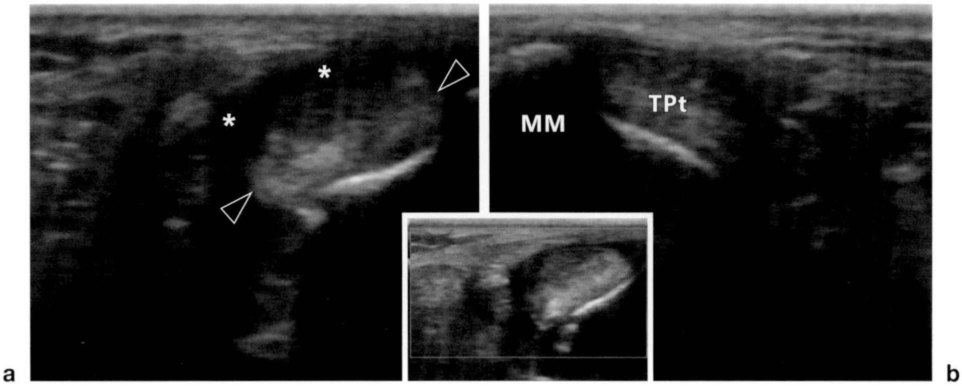

Axial US image over the medial malleolus (**MM**) demonstrates markedly swollen (*arrowheads*) tendon of tibialis posterior (**TPt**) with fluid accumulation (*asterisks*) inside the synovial sheath (**a**). Contralateral normal side (**b**). Note that power Doppler imaging shows no flow signal (*small figure*).

Effusion around the distal tibialis posterior tendon in a patient with ankle pain **11.9**

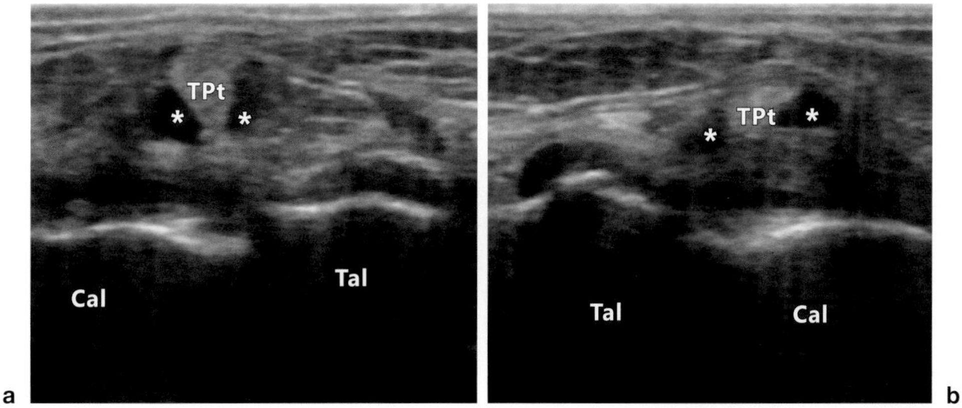

Axial US images show mild effusion (*asterisks*) around the tibialis posterior tendons (**TPt**) on both sides (**a**, **b**).

Cal calcaneus **Tal** talus

Expert note

When searching for local problems of the tendons, imaging throughout their courses is necessary (guided by sono-palpation). Yet, like in this case, the problem might be found in a place which is perhaps not the most common (midway between the medial malleolus and the insertion).

11.10 Tibialis posterior tenosynovitis in an elderly woman after long distance walking

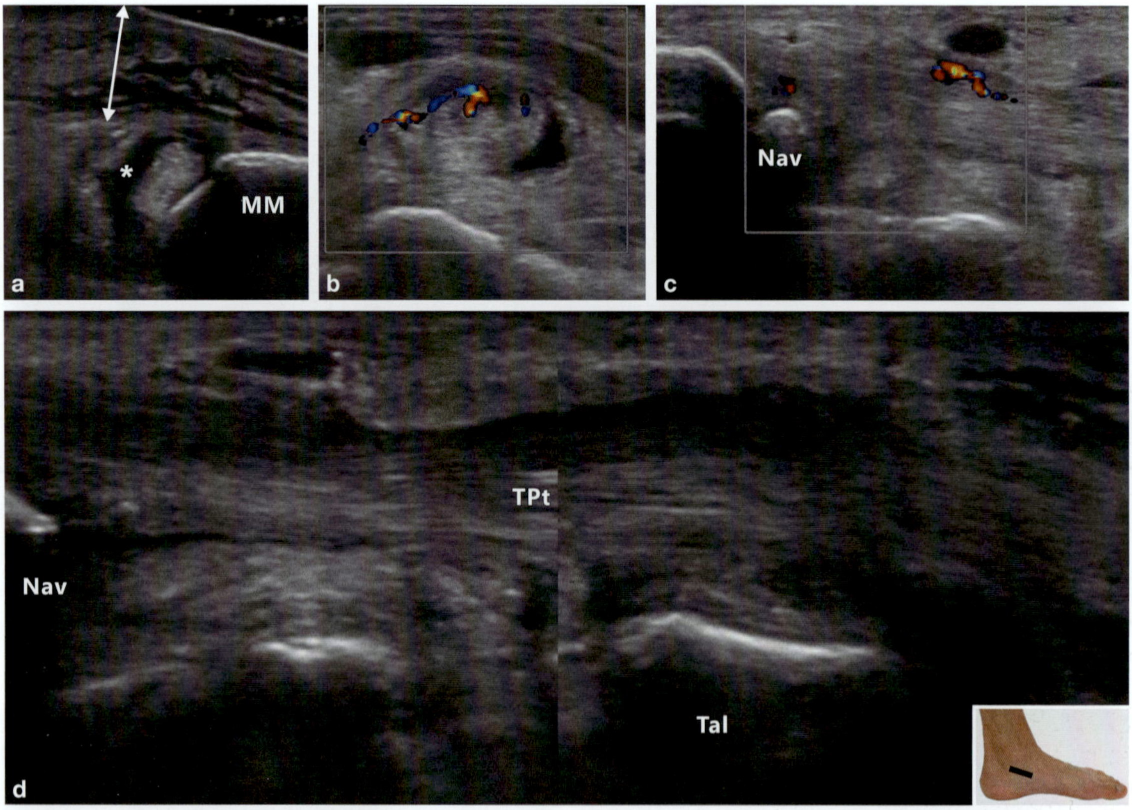

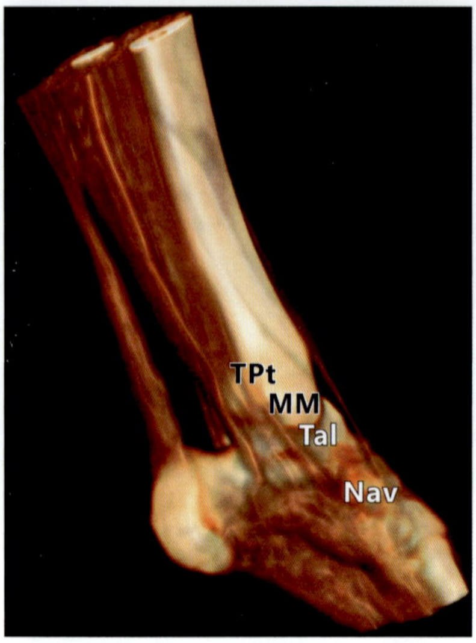

Axial US image demonstrates fluid (*asterisk*) around the tendon and also edema in the subcutaneous tissue (*double arrow*) (**a**). Axial (**b**) and longitudinal (**c**) power Doppler images additionally show the peritendinous inflammation. Longitudinal split-screen view of the tendon distal to the medial malleolus (**MM**) (**d**).

Nav	navicular
Tal	talus
TPt	tibialis posterior tendon

Repaired tibialis posterior tendon rupture in a 34-year-old soldier after mine explosion **11.11**

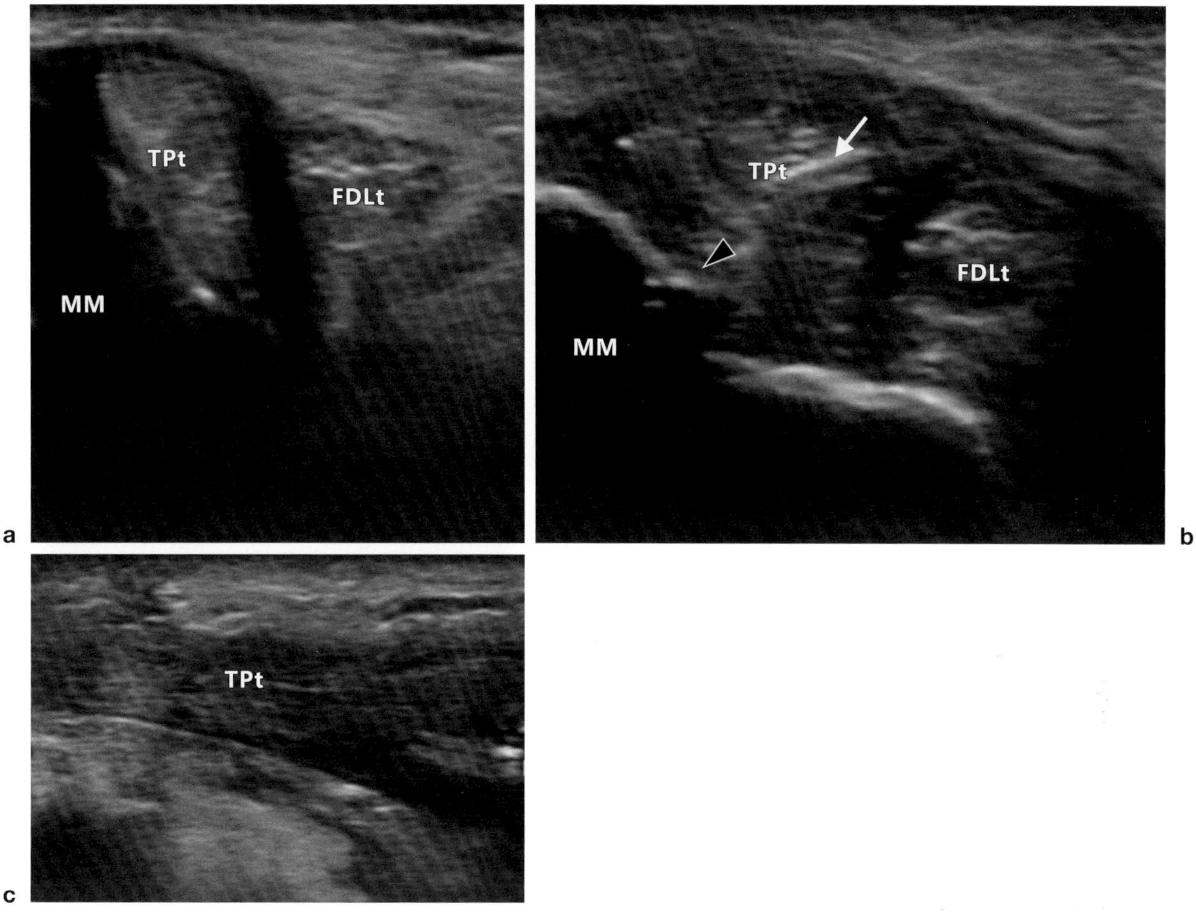

When compared with the normal side (**a**), axial (**b**) and longitudinal (**c**) US images demonstrate partially damaged and repaired tibialis posterior tendon (**TPt**). Aside from the heterogenous and edematous appearance of the tendon, also note the suture material (*arrow*) and the small cortical irregularity (*arrowhead*) on the medial malleolus (**MM**) (**b**).

FDLt flexor digitorum longus tendon

11.12 Fibularis longus tendinopathy in a 33-year-old woman with a snapping sensation at the lateral ankle after an inversion injury

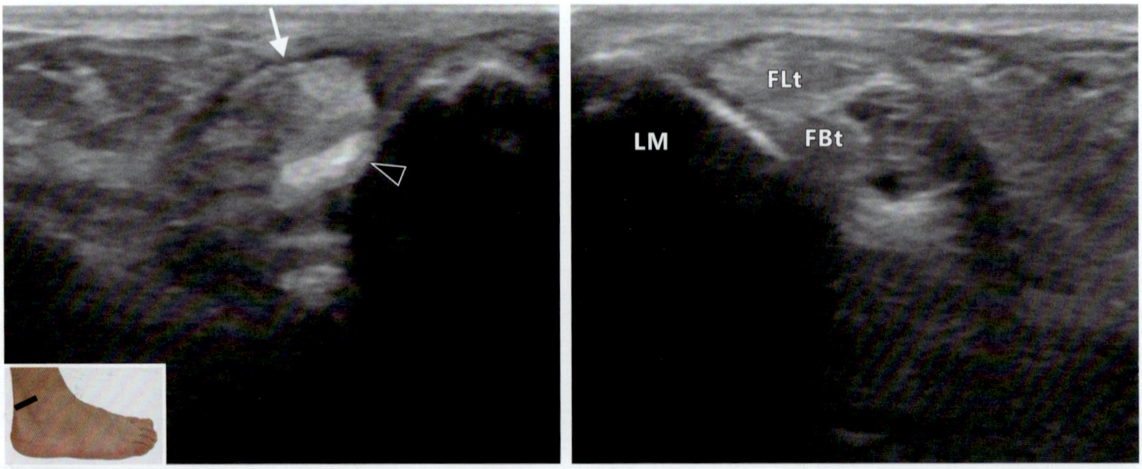

a b

Axial US image (**a**) clearly depicts fibularis brevis tendon (**FBt**) (*arrowhead*) more hyperechoic due to the edema (enhanced through transmission artifact) within the heterogenous fibularis longus tendon (**FLt**) (*arrow*). Normal contralateral side (**b**).

LM lateral malleolus

A thrombosed superficial varicose vein in a 55-year-old woman with ankle swelling

11.13

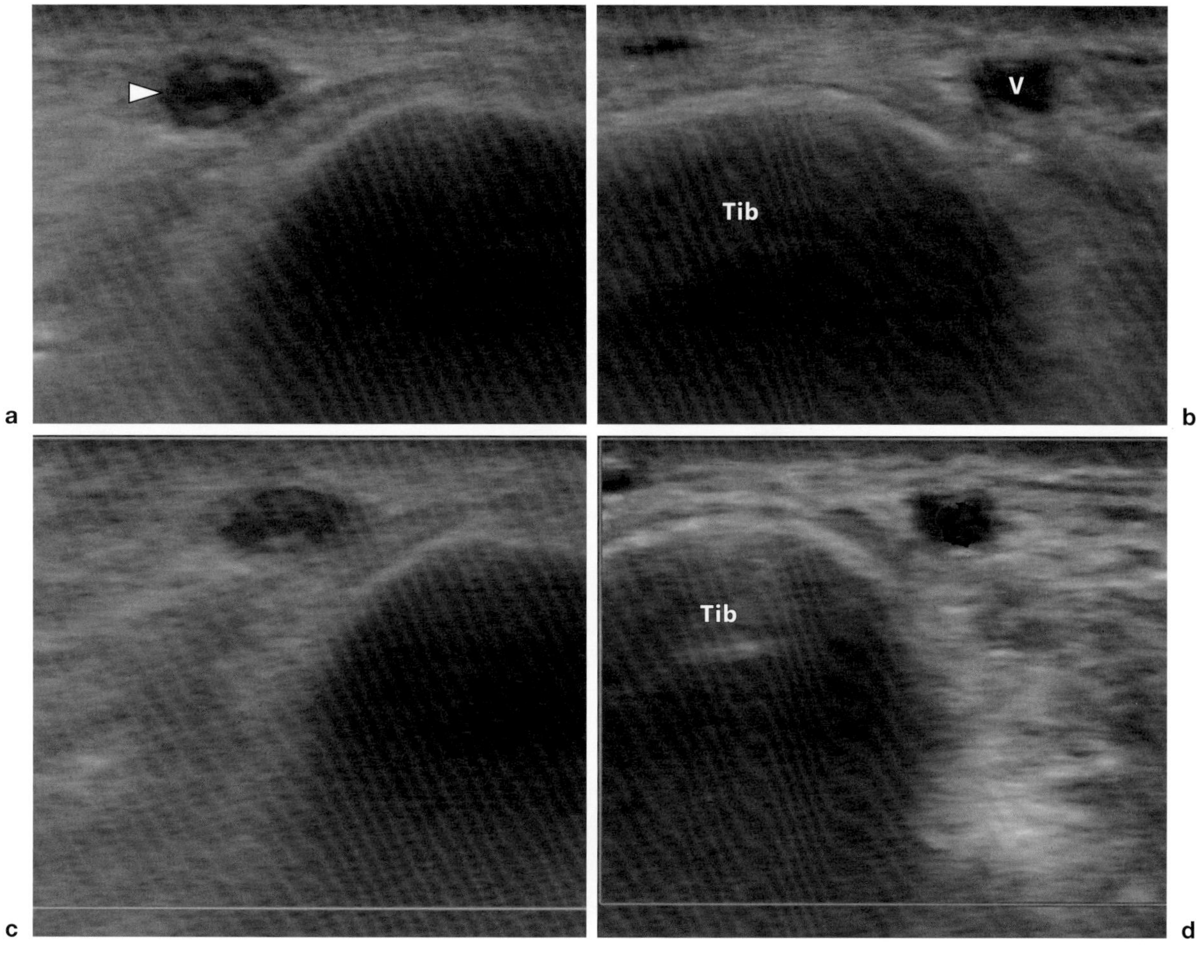

Axial US imaging over the posteromedial side of the lower leg shows a well-defined hypoechoic mass (*arrowhead*) (**a**). Initial suspicion of an occluded vein is confirmed by Doppler imaging (**c**). Corresponding images of the normal side (**b**, **d**).

Tib tibia
V vein

Expert note

Usually veins and arteries can be distinguished even by using the B-mode alone. Yet, the former are more superficially located and compressible while the latter are pulsating and less compressible. Further, if Doppler mode is used, their blood flow patterns will be observed as significantly different.

11.14 Ganglion cyst in a young woman with swelling around the lateral ankle

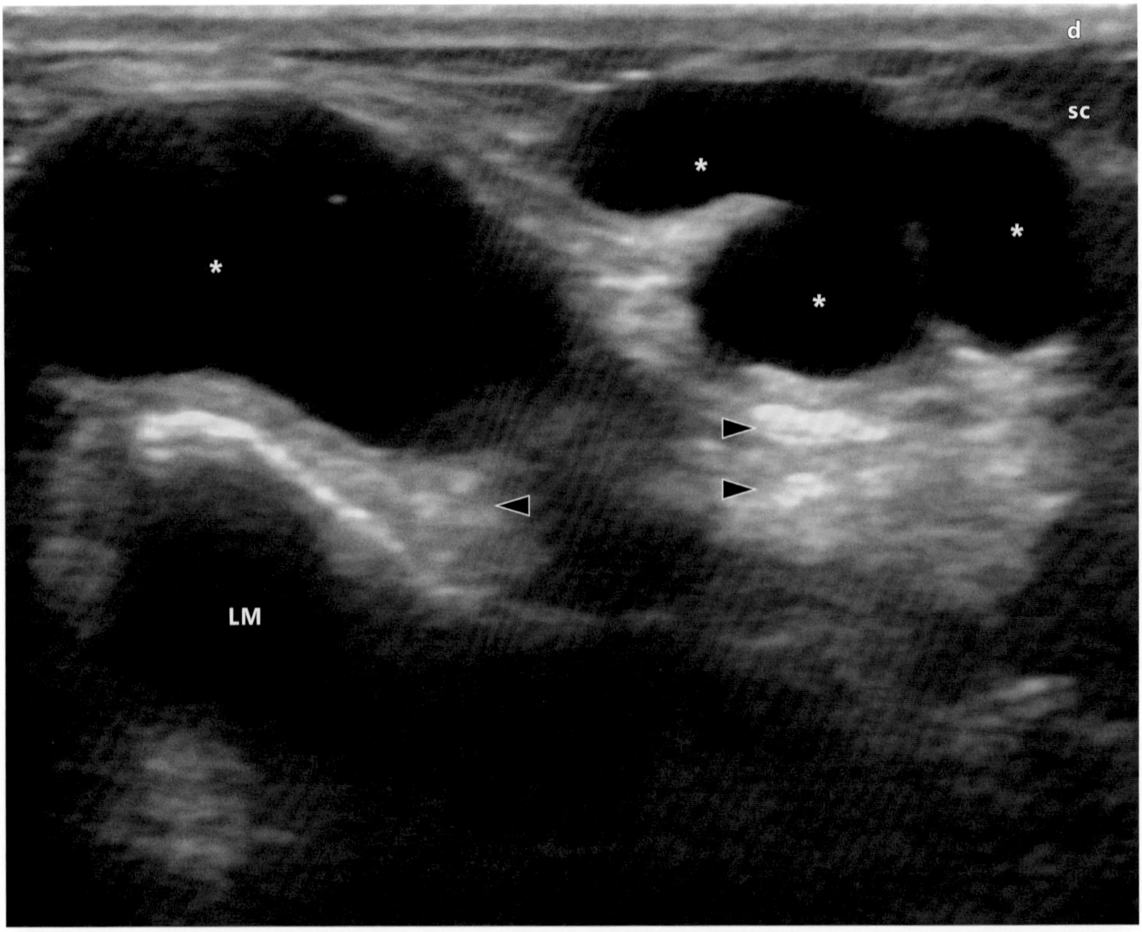

Longitudinal US image obtained over the lateral malleolus (**LM**) demonstrates a big ganglion cyst with multilobular appearance (*asterisks*). Please note enhanced through transmission artifacts (*arrowheads*) deep to the anechoic zones.

d dermis
sc subcutaneous fat

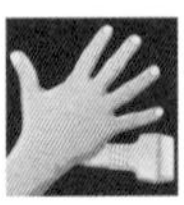

Expert note

In these types of multilobular cysts, US-guidance plays a significant role during the interventions. Yet, the drainage can safely/promptly be performed with multiple trials in different compartments under real-time imaging.

Bursitis in a 55-year-old woman with lateral ankle pain **11.15**

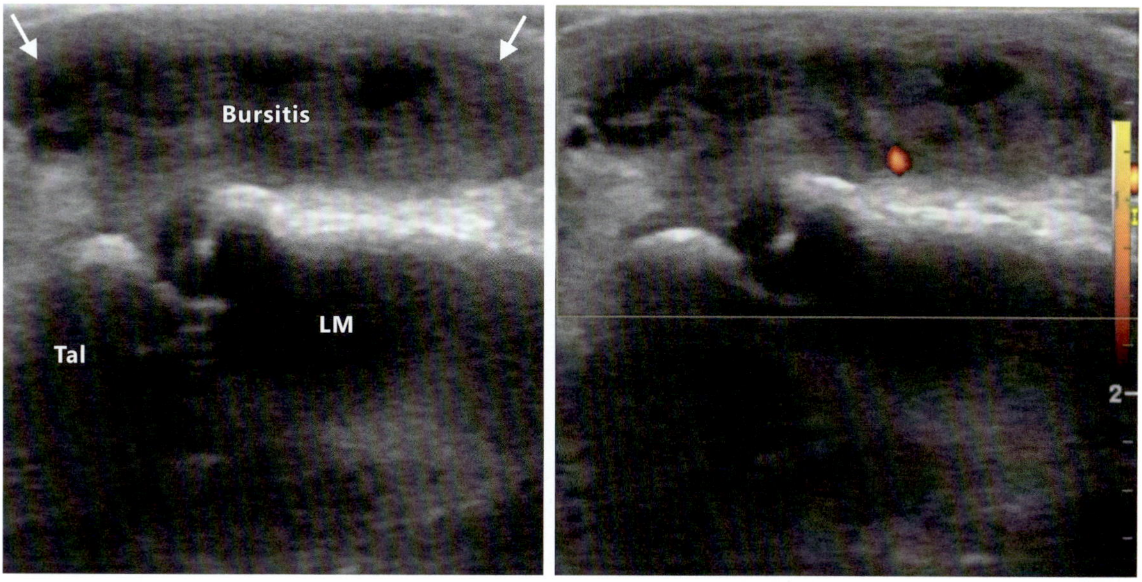

a b

Longitudinal US image reveals hypoechoic swelling of the bursa (*arrows*) within the subcutaneous tissue immediately superficial to the lateral malleolus (**LM**) (**a**). Focal hyperemia is also seen at power Doppler imaging (**b**).

Tal talus

Expert note

Swelling of the perimalleolar region (commonly on the lateral side) is not easily/promptly diagnosed especially in obese subjects. While it is sometimes bursitis, it turns out to be only subcutaneous fat at other times. In this regard, imaging with US is quite helpful for avoiding unnecessary punctures.

11.16 Retrocalcaneal bursitis in a 33-year-old man with chronic posterior heel pain

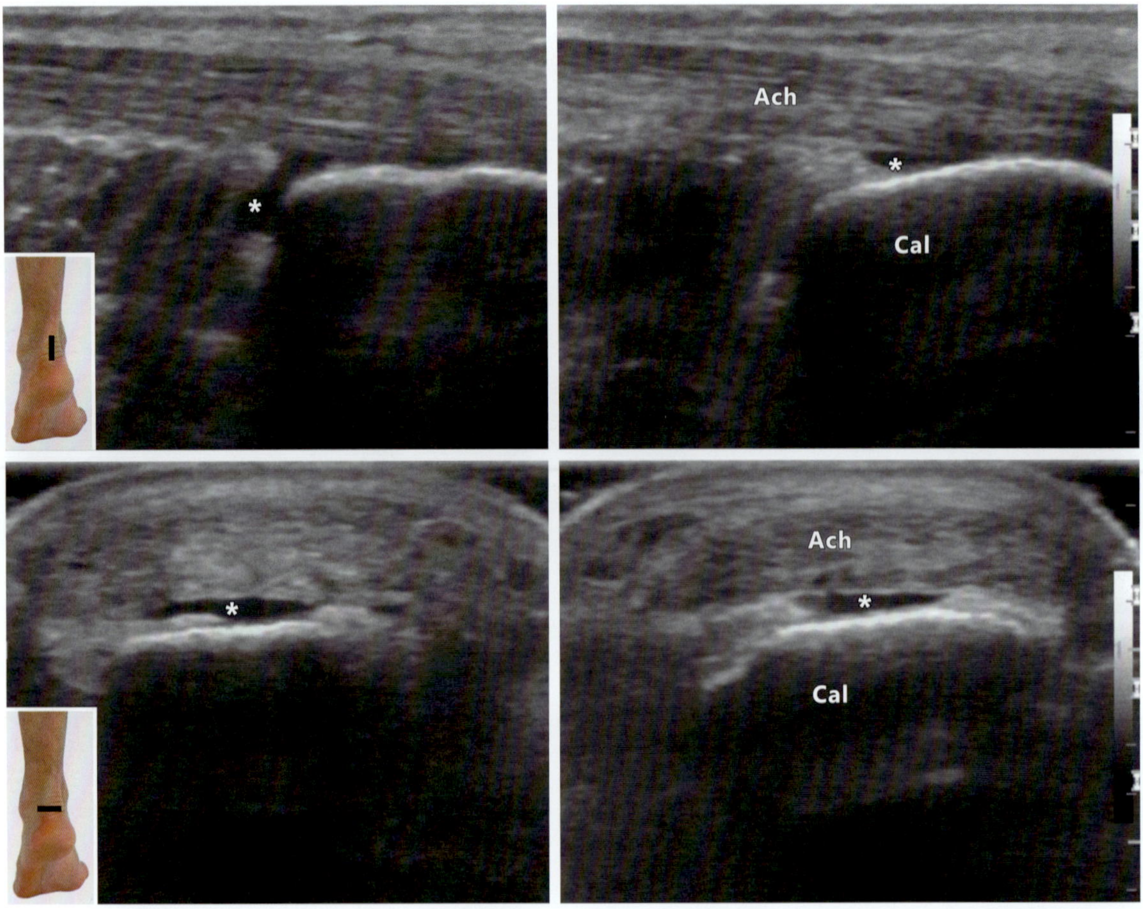

a b c d

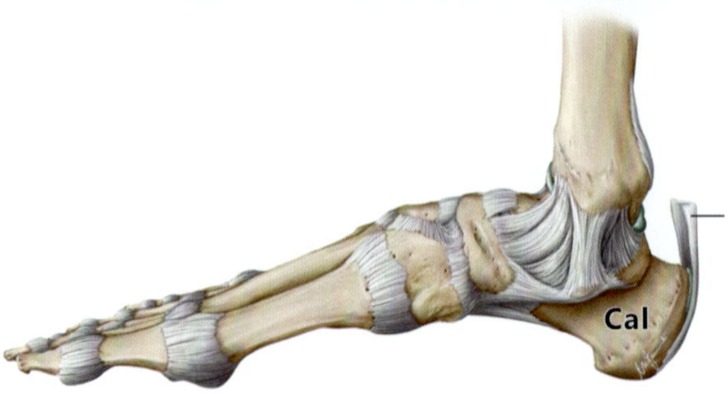

Longitudinal US imaging shows mild swelling of the retrocalcaneal bursa (*asterisk*) deep to the Achilles tendon (**a**). Axial imaging was also confirmatory (**c**). Normal side (**b**, **d**).

Ach Achilles tendon
Cal calcaneus

Expert note

Although the retrocalcaneal bursa can normally be seen with a small amount of (physiologic) fluid (≤3 mm) inside [3]; in case it is symptomatic, looks different from the normal side.

Retrocalcaneal bursitis in a patient with painful heel **11.17**

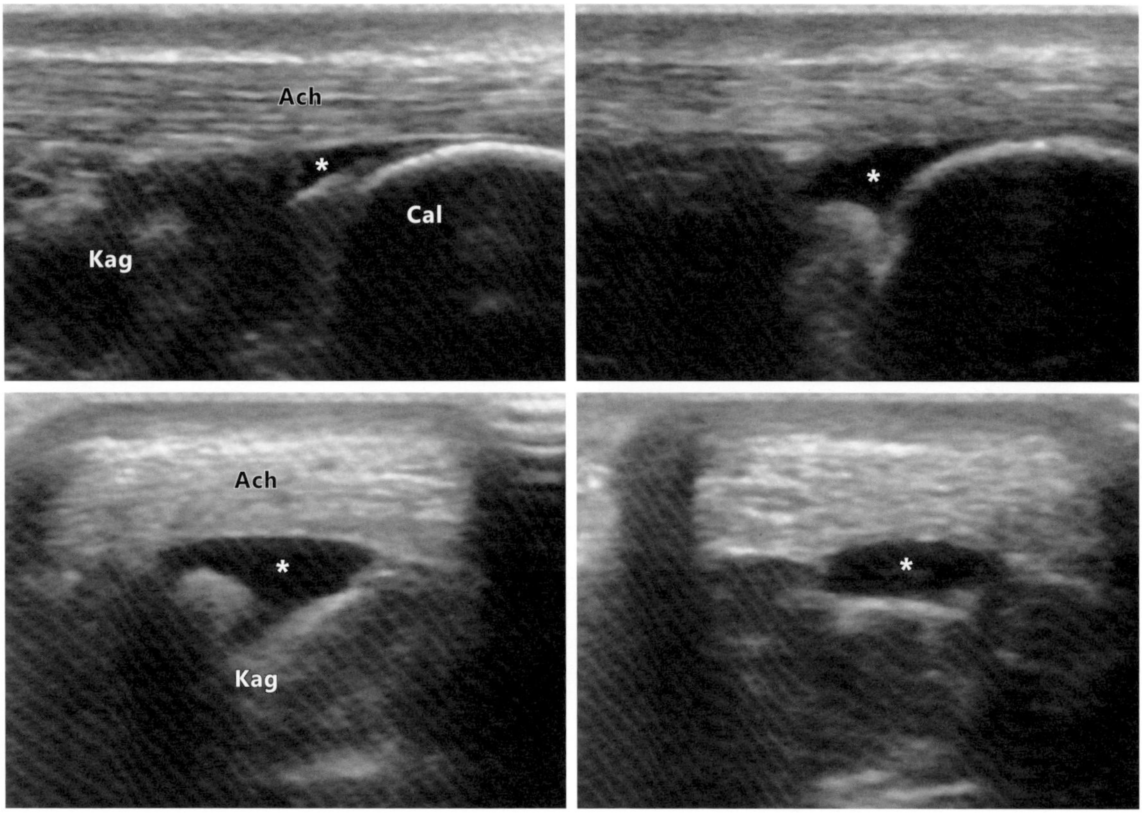

a b c d

When compared with asymptomatic side containing a small amount of effusion (**a**), longitudinal US image reveals effusion filling the retrocalcaneal bursa (*asterisks*) (**b**). Confirmation of effusions are viewed on corresponding axial images as well (**c**, **d**).

Ach Achilles tendon
Cal calcaneus
Kag Kager fat pad

Exper,t note

Since enlargement of the retrocalcaneal bursa can be in any direction/shape that changes during plantar and dorsal flexion of the foot, imaging in different views (also medio-lateral or proximo-distal) is indisputably crucial.

11.18 Achilles tendinopathy and retrocalcaneal bursitis in an elderly patient with bilateral chronic heel pain

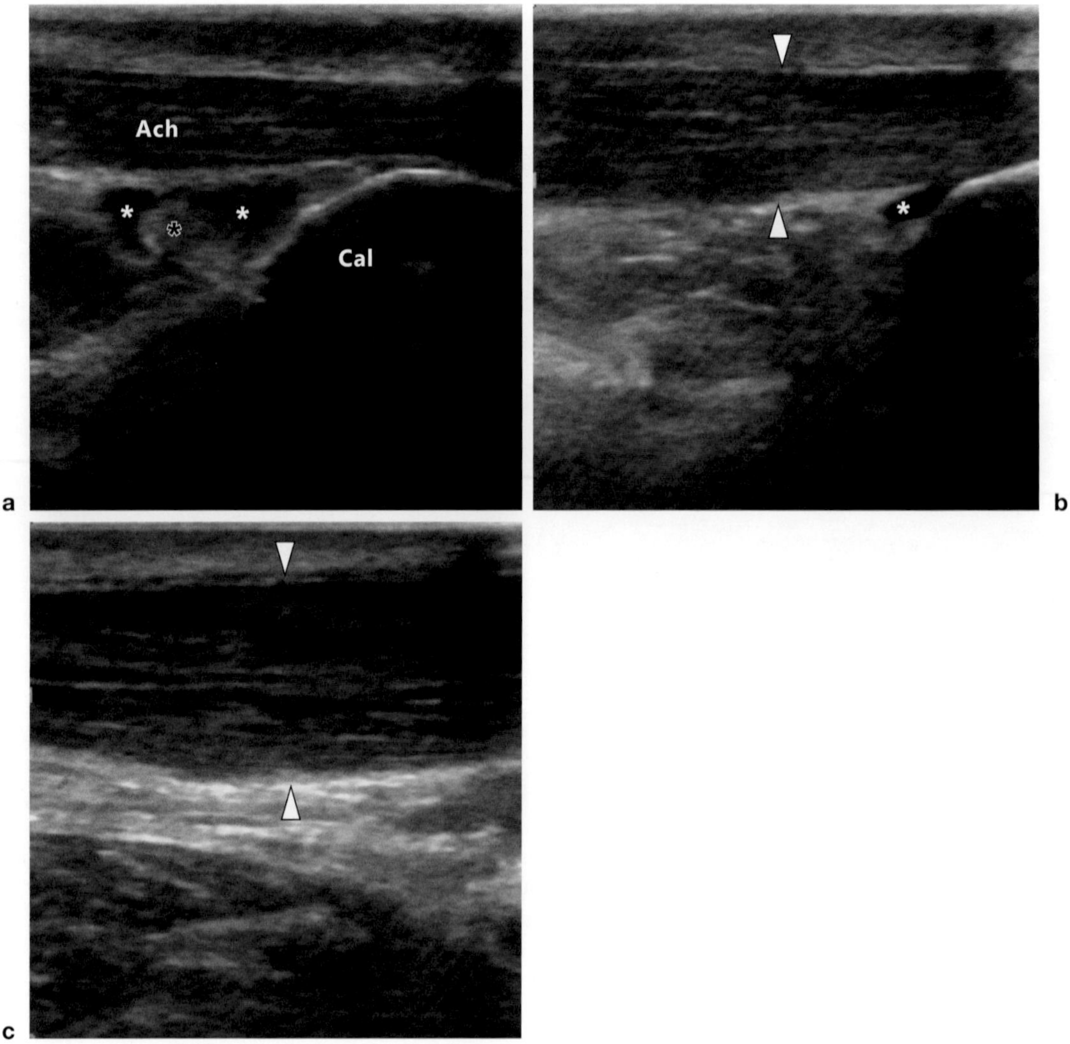

Longitudinal images over the Achilles tendon (**Ach**) illustrate effusion (*white asterisks*) and hypertrophied synovium (*black asterisk*) filling the retrocalcaneal bursa on one side (**a**), and a small amount of bursal effusion (*white asterisk*) but significant proximal thickening of the tendon (*arrowheads*) on the other side (**b**, **c**).

Cal calcaneus

Expert note

In chronic heel pain whereby clinical history and medical examination might not fully help conclude on the exact pathology, US imaging might really guide in the differential diagnosis and onward interventions as well.

RetroAchilles bursitis in a 53-year-old woman with painful and swollen heels **11.19**

a b c d

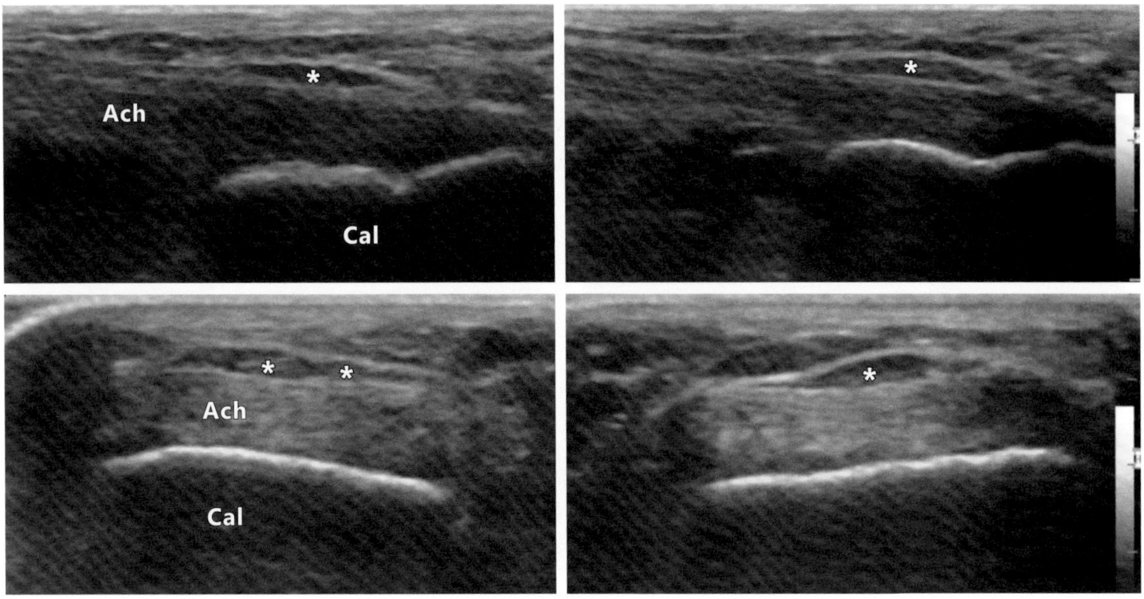

Longitudinal US images show effusion in the retroAchilles bursa (*asterisks*) on both sides (**a**, **b**). Axial images are also confirmatory (**c**, **d**).

Ach Achilles tendon
Cal calcaneus

Expert note

While retrocalcaneal bursitis is more commonplace, fluid accumulation in the retroAchilles bursa can also be found in cases with similar clinical findings. As such, since the bursa is very superficial and the fluid is compressible, the sonographer should avoid unnecessary pressure with the probe which would make the scenario be invisible.

11.20 Calcific entesophytes in a 40-year-old runner with complaints of chronic posterior heel pain and swelling

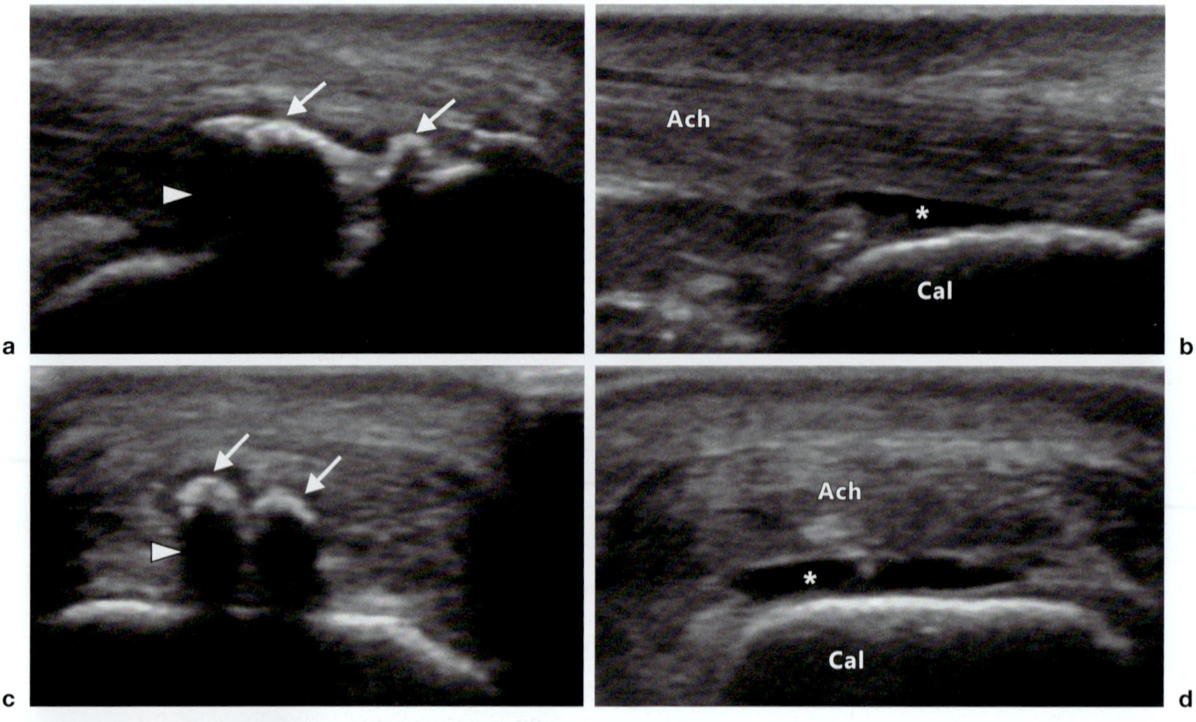

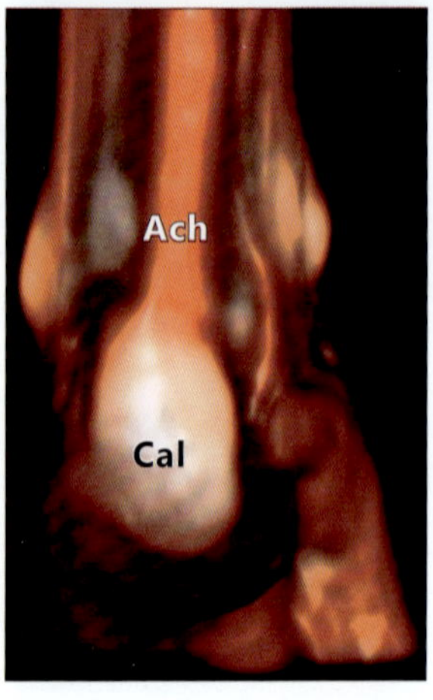

Longitudinal US images reveal calcaneal entesophytes (*arrows*) on the symptomatic side (**a**) and a small amount of effusion in the retrocalcaneal bursa (*asterisk*) on the asymptomatic side (**b**). Corresponding axial images are also confirmatory (**c**, **d**). Please note the posterior acoustic shadowing artifacts (*arrowheads*) caused by entesophytes.

Ach Achilles tendon
Cal calcaneus

Enthesopathy in a 40-year-old ankylosing spondylitis patient with chronic heel pain **11.21**

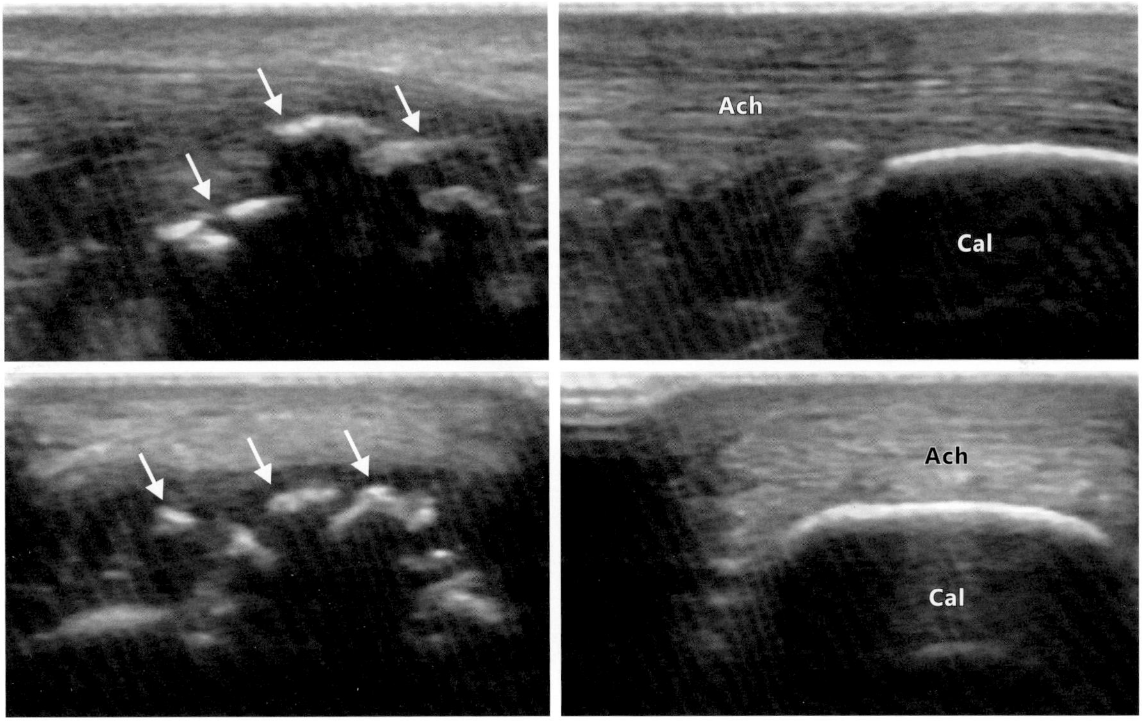

a b c d

Longitudinal (**a**) and axial (**c**) US images of the Achilles tendon (**Ach**) denote marked cortical irregularities (erosions and new bone formation) at the calcaneal insertion (*arrows*) -compatible with inflammatory enthesitis. Corresponding images of the normal side (**b**, **d**).

Cal calcaneus

Expert note

Like in other cases of enthesopathy, axial imaging might give a better overall idea (on the wideness of entheseal involvement) while mediolateral longitudinal imaging would easily fail to illustrate it.

11.22 Calcaneal enthesitis in a 52-year-old man with ankylosing spondylitis

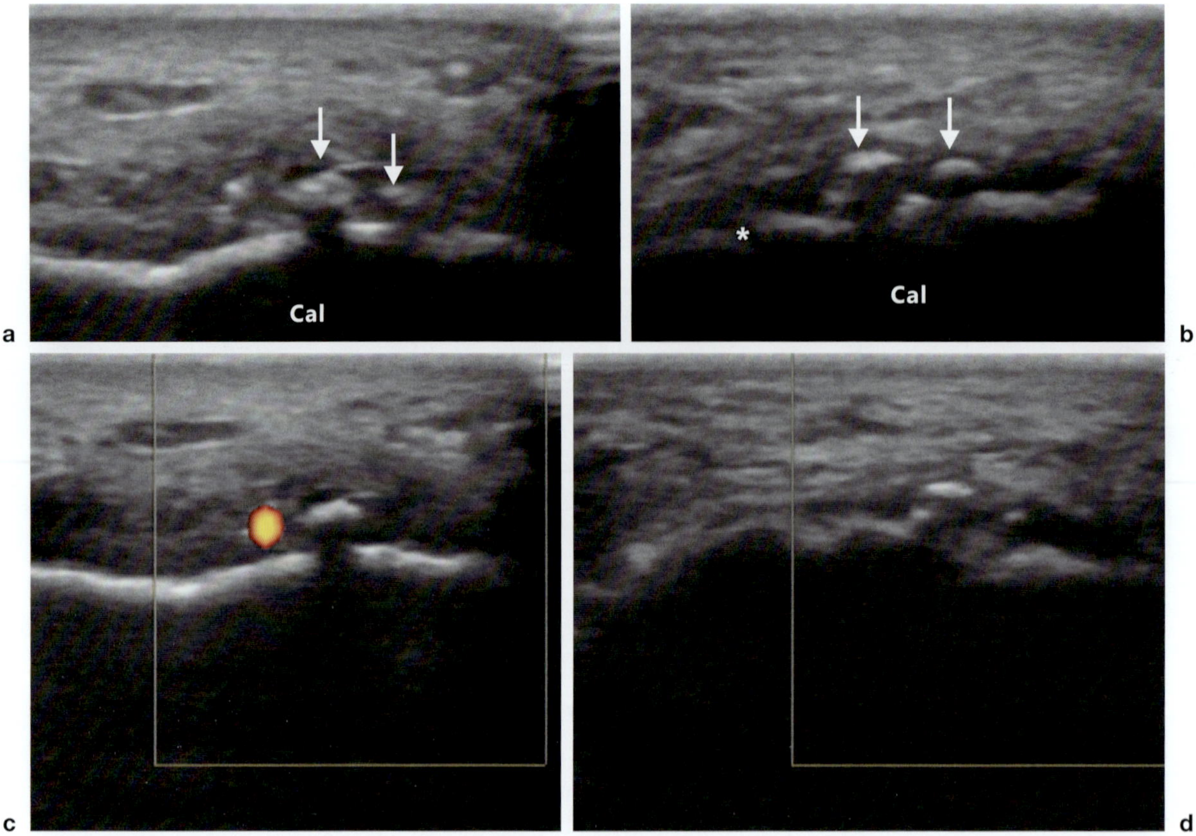

Posterior axial US images (**a**, **b**) demonstrate bony entesophytes (*arrows*) and an erosion (*asterisk*) at the calcaneus (**Cal**). On Doppler imaging, blood flow signal is visible on one side (**c**), not on the other (**d**).

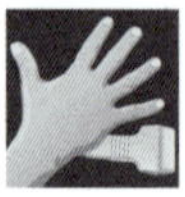

Expert note

Doppler imaging should remain as the prerequisite where inflammatory enthesopathy is to be scanned. For sure, it can further provide an insight into better understanding the disease activity.

Calcific enthesopathy in a reactive arthritis patient presenting with heel pain **11.23**

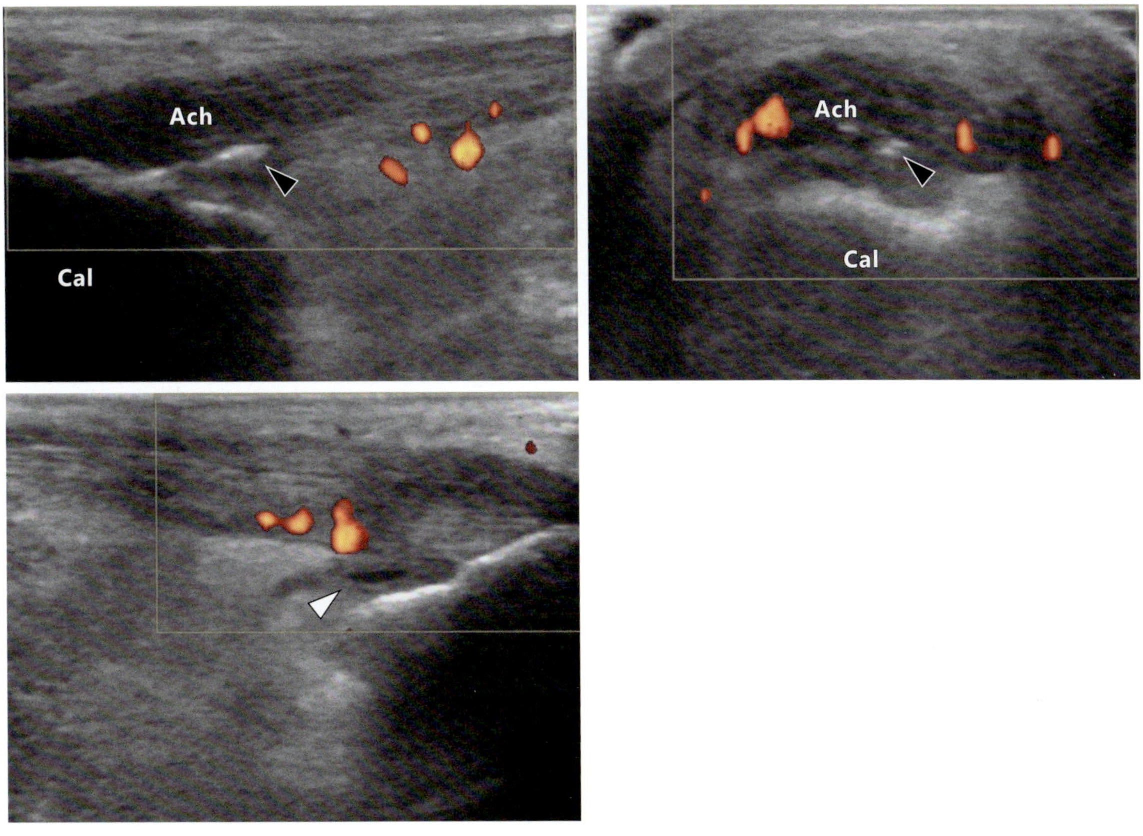

Power Doppler imaging with longitudinal (**a**) and axial (**b**) views through the hindfoot show entesophytes (*black arrowheads*) and flow signals inside the Achilles tendon (**Ach**). Contralateral side demonstrates fluid in the retrocalcaneal bursa (*white arrowhead*) and flow signals within the tendon (**c**).

Cal calcaneus

Expert note

Presence of vascularity should always be evaluated carefully in individual patients. For instance, while the power Doppler signals in this case seems to indicate inflammation (unfavorable disease activity); in another patient with a traumatic injury might well be suggestive for a favorable healing process.
In "classical" tendinosis, the neovascularization will be less diffuse, localized at the anterior (often medial) aspect of the tendon. One should take care not to give passive dorsiflexion, because this can cause a drop in the Doppler flow.

11.24 Partial tear of the Achilles tendon in a 38-year-old man

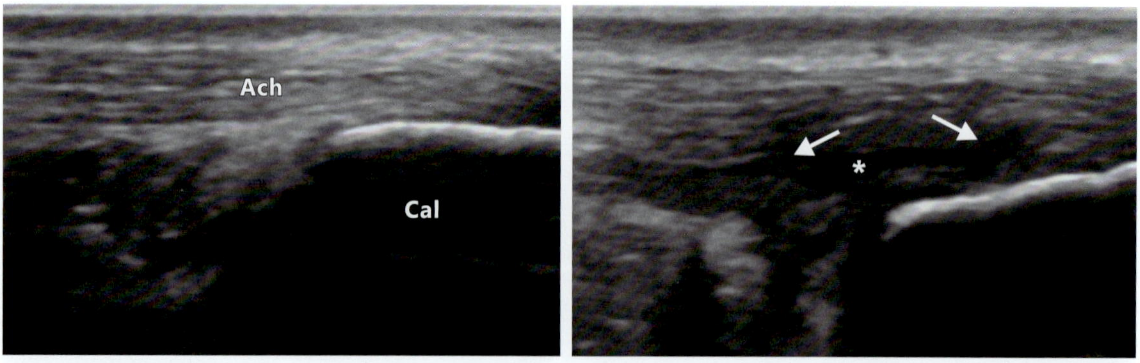

a b

The patient had heel pain, swelling and stiffness causing difficulties during daily life activities.

When compared with the normal side (**a**), longitudinal US image depicts an anechoic gap (*asterisk*) between the detached fibers (*arrows*) of the Achilles tendon (**Ach**) reminiscent of a focal tear (**b**). Please also note the swollen, irregular and hypoechoic pattern of the tendon.

Cal calcaneus

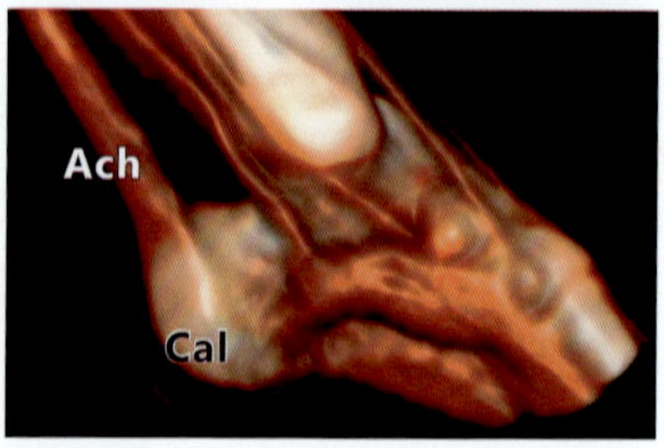

Video 12

Expert note

Like in other cases of tendon ruptures, absence or compressibility of the tendon (at least some parts of it) would surely make the diagnosis straightforward.

Chronic Achilles tendinopathy in a 55-year-old patient with heel swelling and pain exacerbated by running

11.25

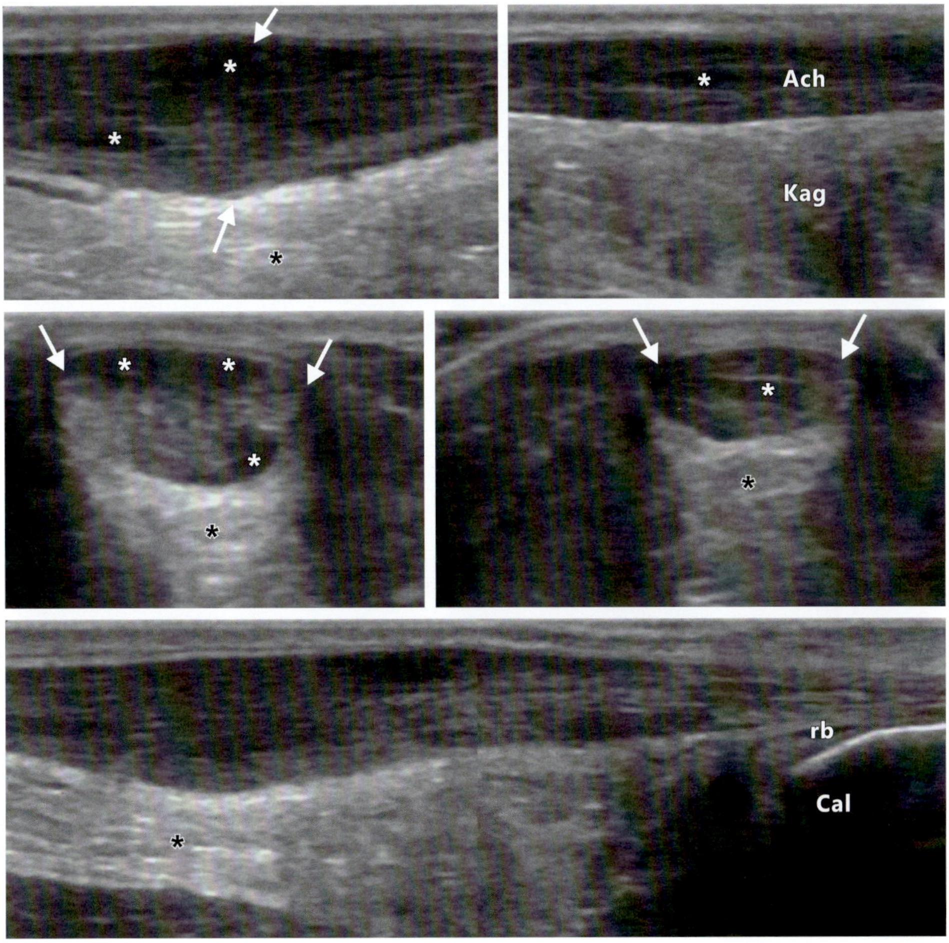

Longitudinal (**a**, **b**) and axial (**c**, **d**) US images of the Achilles tendon (**Ach**) reveal diffuse, fusiform swelling (*arrows*) and hypoechoic appearance (*white asterisks*) at the level of the middle third, more pronounced on the symptomatic side (**a**, **c**). Split-screen view (**e**). Please note enhanced through transmission artifacts (*black asterisks*) reflecting intratendinous edema.

Cal calcaneus
Kag Kager fat pad
rb retrocalcaneal bursa

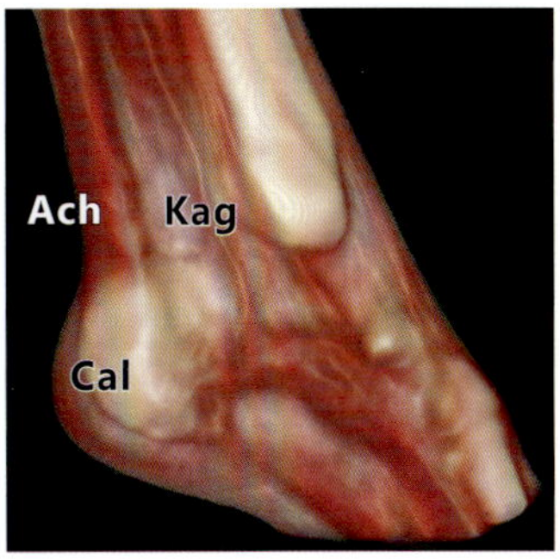

Expert note

In case of multiple intratendinous hypoechoic foci, one should eventually take xanthomatosis into account and check for hypercholesterolemia as well.

11.26 Achilles tendon repair in a patient who had partial rupture of the tendon after jumping

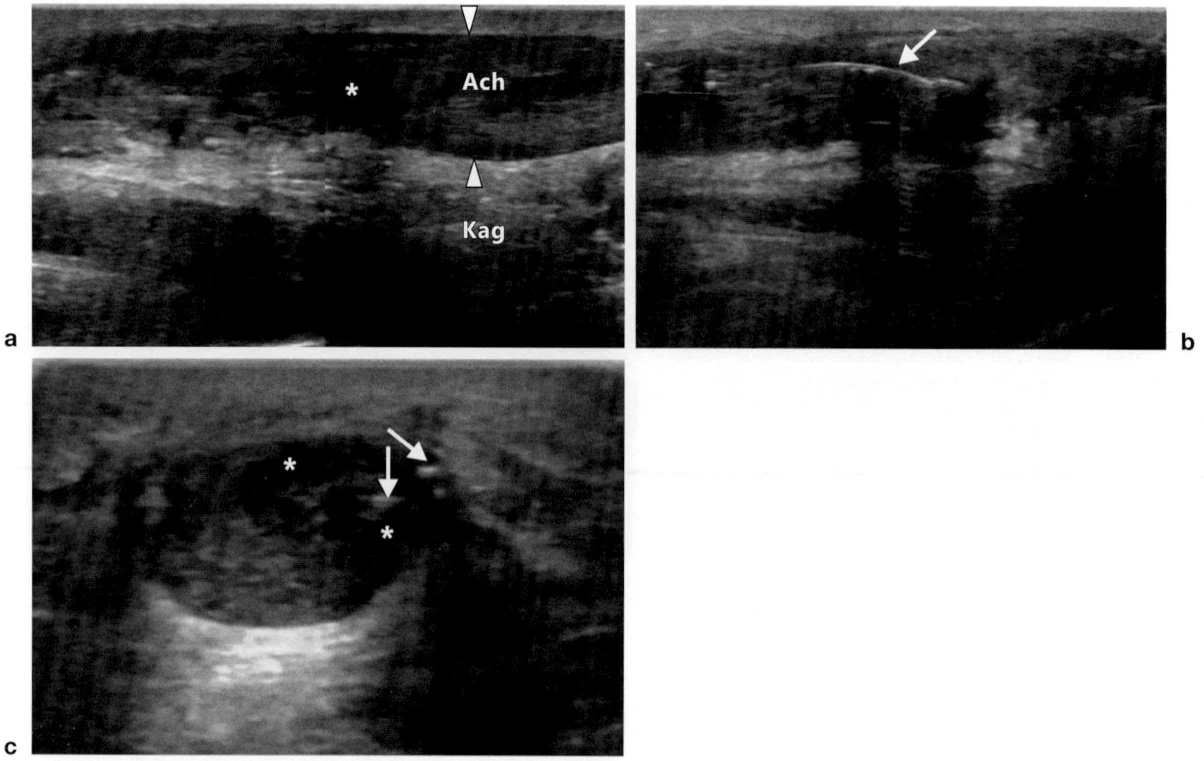

Longitudinal split-screen (**a**, **b**) and axial (**c**) US views over the Achilles tendon (**Ach**) reveal markedly enlarged and heterogeneous appearance (*arrowheads*). Surgical sutures (*arrows*) are seen adjacent to the ruptured areas (*asterisks*).

Kag Kager fat pad

Expert note

Due to its convenience, US imaging can readily be used in the postoperative period of various pathologies. While this would also be contributory in uneventful follow up, in patients with unexpected outcomes, it is definitely more elucidative.

Herewith, it should be kept in mind that tendons seldom seem "normal" postoperatively and that the sonographic appearance is not always proportionate to the clinical outcome. Therefore, serial imaging (if possible) would often be more informative than a once-only evaluation.

Chronic Achilles tendinosis and retrocalcaneal bursitis in a 42-year-old man with chronic posterior heel pain **11.27**

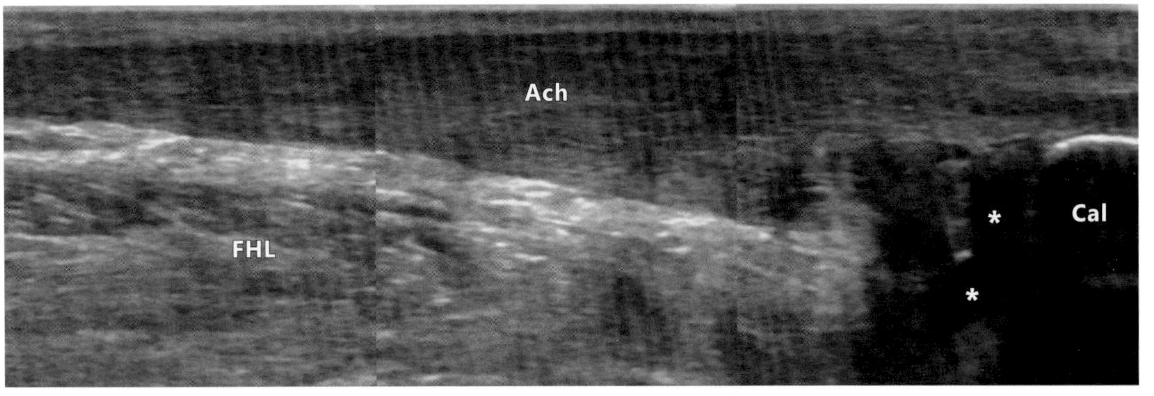

Split-screen longitudinal view demonstrates diffuse hypoechoic distal swelling and thickening of the Achilles tendon (**Ach**) and irregular anechoic fluid in the retrocalcaneal bursa (*asterisks*).

Cal calcaneus
FHL flexor hallucis longus

Repaired Achilles tendon in a 43-year-old man who had recurrent ruptures due to long-distance running **11.28**

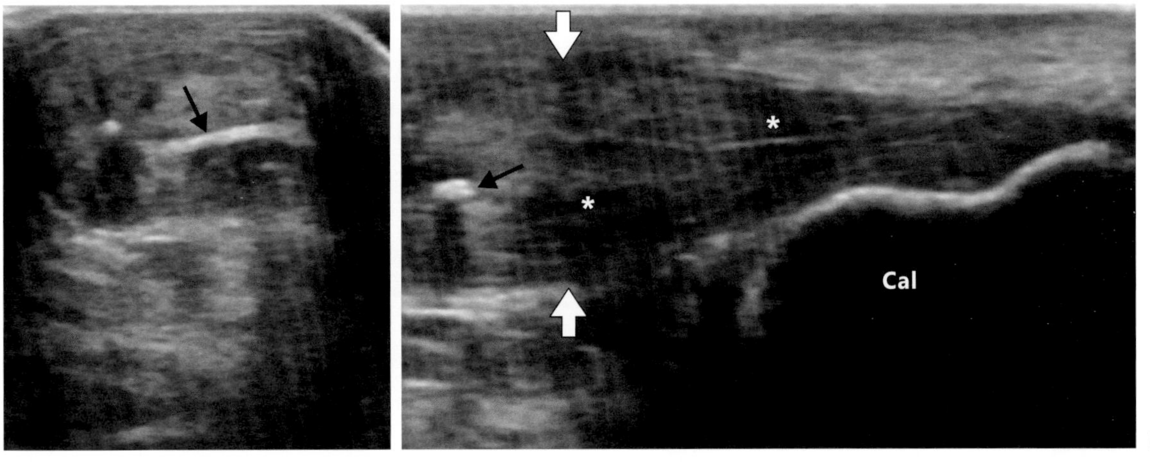

a b

Axial (**a**) and longitudinal (**b**) US images depict sutures (*thin arrows*) as bilaminar bright specular echoes within the markedly enlarged and heterogeneous Achilles tendon (*thick arrows*). Note also the fibrillar pattern loss throughout (*asterisks*).

Ankle and Foot

Video 13

11.29 Chronic operated Achilles tendon tear in a 45-year-old patient with heel pain and swelling

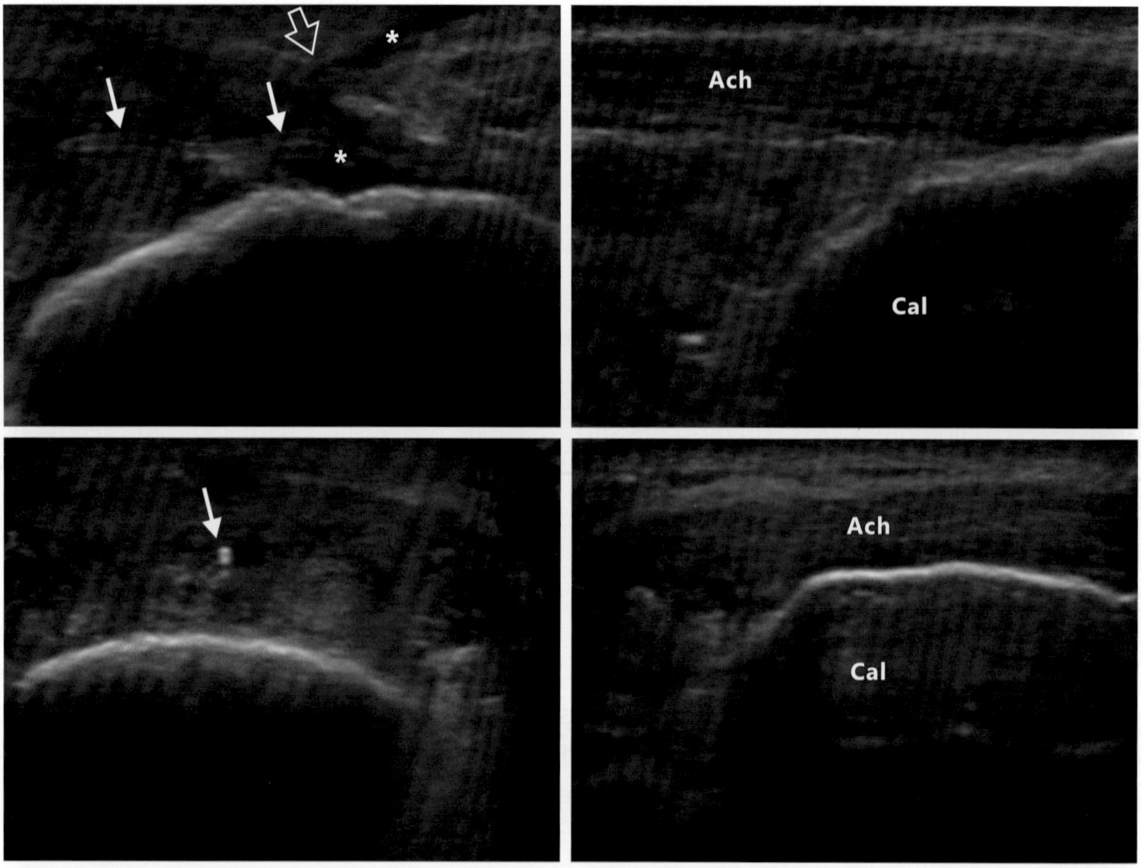

a b c d

Longitudinal (**a**) and axial (**c**) US images over the posterior ankle demonstrate sutures (*thin arrows*) as bright specular echoes within the Achilles tendon (**Ach**) and detachment of its fibrillar pattern (*asterisks*) with a blunted end (*thick arrow*). Normal contralateral side (**b**, **d**).

Cal calcaneus

Expert note

In postoperative cases (especially in the early period); the local tissues are really edematous, making the assessment quite challenging. Like in this case, although the suture materials seem to be intact, dynamic imaging with controlled movements would be really clarifying/necessary as regards the intactness/integrity of the tendons.

Repaired Achilles tendon with paratenonitis in a 55-year-old female tennis-player with chronic heel pain

11.30

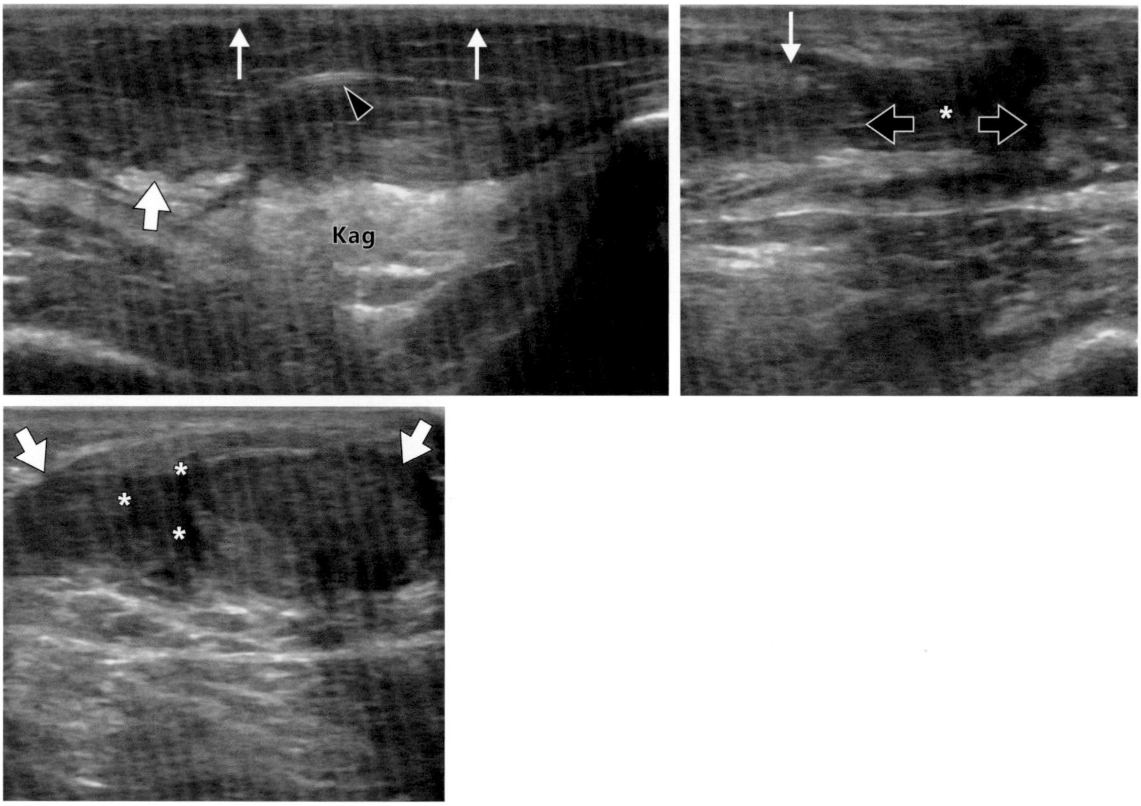

Longitudinal (**a**, **b**) and axial (**c**) images show an irregular and swollen Achilles tendon (*thick white arrows*). The suture material (*arrowhead*) seems to be intact but the hypoechoic rupture zone (*asterisks*) and torn ends (*black arrows*) of the tendon can still be distinguished. Also note the edematous/blurred paratenon (*thin white arrows*) (**a**).

Kag Kager fat pad

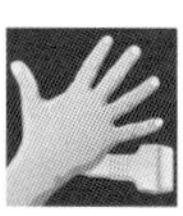

Expert note

A relatively hypovascular area (critical zone) of the Achilles tendon exists 2-6 cm proximal to the calcaneal insertion and ruptures typically occur in most cases at this region [2].

11.31 US-guided platelet-rich plasma injection in a patient with Achilles tendon rupture

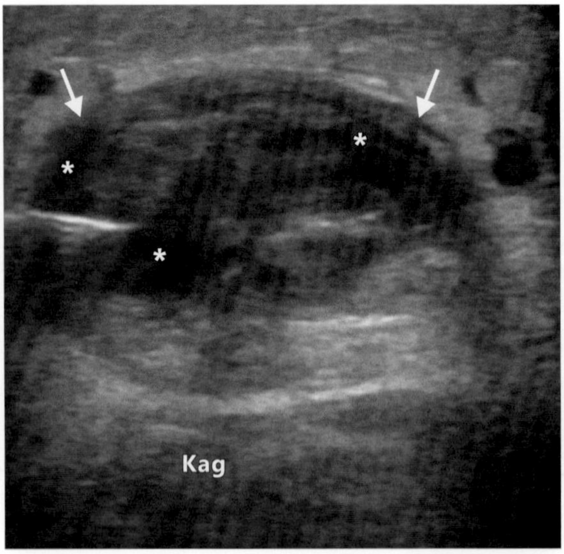

Axial US imaging of the tendon (*arrows*) reveals widespread heterogenous echoes consistent with multiple intratendinous tears (*asterisks*). Hyperechoic needle can also be seen entering from the left side during the intervention (direct in-plane technique).

Kag Kager fat pad

Expert note

Although it is quite difficult and painful to inject inside an otherwise healthy tendon, the injectate is nicely followed to be distributed among/within the torn portions of the relevant tendon.

A 12-year-old boy with heel pain (aggravated by weight-bearing activities) who was eventually diagnosed as Sever disease **11.32**

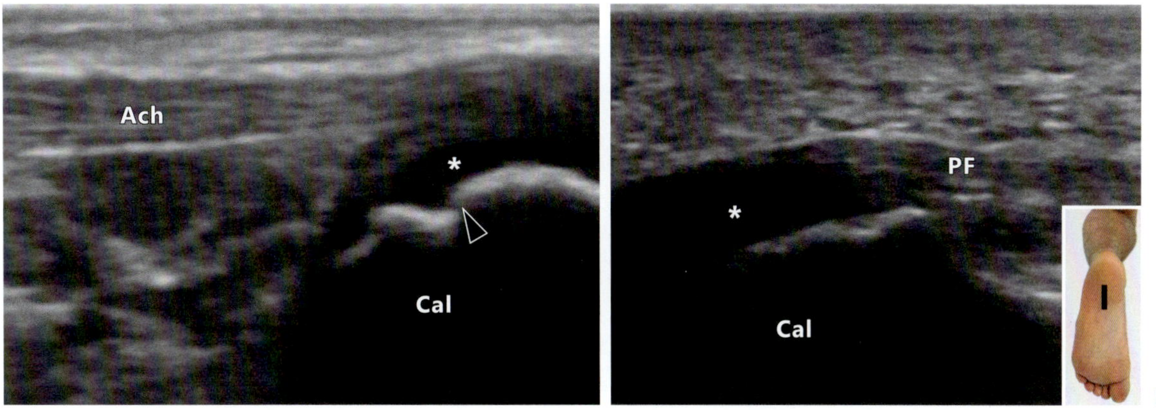

Longitudinal US images obtained over the Achilles tendon (**Ach**) (**a**) and plantar fascia (**b**) illustrate a small irregular cortical area (*arrowhead*) on the calcaneal apophysis (*asterisks*).

Cal calcaneus
PF plantar fascia

Expert note

One should be very cautious in the evaluation of excessive cartilage or the apopyseal plates in children which look quite different than those of the adults. Herein, side-to-side comparison or sono-palpation again appears to be invaluable.
On the other hand, while US cannot depict pathologies inside the bony tissues, in particular cases if they extend to the cortical surface, might give an initial idea at least to suspect.

11.33 Paratenonitis in a patient with posterior ankle pain

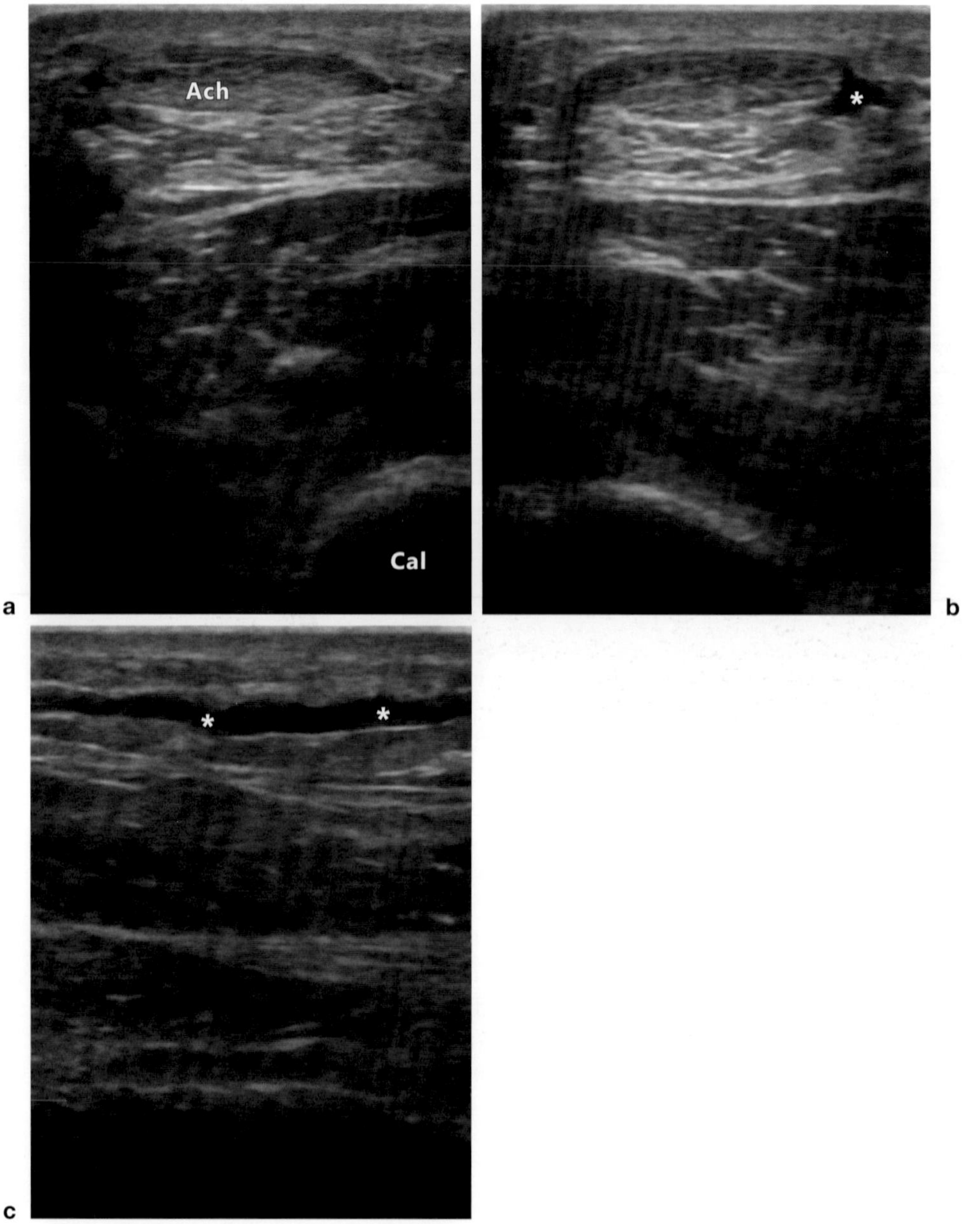

When compared with the normal side (**a**), axial (**b**) and longitudinal (**c**) US images over the Achilles tendon (**Ach**) reveal a small amount of surrounding fluid (*asterisks*).

Cal calcaneus

Paratenonitis of the Achilles tendon in a 57-year-old woman with swelling and pain on the posterior side of the heel

11.34

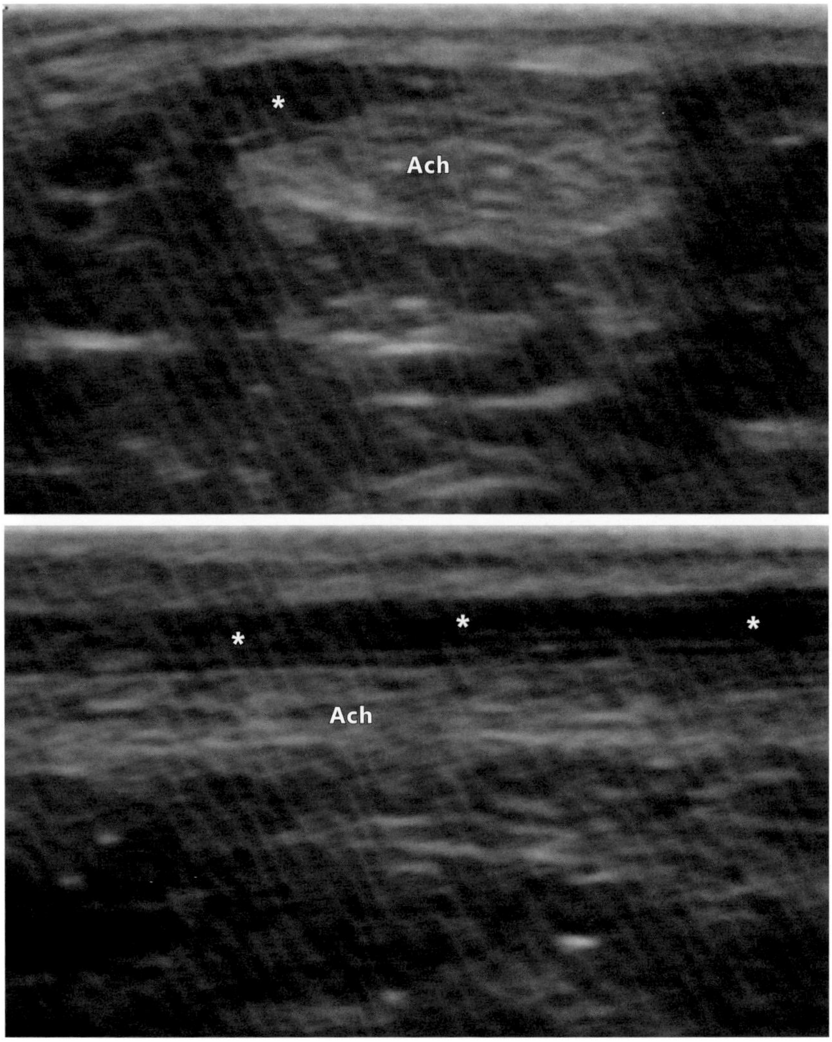

Axial US image reveals hypoechoic appearance (*asterisks*) along the peripheral aspect of the Achilles tendon (**Ach**) (**a**). Corresponding longitudinal view confirms paratenonitis with inhomogenous and blurred superficial margins of the tendon (**b**).

Ankle and Foot

11.35 Achilles tendinosis in a woman with chronic posterior heel pain

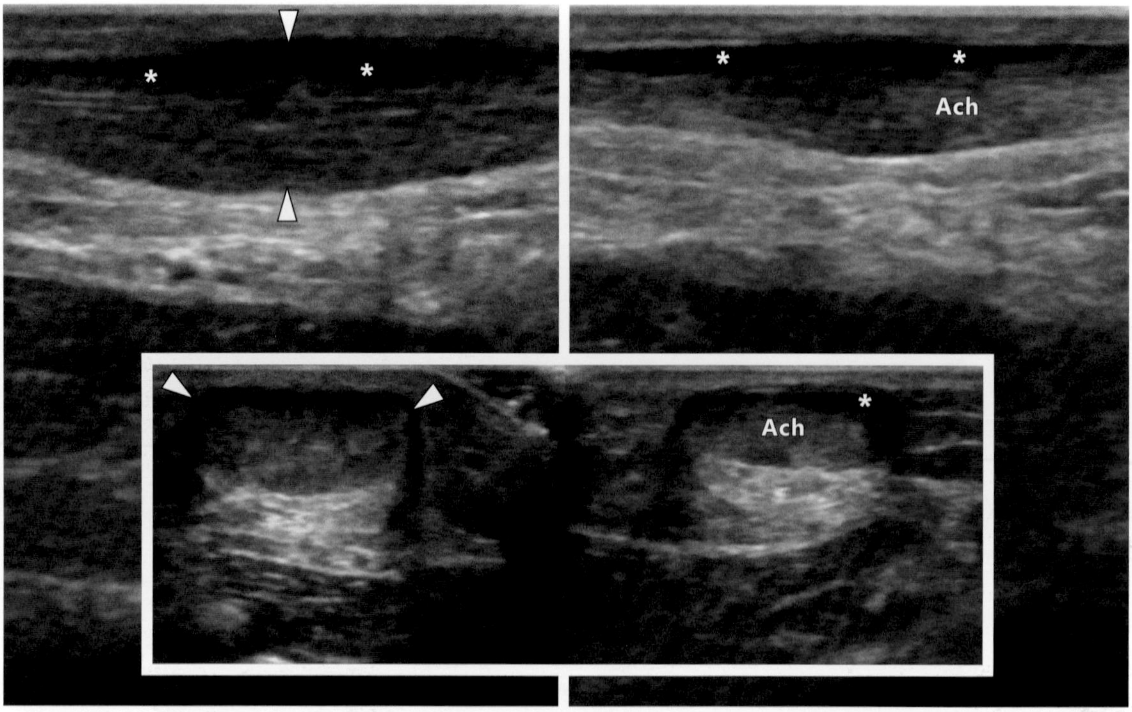

Longitudinal (**a**, **b**) and axial US images (*small figure*) reveal thickening of the paratenons (*asterisks*) surrounding the hypoechoic Achilles tendons (**Ach**) which have marked fusiform swellings, more predominant on one side (*arrowheads*).

Soleus tertius in a 9-year-old girl **11.36**

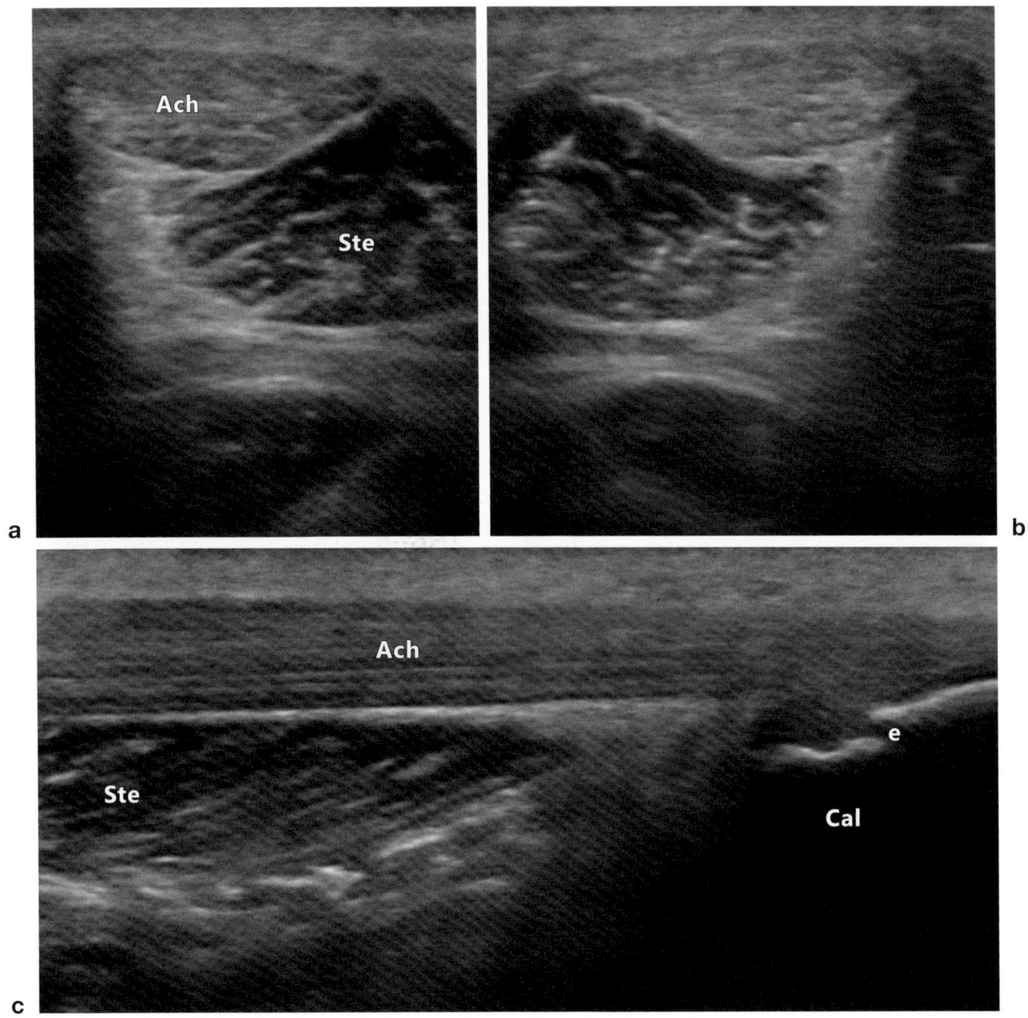

Bilateral axial (**a**, **b**) and unilateral longitudinal (**c**) US images obtained over the posterior aspect of the heel demonstrate the normal epiphysis (**e**) of the proximal calcaneus (**Cal**) and quite distally attaching soleus fibers (accessory soleus muscle or soleus tertius) (**Ste**).

Ach Achilles tendon

Expert note

While the existence of soleus tertius need not be any problematic, in relevant cases, might be considered as one of the potential biomechanical factors causing heel/calf pain. In this sense, US imaging also makes us realize that many anatomical variants exist, most of them being asymptomatic.

11.37 Plantar fasciitis in an obese woman with the complaints of inferior heel pain and tenderness after long distance walks

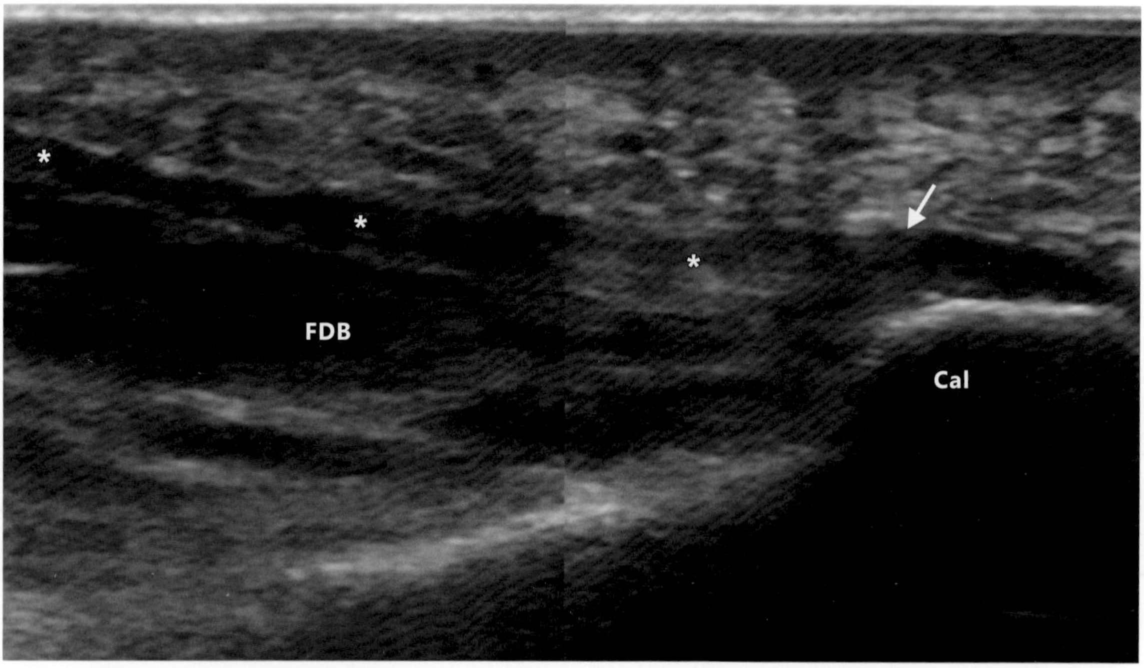

Split-screen longitudinal US imaging shows swollen plantar fascia (*asterisks*) more predominant on the proximal attachment site (*arrow*).

Cal calcaneus
FDB flexor digitorum brevis

Expert note

Delineation of the plantar fascia especially in (obese) subjects with thick calcaneal fat pads might be challenging and necessitate increasing the gain of the US machine -more than that would normally be used in routine imaging.

Plantar fasciitis in a young-aged woman who had complaints of localized pain over the inferomedial aspect of the heel 11.38

a 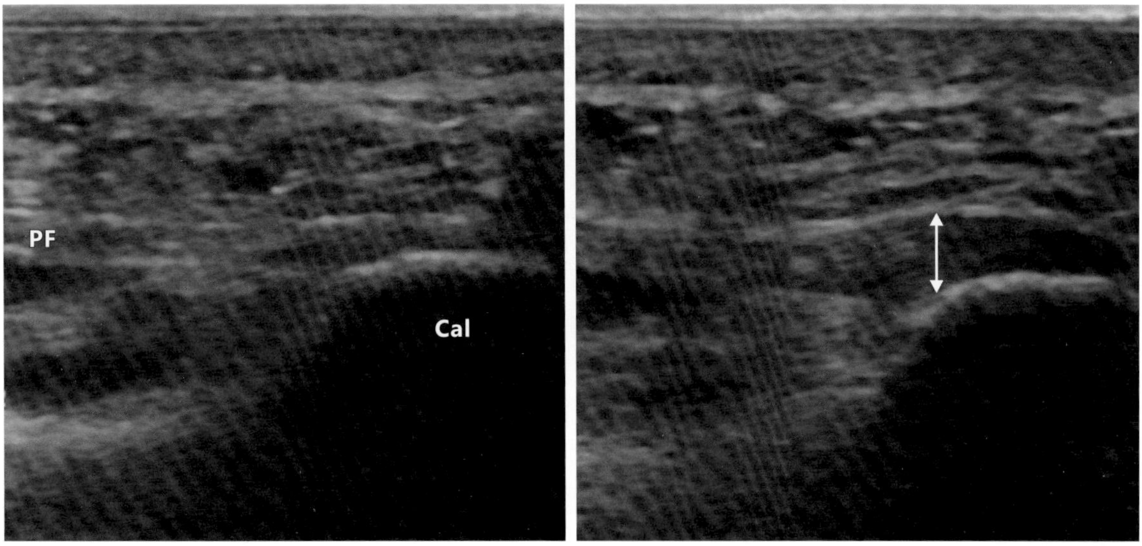 b

The pain worsened in the morning and exacerbated by walking. Physical examination showed tenderness on the medial tubercle of the calcaneus.

When compared with the normal side (**a**), longitudinal US image obtained over the insertion of plantar fascia (**PF**) shows mild thickening and hypoechoic changes (*double arrow*) reflecting edema (**b**).

Cal calcaneus

Expert note

Thickening of the plantar fascia in particular has become an established US criterion for the diagnosis of plantar fasciitis. Asymmetric hypoechoic thickening of the fascia (>4 mm) in the symptomatic patient is consistent with the diagnosis [4, 5].
A difference of >1 mm in fascia thickness between the symptomatic and asymptomatic heel of the same patient is also considered as plantar fasciitis [6].

11.39 Plantar fasciitis in a 55-year-old housewife who was unable to stand or walk for more than 30 minutes without heel pain

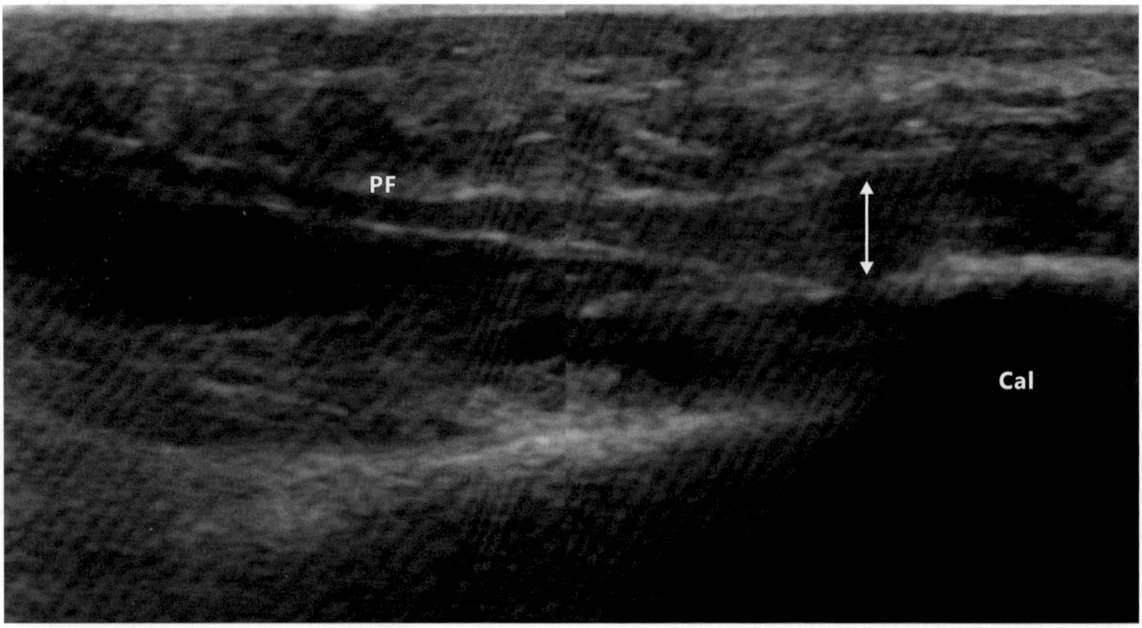

The history included sharp shooting pain and tightness in the right heel and medial arch during weight-bearing.

Longitudinal US image over the plantar fascia (**PF**) shows considerable swelling (*double arrow*) at the proximal insertion point with textural inhomogeneities.

Cal calcaneus

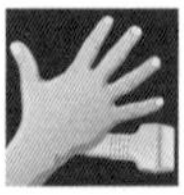

Expert note

Again, the abrupt defect in the calcaneal contour indicates the presence of a bony spur.

Plantar fasciitis in a 55-year-old man with chronic heel pain exacerbated after a jump **11.40**

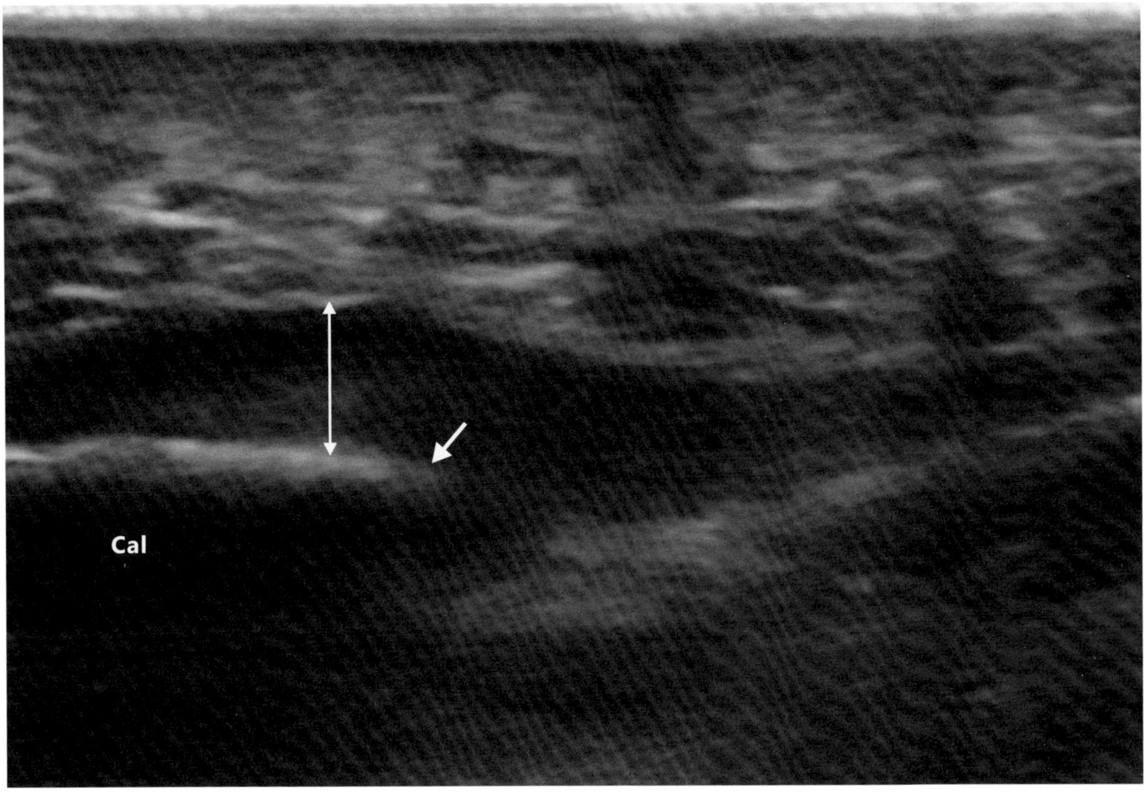

Longitudinal US imaging reveals a thickened and hypoechoic plantar fascia (*double arrow*) and a small bony spur (*arrow*) arising from the calcaneus (**Cal**).

Expert note

When evaluating the cortex of the calcaneus, one should find a continuous line with a curve. On the other hand, when there is an interruption of the line, it is suspicious of an artifact caused by a spur (pseudo-interruption of the cortex).

When evaluating the thickness of the fascia; as always, it is important to compare both sides. The pain of the patient is often more proportionate with the swelling of the fascia than the size of the spur. Hyperemia or neovascularization (positive power Doppler signal) is usually infrequent. Herewith, patients with plantar fasciitis less than 6 months of symptom duration may have hyperemia (40%) associated with high pain levels [7].

11.41 Calcaneal entesophytes and plantar fasciitis in a 60-year-old woman with bilateral chronic inferomedial heel pain

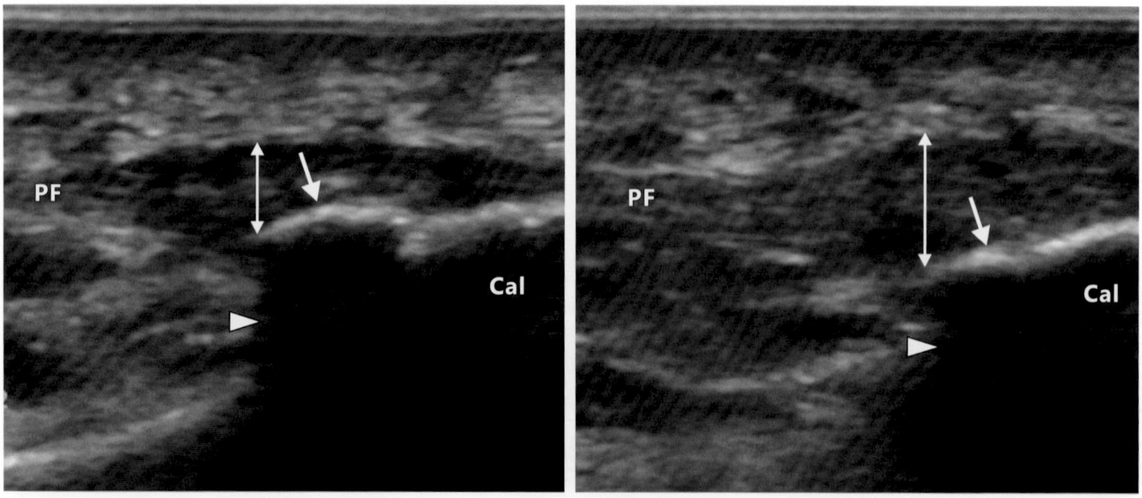

a b

The pain was worse in the morning and during weight-bearing.

Longitudinal US images reveal thickened (*double arrow*) and hypoechoic plantar fasciae (**PF**) at the calcaneal attachment sites. While the calcaneal spur (*arrow*) is more predominant on the right side of the patient (**a**), the plantar fascia is more swollen on the other side (**b**). Note the posterior acoustic shadowing artifacts (*arrowheads*) due to the calcaneal spurs.

Cal calcaneus

Expert note

Although imaging of the calcaneal spurs is not as straightforward as it is with radiography, the strict acoustic shadowings (obliterating the normal/inclined calcaneal contour) might again be confirmatory.

Plantar fasciitis and calcaneal enthesophytes in an elderly woman with chronic heel pain

11.42

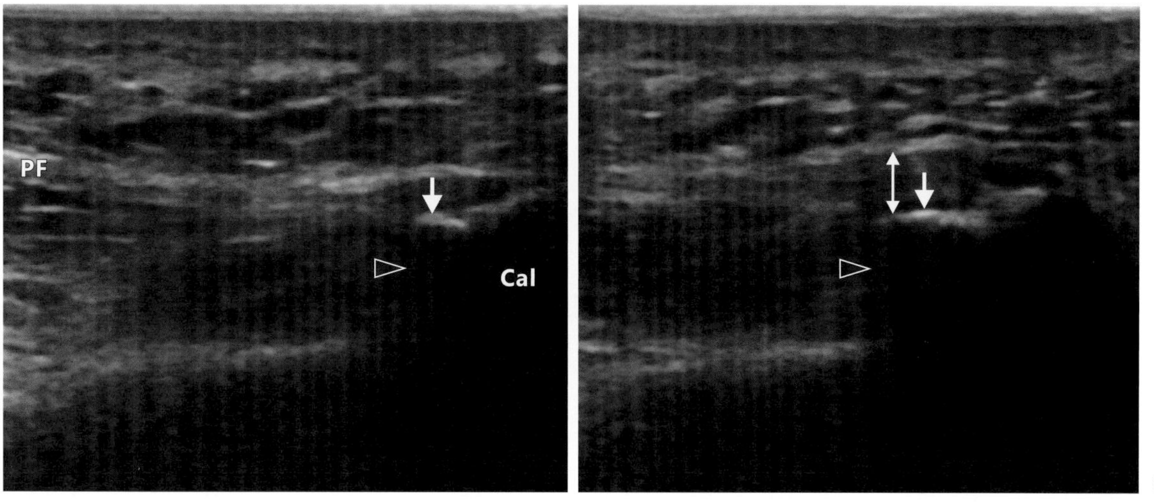

a b

The patient had heel pain particularly with the first weight-bearing step in the morning.

Longitudinal US images illustrate enthesophytes (*arrows*) arising from the inferior aspect of the medial tubercles (**a**, **b**) associated with a sign of insertional fasciitis (*double arrow*) only on one side (**b**). US shows posterior acoustic shadowing artifact as a result of sound-beam refraction (*arrowheads*).

Cal calcaneus
PF plantar fascia

11.43 Plantar fasciitis in a 35-year-old long-distance (marathon) runner

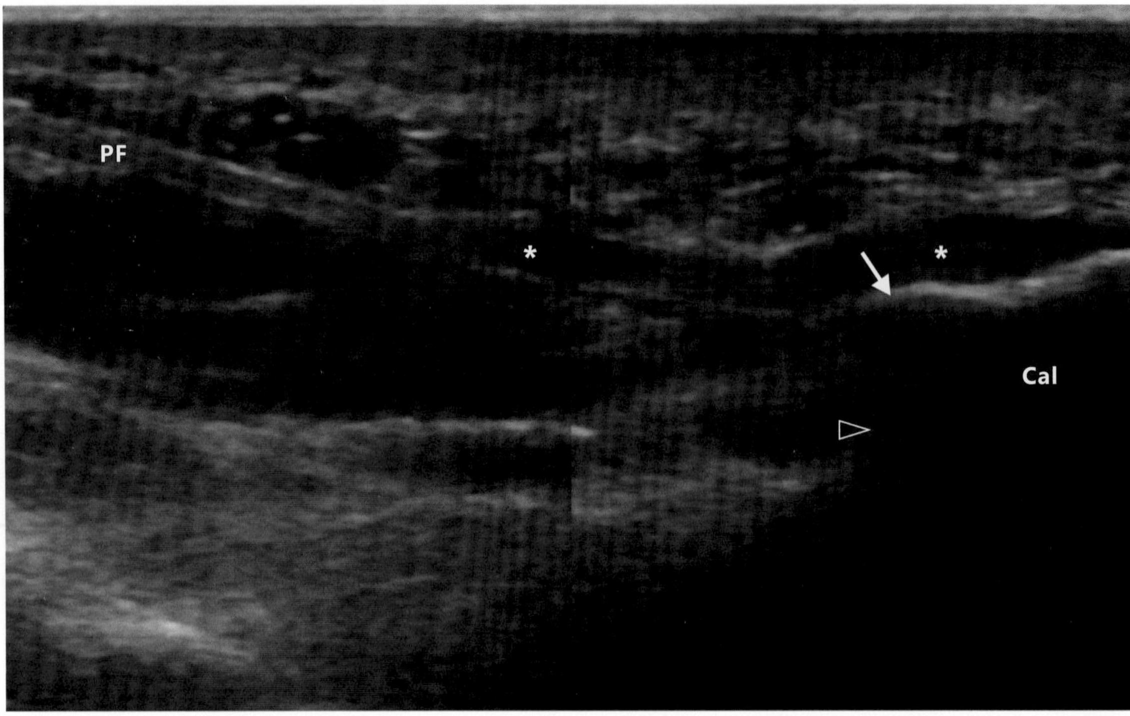

Split-screen longitudinal US image illustrates two (proximal and distal) hypoechoic swellings (*asterisks*) in the plantar fascia (**PF**). A calcaneal spur (*arrow*) is also seen with its posterior acoustic shadowing artifact (*arrowheads*).

Cal calcaneus

Plantar fasciitis in a 63-year-old woman with heel pain

11.44

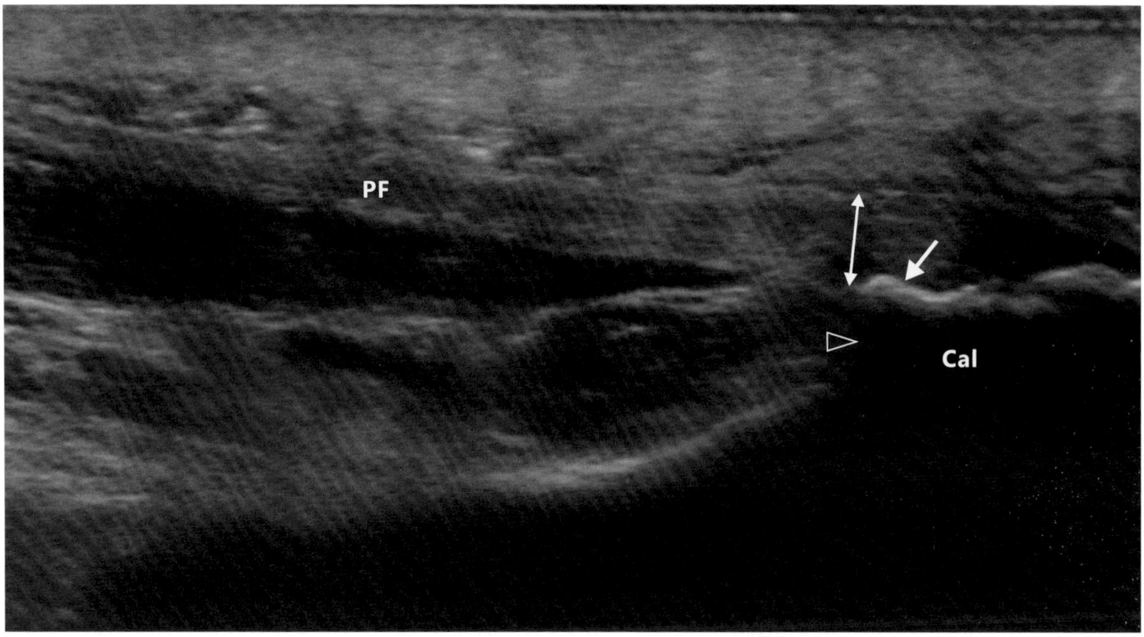

Heel pain was worsened during the first few steps which also caused gait difficulties.

Longitudinal US image reveals hypoechoic swelling (*double arrow*) of the plantar fascia (**PF**) at the calcaneal insertion point with a posterior acoustic shadowing (*arrowhead*) related to a bony spur (*arrow*).

Cal calcaneus

11.45 Plantar fasciitis in an obese woman with chronic heel pain and tenderness

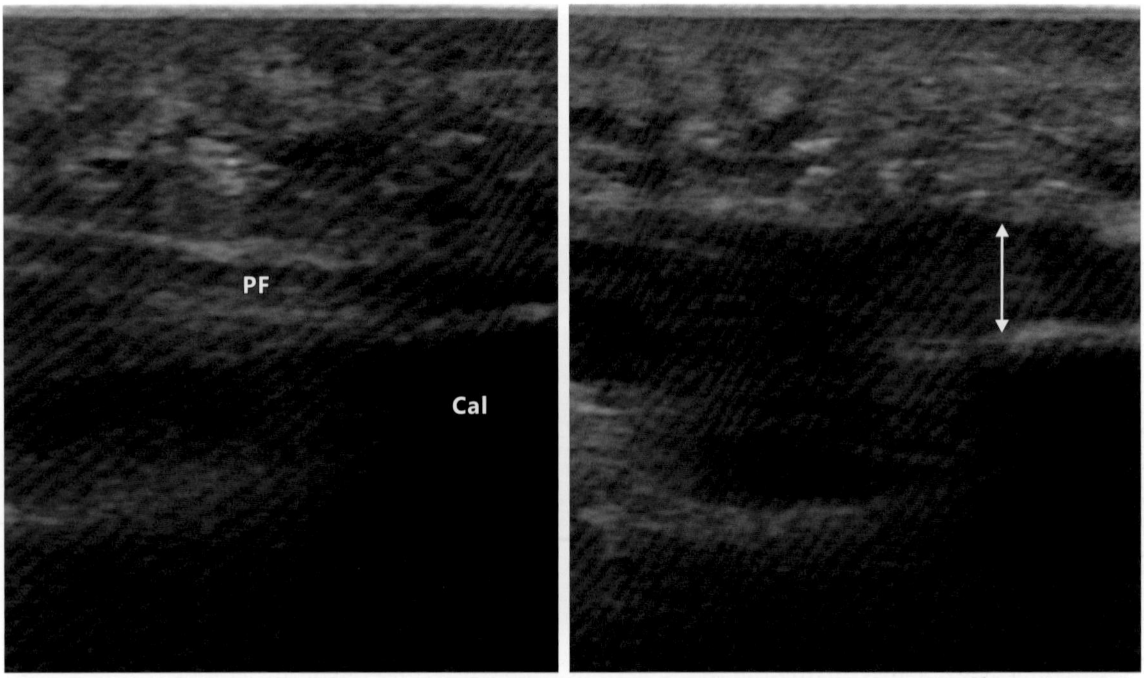

a b

Heel pain increased when getting out of bed, and during initial weight-bearing in the morning.

When compared with the normal side (**a**), longitudinal US image shows a markedly thickened, irregular and hypoechoic plantar fascia (**PF**) at the proximal/insertional portion (*double arrow*) (**b**).

Cal calcaneus

Expert note

Despite increasing the gain of the US machine, prompt imaging would be quite difficult in subjects with prominent fat pads. While the inability to delineate the bony contours "discomforts" the sonographer, controlled compression with the probe is advocated in order not to overlook other likely pathologies -especially pertaining to superficial bursae.

Plantar fasciitis in a 62-year-old man with heel pain exacerbated after wearing an unsupportive, hard-soled shoe

11.46

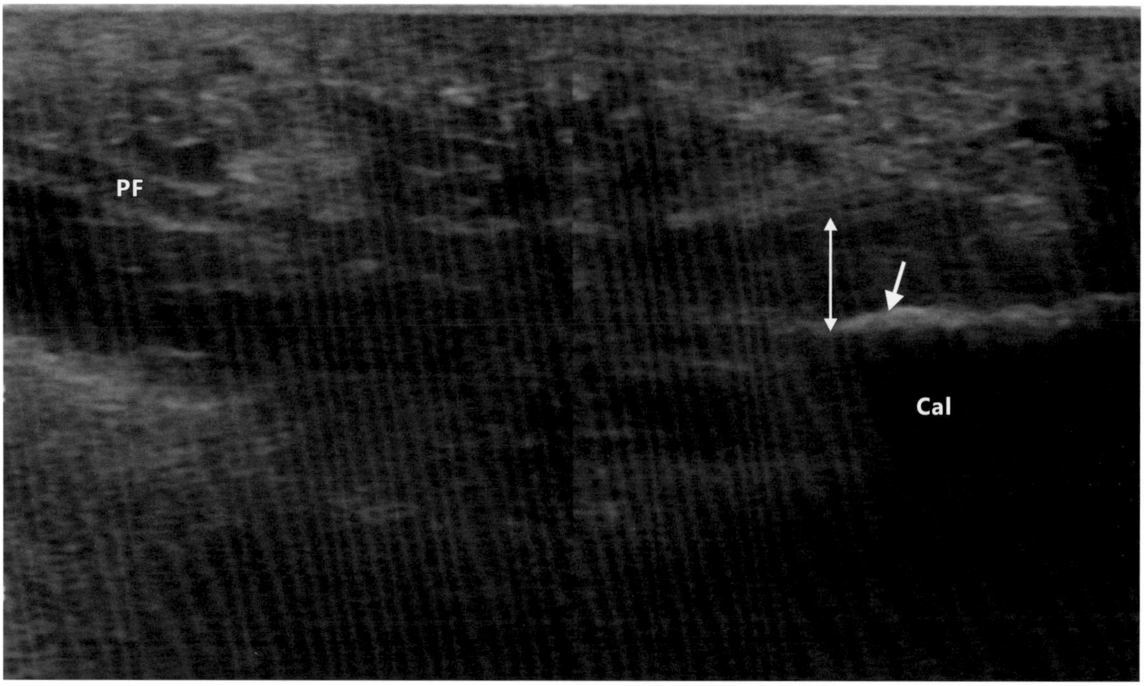

Split-screen longitudinal US imaging demonstrates epin calcanei (*arrow*) and swollen (*double arrow*) plantar fascia (**PF**) on the proximal attachment site.

Cal calcaneus

Expert note

It is important to evaluate the borders of the fascia i.e. especially in case of acute pain, they can be unclear/blurred as in this example.

11.47 Enthesopathy in a 41-year-old ankylosing spondylitis patient with subcalcaneal heel pain

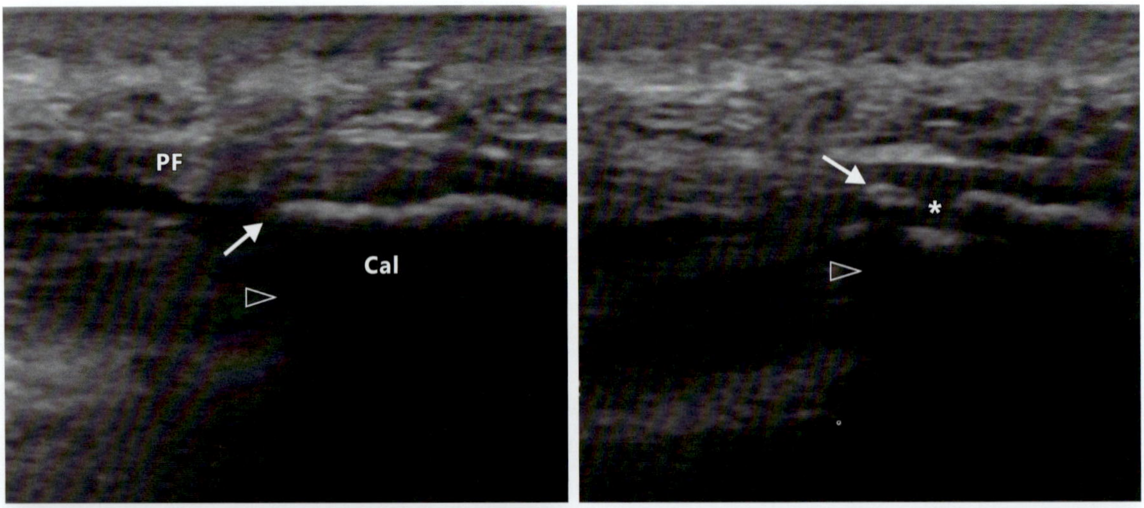

a b

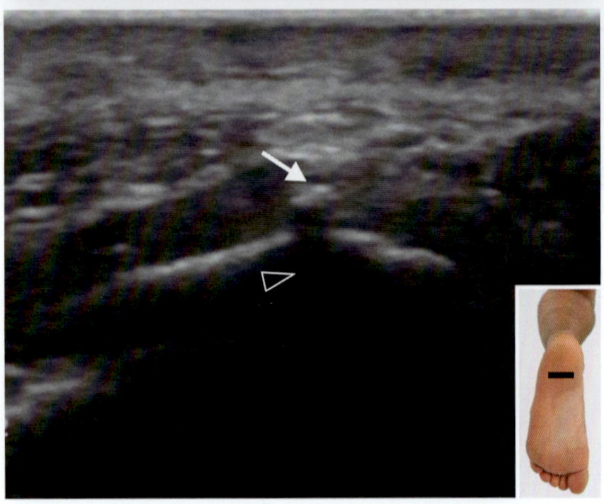

c

When compared with asymptomatic side (**a**), longitudinal (**b**) and axial (**c**) US images demonstrate an irregular entheseal site of the plantar fascia (**PF**) with an erosion (*asterisk*) and ossification (*arrows*). Please note the posterior acoustic shadowing artifacts (*arrowheads*) due to different forms of enthesopathy (*arrows*).

Cal calcaneus

Expert note

Calcaneal attachment of the plantar fascia is one of the most commonly evaluated entheseal sites in seronegative inflammatory diseases. Therefore, the fascia should be scanned for the presence of edema, intraligamentous calcifications and subcalcaneal bursitis, and the bony side for ossifications (enthesophytes) and erosions. Lastly, power Doppler imaging would provide additional information as regards the degree of inflammation (enthesitis).

Plantar fasciitis in a 45-year-old woman with bilateral chronic plantar pain -recently exacerbated with professional activities on one side **11.48**

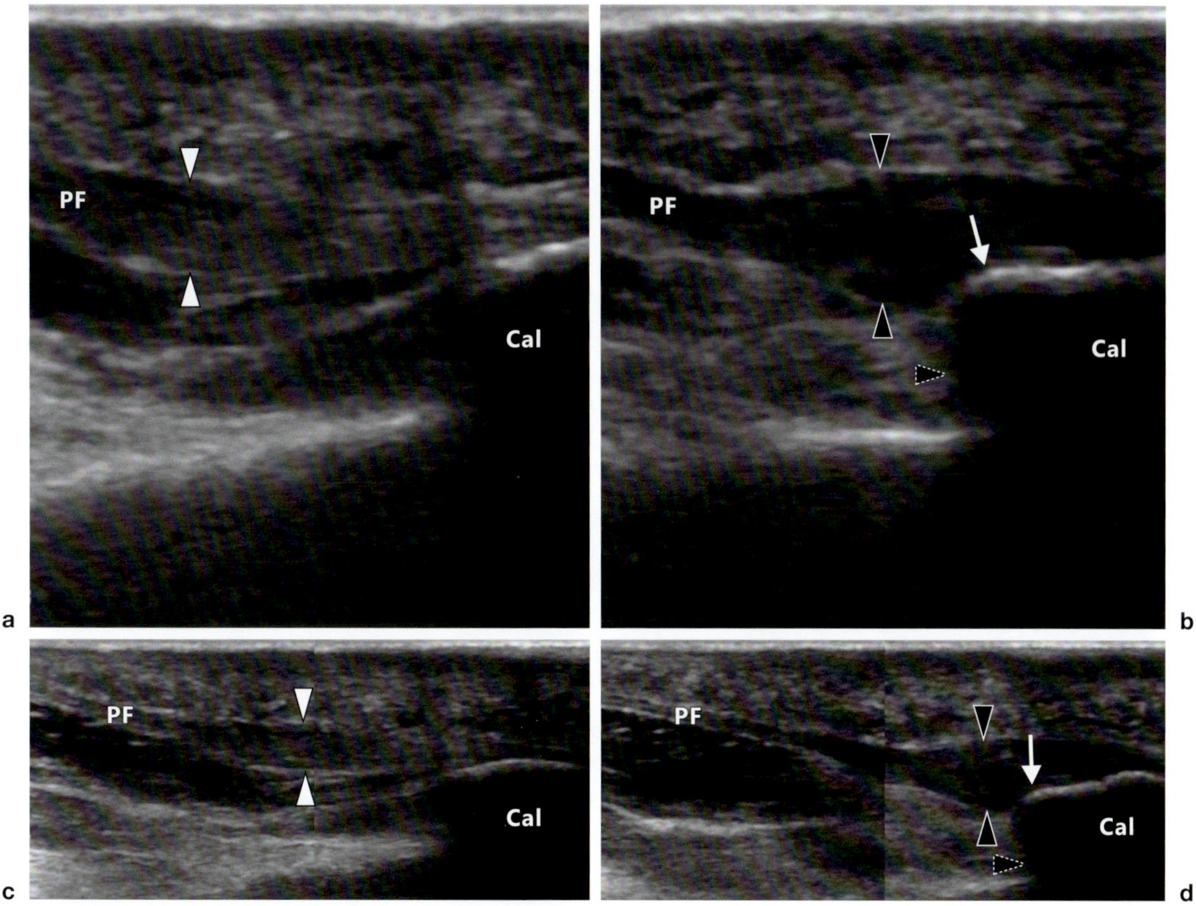

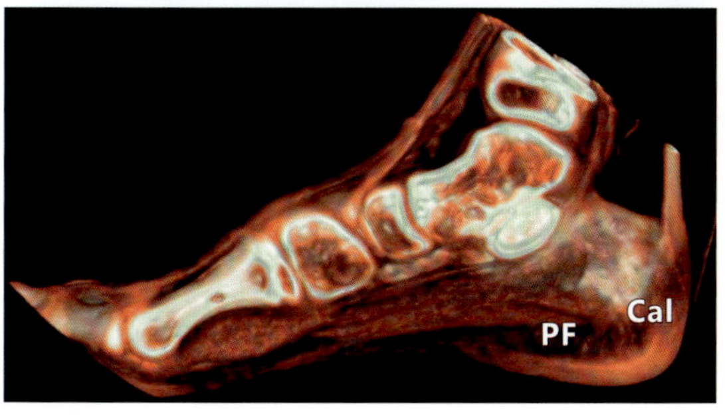

While there is mild, diffuse thickening (*white arrowheads*) of the plantar fascia (**PF**) on the less symptomatic side (**a**), significant hypoechoic swelling (*black arrowheads*) is seen on the acutely exacerbated side (**b**). Corresponding split-screen views (**c**, **d**). Note that the bony spurs (*arrows*) and the pertinent artifacts (*dashed arrowheads*) are better visualized on the painful side (**b**, **d**).

Cal calcaneus

Expert note

Depending on the footprint size of the probe, either split-screen or panoramic views can be used to thoroughly scan the plantar fascia in case it does not suffice.

11.49 Plantar fibromatosis (Ledderhose disease) in a 52-year-old man with a painless lump on the medial aspect of the sole

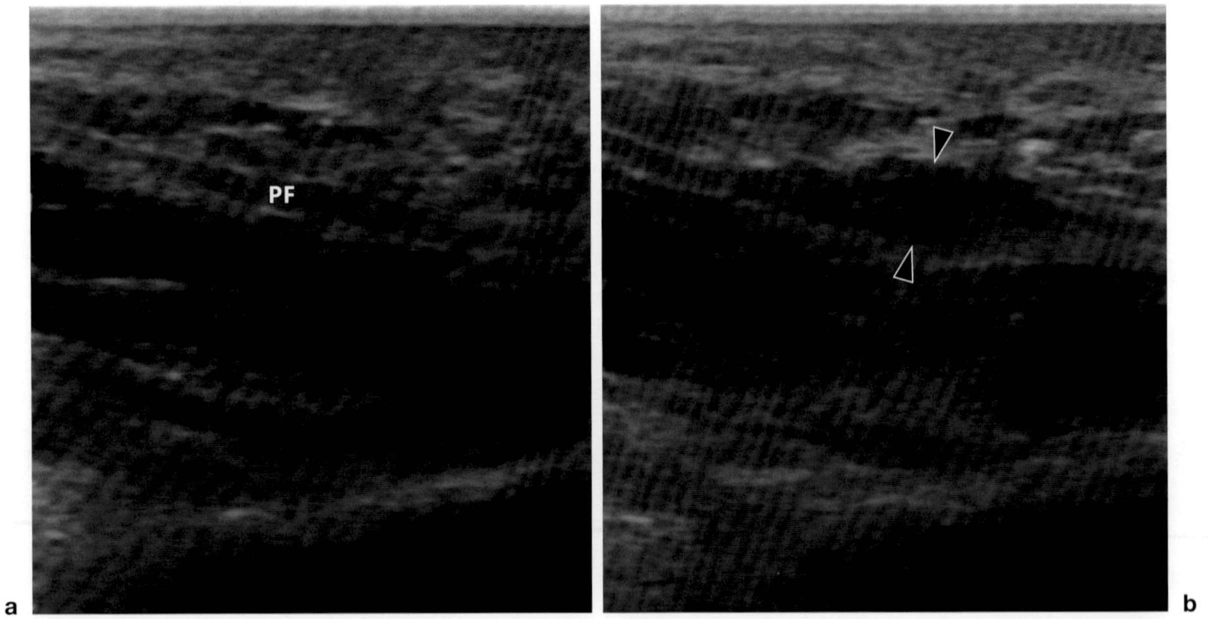

The medical history includes smoking and type 2 diabetes mellitus.

When compared with the normal side (**a**), longitudinal US image of the plantar fascia (**PF**) identifies an oval-shaped hypoechoic nodular thickening (*arrowheads*) (**b**).

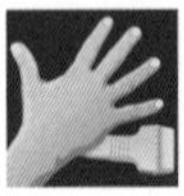

Expert note

If accompanied by positive/likely history, the detection of a fibroma might necessitate further scanning of other sites (e.g. palm) whereby US imaging can readily be used as well [8, 9].

Chronic plantar fasciitis in a 65-year-old man suffering from heel pain for the last six months

11.50

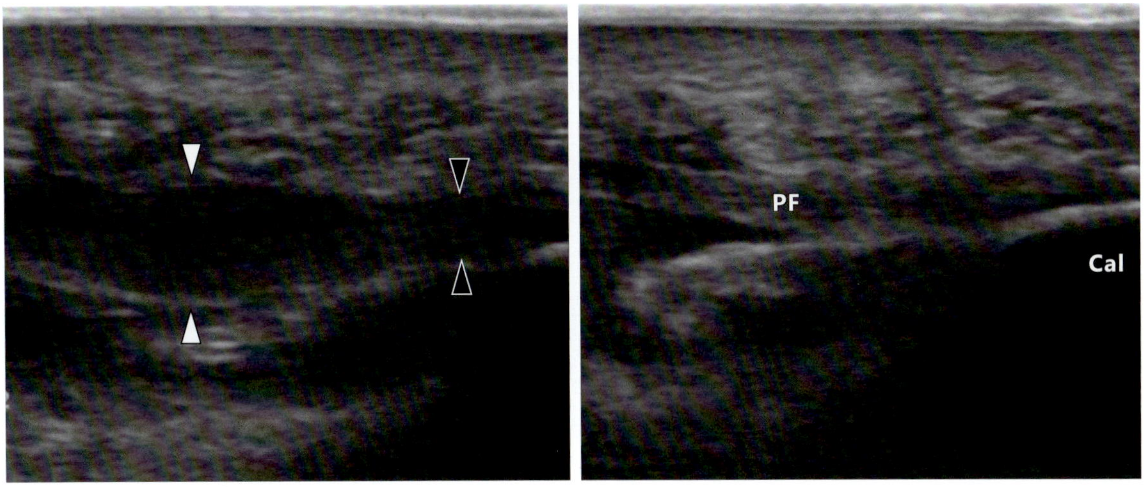

Longitudinal US image reveals diffuse irregular thickening of the fascia (**PF**) at its proximal (*black arrowheads*) and distal (*white arrowheads*) portions with textural inhomogeneities (**a**). Normal side (**b**).

Cal calcaneus

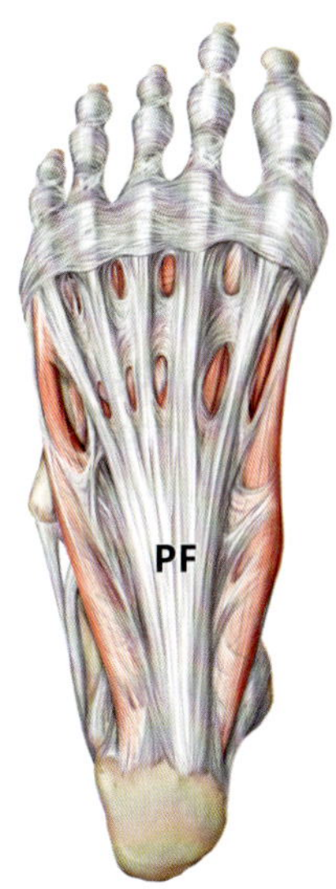

11.51 Ledderhose disease (plantar fibromatosis) in a 51-year-old man with a tender nodule localized at the medial aspect of the sole

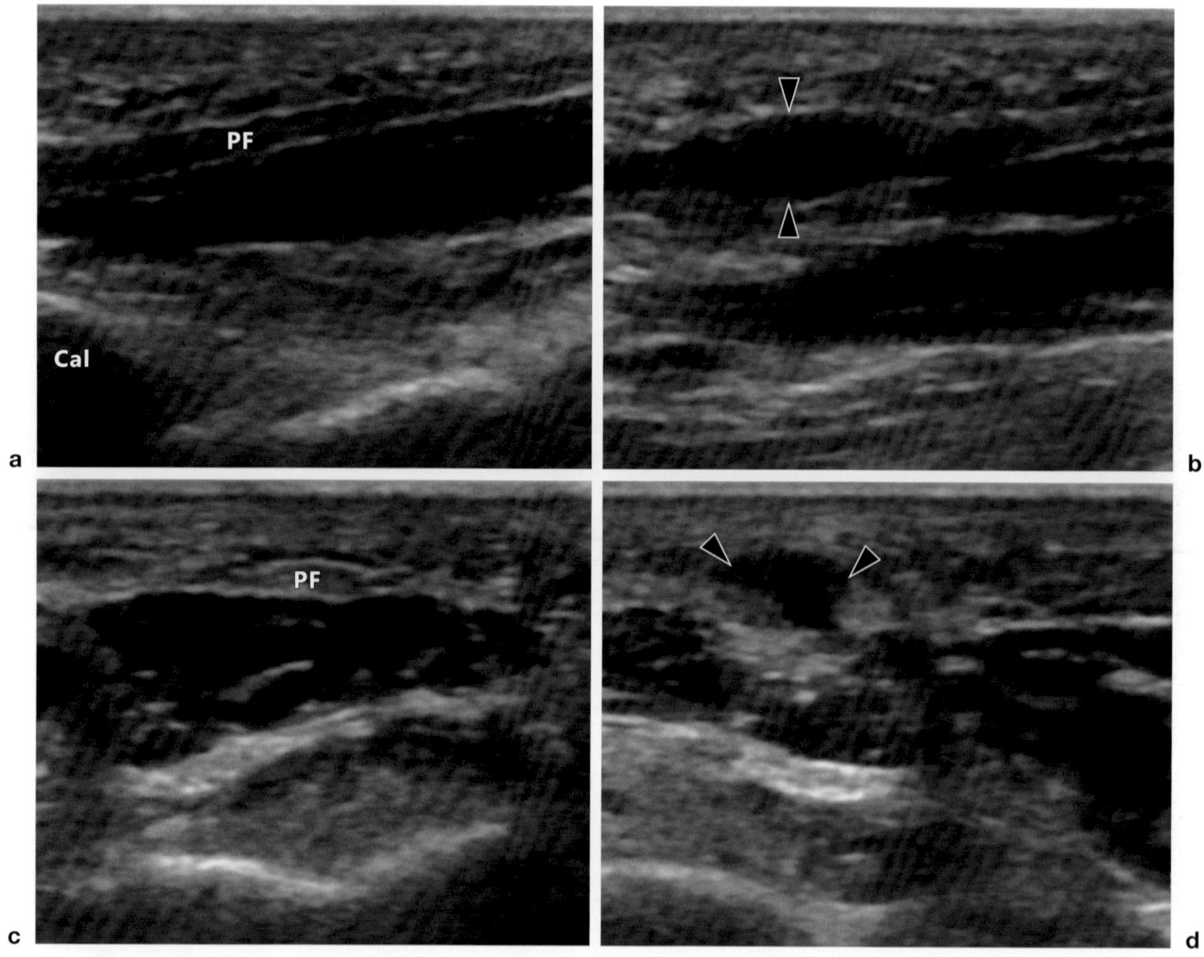

Clinical examination exhibited local pain during passive dorsal extension of the toes.

When compared with the normal side (**a**, **c**) longitudinal (**b**) and axial (**d**) US images demonstrate a well-defined fusiform hypoechoic nodule (*arrowheads*) arising within the superficial and deep fibers of the plantar fascia (**PF**).

Cal calcaneus

Calcified plantar fasciitis in a 45-year-old woman with sole pain and pes planus deformities 11.52

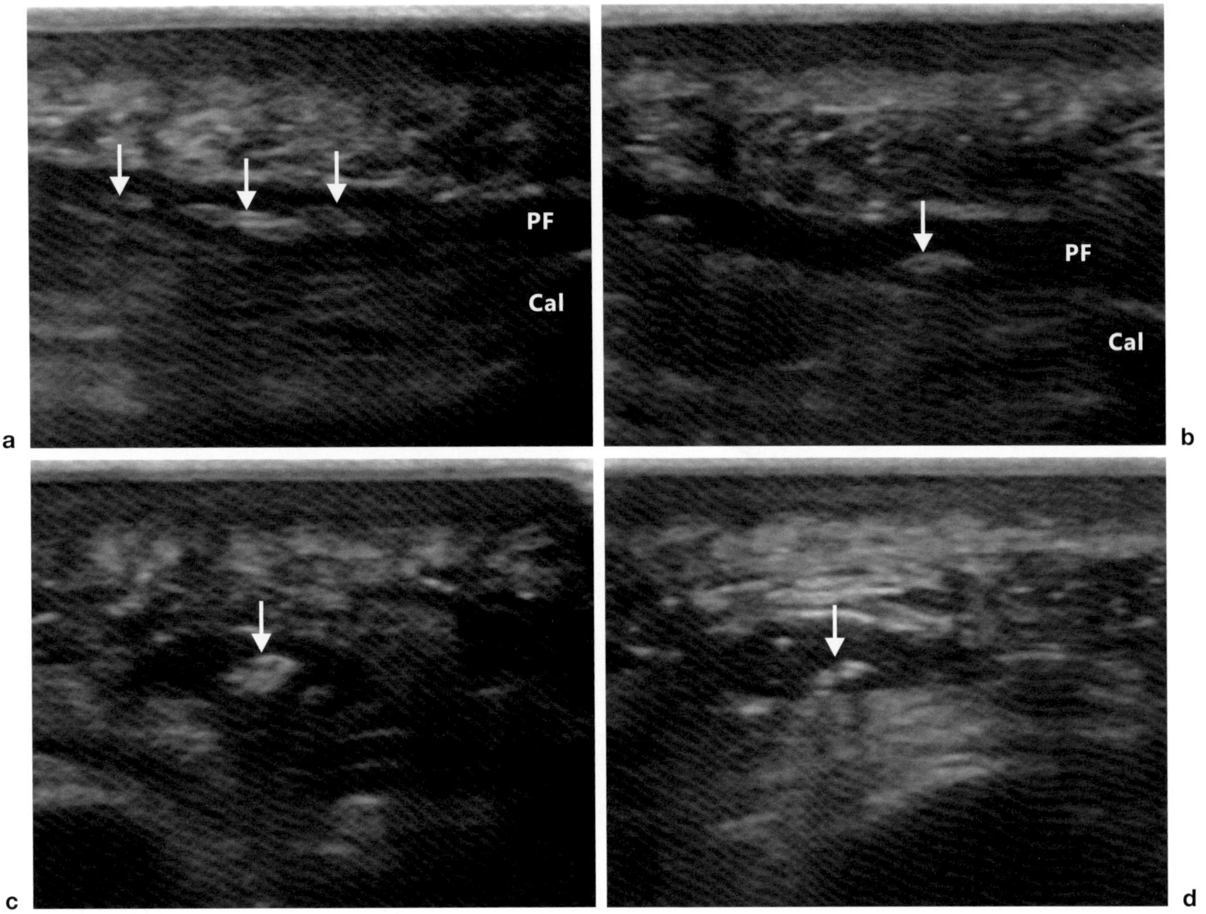

Plantar longitudinal (**a**, **b**) and axial (**c**, **d**) US images demonstrate calcific deposits as hyperechoic echoes (*arrows*) located within the plantar fascia (**PF**).

Cal calcaneus

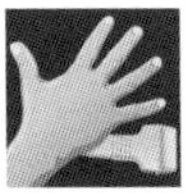

Expert note

Although majority of the plantar fascia pathologies ensue at the calcaneal attachment site, scanning distally should always be performed for complete assessment. For sure, sono-palpation in light of the patient's complaints would be quite subsidiary.

11.53 Callus on the skin in a 13-year-old boy who had a small painful and tender area at the plantar mid-foot

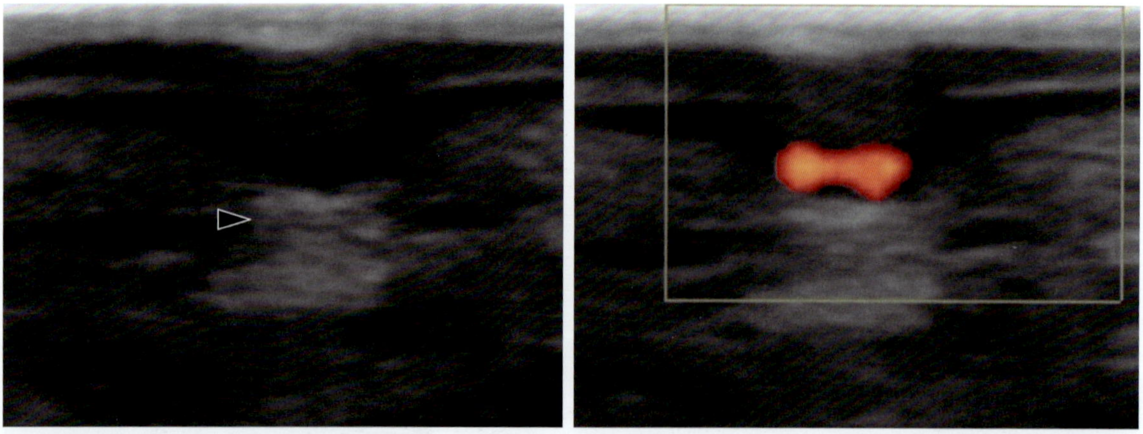

a b

Axial (**a**) and power Doppler (**b**) images show a focal vascular thickening/vascularization of the skin with enhanced through transmission artifact (*arrowhead*).

Expert note

Although majority of the skin lesions are visible in physical examination (inspection), the need for imaging deep layers of the skin or exploring the vascularity of the lesion makes US imaging very important in dermatological diseases.

Ganglion cyst in a woman with pain and a small lump beneath the foot **11.54**

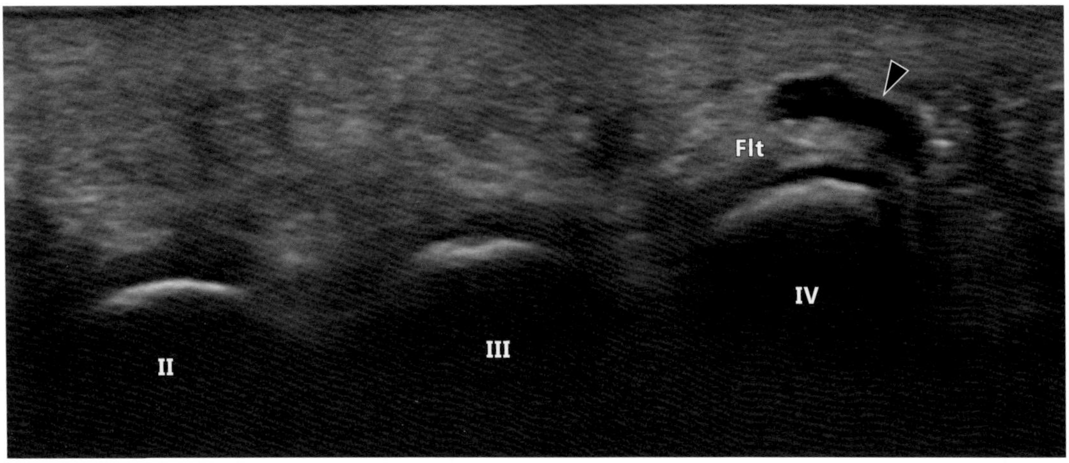

Plantar axial US image demonstrates an anechoic and fusiform cyst (*arrowhead*) over the fourth metatarsal bone, adjacent to the flexor tendon (**Flt**).

Ganglion cyst in a woman with metatarsalgia **11.55**

a 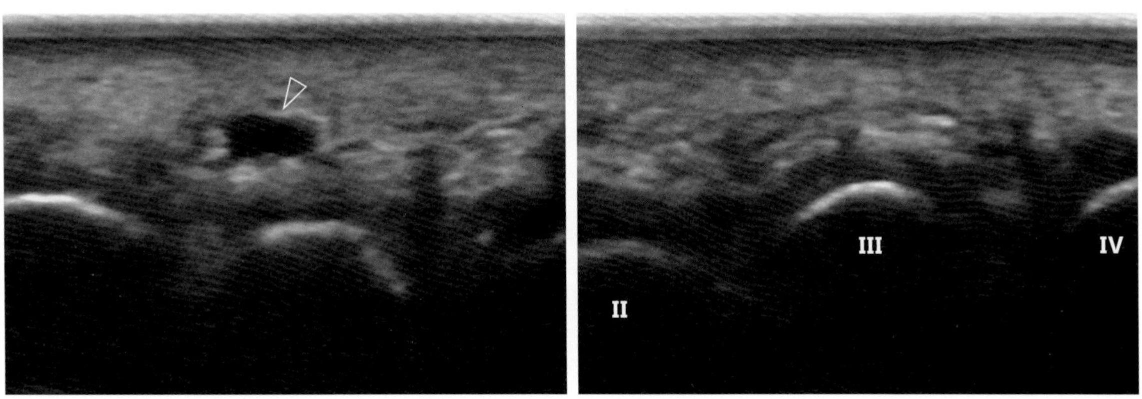 b

Plantar axial US image over the metatarsal heads shows an anechoic, oval-shaped cyst (*arrowhead*) (**a**). Normal side (**b**).

11.56 Anterior talofibular ligament sprain in a 35-year-old woman who had ankle inversion injury

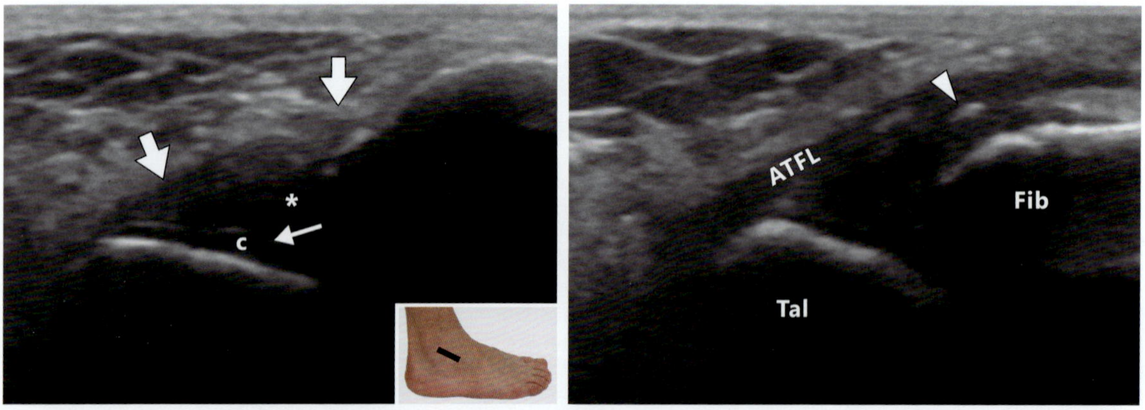

a b

Lateral longitudinal US images reveal thickened (*thick arrows*) anterior talofibular ligament (**ATFL**) with an interface sign (*thin arrow*) on the symptomatic side (**a**), and intraligamentous calcification (*arrowhead*) on the other side (**b**).

c cartilage
Fib fibula
Tal talus

Expert note

The finding of interface sign on the talar cartilage is usually indicative of joint effusion that is accompanying the ATFL injury. Since it can well be present in asymptomatic joints, comparing both sides and correlating with the medical history and clinical exam are always important. When compared with the operative findings; the sensitivity, specificity and accuracy of US imaging for ATFL injury has been found as 98-99%, 92-96% and 84-95%, respectively [2, 10].
The US images can be graded on the basis of severity of the injury as sprain with mild stretching or swollen ligament without tear (grade I), partial tear (grade II), complete ligament tear (grade III) [2, 11].

Partial tear of the anterior talofibular ligament in a female volleyball player with chronic ankle pain **11.57**

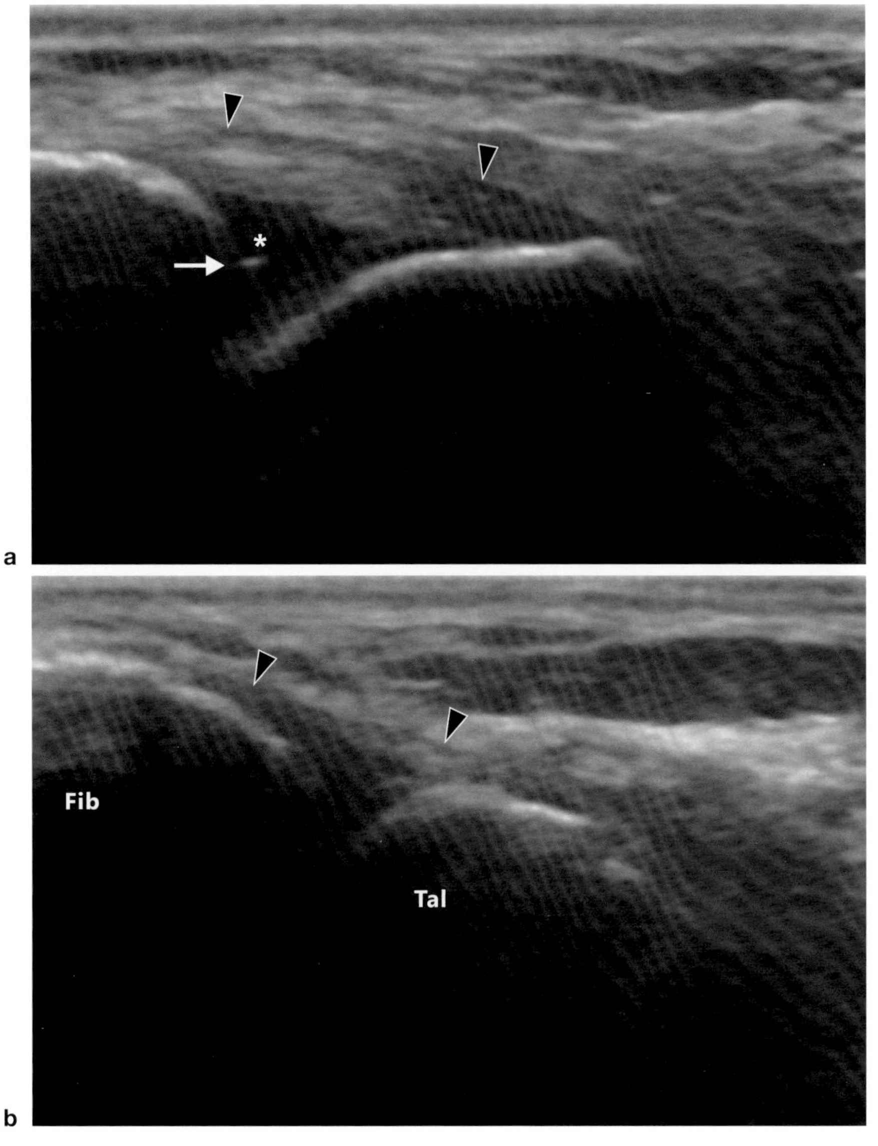

The athlete sustained repetitive inversion blows to the lateral side of the ankle.

Lateral longitudinal US image shows intact but edematous appearance of the anterior talofibular ligament (*arrowheads*), cortical irregularity (*arrow*), and a small amount of fluid (*asterisk*) within the joint (**a**). Contralateral normal side (**b**).

Fib fibula
Tal talus

11.58 Ganglion cyst in a 55-year-old woman with a painless stiff lump on the dorsolateral side of the ankle

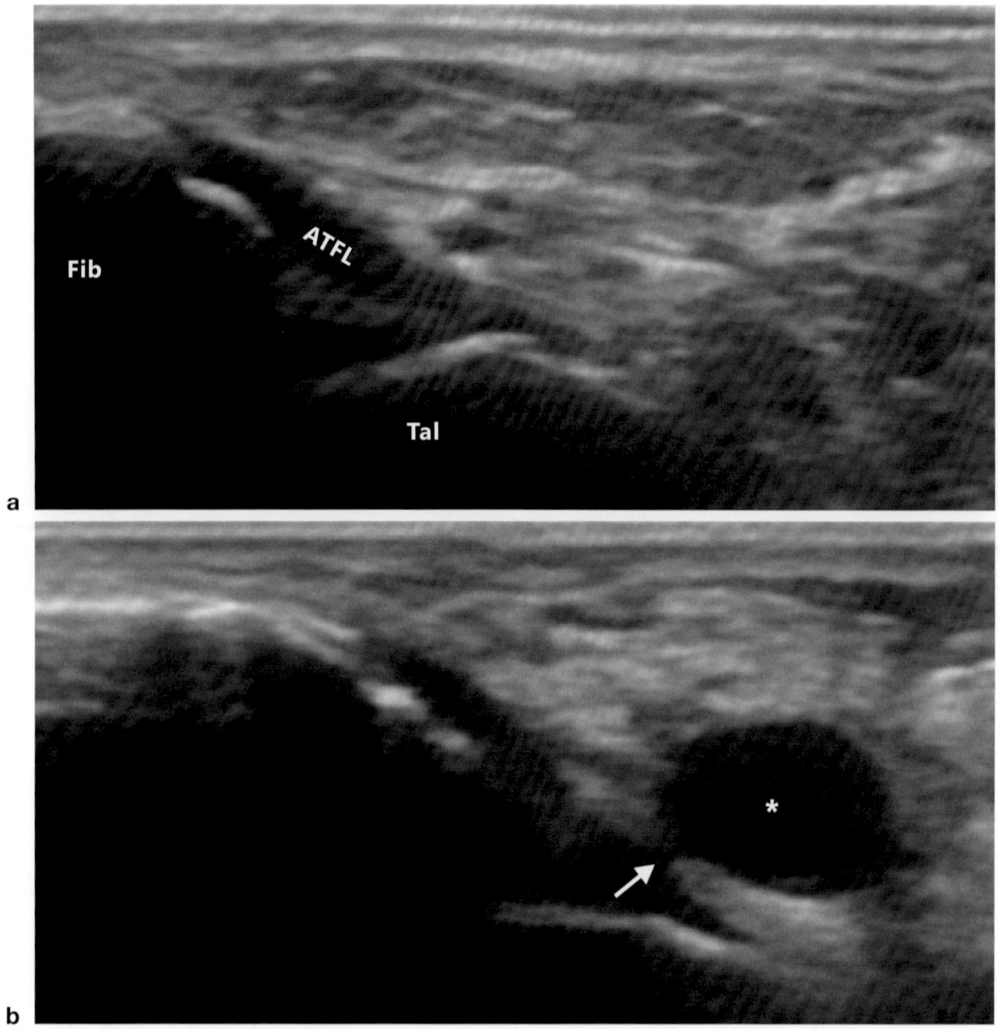

When compared with the normal side (**a**), lateral longitudinal US image (**b**) shows a well-defined, anechoic cyst (*asterisk*) connected with the joint through a small pedicle (*arrow*).

ATFL anterior talofibular ligament
Fib fibula
Tal talus

Expert note

Finding the pedicle of a cyst is usually not easy; as such, applying compression might help widen the pedicle and make it better visible.

Anterior talofibular ligament sprain in a 50-year-old obese patient with lateral ankle pain after an inversion injury

11.59

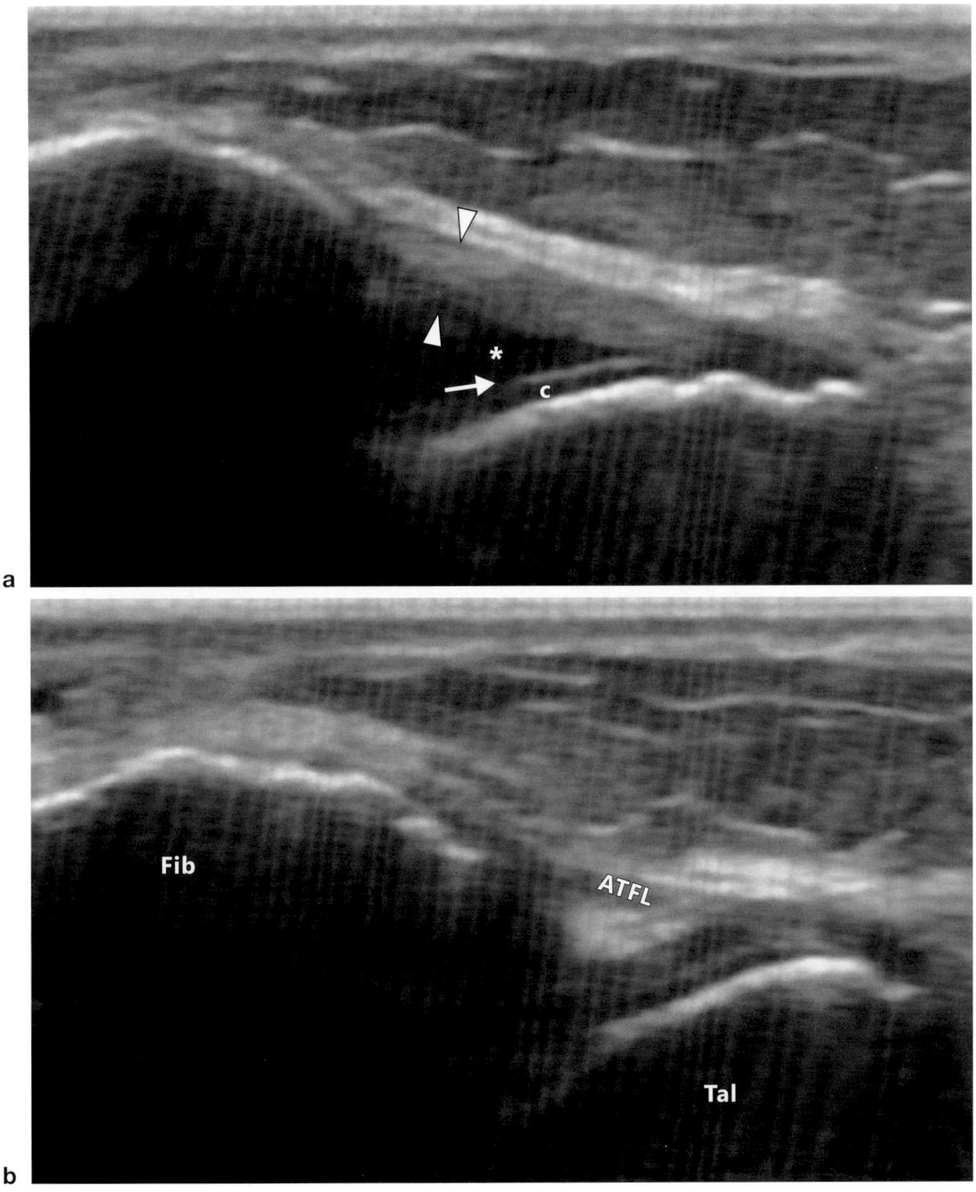

Longitudinal US image reveals intact but thickened (*arrowheads*) anterior talofibular ligament (**ATFL**) and a small amount of effusion (*asterisk*) inside the ankle joint (**a**). Contralateral normal side (**b**). Please note the interface sign (*arrow*) between the effusion and the articular cartilage (**c**).

Fib fibula
Tal talus

11.60 Anterior talofibular ligament sprain in a patient with lateral ankle pain

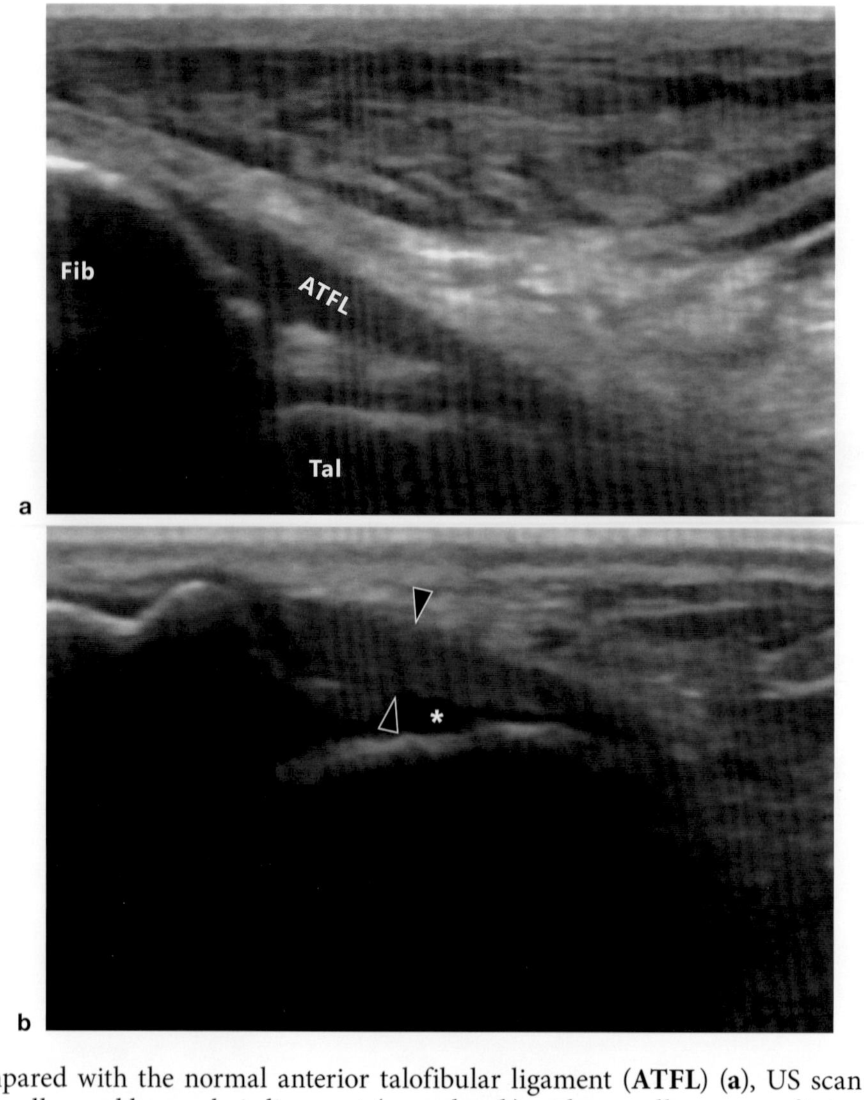

When compared with the normal anterior talofibular ligament (**ATFL**) (**a**), US scan illustrates a markedly swollen and hypoechoic ligament (*arrowheads*) with a small amount of joint effusion (*asterisk*) (**b**).

Fib fibula
Tal talus

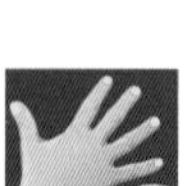

Expert note

The cortex of the fibula is markedly irregular; in other words, bony irregularities are almost always present in the proximal insertion of the ATFL.

Anterior talofibular ligament tear in a patient with ankle pain and swelling after repetitive inversion injuries **11.61**

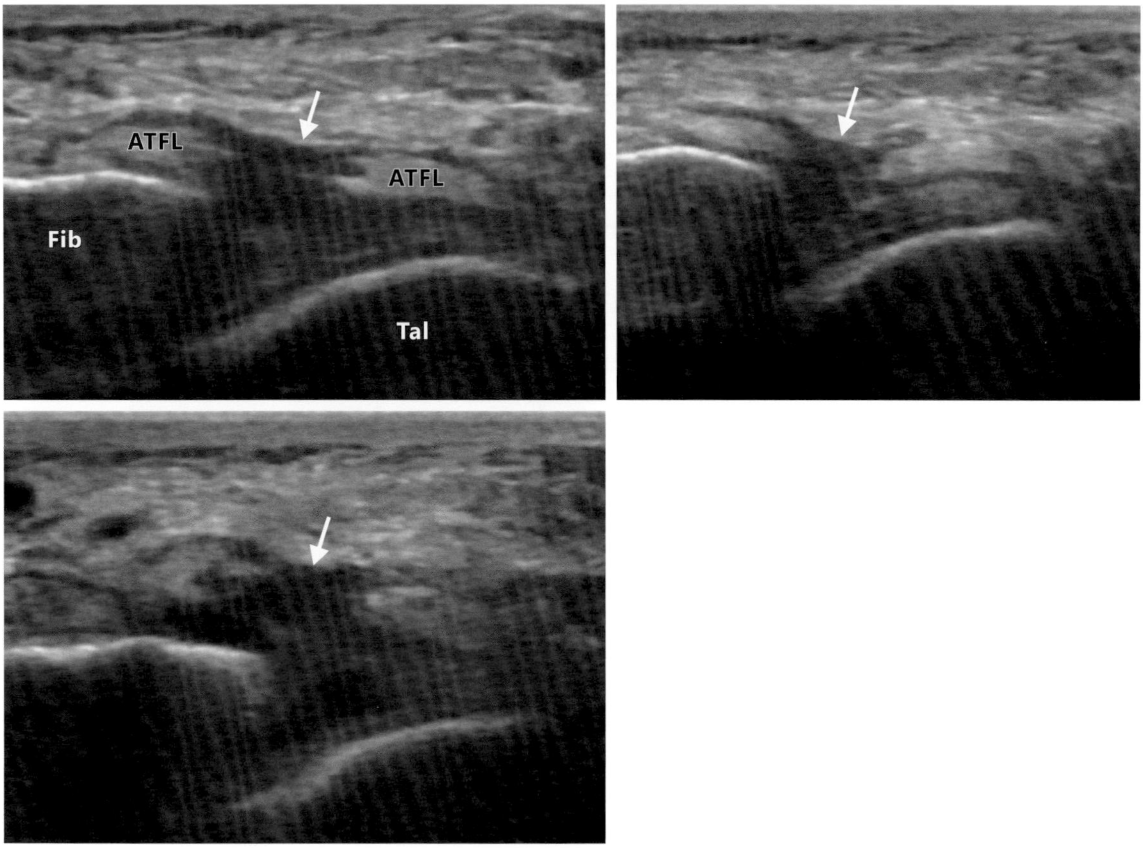

a b c

Lateral longitudinal US imaging with different probe compressions show full thickness rupture (*arrows*) in the anterior talofibular ligament (**ATFL**). Light touch (**a**), during compression (**b**) and removing compression (**c**).

Fib fibula
Tal talus

Expert note

Dynamic imaging -either with passive inversion of the ankle or with probe compression- for the ATFL is of great importance when its rupture is suspected. While the former method can help retract its separated parts, the latter (as shown in this image) will make the overlying soft tissues bulge deep inside the joint. Normally, this "herniation" can never ensue in case of a healthy/intact ATFL. Likewise, this second method can be used to indirectly confirm that the ligament is intact in case ATFL is not well visualized during imaging [12].

Video 14

11.62 Anterior talofibular ligament injuries in a football player with ankle pain, swelling and tenderness

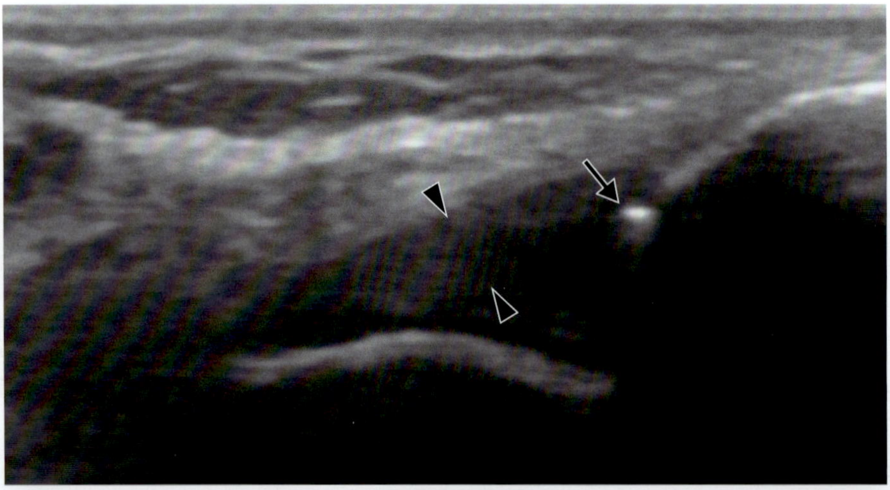
a

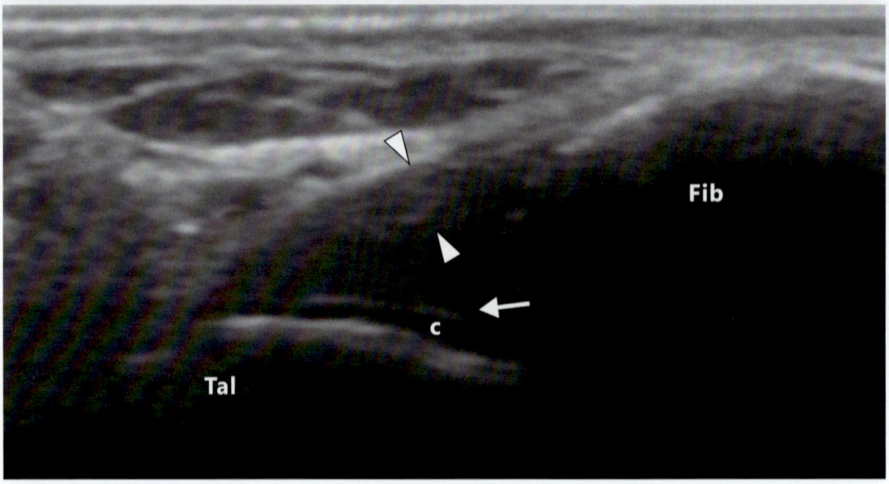

b

Lateral longitudinal US image (**a**) reveals a partial tear of the anterior talofibular ligament (*black arrowheads*) and a small cortical irregularity of the fibula (*black arrow*). A swollen and hypoechoic but intact ligament (*white arrowheads*) with an interface sign (*white arrow*) can be seen on the other side (**b**).

c	talar cartilage	**Tal**	talus
Fib	fibula		

Expert note

Like in other sports (players), finding minor symptomatic or asymptomatic lesions in the ankle of footballers is not uncommon. In this sense, interpretation of the US findings in light of the clinical examination should definitely be considered for treatment or return to sports.

Avulsion fracture at the proximal insertion of the anterior talofibular ligament in a 25-year-old woman with recurrent ankle sprains **11.63**

a

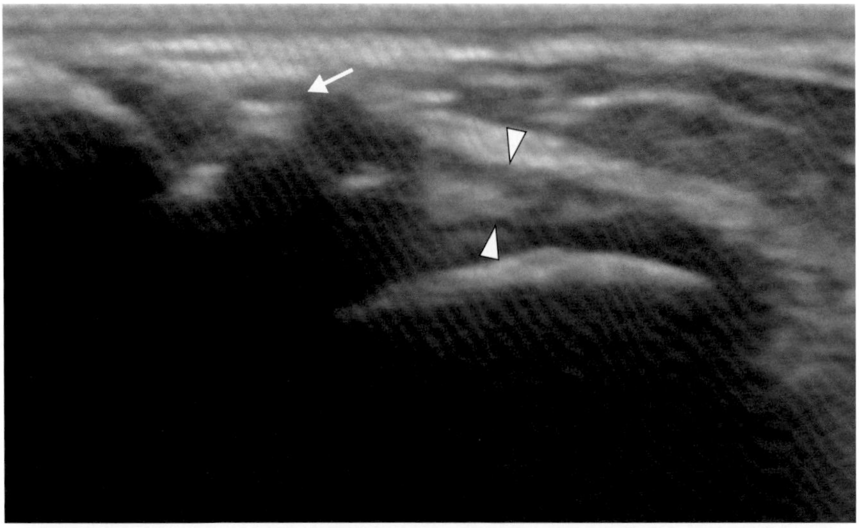

b

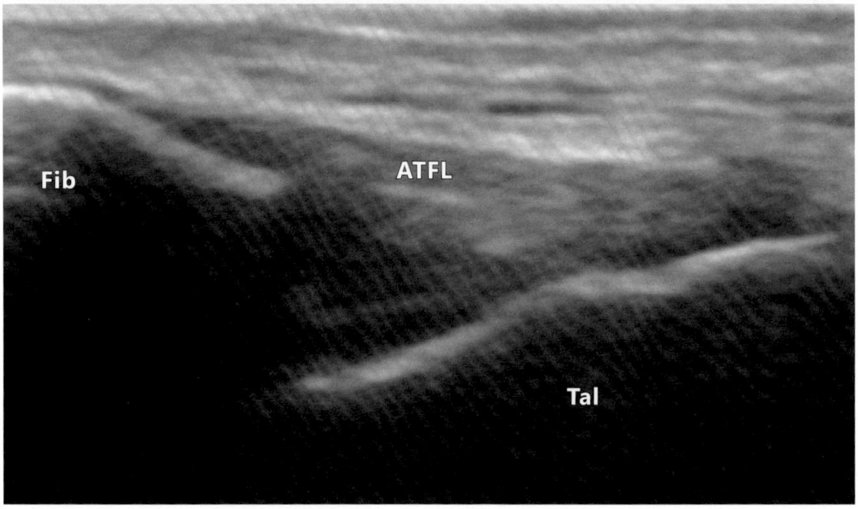

Lateral longitudinal US image over the anterior talofibular ligament (**ATFL**) demonstrates hypoechoic and thickened appearance of the partially ruptured ligament (*arrowheads*) with an irregular hyperechoic fragment (*arrow*) (**a**). Contralateral normal side (**b**).

Fib fibula
Tal talus

Expert note

Similar to bony irregularities, calcifications are mostly found in the proximal insertion of the injured ATFL, which often appear as bony (fibular) avulsion fragments [2].

11.64 Sprain and partial rupture of the anterior talofibular ligament in a 22-year-old woman with ankle pain and swelling

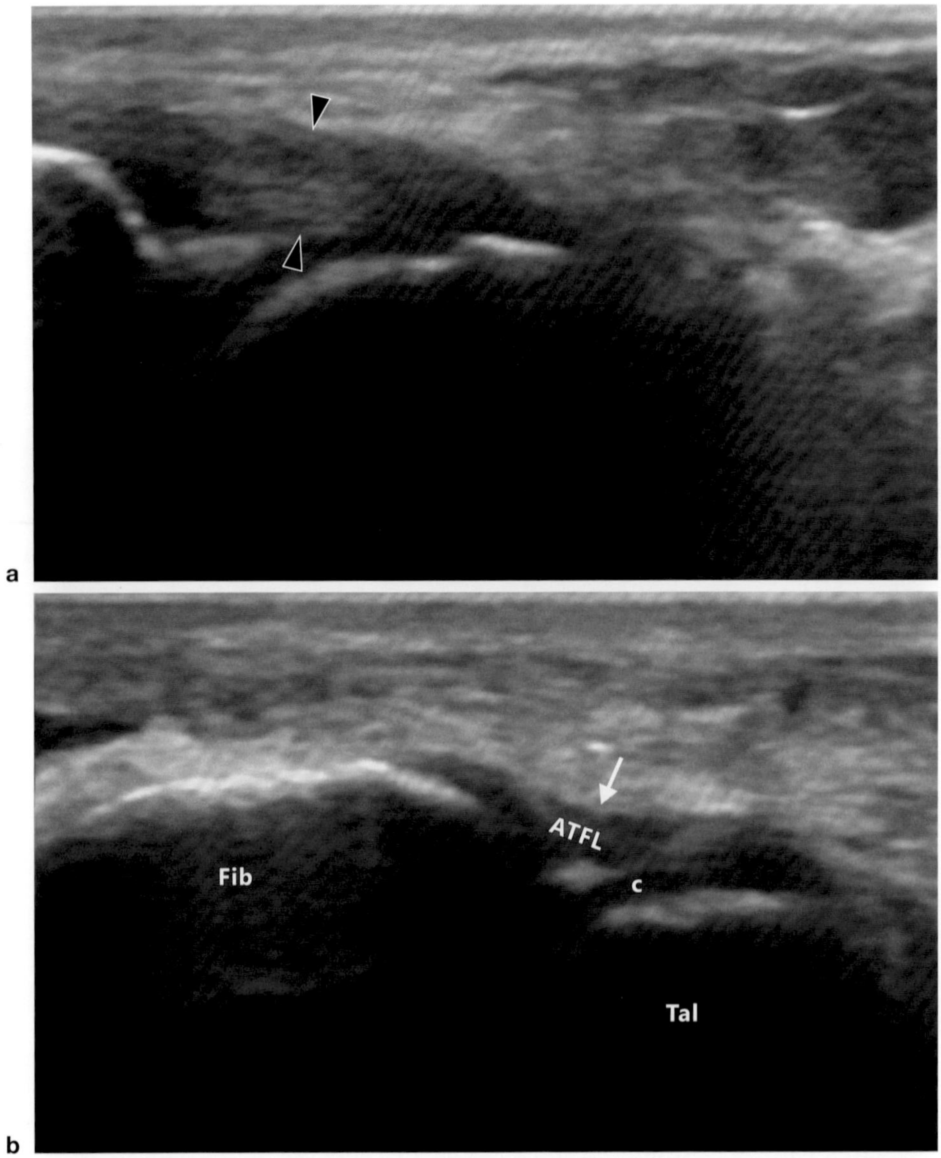

Longitudinal US image over the anterior talofibular ligament (**ATFL**) shows marked enlargement and hypoechogenicity (*arrowheads*) of the ligament (**a**). Contralateral asymptomatic side illustrates mild collapse of the ligament (*arrow*) upon probe compression (**b**).

c talar cartilage
Fib fibula
Tal talus

Anterior talofibular ligament tears in a 35-year-old man with ankle after repetitive sprains

11.65

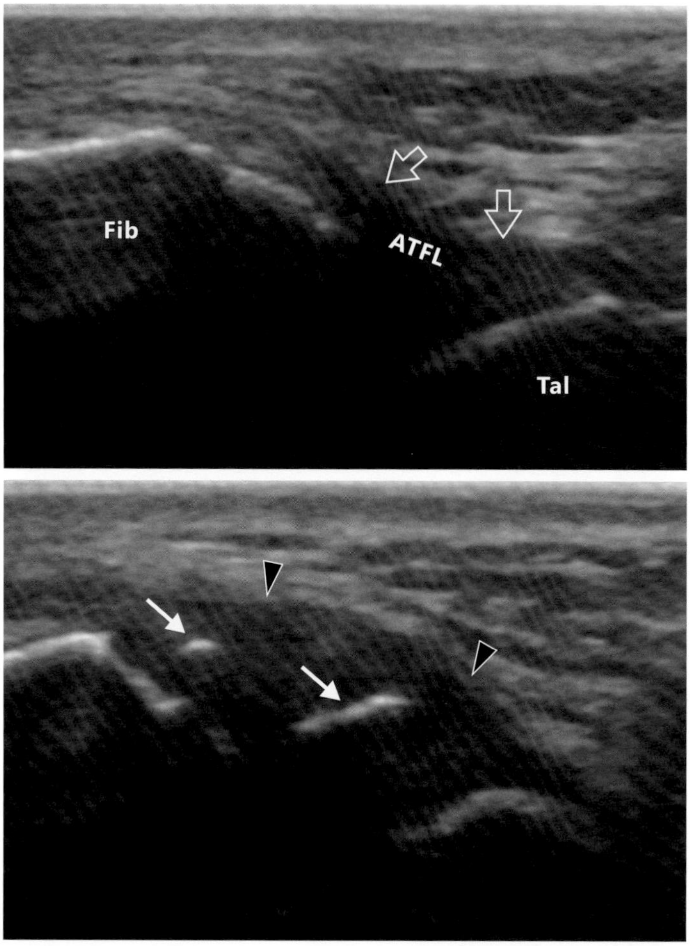

a

b

Unlike the regular compact structure of the anterior talofibular ligament (**ATFL**), longitudinal US image under the probe compression exhibits a mild concave deformation of the ligament (*thick arrows*) (**a**). Contralateral side shows partial ligament tear with irregular thickening (*arrowheads*) and two hyperechoic fragments (*thin arrows*) beneath the ligament (**b**).

Fib fibula
Tal talus

Expert note

Avulsion fractures in the ATFL like many other tendinous/ligamentous areas can be kept in mind especially when patients describe trauma. In this case, as the US imaging could not show all the bony surfaces thoroughly, magnetic resonance imaging was performed and it showed a minor fibular fracture.

11.66 Partial rupture of the anterior talofibular ligament in an 18-year-old ballet with chronic ankle pain

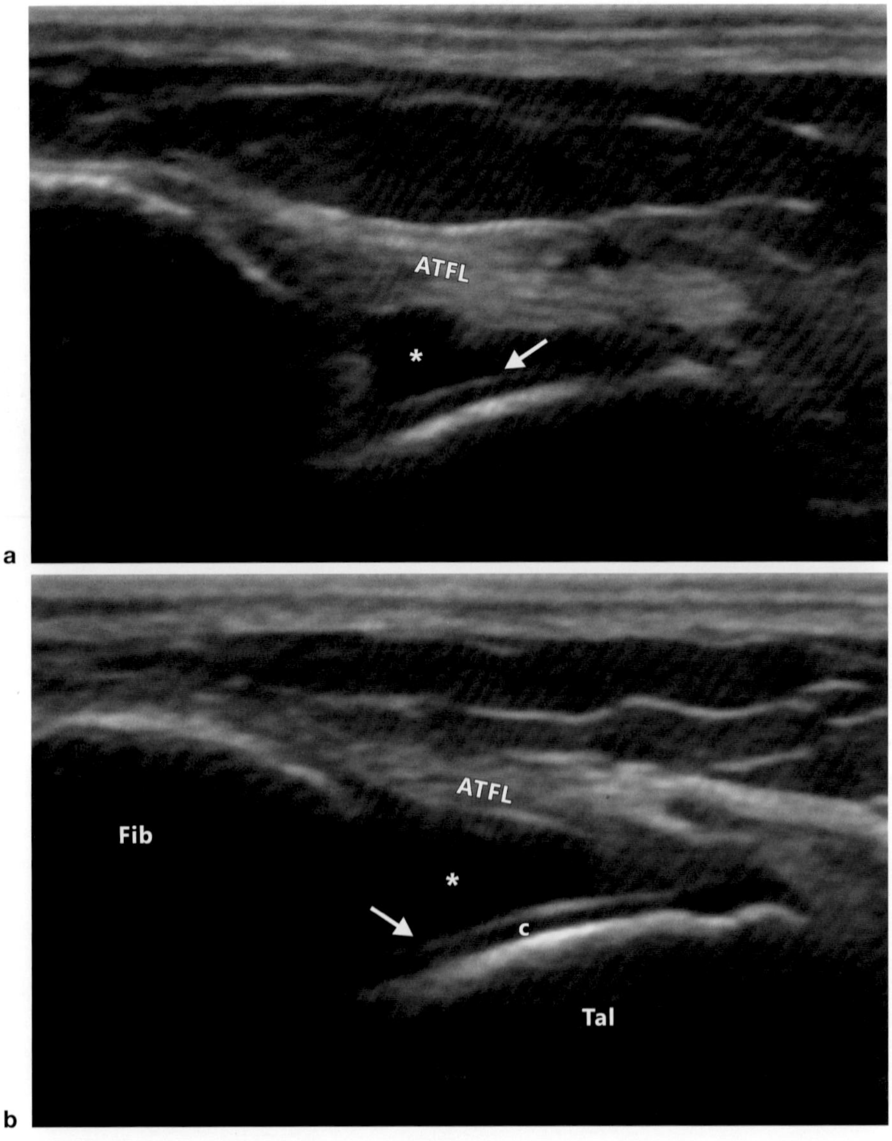

Longitudinal US images over the anterior talofibular ligament (**ATFL**) illustrate anechoic effusions (*asterisks*) extending along the lateral side of the ankle joints. While the ATFL is thickened with a partial tear on one side (**a**), joint effusion seems to be more predominant on the other side (**b**). Note the acoustic interface signs as bright linear echoes (*arrows*) between the fluid and articular cartilage (**c**).

Fib fibula
Tal talus

Anterior talofibular ligament sprain in a patient with ankle pain after an inversion injury 11.67

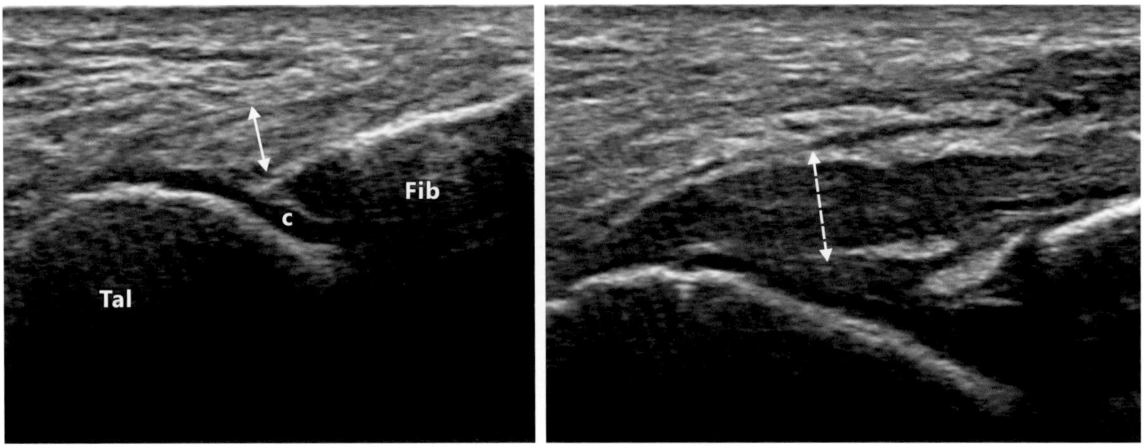

a b

The anterior drawer test corroborated ligament sprain.

When compared with normal view of the anterior talofibular ligament (*double arrow*) (**a**), longitudinal US image (**b**) shows markedly swollen and edematous appearance (*dashed arrow*) of the ligament.

c	talar cartilage
Fib	fibula
Tal	talus

11.68 Deltoid ligament sprain in a woman with ankle pain after repetitive eversion injuries

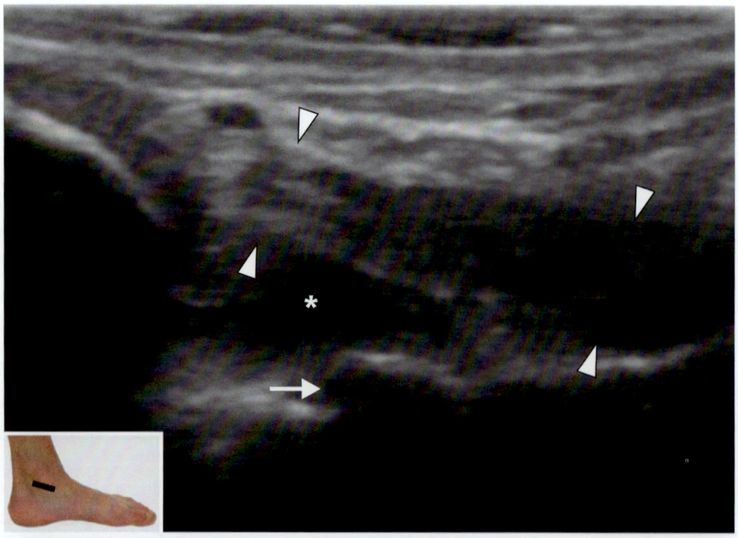

a

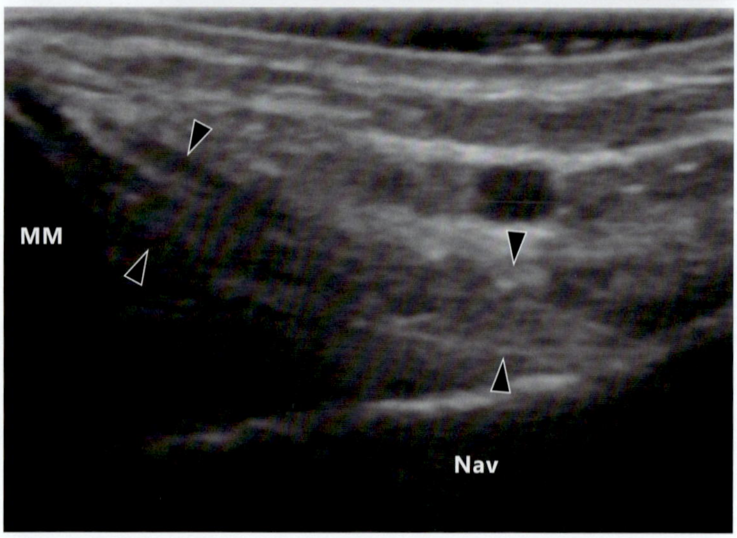

b

Medial longitudinal US image (**a**) shows intact but swollen and hypoechoic deltoid ligament (*white arrowheads*), effusion (*asterisk*) and cortical irregularity (*arrow*). Normal view of the ligament (*black arrowheads*) on the contralateral side (**b**).

MM medial malleolus **Nav** navicular

Expert note

When scanning around the medial malleoli, owing to the irregular contours, extra gel is usually necessary between the skin and probe for optimal imaging.

Anterior tibiofibular ligament rupture in a 35-year-old girl who had ankle injury after athletic play **11.69**

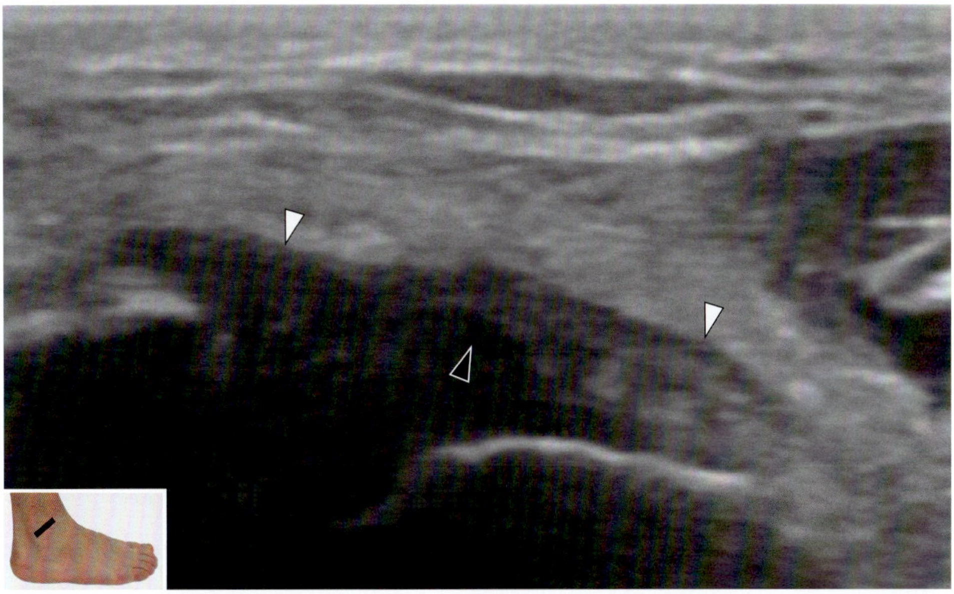

a

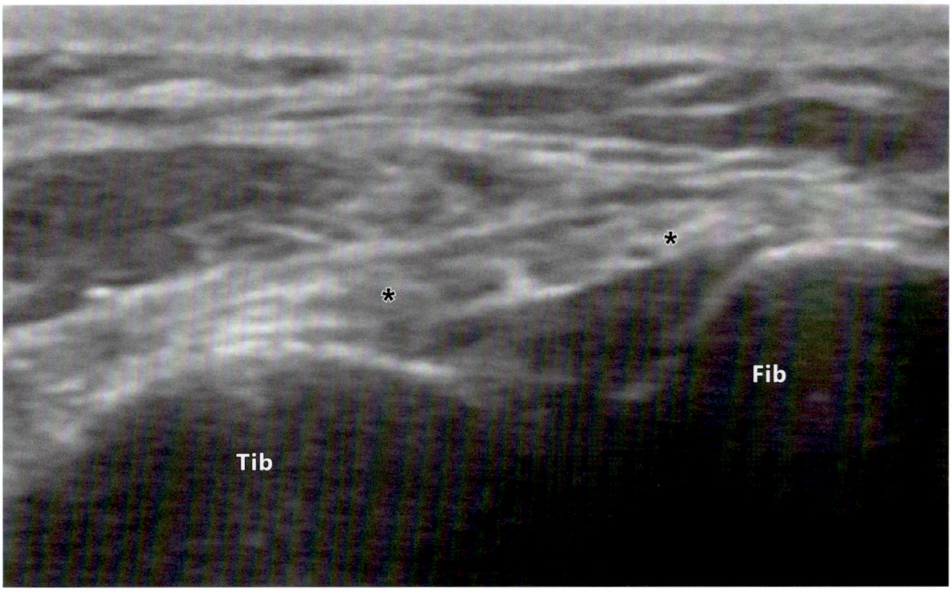

b

Longitudinal US image shows hypoechoic, swollen (*white arrowheads*) and partially torn (*black arrowhead*) anterior tibiofibular ligament (**a**). Normal view (**b**) of the ligament with nice fibrillary appearance (*asterisks*).

Fib fibula
Tib tibia

11.70 Metatarsophalangeal joint osteoarthritis in a 50-year-old man with pain and limitation in the great toe

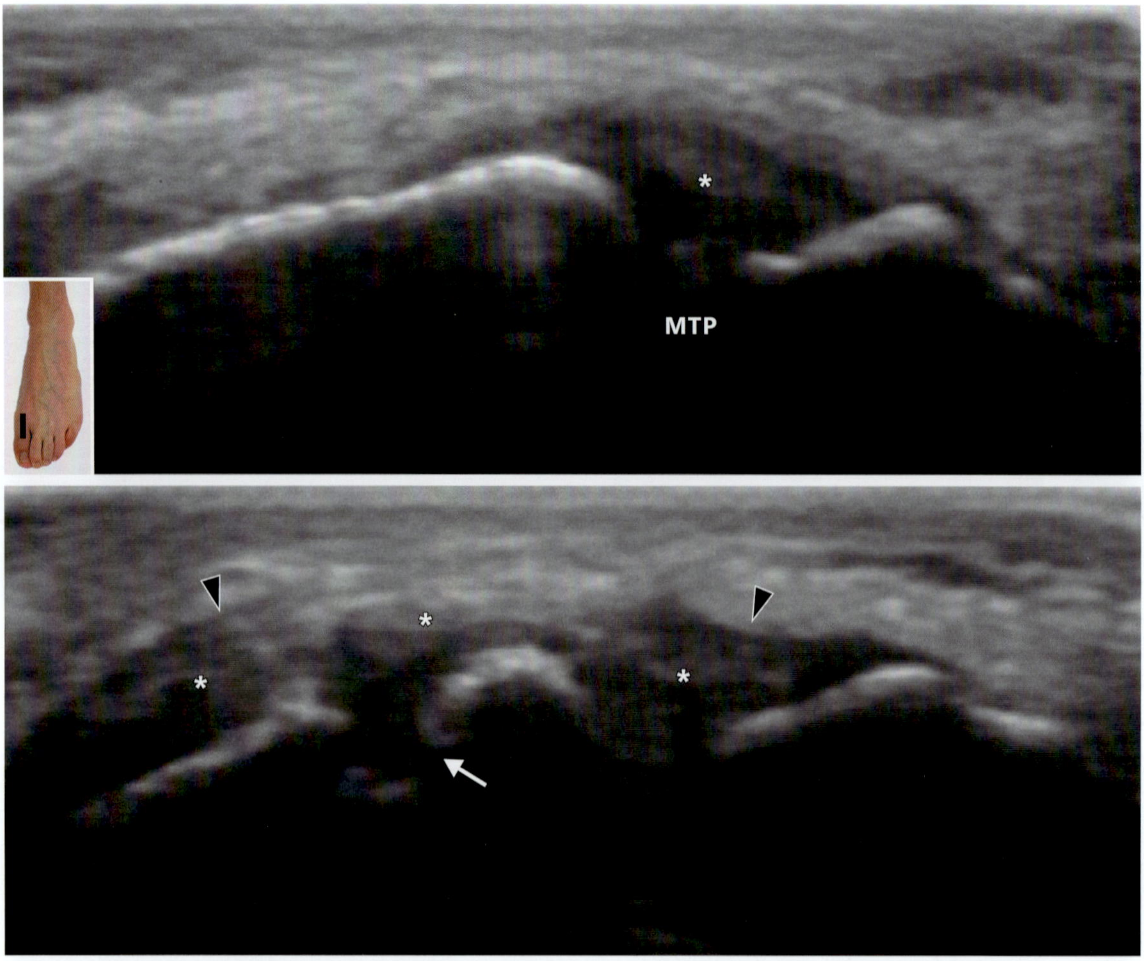

When compared with the asymptomatic side (**a**), longitudinal US image (**b**) of the first metatarsophalangeal joint (**MTP**) shows a markedly distended joint capsule (*arrowheads*) due to synovial hypertrophy (*asterisks*). Note the cortical irregularity (*arrow*) on the metatarsal head.

Expert note

Like elsewhere, finding these cortical irregularities would be quite easy with the use of sonopalpation. This would be quite in contrast to conventional radiographs whereby these lesions can easily be missed.

First metatarsophalangeal joint degenerative osteoarthritis in a 60-year-old man **11.71**

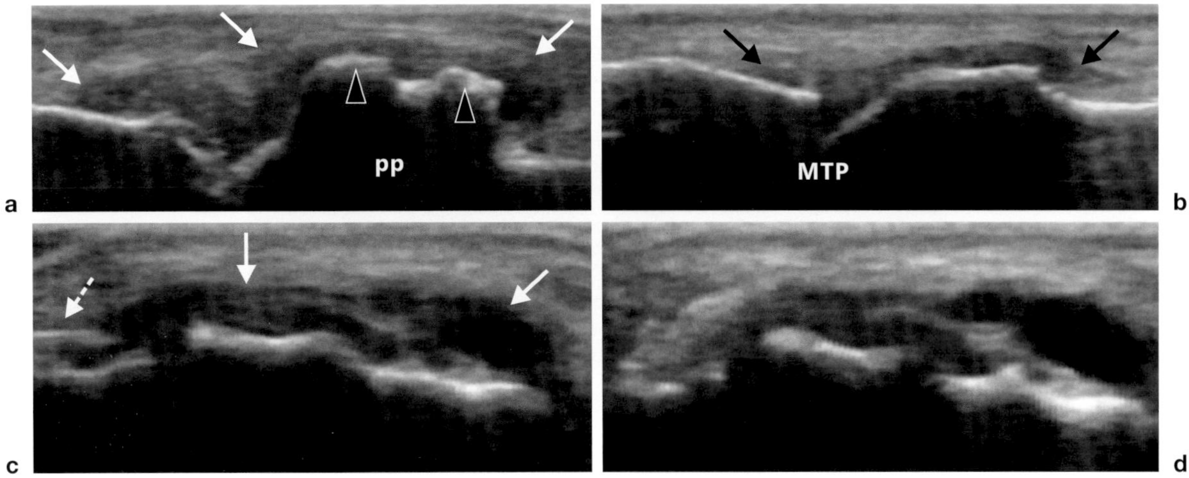

The patient had painful and limited dorsiflexion of the great toe.

Longitudinal US image demonstrates enlargement of the joint capsule (*white arrows*) and osteophytes (*arrowheads*) on the proximal phalanx (**pp**) (**a**). Normal joint capsule (*black arrows*) on the asymptomatic side (**b**). A 26-G needle (*dashed arrow*) can be seen during the US-guided injection of the joint (direct in-plane technique) (**c**). Please also note the hyperechoic appearance of the injectate (corticosteroids) thereafter (**d**).

MTP metatarsophalangeal joint

Expert note

Since these joints are very superficially localized and US can provide precise guidance; it is quite possible that tiny needles can be used during the intervention which would definitely be comfortable for the patient and the physician alike.

11.72 Metatarsophalangeal joint arthritis in a 17-year-old girl diagnosed with juvenile idiopathic arthritis

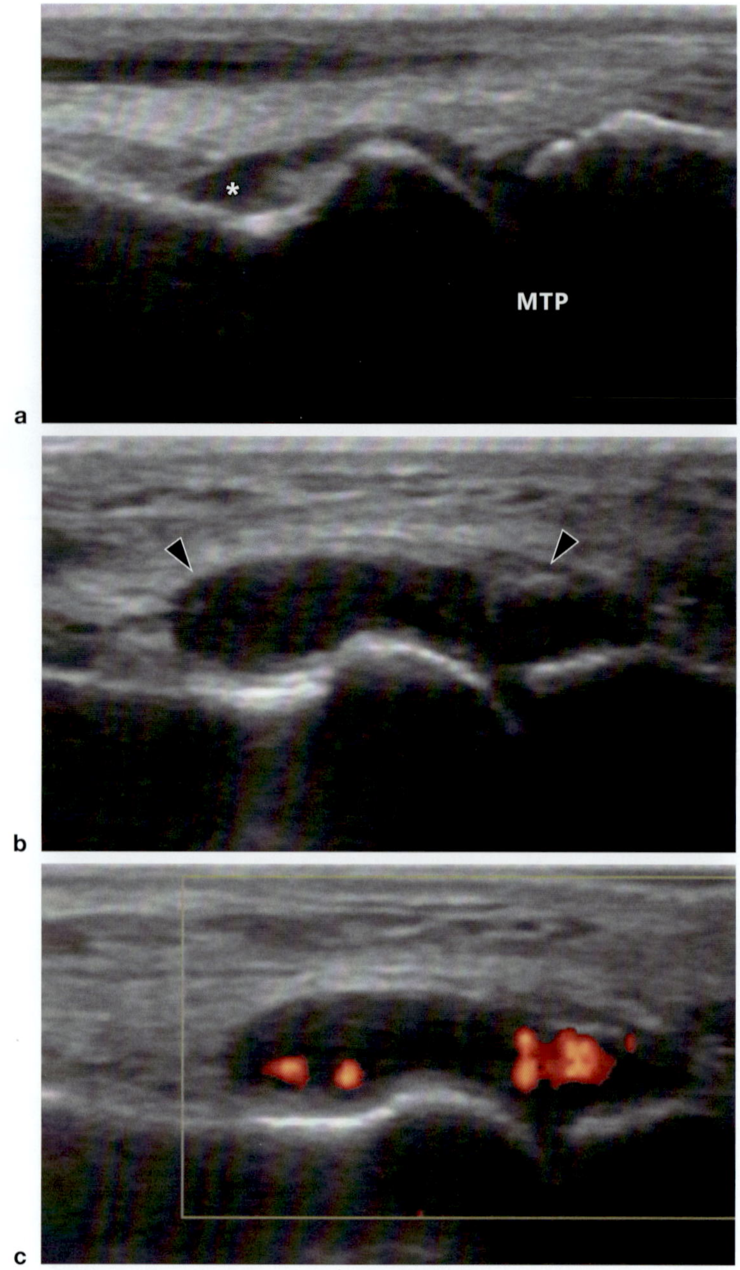

Video 15

When compared with the asymptomatic side including mild fluid (*asterisk*) in the first metatarsophalangeal joint (**MTP**) (**a**), longitudinal US image shows synovial hypertrophy distending the joint capsule (*arrowheads*) (**b**). Power Doppler imaging reveals increased blood flow (Grade II) in the synovial tissue (**c**).

Metatarsophalangeal joint ostheoartritis in an elderly woman with great toe pain and swelling

11.73

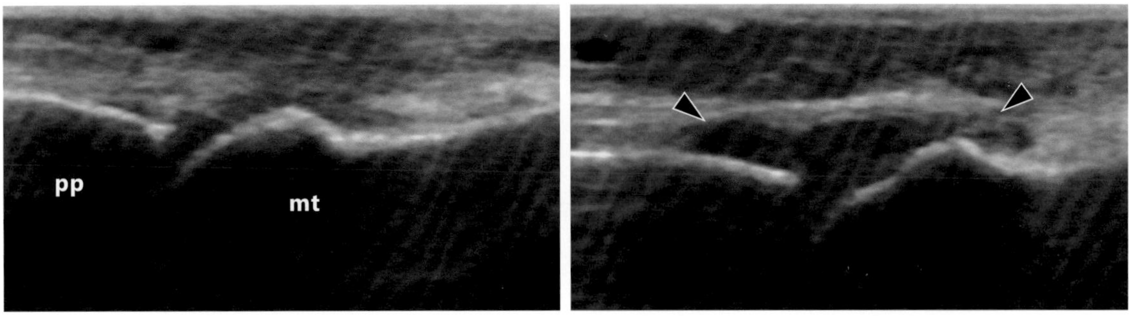

When compared with the normal side (**a**), longitudinal US image of the metatarsophalangeal joint shows a distended joint capsule (*arrowheads*) suggesting non-inflammatory arthritis (**b**).

mt metatarsal bone
pp proximal phalanx

11.74 Tophaceous gout in a 49-year-old man who had pain and soft tissue swelling at the great toe

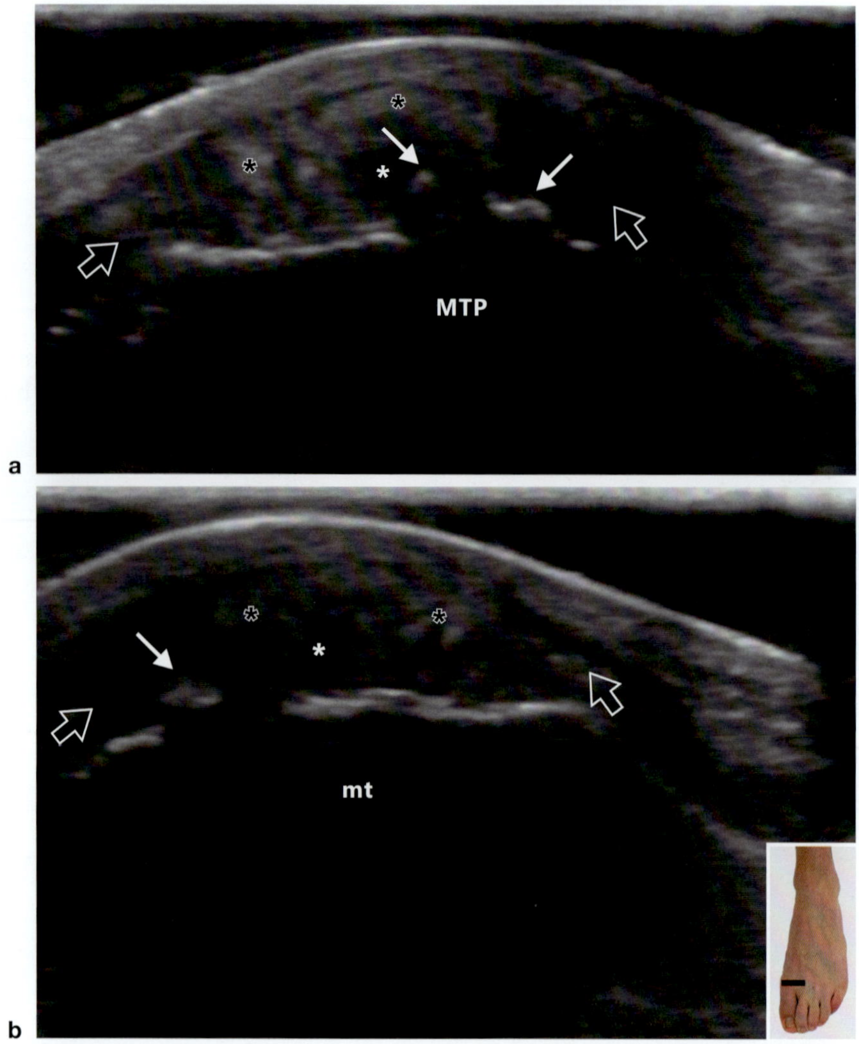

Axial (**a**) and lateral longitudinal (**b**) US images over the first metatarsophalangeal joint (**MTP**) reveal a heterogeneous tophus (*thick arrows*) that contains hypoechoic areas (*white asterisks*) related to chalky liquid material surrounded by hyperechoic tissue (*black asterisks*).
Please also note the degenerative changes in the joint (*thin arrows*).

mt metatarsal bone

Expert note

Due to the significant/possible distortion of the joint morphology, the use of extra gel (or insertion of the foot inside water) is necessary for optimal scanning (as seen in these images).

Degenerative osteoarthritis of the second metatarsophalangeal joint in a 57-year-old man **11.75**

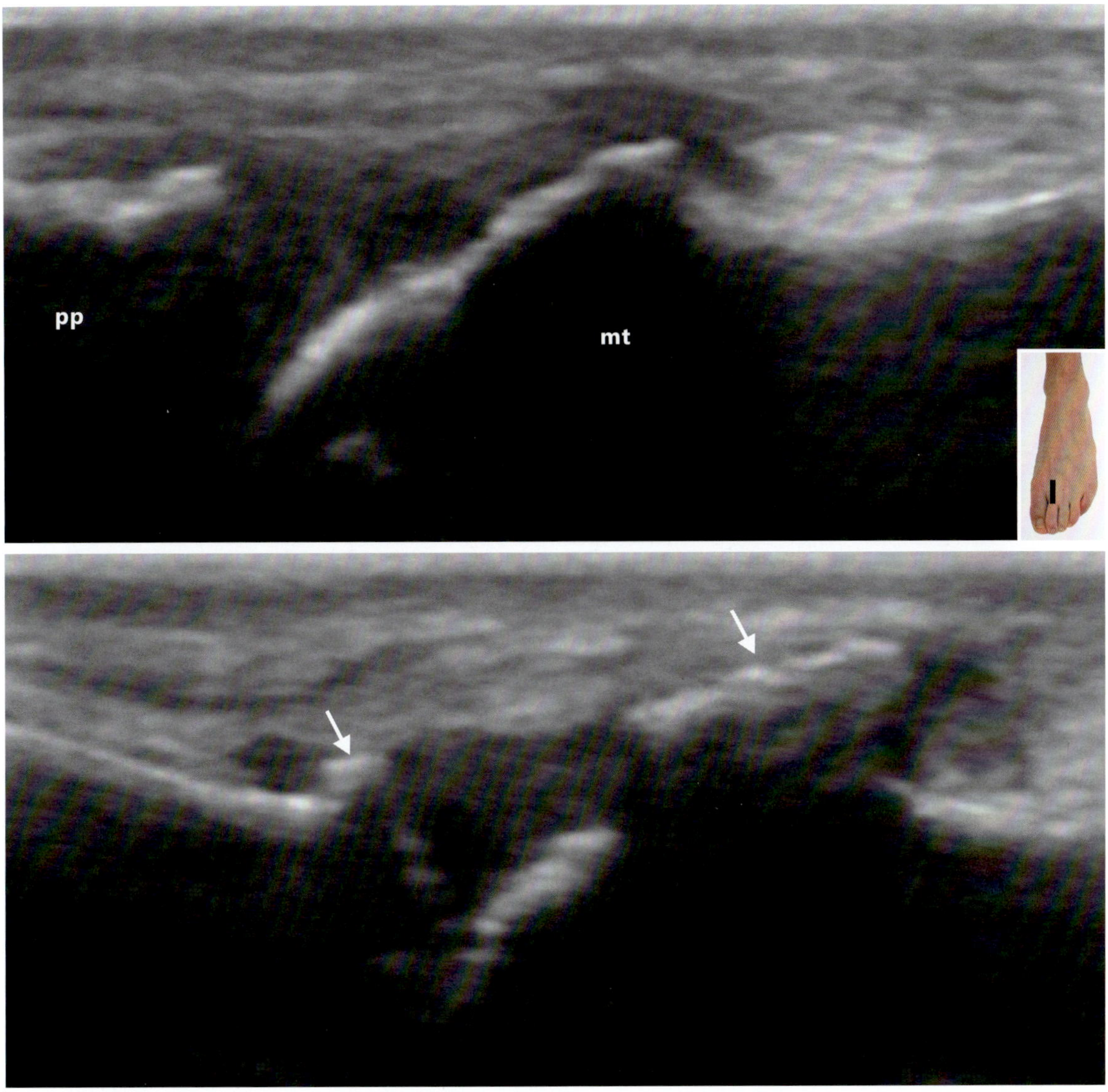

a

b

When compared with the asymptomatic side (**a**), longitudinal US image (**b**) obtained over the dorsal aspect of the 2nd toe reveals osteophytes (*arrows*) on the articular surfaces.

mt metatarsal bone
pp proximal phalanx

11.76 Degenerative osteoarthritis in a 66-year-old woman with foot pain during weight-bearing activities

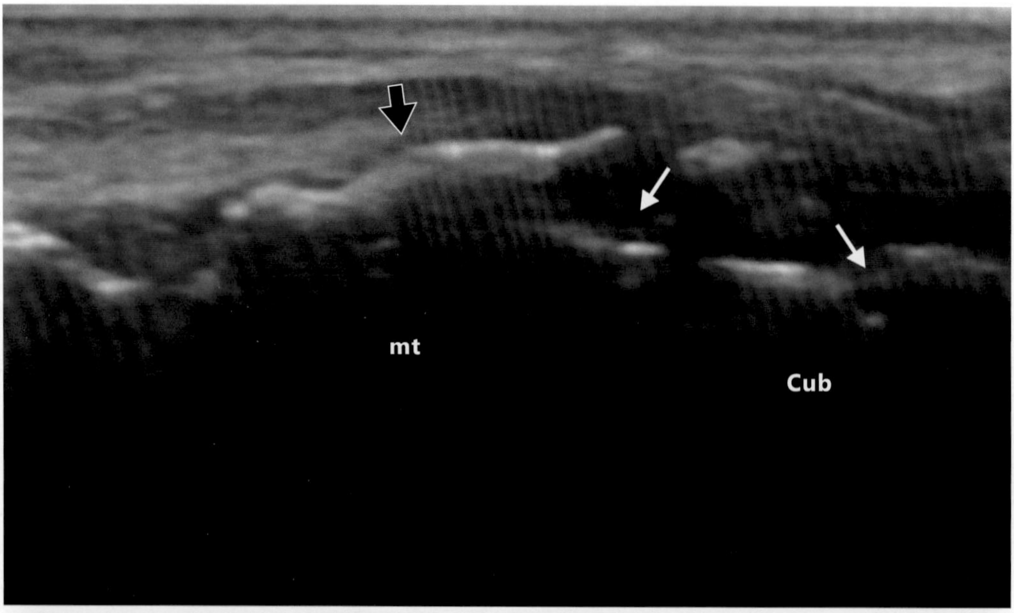

a

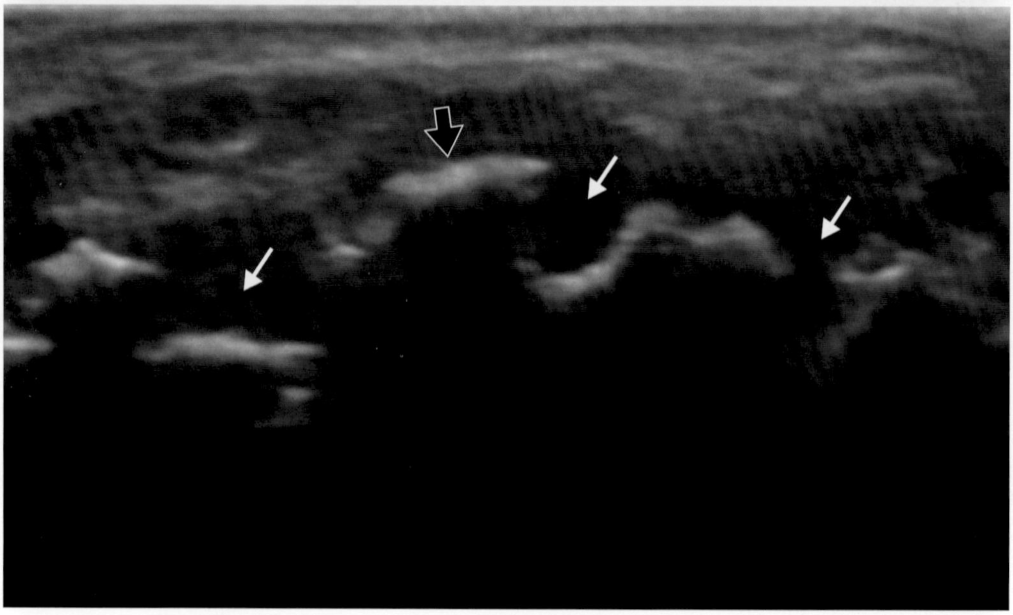

b

Longitudinal (**a**) and axial (**b**) US images show degenerative changes affecting the metatarsal base (**mt**) and cuboid bone (**Cub**) with several/marked osteophytes (*thick arrows*) and erosions (*thin arrows*).

Chronic abductor hallucis longus strain in a 45-year-old obese patient with sole pain

11.77

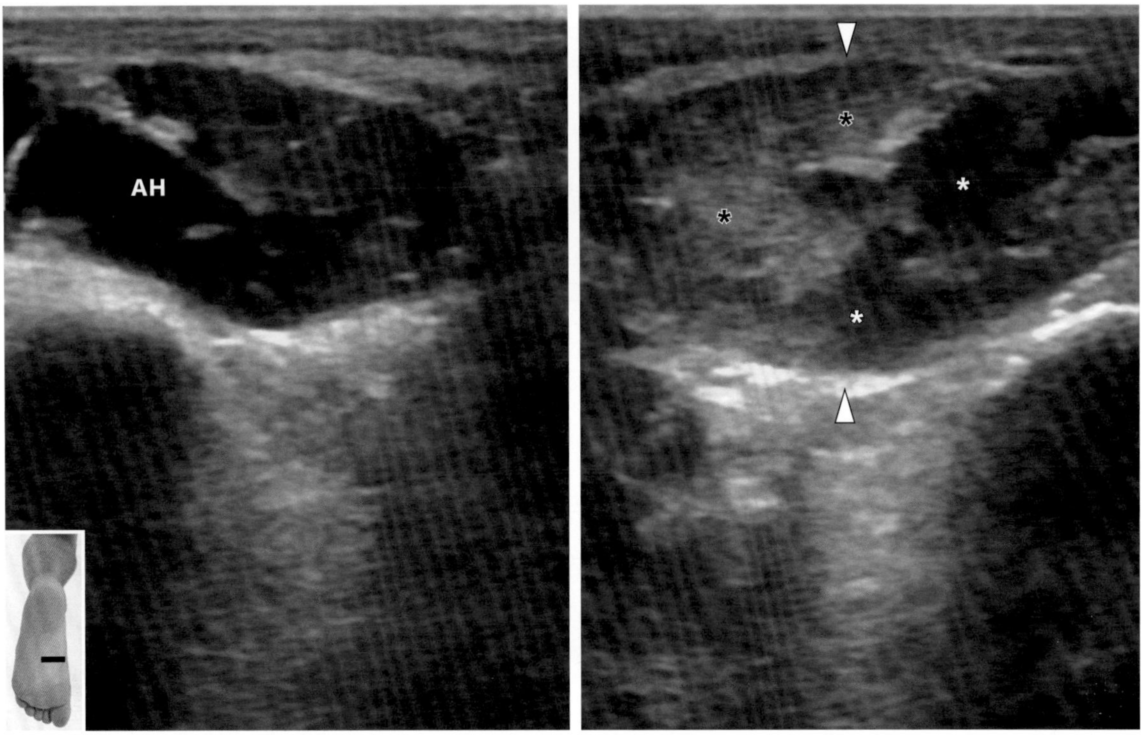

He had pain and swelling inside the medial arch of the foot due to repetitive prolonged walking.

When compared with the normal side (**a**), axial US image (**b**) demonstrates irregularly swollen muscle (*arrowheads*) with heterogenous areas of interstitial edema (*white asterisks*) and incomplete healing process (*black asterisks*).

AH abductor hallucis

11.78 Submetatarsal bursitis in a 45-year-old woman with forefoot pain during weight-bearing

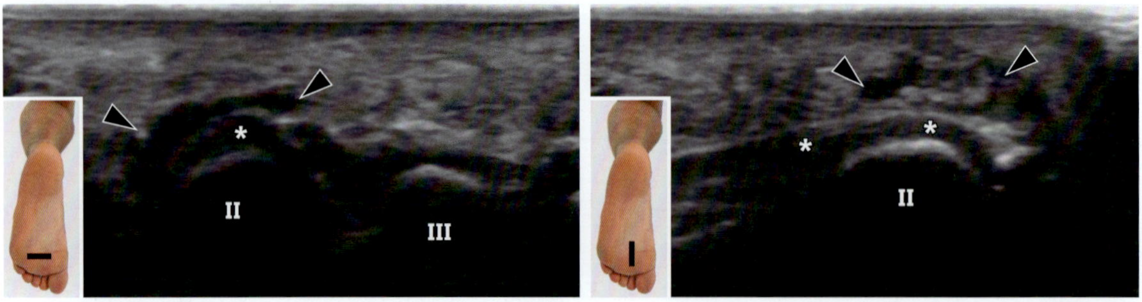

a b

Axial (**a**) and longitudinal (**b**) US images obtained from the plantar approach show bursitis (*arrowheads*) as a heterogenous hypoechoic mass (fluid & synovium) over the second metatarsal head (**II**) and the flexor tendon (*asterisks*).

11.79 Submetatarsal bursitis in a middle-aged woman who had severe pain on walking and during the squeeze test

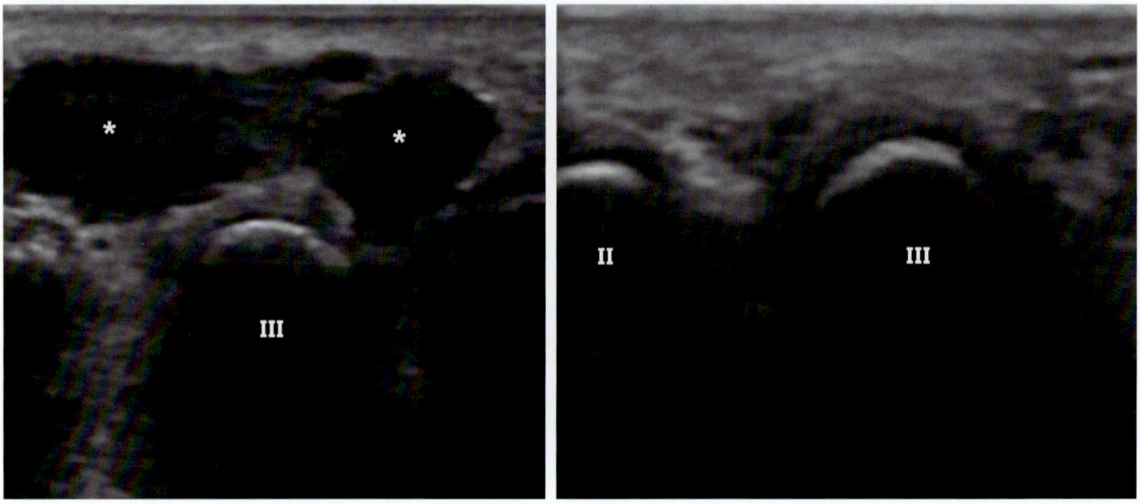

a b

Axial US image obtained from the plantar view (**a**) illustrates hypoechoic fluid distension in the bursa (*asterisks*) overlying the 3rd metatarsal heads (**III**). Normal side (**b**).

Healing metatarsal fracture three months after prolonged walking in a postmenopausal woman **11.80**

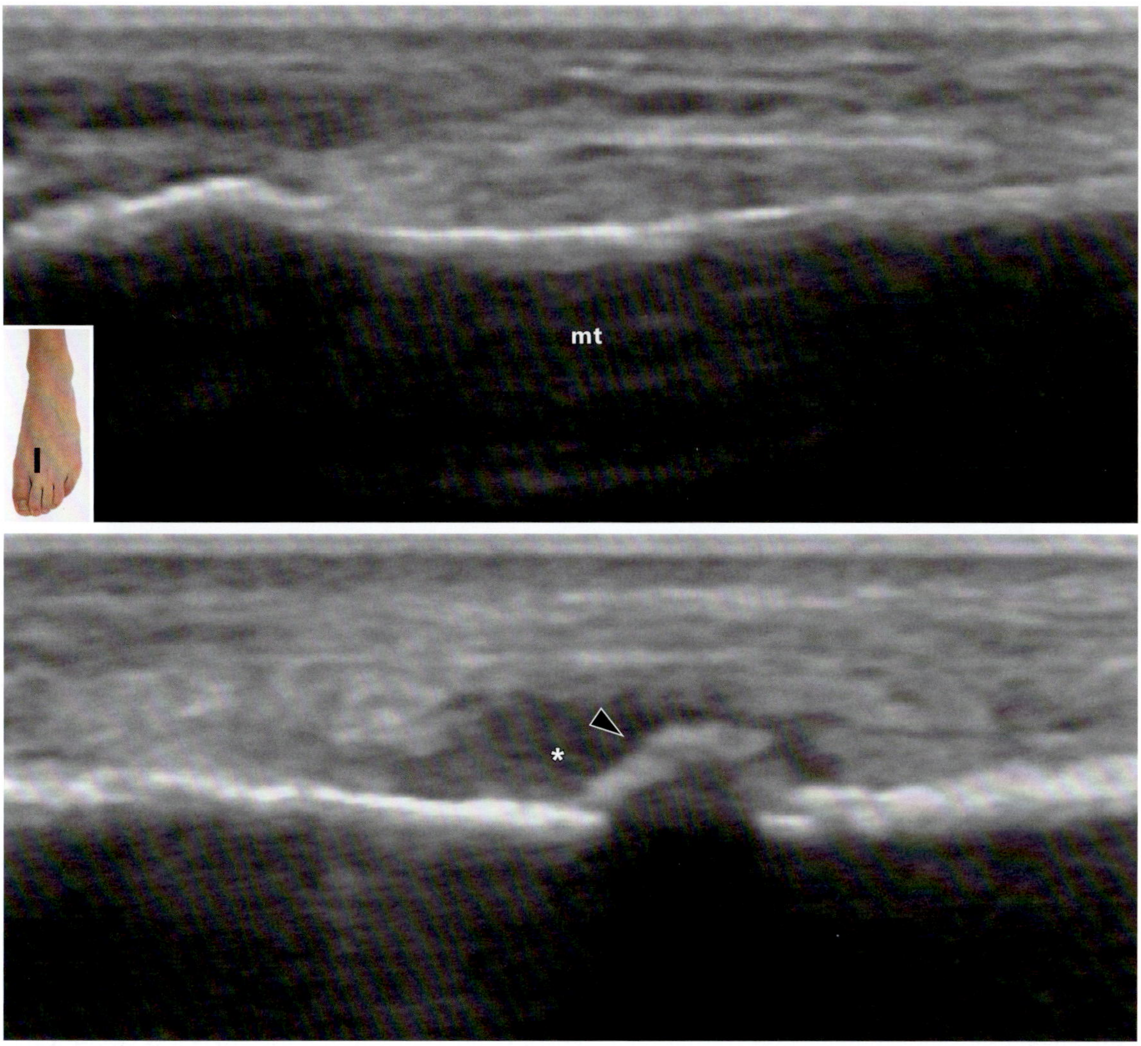

a
b

When compared with the normal side (**a**), longitudinal US image (**b**) depicts a focal periosteal hyperechoic rim (*arrowhead*) surrounded by a small semicircular hypoechoic zone (*asterisk*) on the second metatarsal bone (**mt**).

Expert note

Sono-palpation is again paramount in these cases where X-rays would generally be inconclusive/unremarkable.
In the acute phase, the "micro-massage" during the passage of the probe (without pushing or even palpating) can be enough to elicit pain. In this acute phase, a small interruption of the cortex with overlying edema can be visible.

11.81 Extensor hallucis longus tendinitis in a patient who had recent onset of pain during extension of the great toe

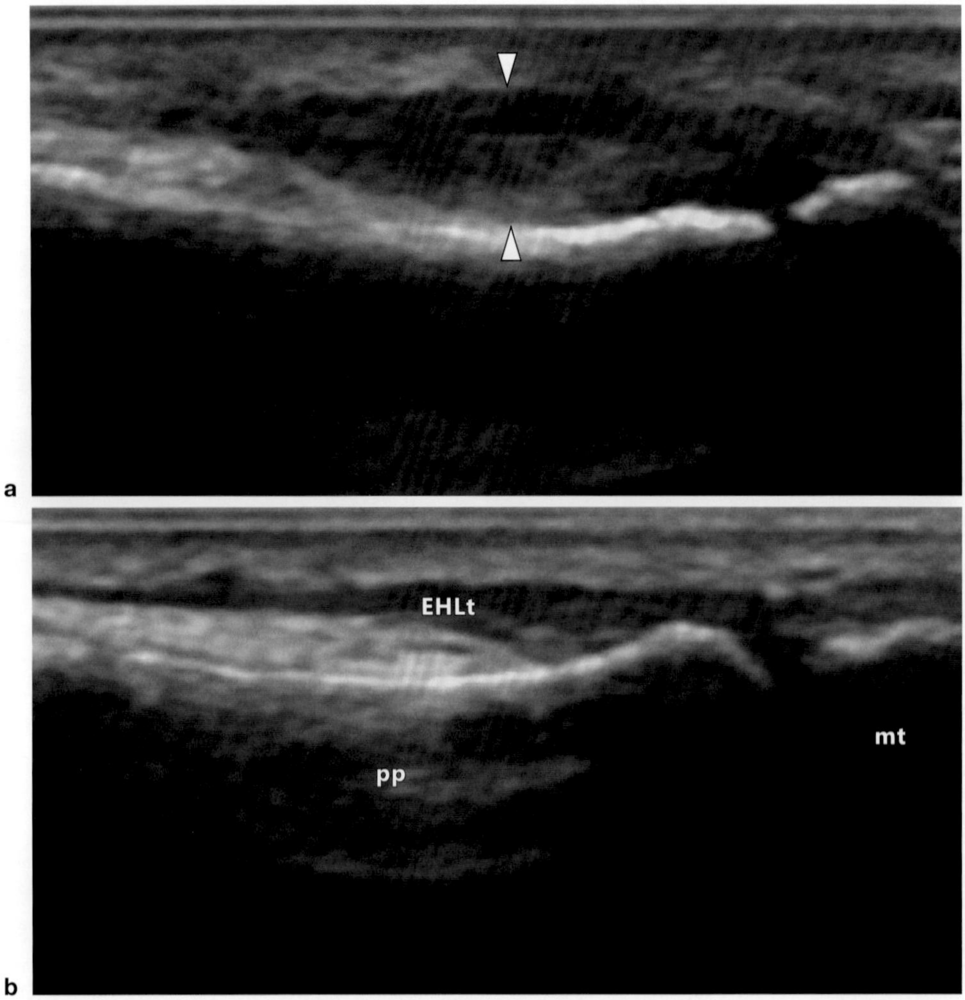

Dorsal longitudinal US image reveals that the extensor hallucis longus tendon (**EHLt**) is swollen and hypoechoic (*arrowheads*) over the proximal phalanx (**pp**) (**a**). Normal contralateral side (**b**).

mt metatarsal bone

Extensor tenosynovitis in a Charcot-Marie-Tooth patient with recurrent inversion injuries **11.82**

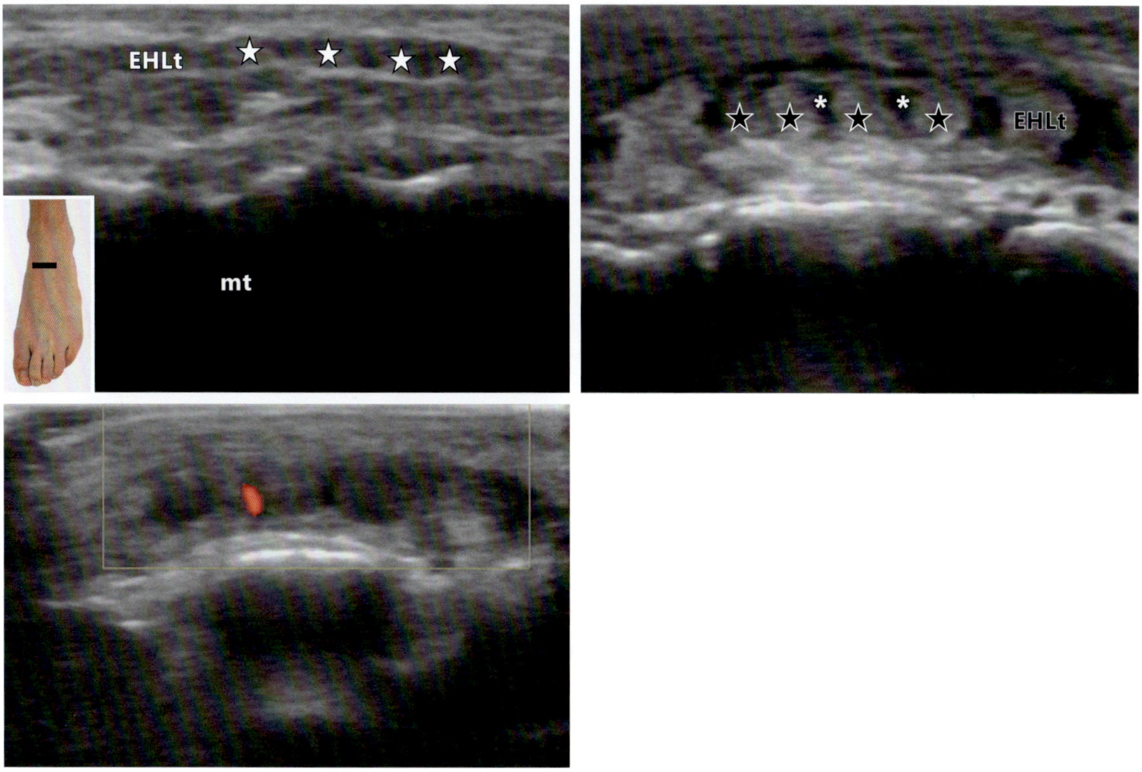

a b c

When compared with the normal side (**a**), axial US images obtained over the dorsal foot demonstrate markedly thickened extensor digitorum longus (*stars*) (**EDLt**) and extensor hallucis longus tendons (**EHLt**) with mild fluid (*asterisks*) (**b**) and hyperemia on power Doppler imaging (**c**).

mt metatarsal bone

11.83 Ganglion cyst in a 65-year-old man with painless lump of the great toe

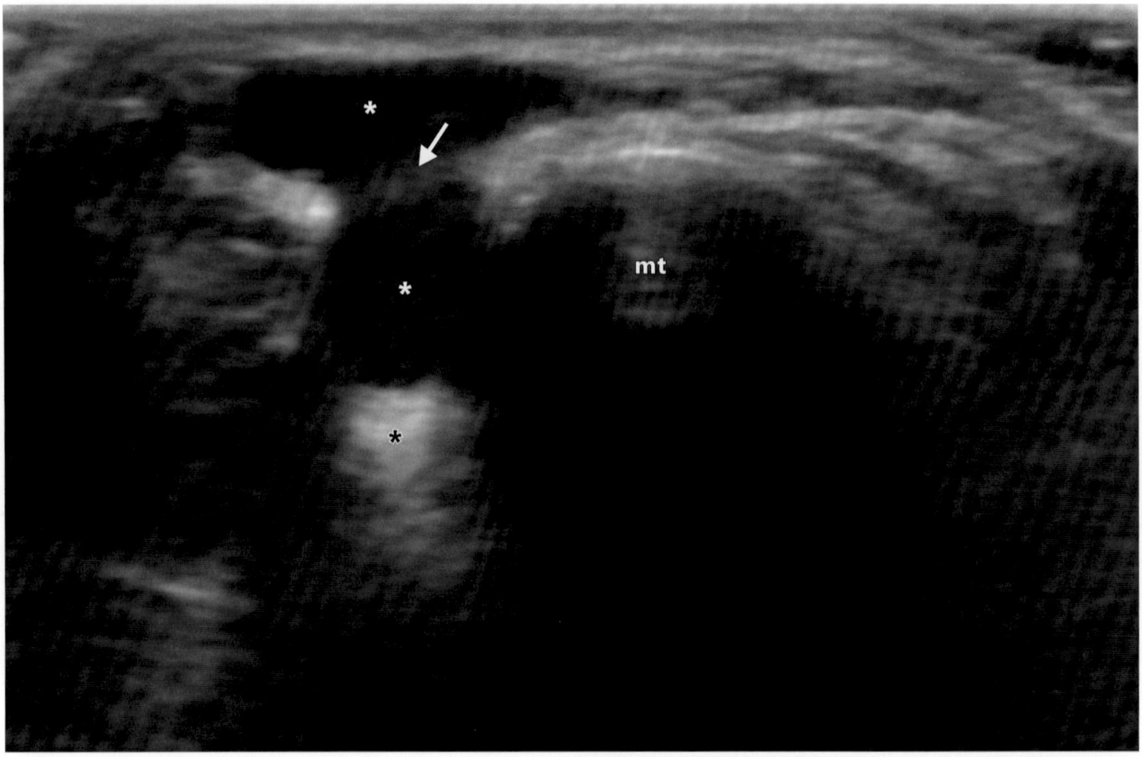

Axial US image on the dorsal aspect of the first metatarsal bone (**mt**) shows a lobulated ganglion cyst (*white asterisks*) with an internal septum (*arrow*). Note the enhanced through transmission artifact (*black asterisk*).

REFERENCES

1. Schmidt WA, Schönau V, Reiche BE, Oberdorfer PD, Ohrndorf S, Backhaus M. Grading of ultrasound Doppler signals in synovitis: does it need an update? Rheumatology (Oxford). 2015; 54: 1897-903.
2. Martinoli C, Bianchi S. Ankle: Bianchi S, Martinoli C, editors. Ultrasound of the musculoskeletal system. Berlin: Springer; 2007. p. 773-834.
3. Nazarian LN, Rawool NM, Martin CE et al. Synovial fluid in the hindfoot and ankle: detection of amount and distribution with US. Radiology 1995; 197: 275-8.
4. Sabir N, Demirlenk S, Yagci B, Karabulut N, Cubukcu S. Clinical utility of sonography in diagnosing plantar fasciitis. J Ultrasound Med. 2005; 24: 1041-8.
5. Fessell DP, Van Holsbeeck M. Sonography of the Ankle and Foot. In: Van Holsbeeck M, Introcaso JH (editors). Musculoskeletal ultrasound. 2nd ed. St Louis: Mosby, 2001. p.605-24.
6. Kane D, Greaney T, Shananhan M, Duffy G, Bresnihan B, Gibney R. The role of ultrasonography in the diagnosis and management of idiopathic plantar fasciitis. Rheumatology (Oxford). 2001; 40: 1002-8.
7. Walther M, Radke S, Kirschner S, Ettl V, Gohlke F. Power Doppler findings in plantar fasciitis. Ultrasound Med Biol. 2004; 30: 435-40.
8. Çapkın E, Karakucak M. Ultrasound evaluation of the ankle and foot. In: Özçakar L, De Muynck M, editors. Musculoskeletal ultrasound in physical and rehabilitation medicine. Milan: Edi.Ermes; 2014. p. 111-21.
9. Bianchi S, Martinoli C. Foot. In: Bianchi S, Martinoli C, editors. Ultrasound of the musculoskeletal system. Berlin: Springer; 2007. p. 835-89.
10. Hua Y, Yang Y, Chen S, Cai Y. Ultrasound examination for the diagnosis of chronic anterior talofibular ligament injury. Acta Radiol. 2012; 53: 1142-5.
11. Cheng Y, Cai Y, Wang Y. Value of ultrasonography for detecting chronic injury of the lateral ligaments of the ankle joint compared with ultrasonography findings. Br J Radiol. 2014; 87: 20130406.
12. Özçakar L, Kara M, Chang KV, Bayram Çarli A, Hung CY, Tok F, et al. EURO-MUSCULUS/USPRM basic scanning protocols for ankle and foot. Eur J Phys Rehabil Med. 2015; 51: 647-53.

Section 4
NERVES

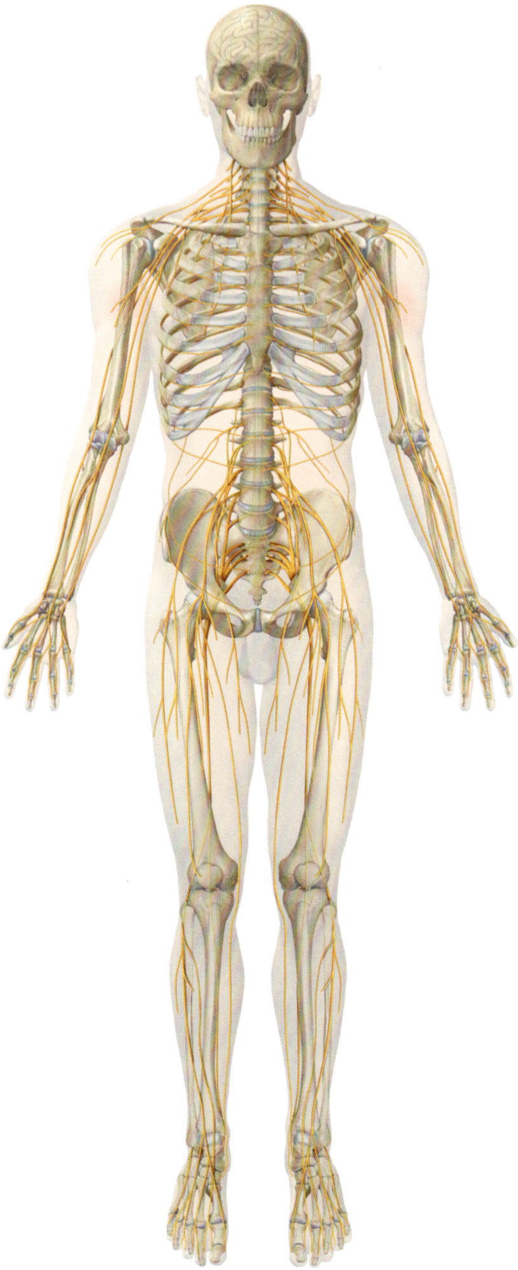

Nerves 12

- **Optic nerve**
- **Brachial plexus**
- **Suprascapular nerve**
- **Long thoracic nerve**
- **Radial nerve**
- **Posterior interosseous nerve**
- **Ulnar nerve**
- **Median nerve**
- **Lateral femoral cutaneous nerve**
- **Sciatic nerve**
- **Tibial nerve** - Popliteal
- **Common fibular nerve**
- **Superficial fibular nerve**
- **Tibial nerve** - Ankle
- **Sural nerve**
- **Interdigital nerve** - Foot

12.1 Normal eye view of a 40-year-old man

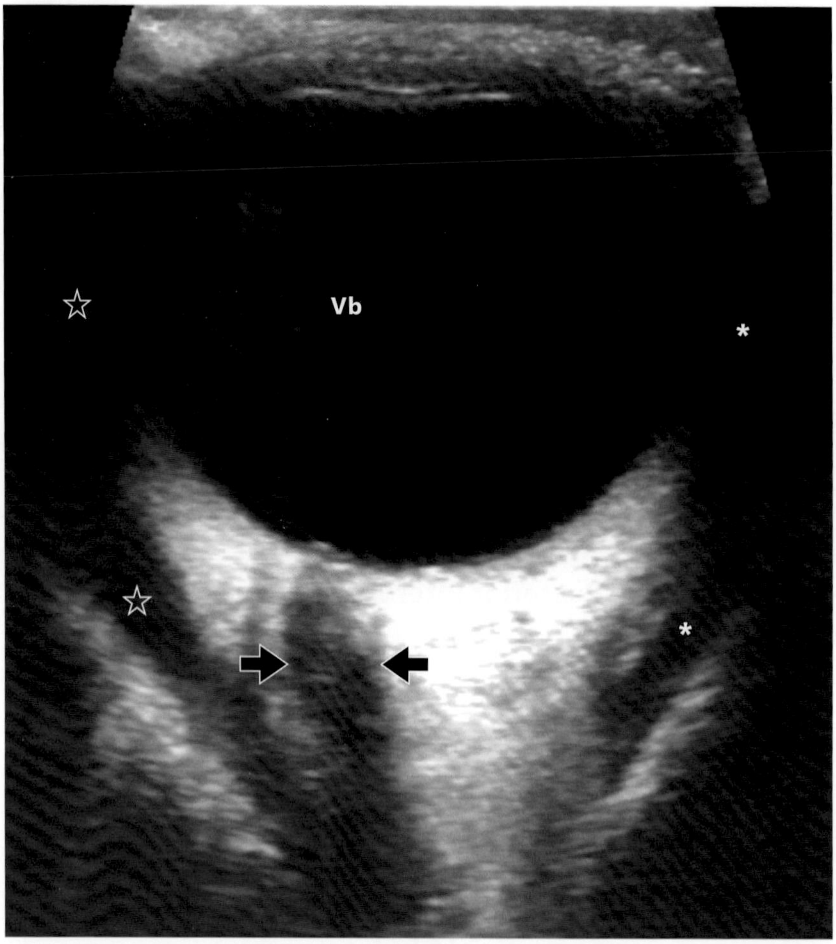

Axial US image reveals rectus medialis (*stars*) and rectus lateralis (*asterisks*) muscles and the optic nerve (*arrows*).

Vb vitreous body

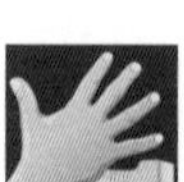

Expert note

Peripheral nerve imaging using US is not only limited to the extremities i.e. the general rule of "anything outside the bone can be visualized" is also applicable here.
Closing the eye lid and using enough gel (while the patient is lying supine) is very convenient for optic nerve imaging. Main clinical indication is increased intracranial pressure whereby detection of edema around the optic nerve is incomparable to any other imaging modality. Yet, especially in children, the clinical scenario is an important emergency which is otherwise very difficult to technically diagnose.

Radiation induced brachial plexopathy in a 48-year-old patient with lymphoma

12.2

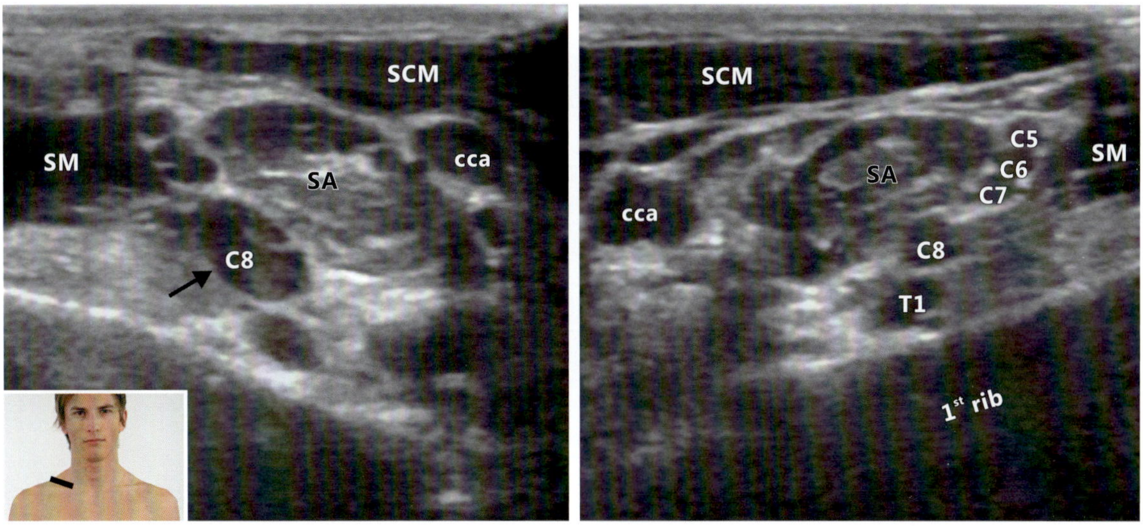

Axial US image over the interscalene region shows edematous roots (C5-T1), particularly at the C8 nerve root (*arrow*) (**a**). Normal brachial plexus view between the scalenus anterior (**SA**) and medius (**SM**) muscles (**b**).

cca common carotid artery
sa subclavian artery
SCM sternocleidomastoid
SP scalenus posterior

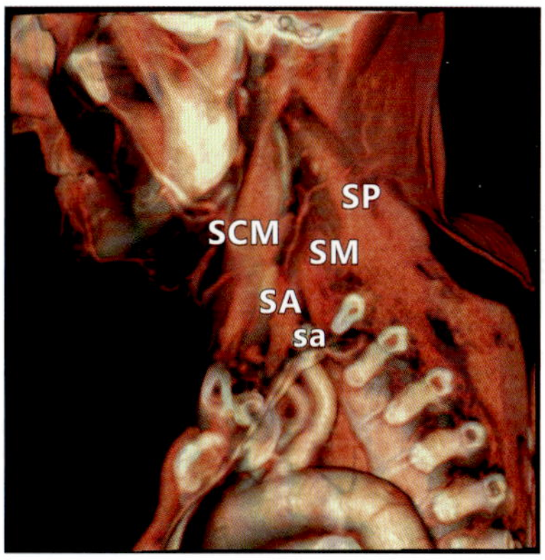

Expert note

Imaging of the brachial plexus starting from the root level is possible in the supraclavicular region and distally thereafter. Like in many other peripheral nerve problems, the morphological changes in the nerve or the related soft tissue problems can readily be scanned with US imaging. The use of "sono-Tinel" would, for sure, be of much additional value [1].

12.3 Parsonage-Turner syndrome in a 54-year-old man with sudden severe shoulder pain

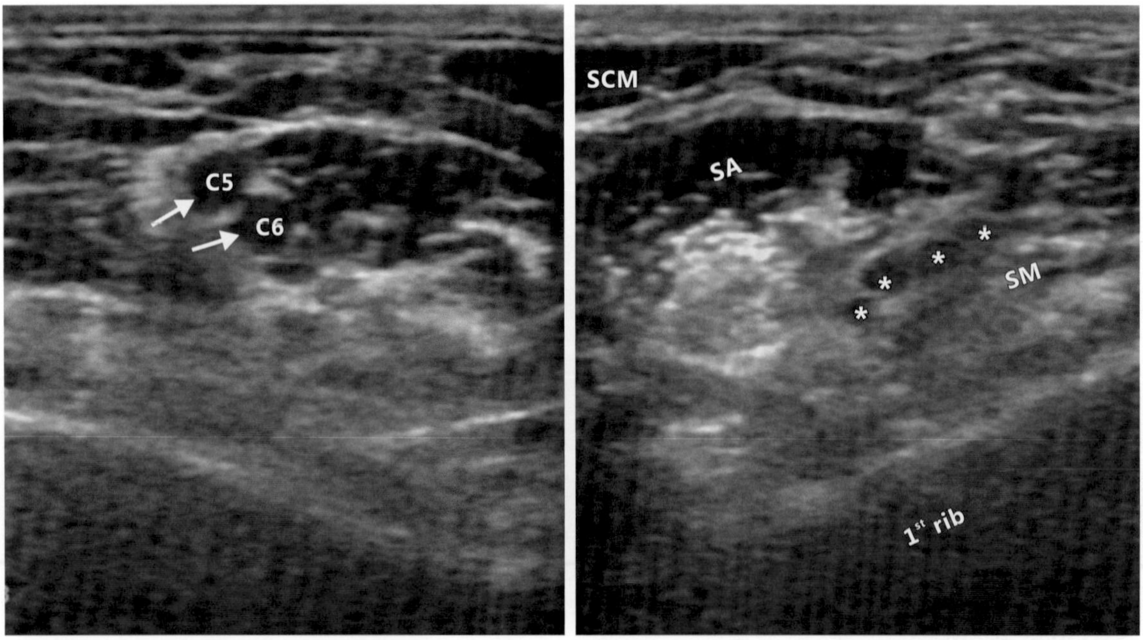

a b

The pain was followed by muscle weaknesses in the shoulder girdle and upper arm.

Axial US image obtained over the interscalene region shows edematous upper trunk of the brachial plexus (*arrows*) (**a**). Contralateral side with normal brachial plexus view (*asterisks*) (**b**).

SA scalenus anterior
SCM sternocleidomastoid
SM scalenus medius

Brachial plexopathy in a 47-year-old woman who had a 3-month history of ovarian cancer without radiation therapy **12.4**

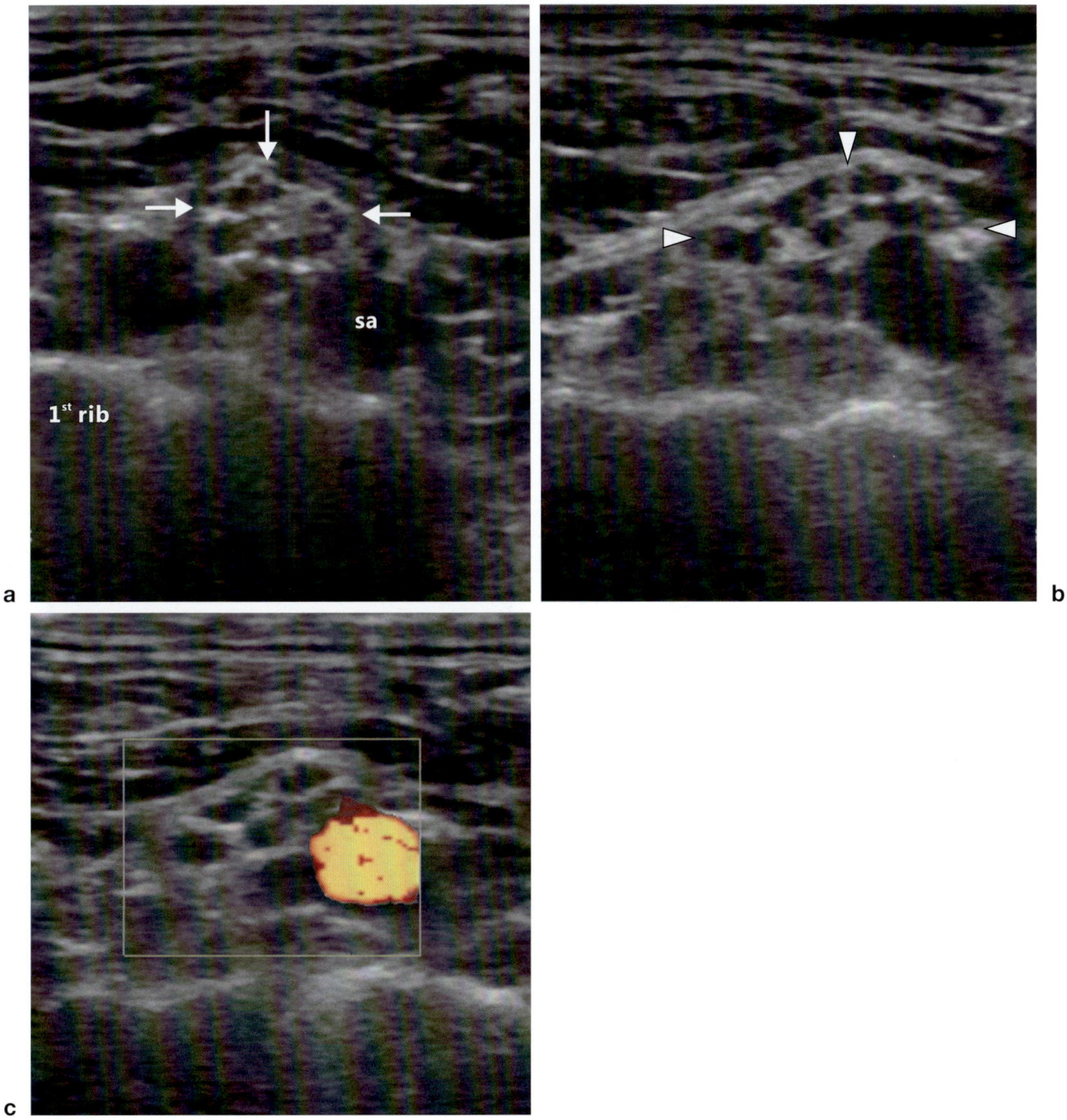

She presented with complaints of burning-like pain and weakness in the arm during the day.

When compared with normal view of the brachial plexus (*arrows*) on the healthy side (**a**), axial US scan over the brachial plexus demonstrates swelling of nerve trunks/fascicles (*arrowheads*) as they course superficial to the subclavian artery (**sa**) (**b**). Power Doppler image demonstrates the normal arterial flow without any involvement of the plexus (**c**).

12.5 Imaging for suprascapular nerve blockage in a 44-year-old woman patient with painful adhesive capsulitis

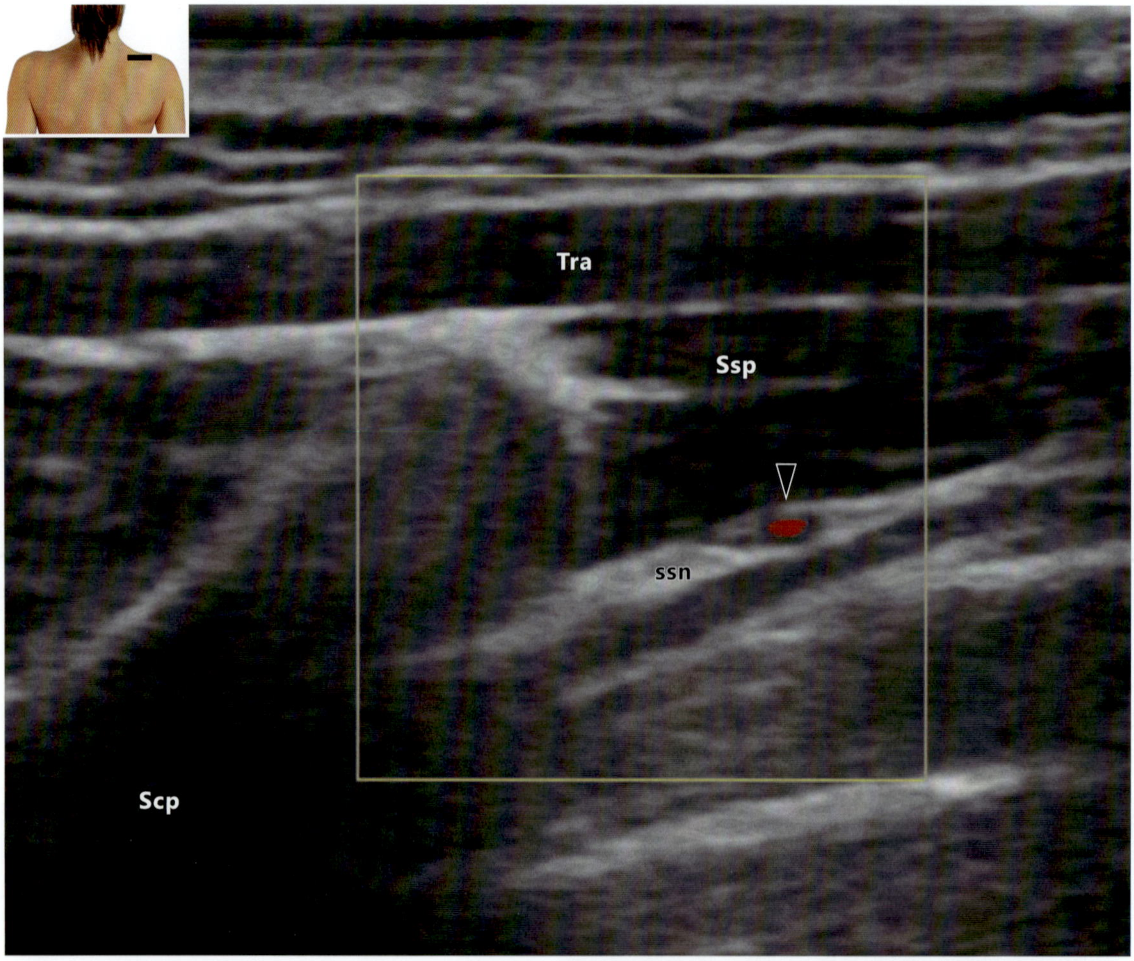

Axial Doppler US image obtained over the posterior shoulder demonstrates the suprascapular artery (*arrowhead*) and the adjacent suprascapular nerve (**ssn**).

Scp scapula
Ssp supraspinatus
Tra trapezius

Expert note

Like elsewhere, detection of the accompanying artery/vessel using Doppler imaging is always helpful for localizing the peripheral nerve of interest.

Long thoracic nerve injury in a 28-year-old hairdresser who presented with difficulty of elevating her arm after weight training

12.6

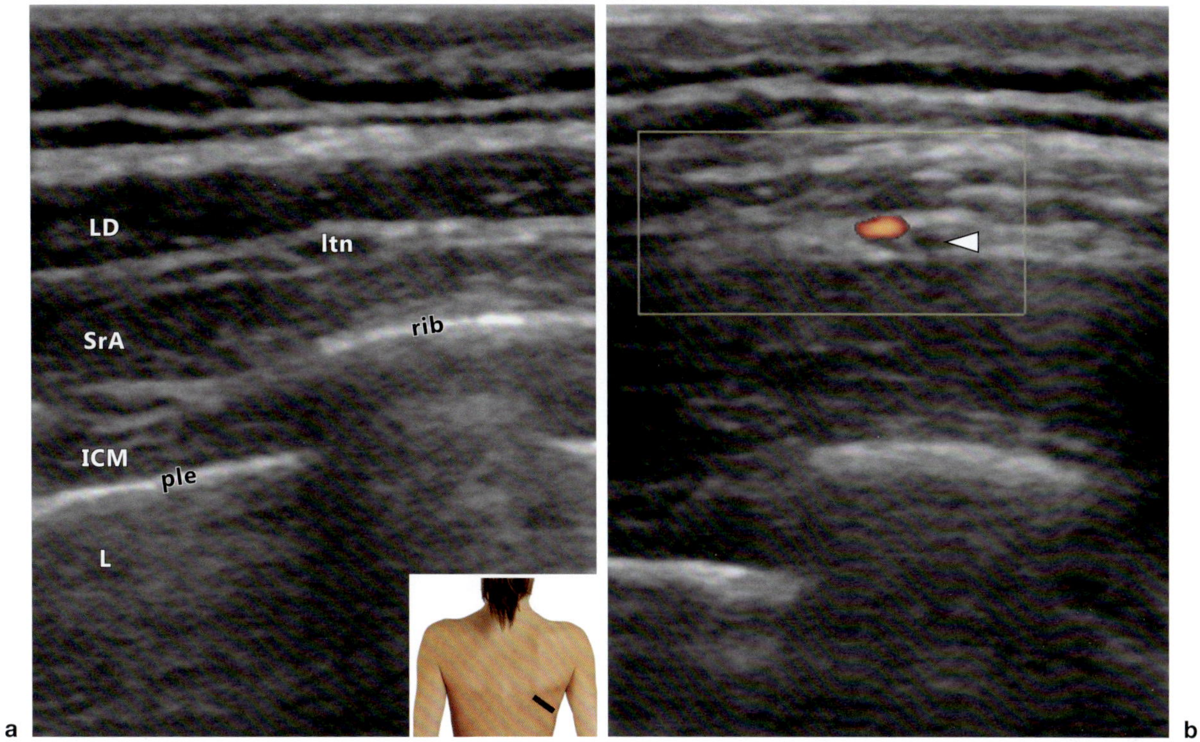

Axial US image illustrates edematous swelling of the long thoracic nerve (*arrowhead*) (**a**) and its close relationship with the thoracodorsal artery at power Doppler imaging (**b**).

ICM	intercostal muscle
L	lung
LD	latissimus dorsi
ple	pleura
SrA	serratus anterior

Expert note

Not only for particular nerves but in general; the sonographer only finds what he/she is looking for and that is only what he/she knows. Accordingly, it is important to keep in mind that unless inside/under a bone, any structure can be seen using US imaging with optimal technical settings.

12.7 Radial nerve entrapment in a 33-year-old woman who frequently uses computer

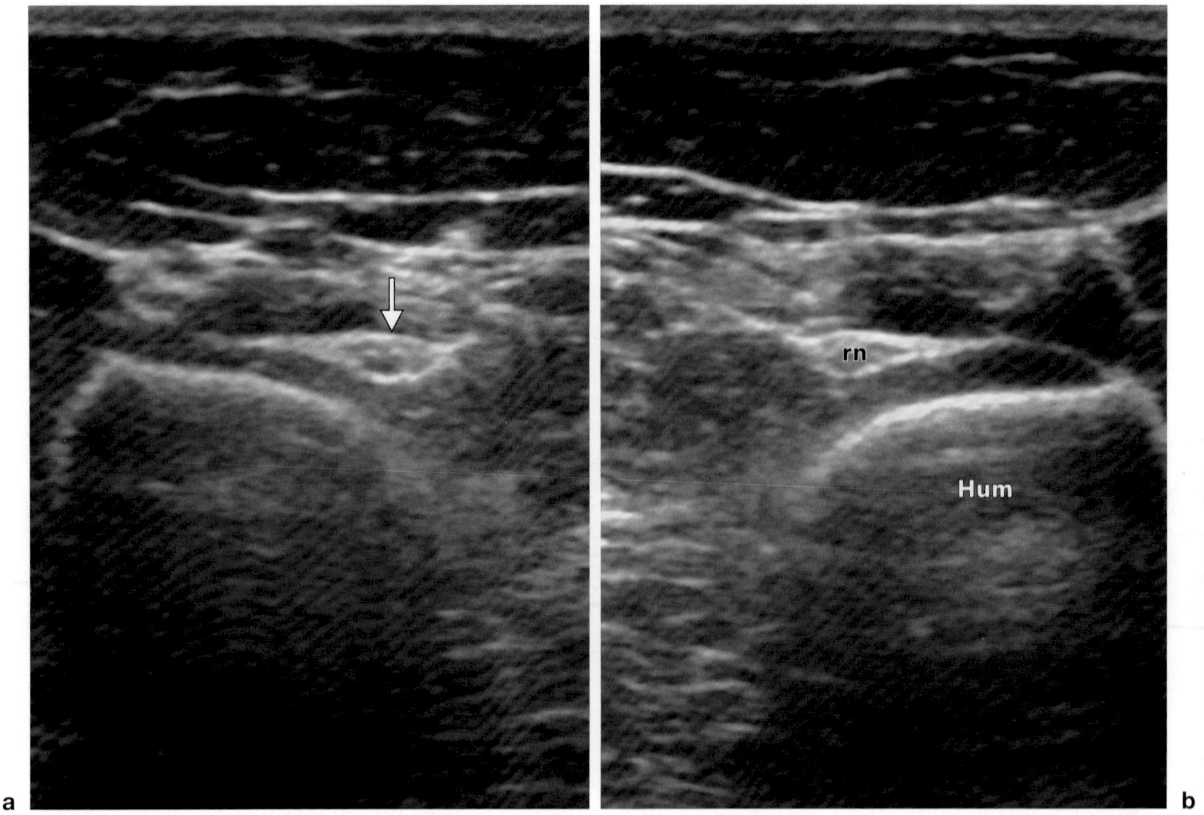

Axial US image over the spiral groove demonstrates mild edema and swelling of the radial nerve (*arrow*) (**a**). On the contralateral normal side, the radial nerve (**rn**) shows a relatively normal hyperechoic appearance at the same level.

Hum humerus

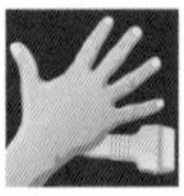

Expert note

No need to mention that (mild) swelling in a peripheral nerve might not always indicate a dysfunction; electrophysiological assessment is always complementary [2].

A 13-year-old boy had limitations in the range of motion at the elbow joint after a humeral shaft fracture

12.8

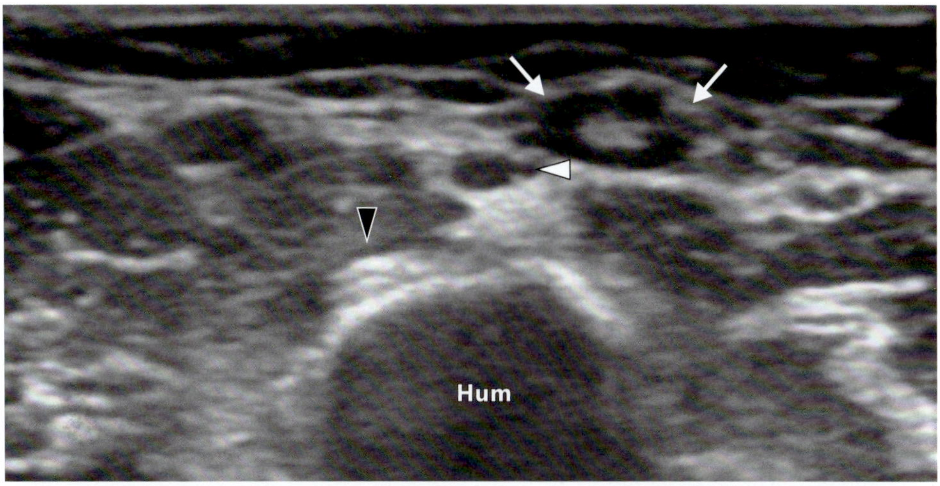

a

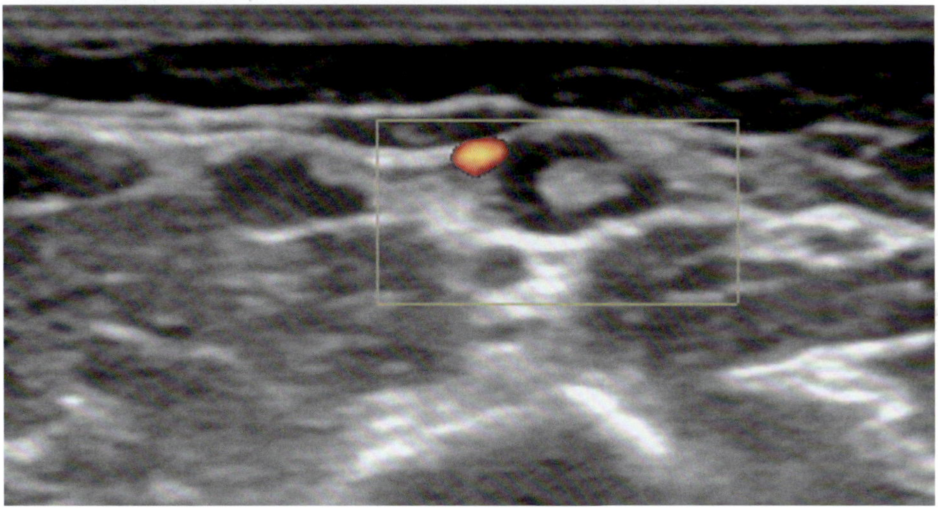

b

Axial US image obtained over the spiral groove shows the localization of the radial nerve (*white arrowhead*) in between the cortical callus (*black arrowhead*) and a nearby lymph node (*arrows*) (**a**). Power Doppler shows the vascular entry into the lymph node (**b**).

Hum humerus

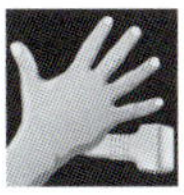

Expert note

One of the superiorities of US imaging for peripheral nerve entrapments is the possibility to uncover the precise relationship between the nerves and the surrounding structures [3]. In this case, although the patient is currently asymptomatic, there seems to be two potential factors to cause an irritation on the radial nerve.

12.9 Radial nerve injury after humeral shaft fracture in a 28-year-old man

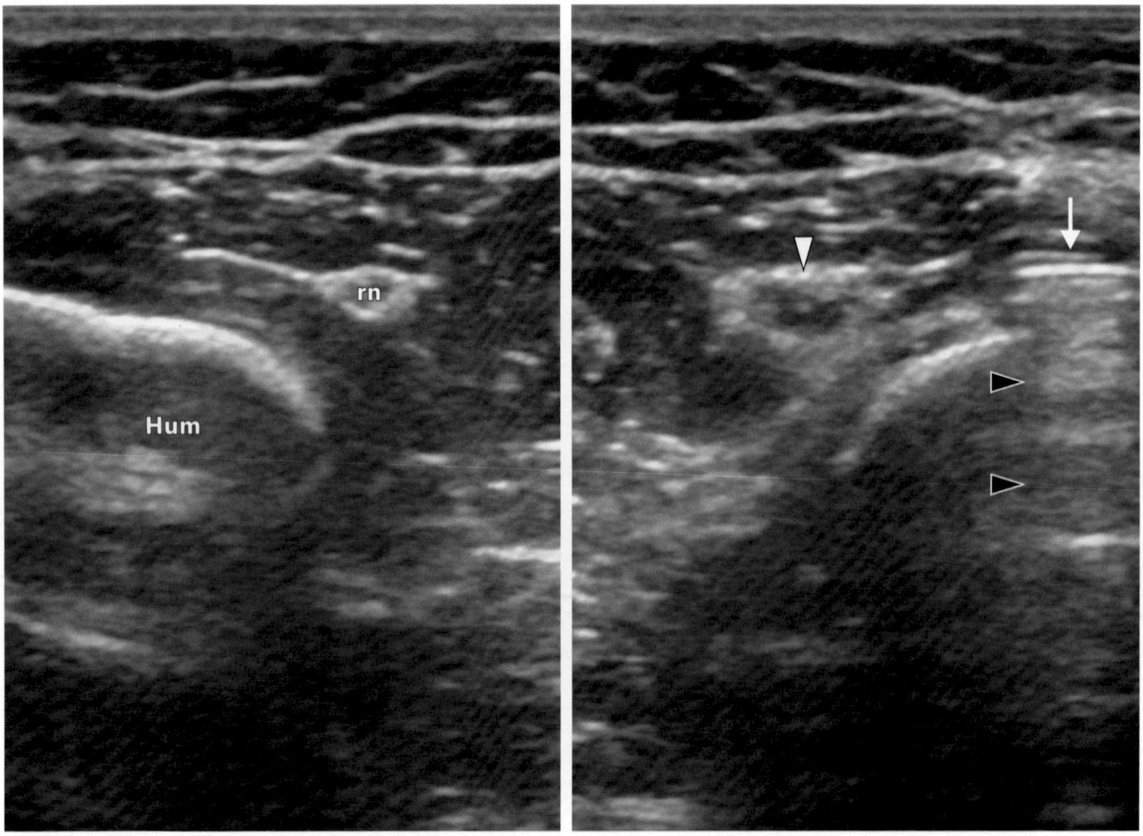

a b

The patient had complaints of pain and numbness at the dorsal side of the hand.

Video 16

When compared with the normal radial nerve (**rn**) (**a**), axial US image obtained over the mid-arm level illustrates that the radial nerve (*white arrowhead*) is more hypoechoic and enlarged. Please note the metal plaque (*arrow*) and its comet-tail artifact (*black arrowheads*).

Hum humerus

Expert note

Aside from static imaging, dynamic scanning from proximal to distal (using sono-Tinel) and also during particular movements of the extremity (especially during which the patient describes symptoms) is always possible and definitely enlightening with US [4]. Further, in postoperative cases like this one, relevant findings might/need to guide the surgeon as well.

Radial nerve injury in a 38-year-old man who had weakness of wrist extension after an antecedent surgery for humerus fracture **12.10**

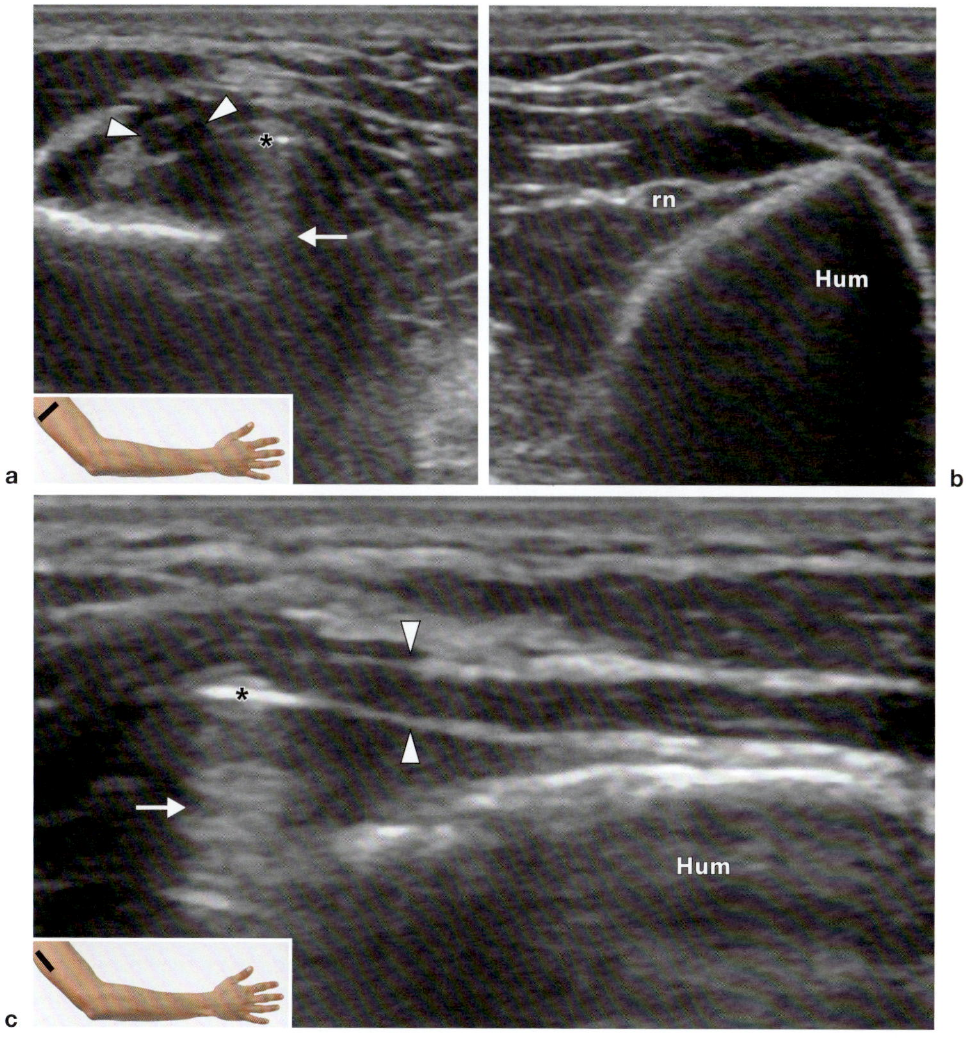

Axial (**a**) and longitudinal (**c**) US images demonstrate the metallic pin (*asterisks*) as bright straight echoes with comet-tail artifacts (*arrows*) together with (and very close to the) swollen and hypoechoic (*arrowheads*) radial nerve (**rn**). Normal side (**b**).

Hum humerus

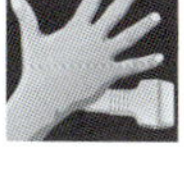

Expert note

Surgeons usually want to know if there is continuity of the nerve or what exactly the relation with the fracture/osteosynthesis material is.

12.11 Radial nerve entrapment in the spiral groove after repair of a midshaft fracture of the humerus in a 50-year-old man

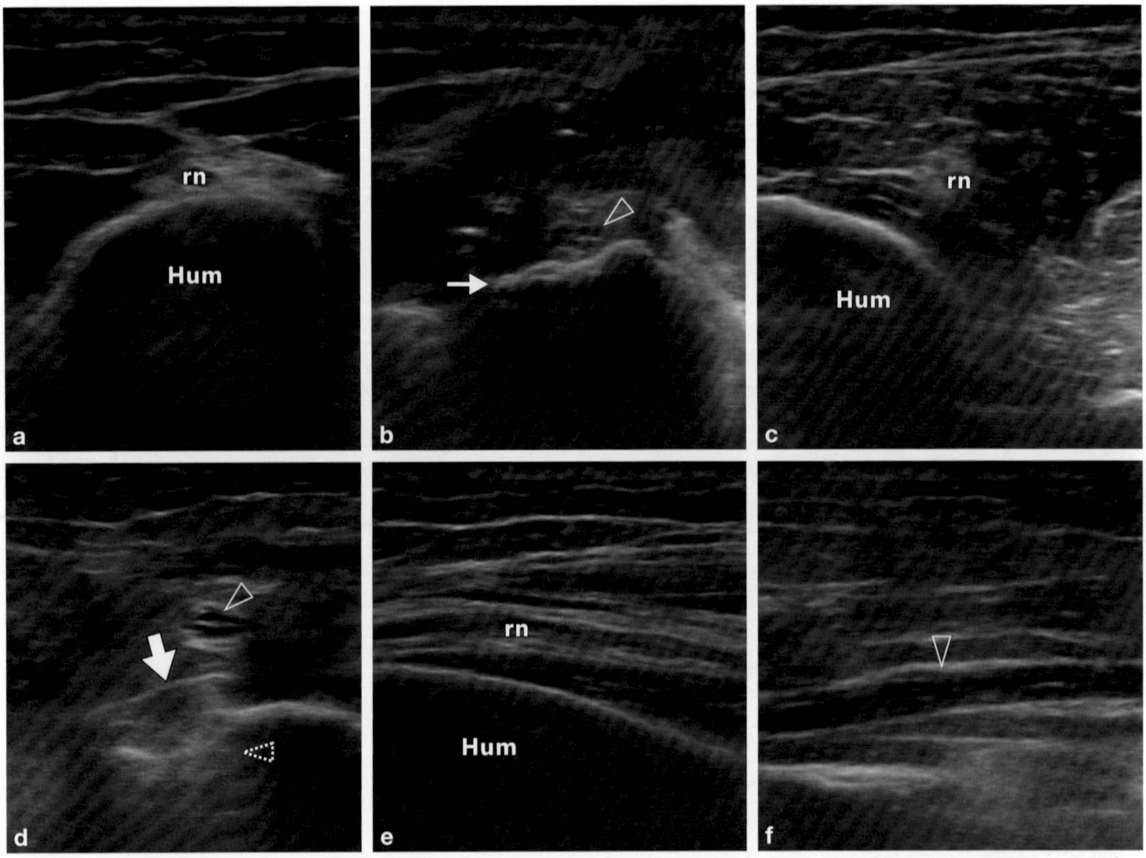

The patient has currently drop hand.

When compared with the normal side (**a**, **c**), axial US images obtained over the spiral groove (**b**) and distally over the internal fixator (*thick arrow*) (**d**) demonstrate cortical irregularity (*thin arrow*) of the humerus (**Hum**), posterior reverberation artifact (*dashed arrowhead*) and swollen/hypoechoic (*arrowheads*) radial nerve (**rn**). Corresponding longitudinal images (**e**, **f**) confirm the nerve swelling (*arrowhead*).

Radial neuropathy in a young patient who has been using axillary crutches for 5 years **12.12**

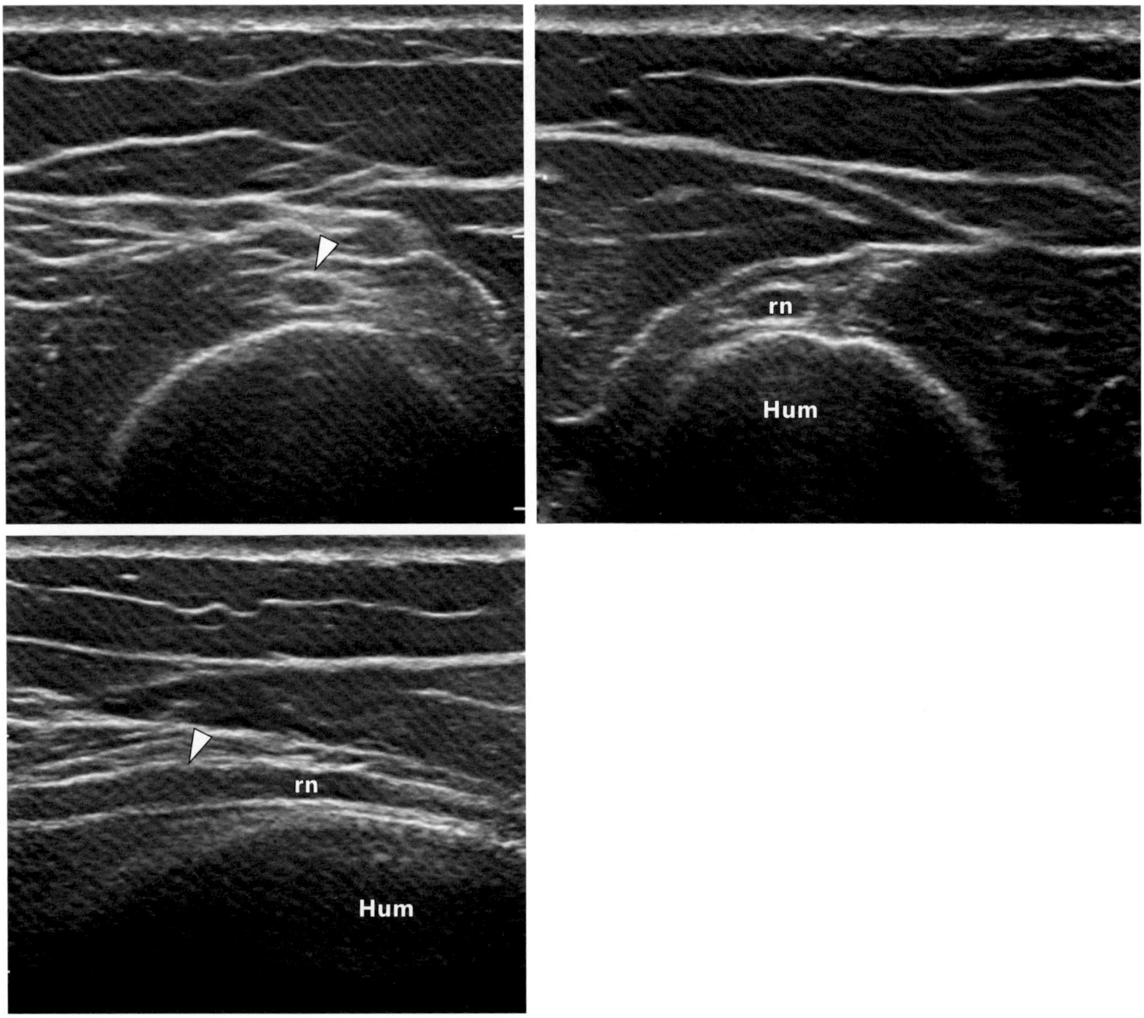

Axial US images obtained over the proximal (**a**) and distal (**b**) spiral groove reveal mild swelling (*arrowhead*) of the radial nerve (**rn**). Corresponding longitudinal US image confirms the swollen appearance (*arrowhead*) (**c**).

Hum humerus

Expert note

When the swelling is mild, it might be quite difficult to distinguish the exact area on axial imaging (unless serial measurements are done). Herewith, although it is not appropriate to perform any thickness measurements on them, long-axis views would be much more demonstrative in this sense.

12.13 Saturday night palsy in a 34-year-old man

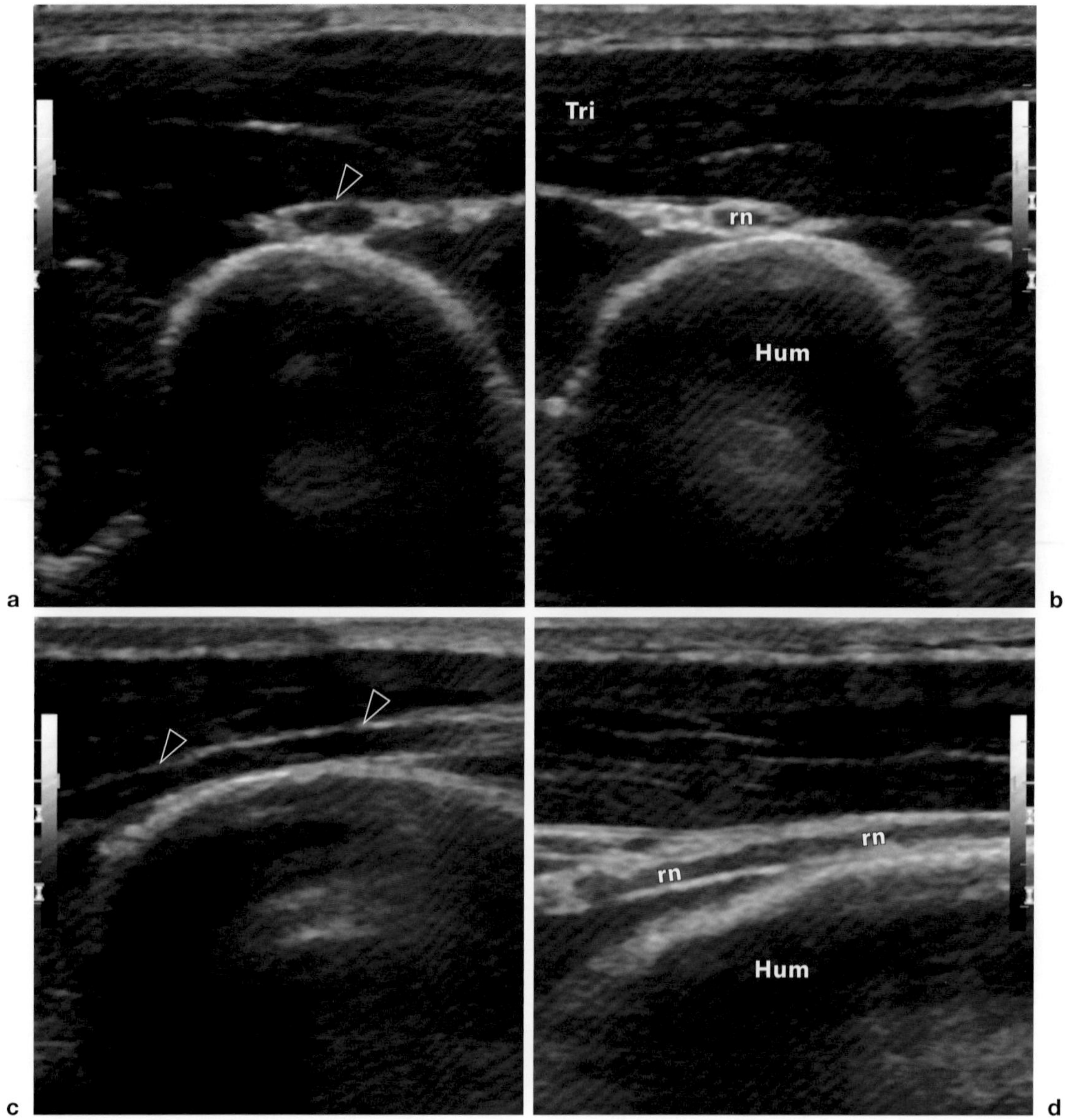

The patient injured his upper arm during sleeping and had inability to extent his wrist and thumb.

Axial (**a**) and longitudinal (**c**) US images at the spiral groove reveal focally swollen and hypoechoic radial nerve (*arrowheads*). Normal views of the radial nerve (**rn**) on the other side (**b**, **d**).

Hum humerus
Tri triceps

Radial neuropathy in a 45-year-old man after a trauma without any fracture/dislocation **12.14**

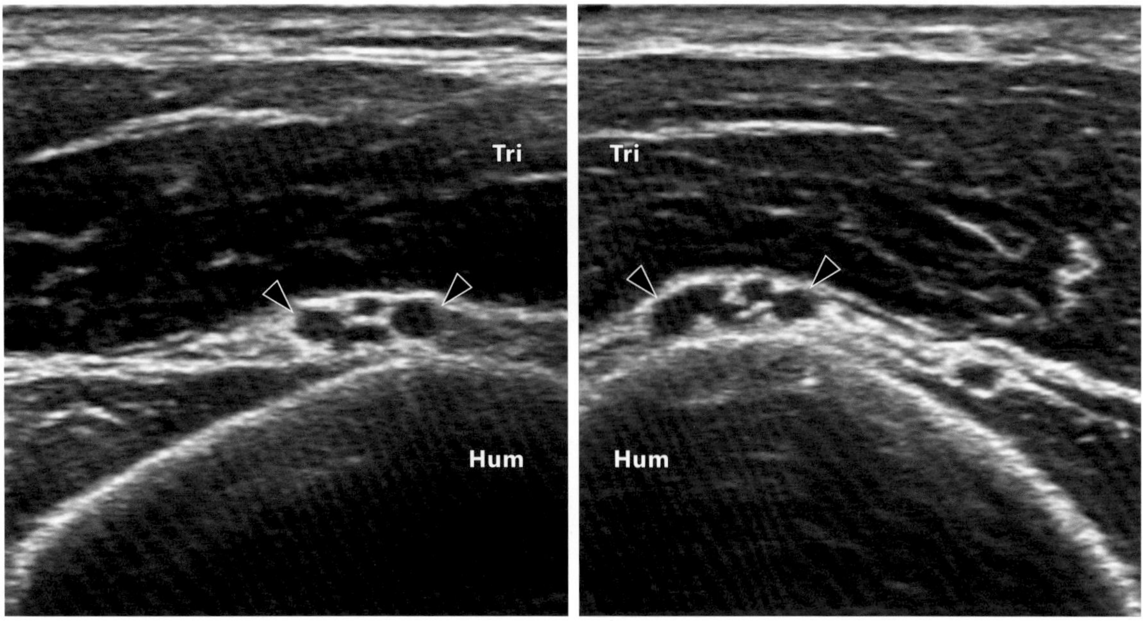

a b

Axial US images at the spiral groove exhibit abnormally swollen fascicles of the radial nerve (*arrowheads*) on both sides (**a**, **b**).

Hum humerus
Tri triceps

Expert note

Although fascicular swelling might well be suggestive for nerve entrapment, various polyneuropathies (e.g. Charcot-Marie Tooth disease) or mass lesions (e.g. neurofibromatosis) also need to be considered in the differential diagnosis.

12.15 Charcot-Marie-Tooth disease in a 23-year-old patient with vague weakness in the radial nerve innervated muscles

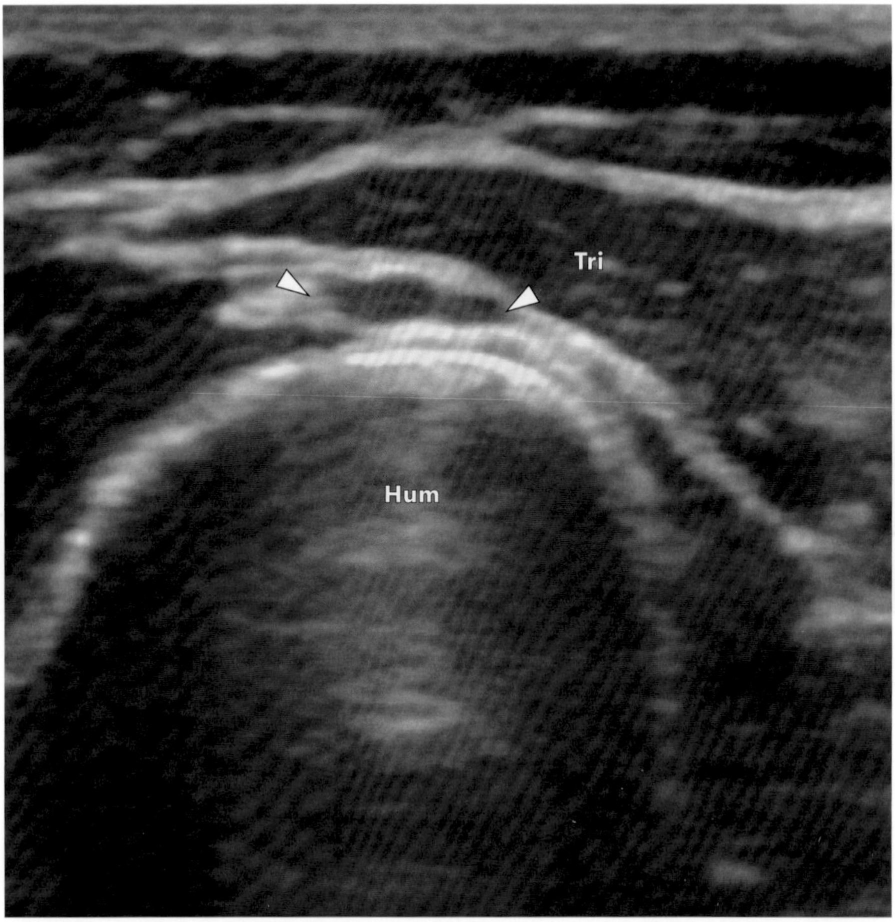

Axial US image obtained over the spiral groove shows that the radial nerve is mildly swollen and more hypoechoic (*arrowheads*).

Hum humerus
Tri triceps

Schwannoma of the radial nerve in a 45-year-old man with pain and progressive weakness in wrist extension 12.16

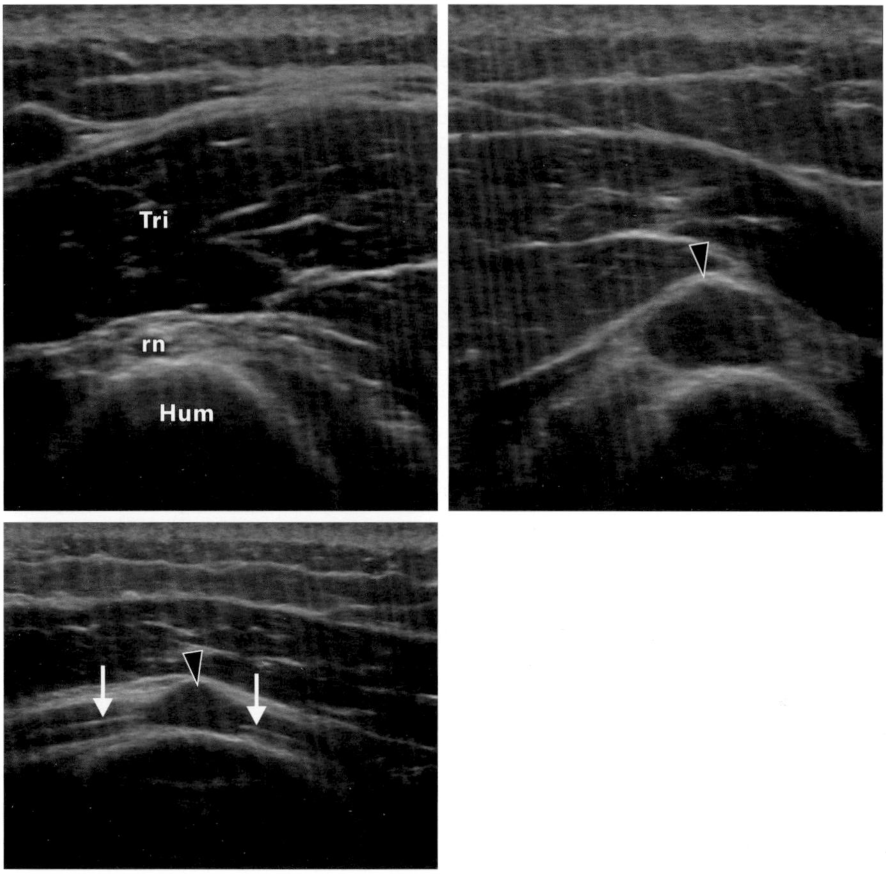

a b c

When compared with the normal radial nerve (**rn**) over the spiral groove (**a**), axial (**b**) and longitudinal (**c**) US images show the schwannoma as a hypoechoic, thickened oval-shaped mass (*arrowheads*). Please note the “rat tail” appearance on either side of the mass (*arrows*).

Hum humerus
Tri triceps

Expert note

Although it is not always possible to conclude specifically on the pathology and it is better to define/explain what is seen on the image; sometimes certain appearances help us diagnose particular conditions. For instance, due to their eccentric localizations on the nerve trunk, “rat tail” appearance is quite pathognomonic for schwannomas. Additionally, their vascularity on Doppler imaging can also help differentiate them from neurofibromas [3-5].
In this patient, sono-Tinel was significantly positive on the lesion and the patient described severe pain as exactly as he reported to suffer intermittently during his daily life.

12.17 Posterior interosseous nerve syndrome in a patient who had deficit of abduction and extension of the thumb

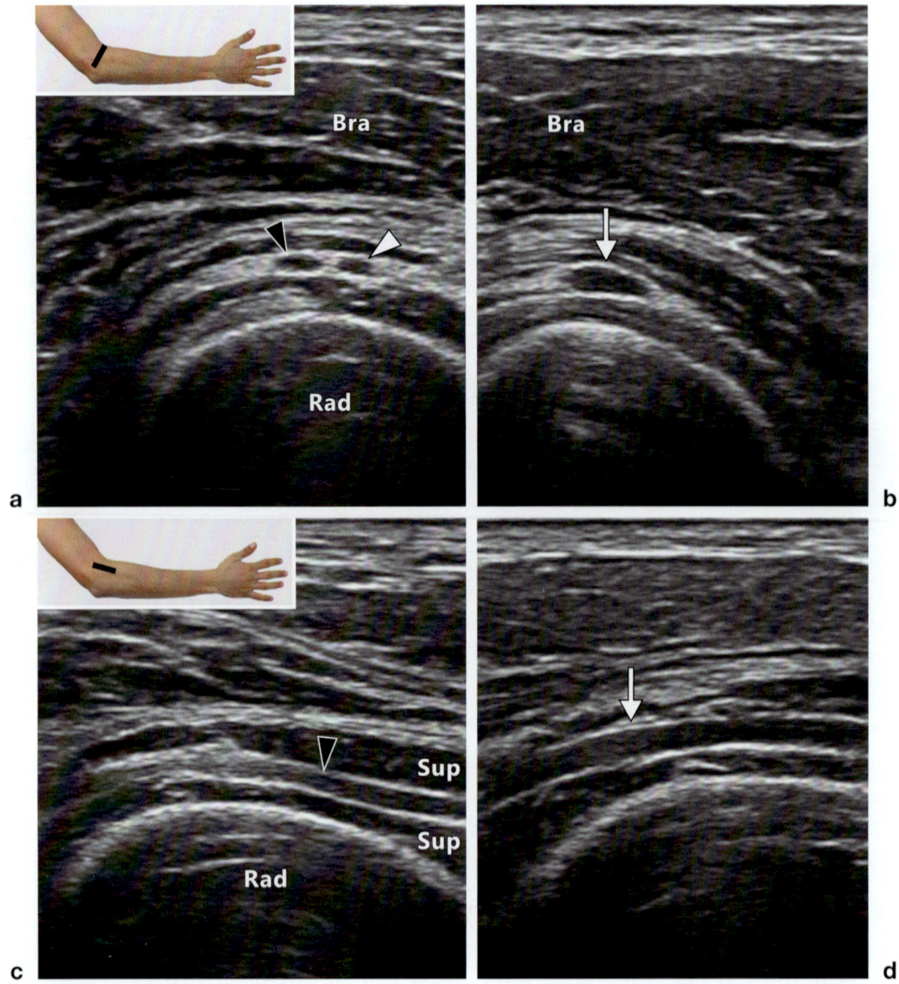

When compared with the normal side (**a**) where the posterior interosseous nerve seems to be bifid (*arrowheads*), axial US image (**b**) obtained over the proximal forearm shows that the nerve is markedly thickened (*arrow*) where it traverses the supinator muscle (**Sup**). Corresponding longitudinal views are also confirmatory (**c**, **d**).

Bra brachioradialis
Rad radius

Expert note

When the nerve comprises two fascicles; during long-axis view, the sonographer should be cautious that only one of them can be scanned at a particular position/window.

Radial tunnel syndrome in a 37-year-old man who presented with weakness in extending his fingers **12.18**

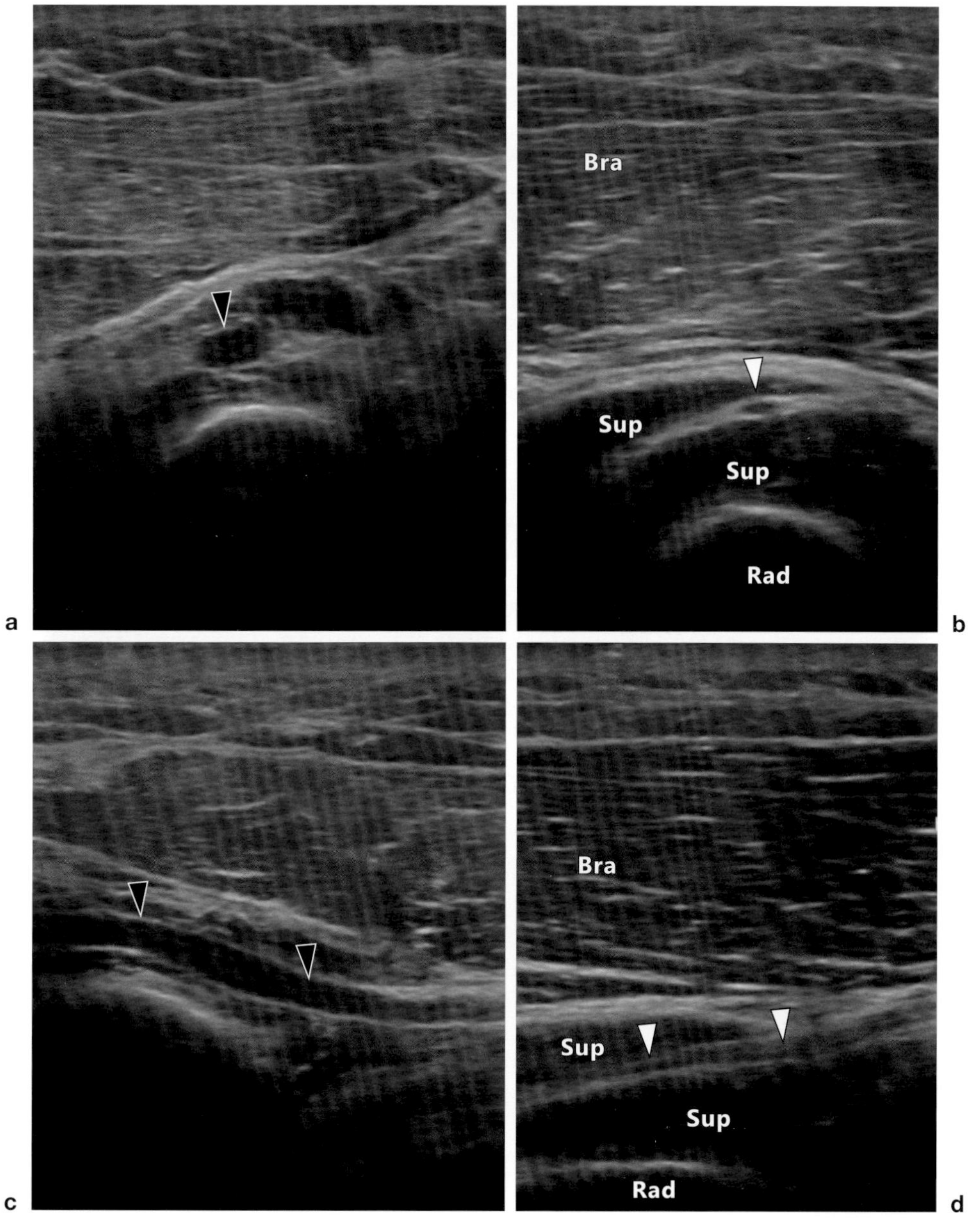

Axial (**a**) and longitudinal (**c**) US images obtained over the proximal forearm show that the posterior interosseous nerve is swollen and hypoechoic (*black arrowheads*) within the supinator muscle (**Sup**). Normal views of the nerve (*white arrowheads*) on the contralateral side (**b**, **d**).

Bra brachioradialis

Rad radius

12.19 Posterior interosseous neuropathy in a 40-year-old woman who had burning pain and tenderness over the lateral elbow

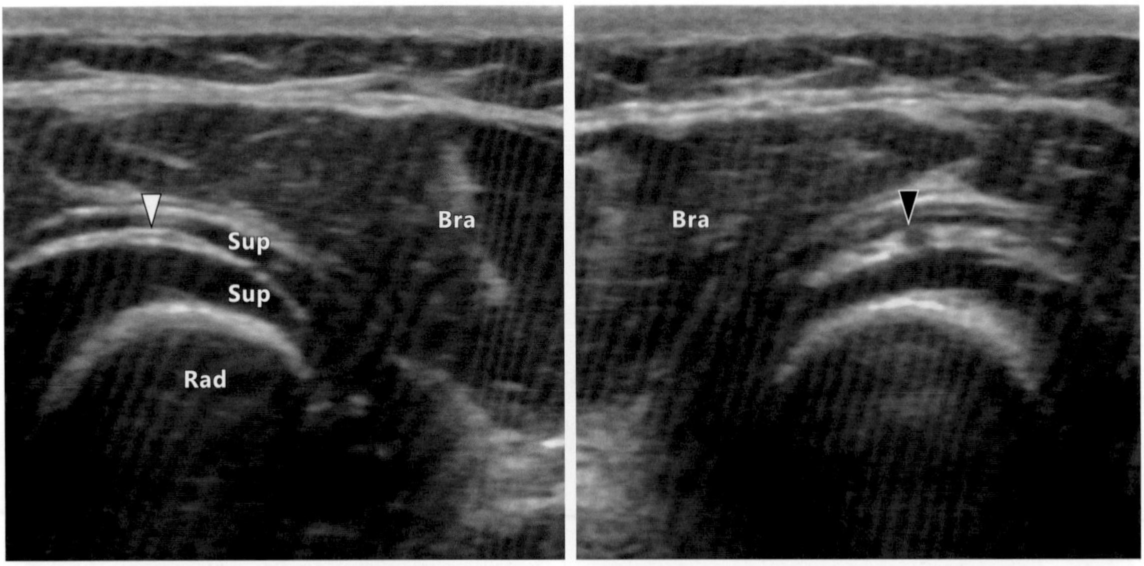

a b

When compared with the normal posterior interosseous nerve (*white arrowhead*) within the two heads of the supinator muscle (**Sup**) (**a**), axial US image of the proximal forearm demonstrates swollen nerve with hypoechoic view (*black arrowhead*) (**b**).

Bra brachioradialis
Rad radius

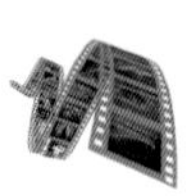
Video 17

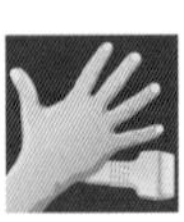

Expert note

Like in other nerves, it is usually quite easy to follow the radial nerve or its distal branches from proximal to distal or vice versa. Since the peripheral nerves do not lie "very straight" in an extremity (i.e. sometimes deep/superficial and sometimes medial/lateral), axial follow up is always/initially preferred throughout a long course. Herewith, in case of a suspicion, long-axis view is definitely/immediately performed [6].

Finger drop which developed after the injection of botulinum toxin in a man with previous stroke 12.20

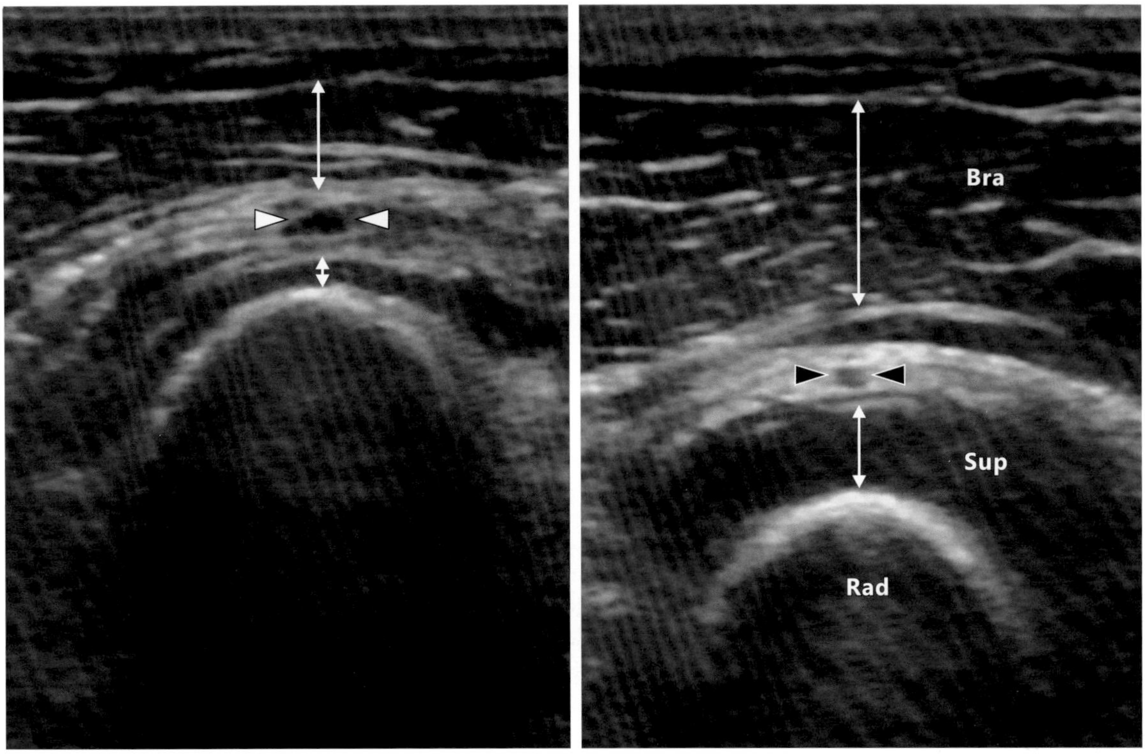

Axial US image over the proximal radius shows swelling of the posterior interosseous nerve (*white arrowheads*) together with atrophy in the supinator and brachioradialis muscles (*arrows*) (**a**). Normal nerve (*black arrowheads*) on the contralateral side (**b**).

Bra brachioradialis
Rad radius
Sup supinator

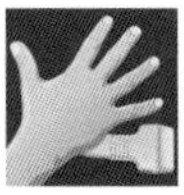

Expert note

Independent of the radial nerve palsy, US imaging also gives idea regarding the impact of stroke/spasticity on the hemiplegic side muscles [7]. In case of posterior interosseous neuropathy, one would not expect atrophy of brachioradialis, the muscle is thin, but not hyperechoic. This could be due to central and not to peripheral neurological pathology.

12.21 Posterior interosseous neuropathy in a 50-year-old patient with weakness of the thumb after surgery for proximal radial fracture

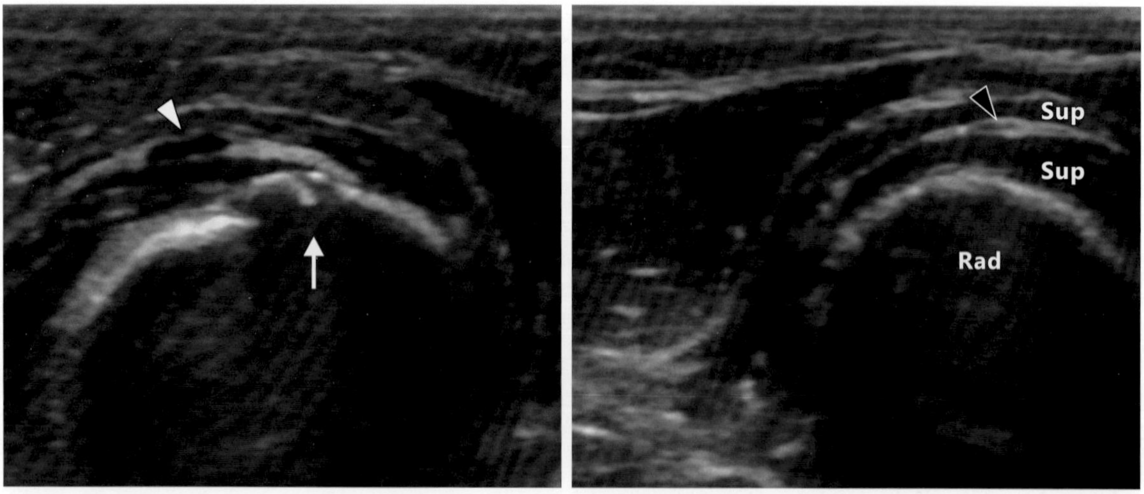

a b

Axial US image obtained over the proximal forearm illustrates the impingement of the posterior interosseous nerve (*white arrowhead*) with swollen and hypoechoic appearance just above the healing cortical zone (*arrow*) (**a**). Normal view of the nerve (*black arrowhead*) and supinator muscle (**Sup**) on the contralateral side (**b**).

Rad radius

Posterior interosseous nerve injury after repair of a proximal radial fracture 12.22

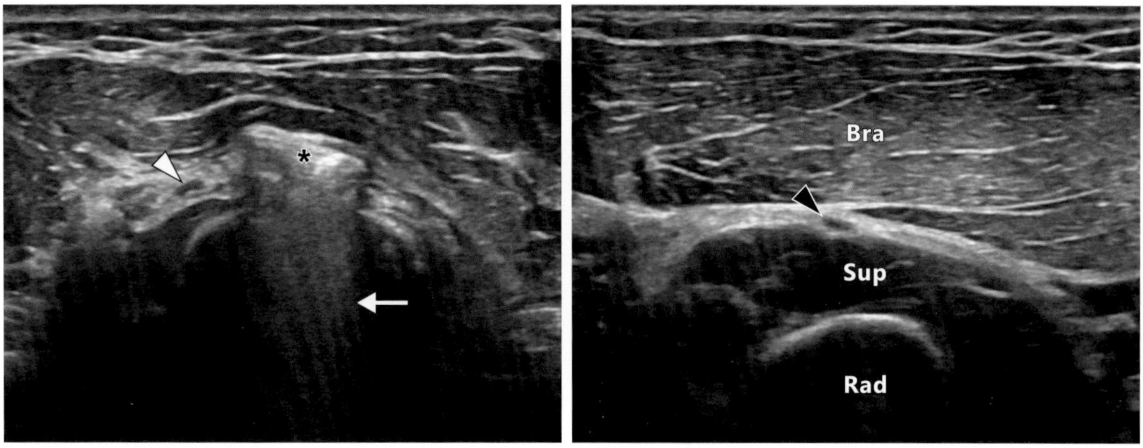

a b

Axial US image shows the posterior interosseous nerve as flattened and compressed (*white arrowhead*) adjacent to the tip of the metallic plate (*asterisk*). US depicts the plate as a thin, linear and bright hyperechoic structure giving a posterior reverberation artifact (*arrow*) (**a**). Normal appearance of the nerve (*black arrowhead*) on the contralateral side (**b**).

Bra brachioradialis
Rad radius
Sup supinator

Expert note

Although the nerve is not much swollen when compared with the normal side; the combination of his complaints, clinical presentation and imaging helps to reach a diagnosis/decision.

12.23 Charcot-Marie-Tooth disease in an adult man with claw hand deformity

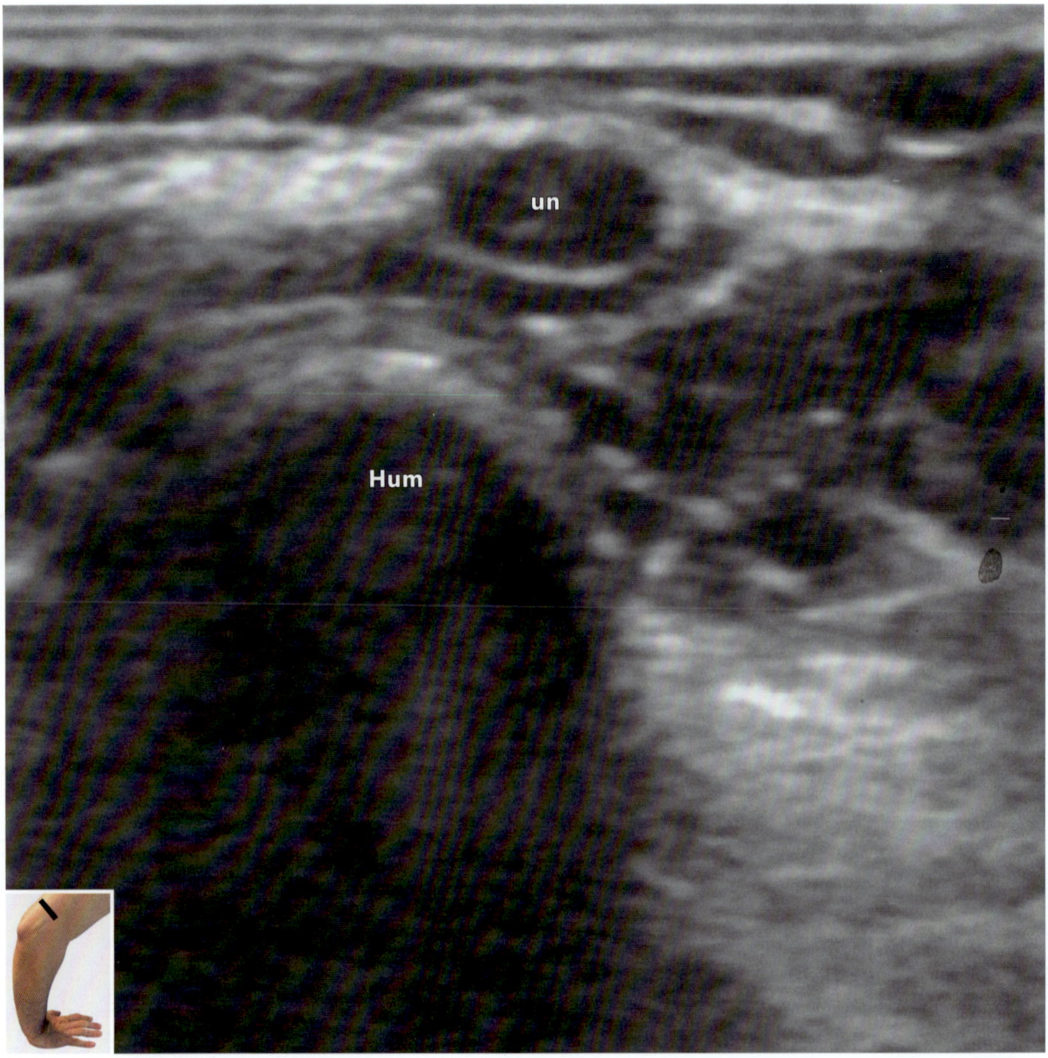

Axial US image obtained over the distal humerus (**Hum**) exhibits a swollen hypoechoic ulnar nerve (**un**).

Expert note

Instead of individual fascicle swellings, diffuse enlargement of the nerve itself can also be seen in patients with Charcot-Marie-Tooth disease.

Cubital tunnel syndrome in a 28-year-old patient with elbow pain radiating down to the medial forearm and hand

12.24

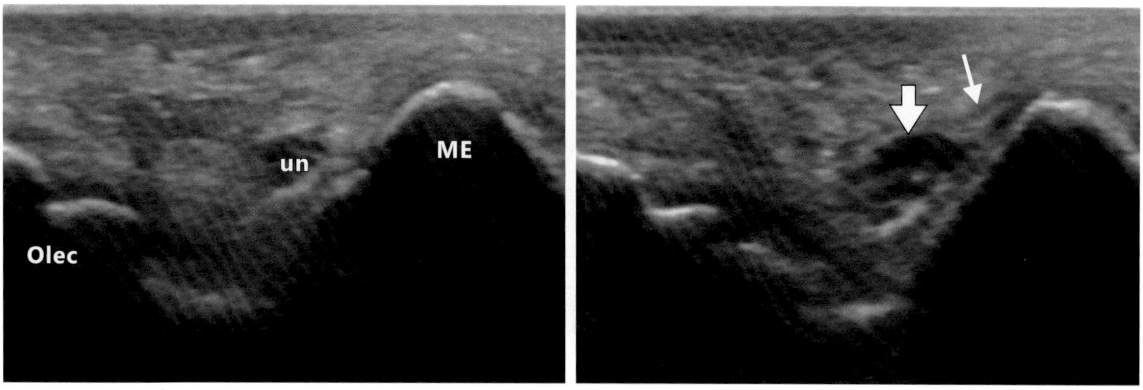

a b

When compared with the normal side (**a**), axial US image at the condylar groove level reveals swollen and hypoechoic (*thick arrow*) ulnar nerve (**un**) under the Osborne ligament (*thin arrow*) on the symptomatic side (**b**).

ME medial epicondyle
Olec olecranon

Expert note

Independent of the terminology differences as regards cubital tunnel syndrome (i.e. site of compression), US imaging can readily show where exactly the nerve looks like to be entrapped -at the bony tunnel, between the heads of the flexor carpi ulnaris muscle etc. [8]. In this case, the nerve is swollen at the level of the medial epicondyle and olecranon.

12.25 Cubital tunnel syndrome in a 35-year-old man with a positive Tinel's sign at the elbow, and hypoesthesia in the medial forearm and fingers

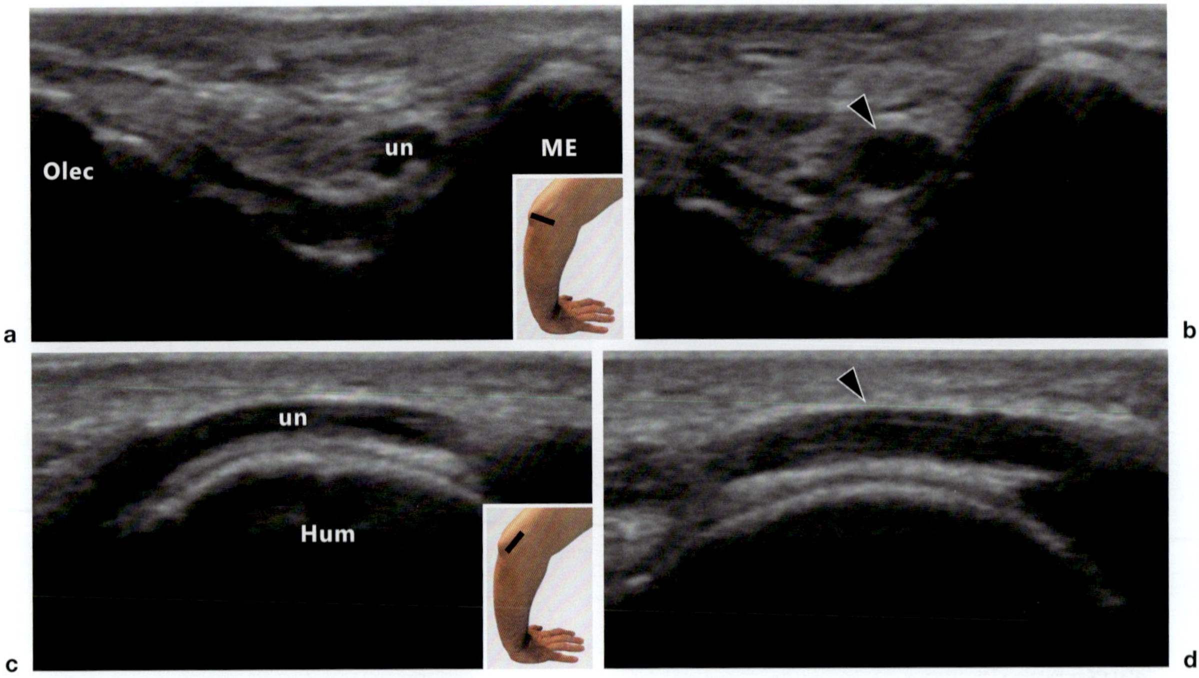

When compared with the normal side (**a**, **c**), axial (**b**) and longitudinal (**d**) US images show the swollen (*arrowheads*) ulnar nerve (**un**) at the proximal cubital tunnel.

Hum humerus
ME medial epicondyle
Olec olecranon

Cubital tunnel syndrome in a 55-year-old man **12.26**

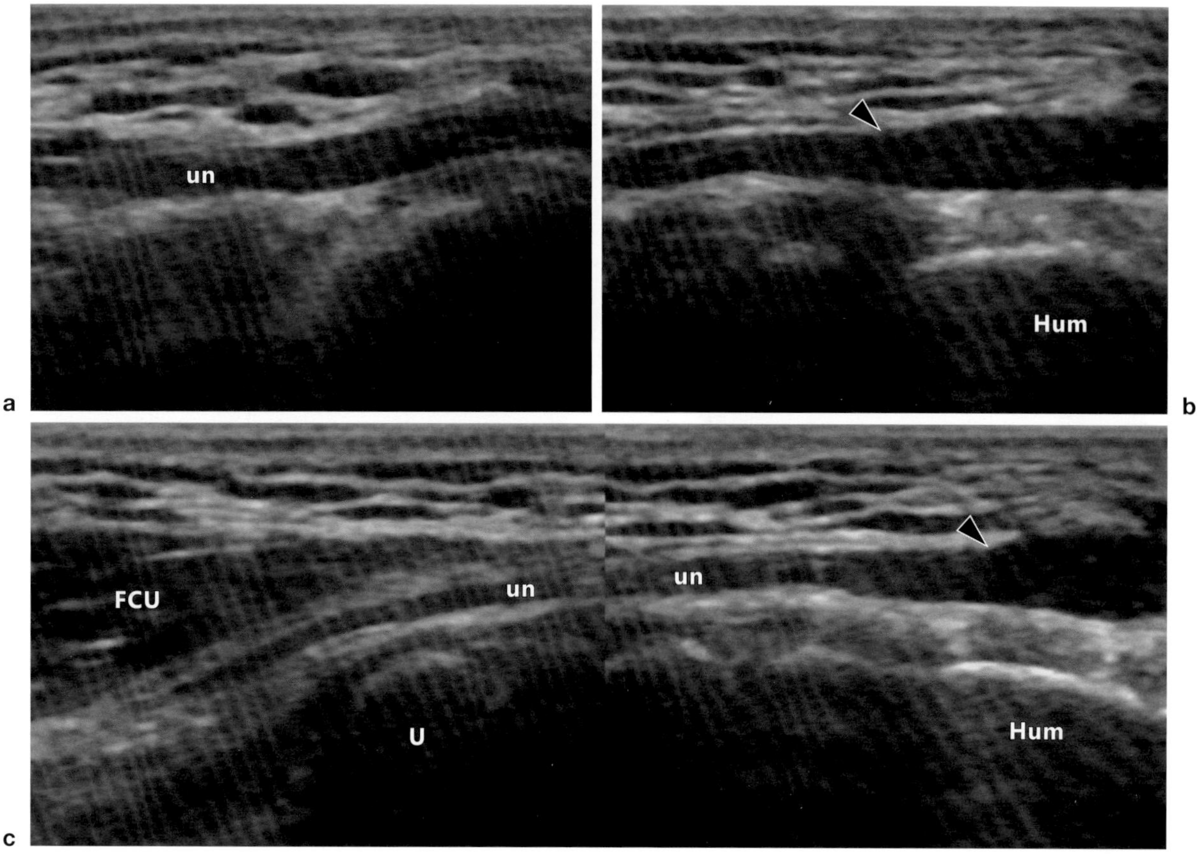

The patient had posteromedial elbow pain and hand tingling sensation on the ulnar innervated fingers.

When compared with the normal side (**a**), longitudinal (**b**) and split-screen longitudinal (**c**) US images show the swollen (*arrowheads*) ulnar nerve (**un**) just proximal to the cubital tunnel.

FCU flexor carpi ulnaris
Hum humerus
U ulna

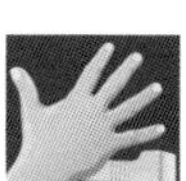

Expert note

In case of nerve entrapment, one can see a "bottle neck" phenomenon, with enlargement often proximal to the entrapment site.

12.27 Cubital tunnel syndrome in a 35-year-old woman with complaints of medial elbow pain and paresthesia for two months

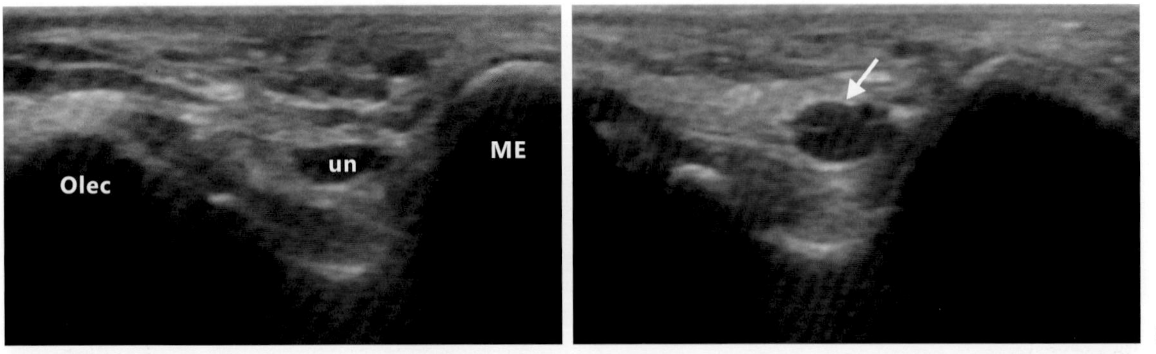

a b

She had a positive Tinel's sign over the cubital tunnel and hypoesthesia in the fourth and fifth fingers.

When compared with the normal side (**a**), axial US image shows swollen and hypoechoic (*arrow*) ulnar nerve (**un**) at the proximal cubital tunnel (**b**).

ME medial epicondyle
Olec olecranon

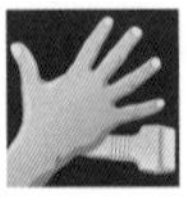

Expert note

One should always perform a dynamic exam i.e. looking for luxation of the ulnar nerve during passive flexion of the elbow [9]. (Sub)luxation can be found in asymptomatic people, but it can be a predisposition for neuropathy.

Cubital tunnel syndrome in a 67-year-old man with poor hand dexterity after a distal humeral fracture 12.28

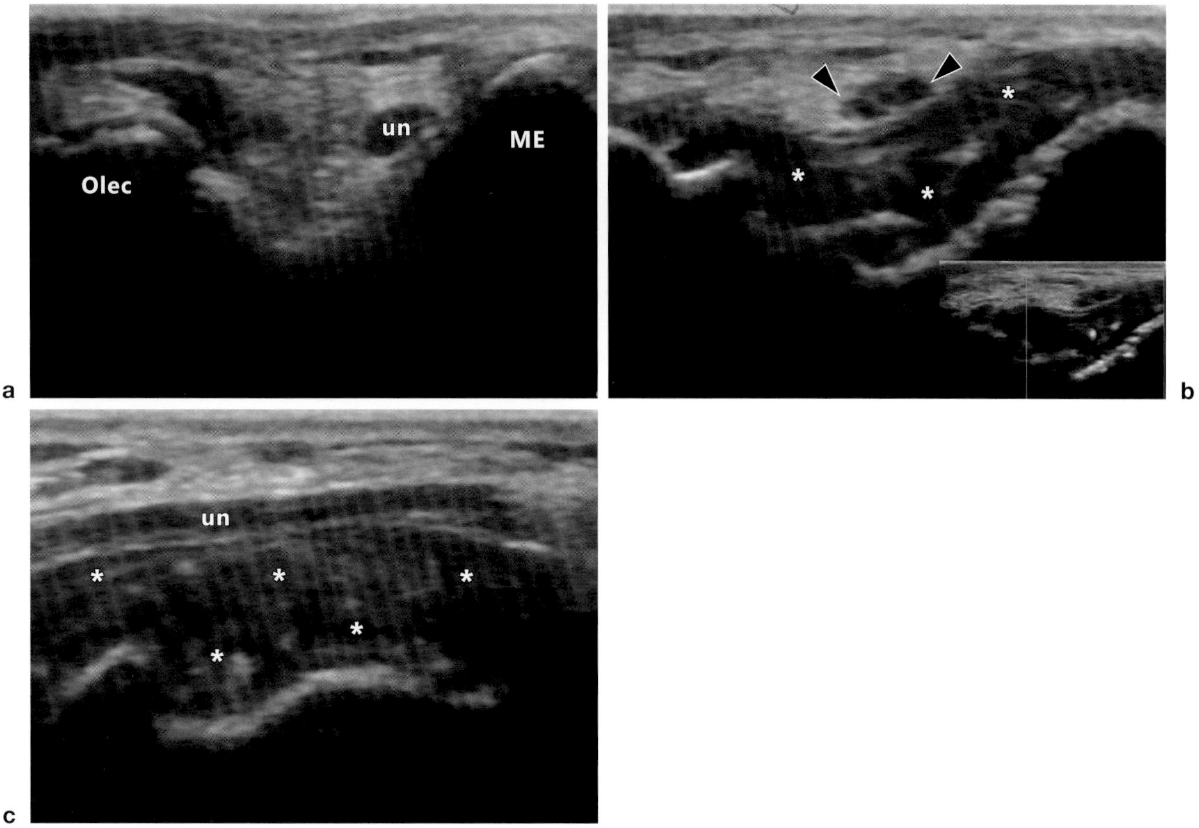

When compared with the normal side (**a**), axial (**b**) and longitudinal (**c**) US images reveal synovial hypertrophy (*asterisks*) and cortical irregularities subluxating and stretching the ulnar nerve (**un**) (*arrowheads*). Power Doppler imaging demonstrates slow blood flow (*small figure*).

ME medial epicondyle
Olec olecranon

12.29 Bilateral cubital tunnel syndrome in an elderly patient with complaints of hand weakness and paresthesia

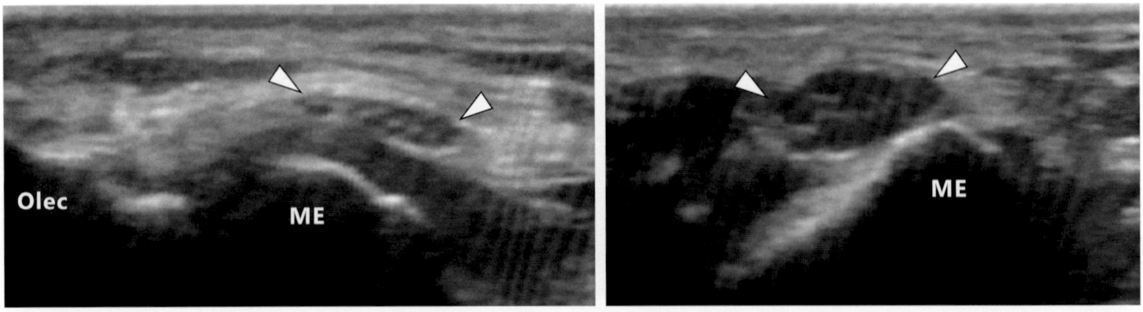

a b

Axial US image at the proximal cubital tunnel demonstrates flattened and subluxated ulnar nerve (*arrowheads*) (**a**). Contralateral side reveals a more hypoechoic ulnar nerve with markedly swollen fascicles (*arrowheads*) (**b**).

ME medial epicondyle
Olec olecranon

Expert note

While the size of nerve swelling is generally in correlation with the patient's complaints or the functional deterioration; "asymptomatic but swollen" or "functionally normal but swollen" nerves should not be unexpected in clinical practice. In this sense, US and electrodiagnostic testing might necessarily be used as complementary. Yet, the former is a morphological and the latter is a physiological assessment tool [4].

Cubital tunnel syndrome in a 40-year-old man with clinical symptoms of ulnar neuropathy **12.30**

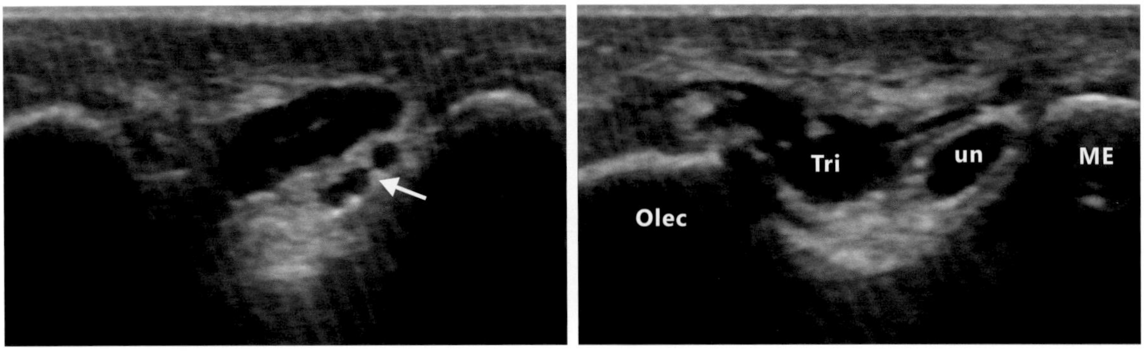

a b

While axial US image of the asymptomatic side demonstrates multifascicular ulnar nerve (*arrow*) (**a**), symptomatic side at the proximal cubital tunnel shows enlarged ulnar nerve (**un**) with a hypoechoic appearance (**b**).

ME medial epicondyle
Olec olecranon
Tri triceps

Expert note

While anatomic variations do not always indicate nerve pathology or might not be associated with any preponderance to entrapment syndromes, US imaging is very important to unmask "all details of the story" [10].
One important note concerning area measurements in such cases would be the need for separate measurements for each fascicle and adding them eventually.

12.31 Ulnar nerve entrapment due to heterotopic ossification after traumatic brain injury in a 50-year-old man

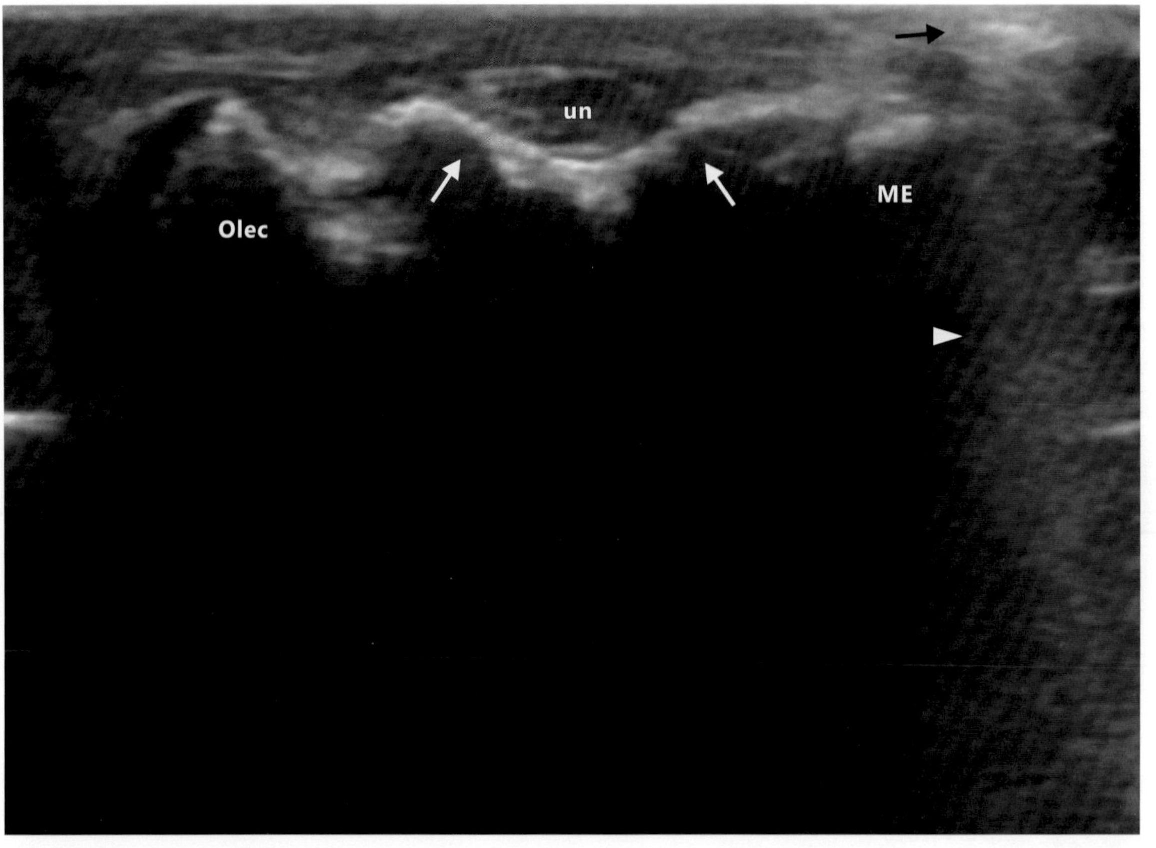

On physical examination, the patient had severe spasticity on the upper extremity, limitation of elbow motions and also claw hand deformity.

Axial US image demonstrates edematous and subluxated ulnar nerve (**un**) caused by the ossification (*white arrows*). Also note the comet-tail artifact (*arrowhead*) deep to the metallic implant (*black arrow*) which had been used for the humeral fracture.

ME medial epicondyle
Olec olecranon

Expert note

Aside from prompt imaging for ulnar nerve entrapment, early diagnosis for heterotopic ossification would indisputably be an additional benefit of US imaging [11].
In the presence of osteosynthesis materials, metal artifacts are problem for MRI, not for US.

Bilateral traumatic ulnar nerve injuries in a 43-year-old woman after a traffic accident

12.32

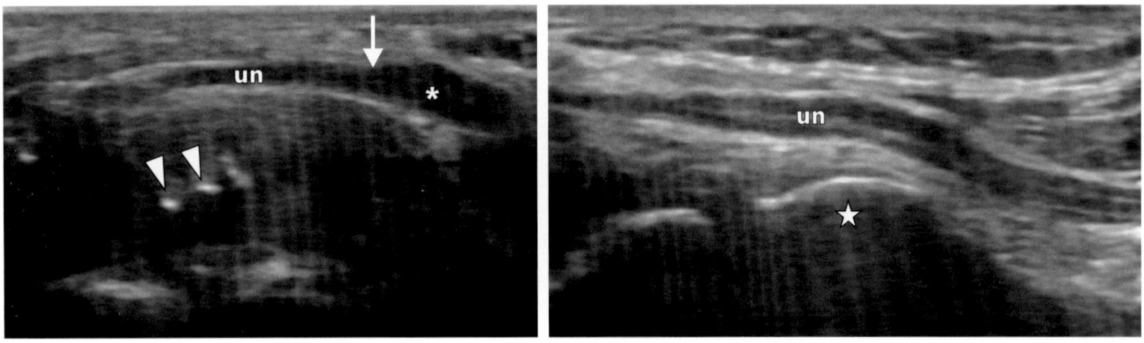

Longitudinal US image demonstrates a markedly hypoechoic and swollen (*asterisk*) ulnar nerve (**un**) just proximal to the compression level (*arrow*) (**a**). Note the non-absorbable suture materials as bright linear echoes (*arrowheads*) within the irregular/healing soft tissues (**a**). Contralateral side reveals diffusely enlarged nerve due to callus formation (*star*) (**b**).

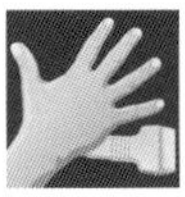

Expert note

As always, when evaluating a nerve, one should look for changes in shape and echogenicity of the nerve itself and for possible "extrinsic" structures compressing the nerve as well.

12.33 Cubital tunnel syndrome in an elderly patient with elbow flexion contracture and claw hand deformity

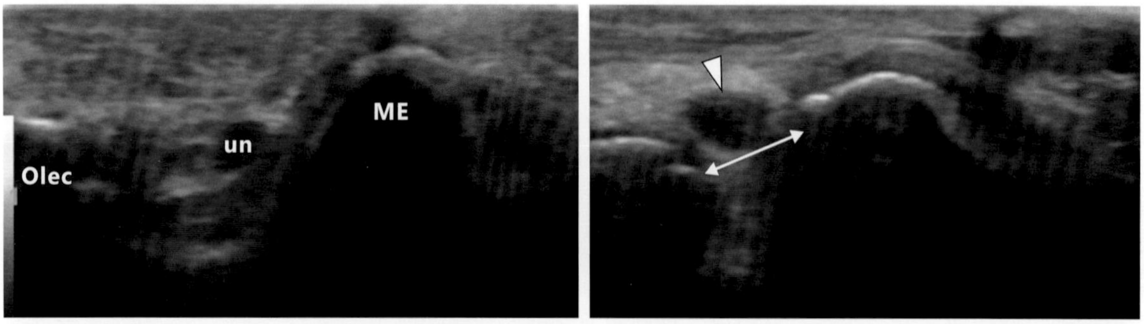

a b

When compared with the normal side (**a**), axial US image reveals a swollen and hypoechoic (*arrowhead*) ulnar nerve (**un**) within the narrowed (*double arrow*) condylar groove (**b**).

ME medial epicondyle
Olec olecranon

Expert note

In patients with degenerative problems, it is not uncommon to find various pathologies as regards the bony sides of the tunnel (e.g. spurs, cortical irregularities). It is quite valuable to understand their dynamic relationship with the entrapped nerve not only for diagnosis but also for planning a corrective surgery in severe cases.

Cubital tunnel syndrome in a 57-year-old man with ulnar claw hand **12.34**

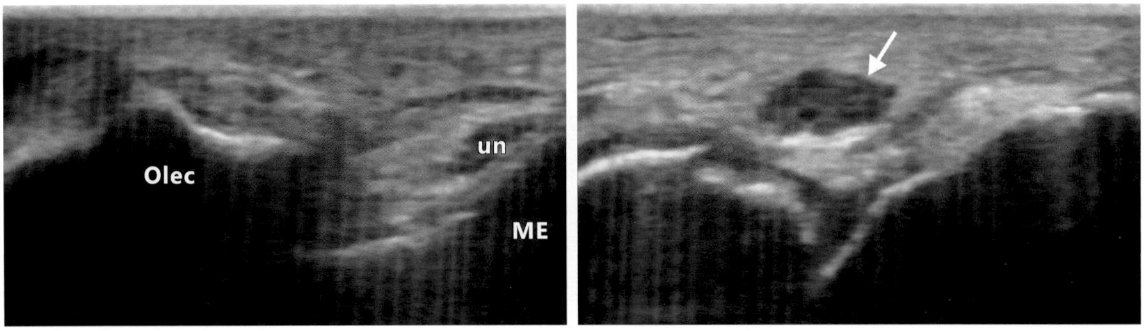

a b

When compared with the normal side (**a**), axial US image over the condylar groove demonstrates a markedly edematous ulnar nerve (**un**) (*arrow*) (**b**). Please note the narrowing of the bony tunnel which seems to push the nerve outwards.

ME medial epicondyle
Olec olecranon

Expert note

Electrodiagnosis is definitely needed to differentiate between conduction problems and neuropathy with axonal loss. Herewith, during the US exam, one can image the muscles in the territory of the nerve to explore fatty degeneration. They generally become thinner and hyperechoic and this is an indirect evaluation of the nerve pathology.

12.35 Cubital tunnel syndrome in a 7-year-old girl after a blunt trauma to her elbow

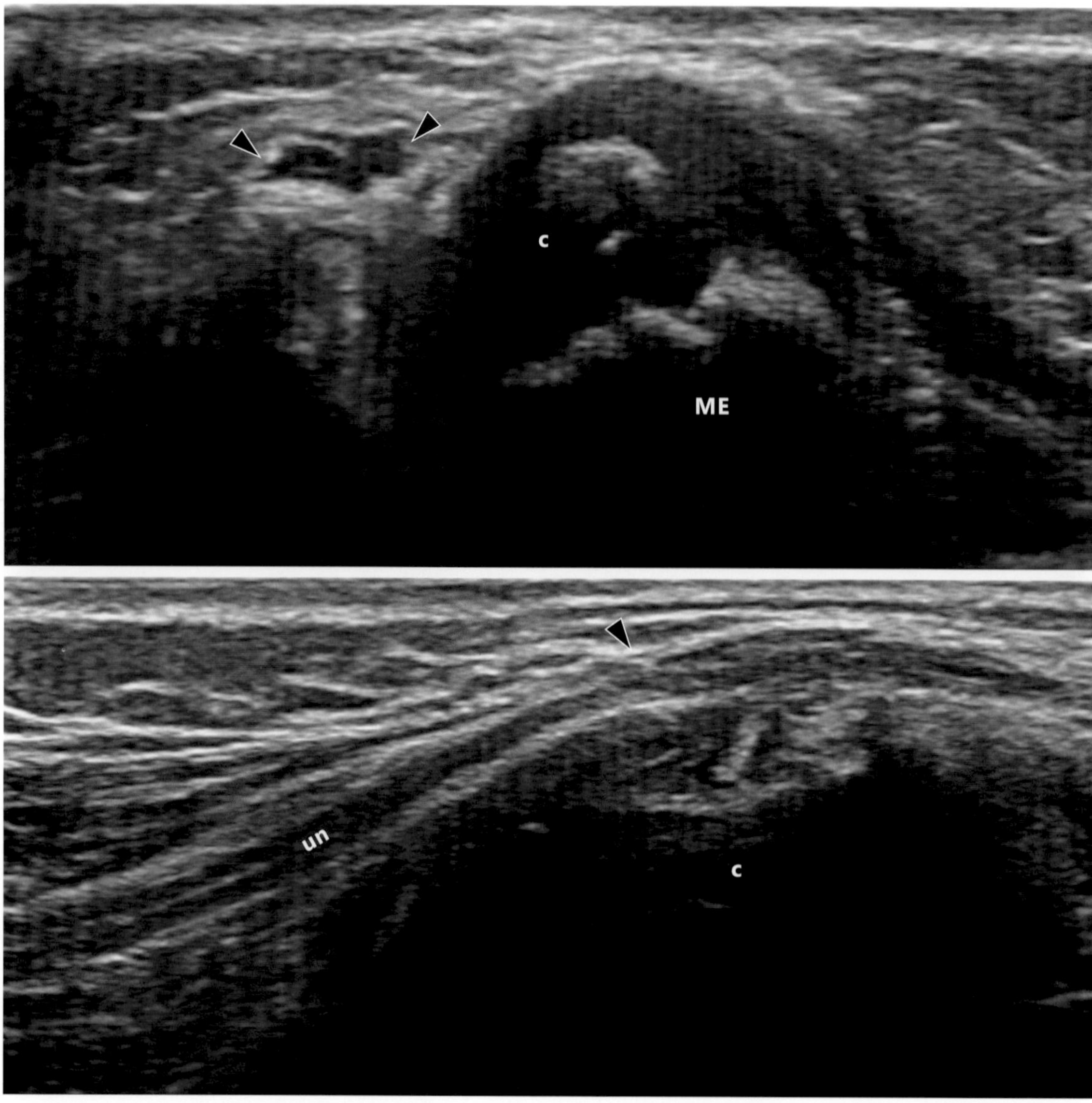

Axial (**a**) and longitudinal (**b**) US images over the proximal cubital tunnel reveal swollen and hypoechoic ulnar nerve (**un**) (*arrowheads*). Please note the irregular cartilaginous growth plate (**c**) as compared to normal appearance of the medial epicondyle (**ME**).

Cubital tunnel syndrome in a 45-year-old man with complaints of medial elbow pain radiating down to the hand

12.36

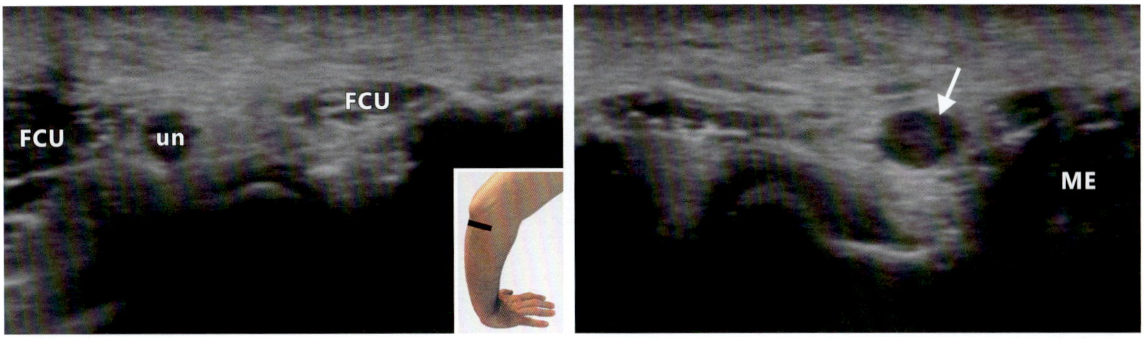

Axial US image shows normal appearance of the ulnar nerve (**un**) between the two heads of the flexor carpi ulnaris muscle (**FCU**) distally (**a**). The nerve seems to be enlarged and hypoechoic (*arrow*) at the proximal cubital tunnel (**b**).

ME medial epicondyle

12.37 Cubital tunnel syndrome in an adult patient with clumsiness and paresthesia in his hand

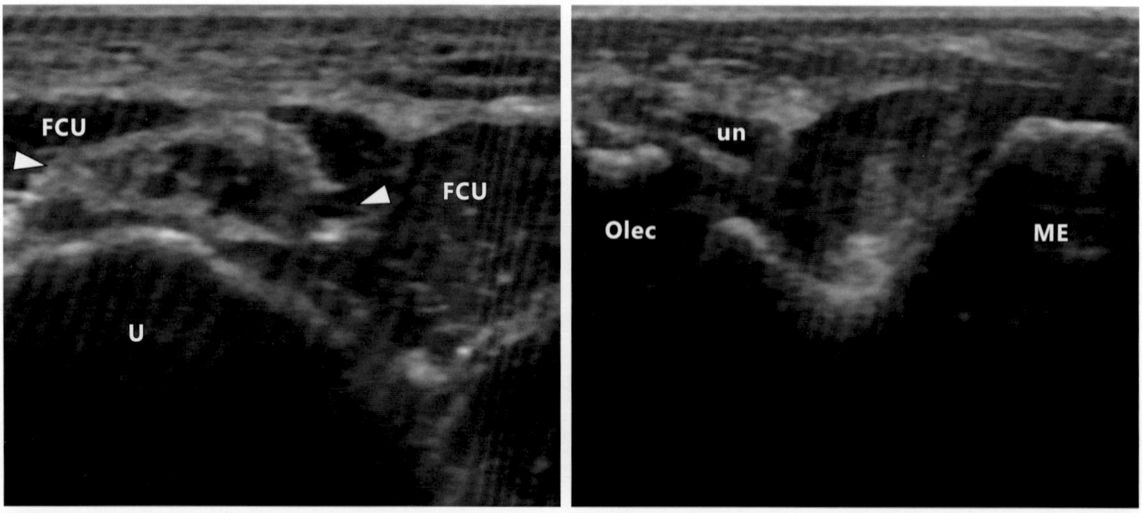

a b

Axial US image shows a significantly swollen (*arrowheads*) ulnar nerve (**un**) with heterogenous echogenicities between the two heads of the flexor carpi ulnaris muscle (**FCU**) (**a**).
The nerve is seen in normal appearance at the proximal cubital tunnel on the contralateral side (**b**). Note that the FCU muscle extends quite proximally.

ME medial epicondyle
Olec olecranon
U ulna

Expert note

Sometimes epitrochlearis or hypertrophic portions of triceps muscles can also give the same appearance. Dynamic imaging from proximal to distal and vice versa usually helps to clarify such anatomical variations.

Repaired ulnar artery in a girl who injured her forearm with a scissor

12.38

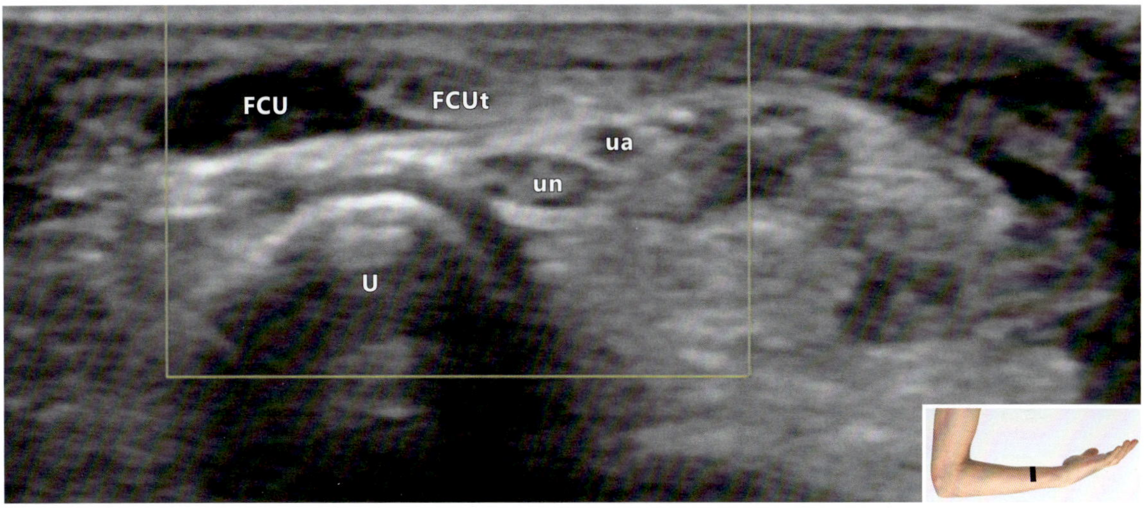

Axial US image demonstrates the ulnar artery (**ua**) and nerve (**un**) passing through the volar compartment of the distal forearm. The nerve contains a few internal hypoechoic fascicles. Although the artery was repaired, blood flow is not patent on Doppler imaging.

FCU flexor carpi ulnaris
FCUt FCU tendon
U ulna

12.39 Repaired ulnar nerve injury in a 45-year-old man who had neuropathic pain on the 4th and 5th fingers

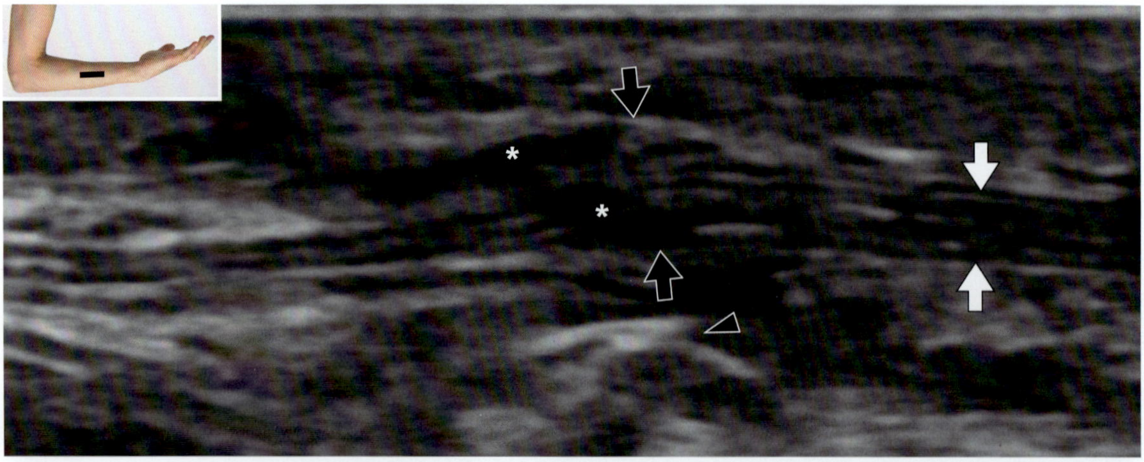

Longitudinal US image of the ulnar nerve (*white arrows*) at the level of mid-forearm demonstrates irregular hypoechoic bands (*asterisks*) and focal enlargement (*black arrows*) of the nerve. Also note the hyperechoic suture material (*arrowhead*) beneath the zone of injury.

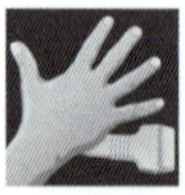

Expert note

For sure, serial follow up -especially in symptomatic cases- would be quite elucidative for nerve healing (or neuroma formation) [12]. Allodynia can make the exam very difficult. One should use a lot of gel, or eventually prepare the patient using local anaesthetic gel.

Surgical transposition of the ulnar nerve in a 38-year-old man with medial elbow pain

12.40

a 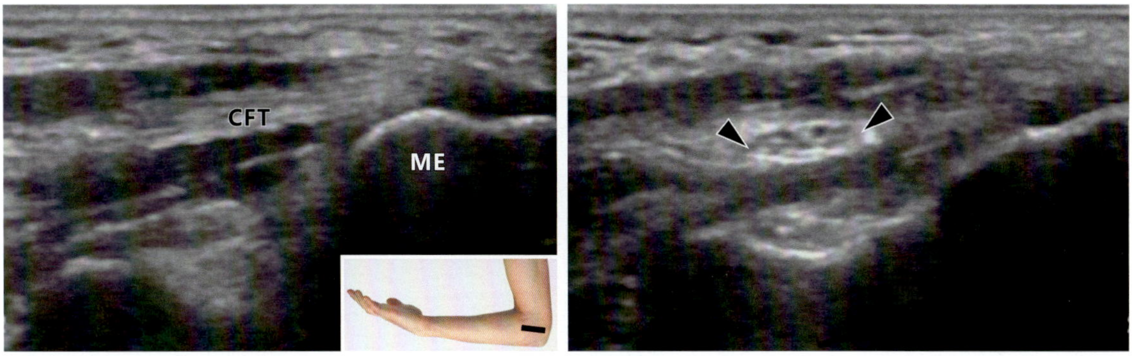 b

When compared with the normal side (**a**), medial longitudinal US image shows the anteriorly transposed ulnar nerve (*arrowheads*) near the common flexor tendon (**CFT**) (**b**).

ME medial epicondyle

Expert note

US imaging can readily be performed during the postoperative follow up of nerve entrapments especially in cases where the surgical outcome is unfavorable [13]. Herein, the details of the surgical procedure should definitely be known for prompt imaging i.e. in order to avoid misinterpretations as regards the changes in the normal anatomy.

In case of unfavorable outcome after anteriorization of the ulnar nerve, one should look for a short bend, turning or snapping of the nerve in the forearm and carefully ask for the presence of a sono-Tinel.

Video 18

12.41 Bilateral carpal tunnel syndrome in a 45-year-old woman with numbness in the palm of the hand, thumb and index finger

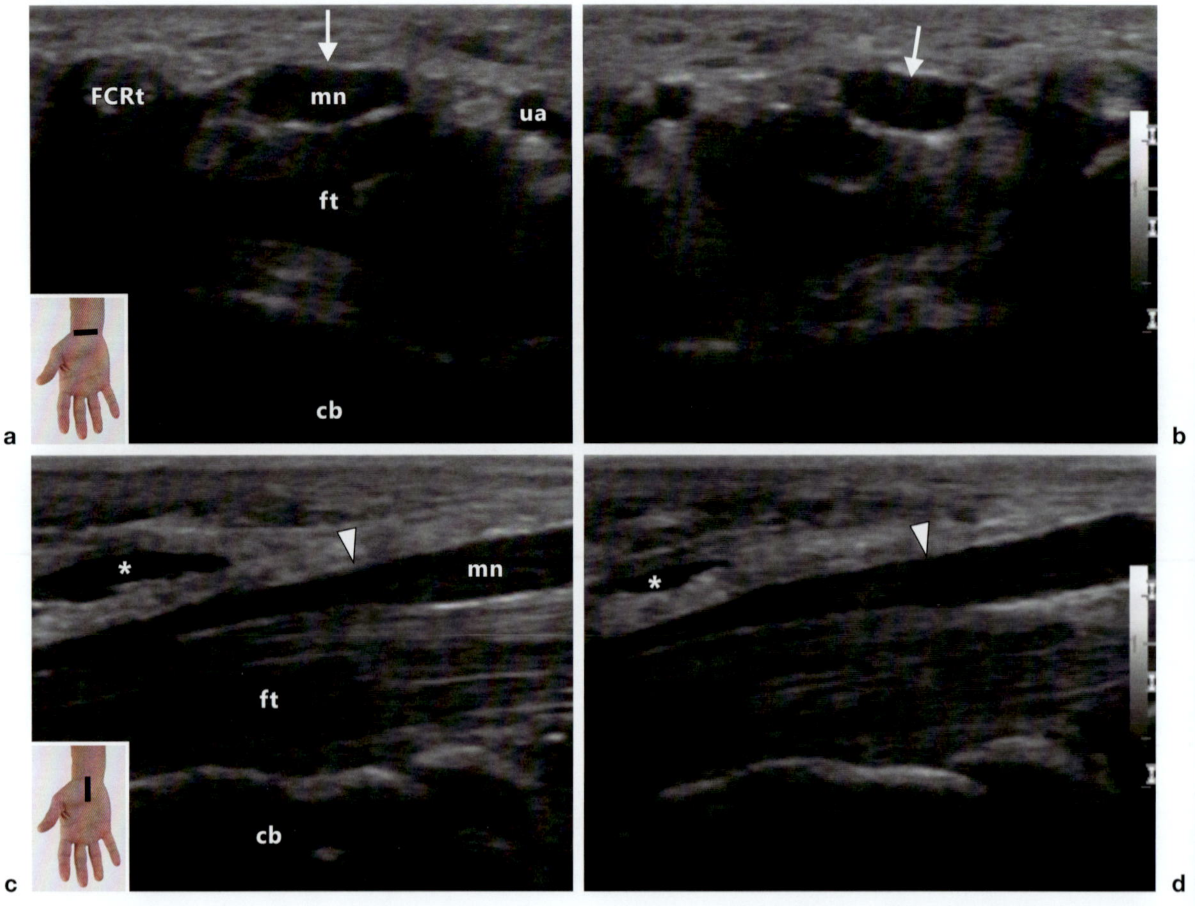

US images exhibit diffuse anechoic enlargement (*arrows*) of the median nerve (**mn**) in the axial views (**a**, **b**), and abrupt changes in the nerve size at the proximal carpal tunnel level (*arrowheads*) in the longitudinal views (**c**, **d**).
Note the close relationship of the nerve with the flexor tendons (**ft**) in the tunnel and with the flexor carpi radialis tendon (**FCRt**) outside the tunnel.

cb carpal bones
ua ulnar artery
* muscle

Expert note

Peripheral nerve entrapment syndromes can be very effectively evaluated with US imaging. First, morphological confirmation of the entrapment can be done (i.e. with swelling of the nerve usually proximal to the site of compression). Second, a possible underlying cause (e.g. aberrant/pathological structure) can be uncovered. Third, if needed, an intervention can simply be performed under US guidance. Fourth, in case of surgery, the surgeon can be “navigated” in advance i.e. where exactly to dissect. Last but not least, close (postoperative) follow up is always possible due to its convenience [3].

The application of sono-palpation is also referred as “sono-Tinel” in peripheral nerve imaging.

One can also do a dynamic exam, to check the mobility of the median nerve. In transverse view, when the flexor pollicis longus is moved passively, the median nerve should “swing” a little bit. In longitudinal view, when the fingers are moved (flexion/extension) passively, the nerve should also “glide” up and down. In carpal tunnel syndrome, the nerve becomes less mobile.

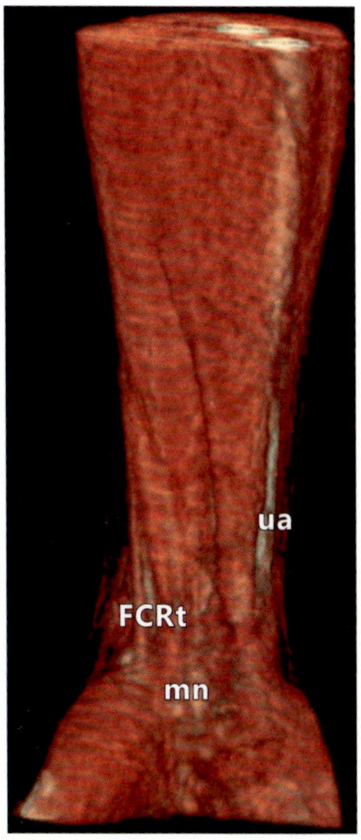

12.42 Bilateral carpal tunnel syndrome in a 57-year-old auto mechanic who felt pain during the day and paresthesias during the night

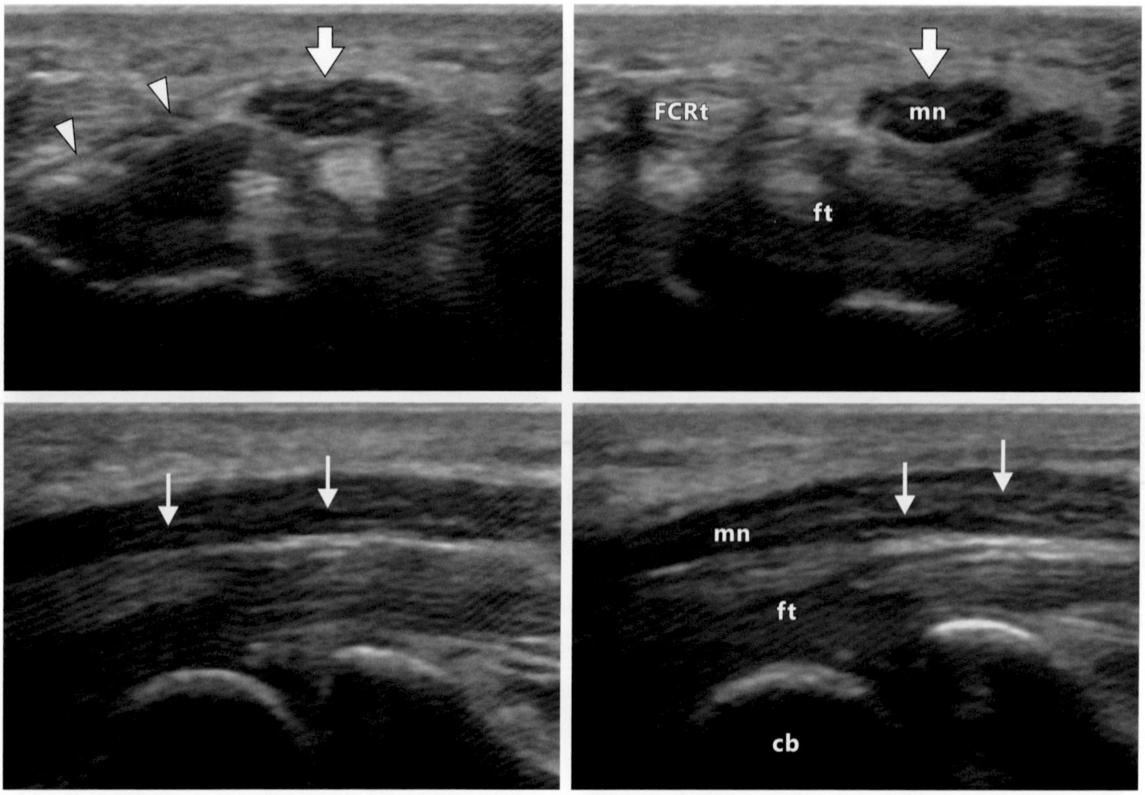

Axial US images show swollen (*thick arrows*) median nerves (**mn**) under the flexor retinaculum (*arrowheads*) (**a**, **b**). Longitudinal views demonstrate diffusely swollen fascicles (*thin arrows*) within the nerves (**c**, **d**).

cb carpal bones
FCRt flexor carpi radialis tendon
ft flexor tendons

Expert note

The usual appearance of nerves is that of fascicular pattern (in contrast to tendons which display a fibrillar pattern). Typically, peripheral nerves seem to be anechoic when they are superficially localized and more hyperechoic as they course deep in the muscle compartments [3]. Nerves generally get enlarged (due to edema) when they are entrapped. This swelling can be detected either diffusely or can at times be observed even within individual fascicles [4].

Carpal tunnel syndrome in a 55-year-old man who had a 3-month history of intermittent numbness and burning pain in the three radial digits

12.43

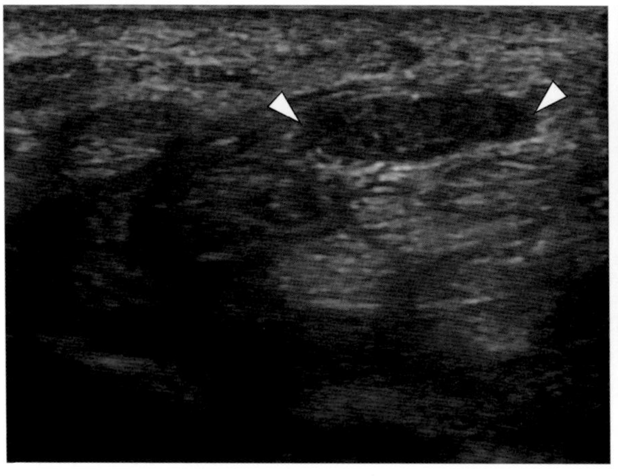

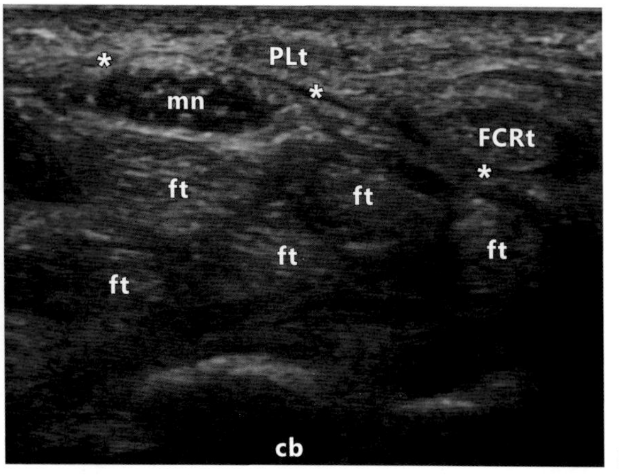

Axial US image over the volar wrist shows swelling of the median nerve (*arrowheads*) with loss of the fascicular echotexture (**a**). Normal findings of the median nerve (**mn**) and adjacent tissues (**b**).

cb	carpal bones
FCRt	flexor carpi radialis tendon
ft	flexor tendons
PLt	palmaris longus tendon
*	flexor retinaculum

12.44 Bilateral carpal tunnel syndrome in a young girl

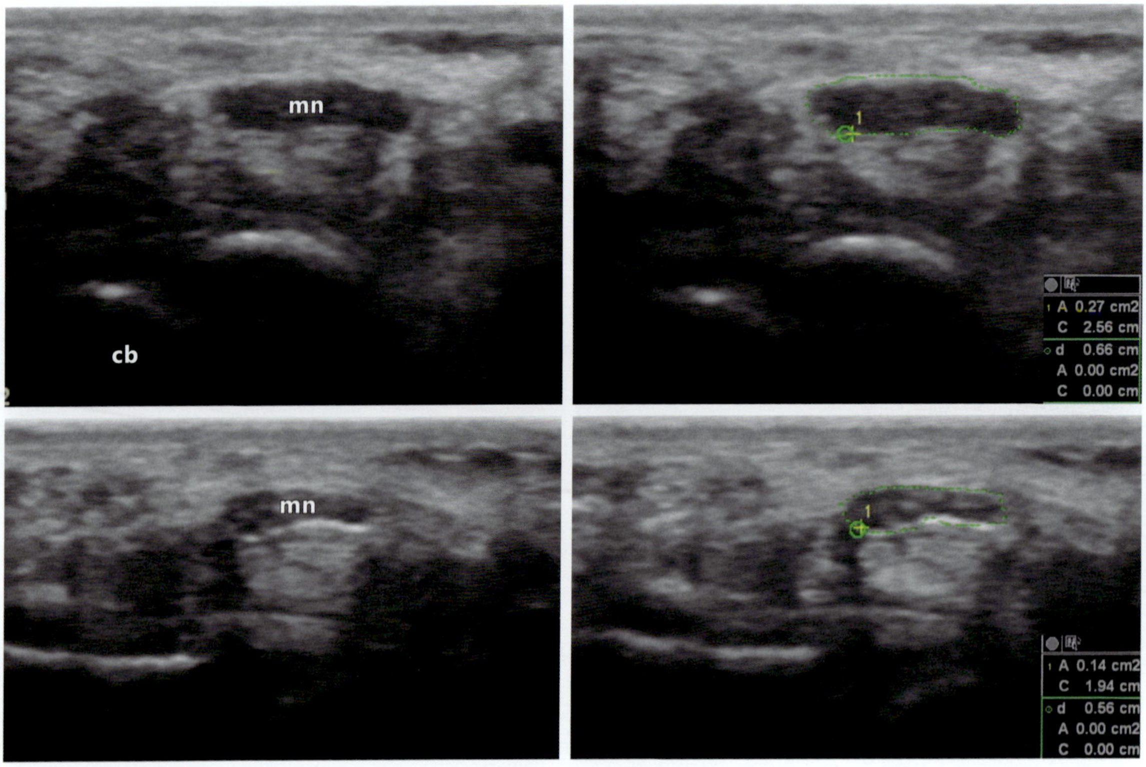

a b c d

She had paresthesia and pain on the volar side of the wrists extending along the first three fingers.

Axial US images (**a**, **c**) over the proximal carpal tunnel demonstrate hypoechoic and swollen appearances of the median nerves (**mn**), more prominent on one side (**a**). Corresponding views illustrate the cross-sectional area measurements (**b**, **d**).

cb carpal bones

Expert note

Aside from general morphological assessment, US imaging can also provide quantification (usually as regards cross-sectional area measurements). Although cut-off values do not exist for each and every nerve, certain measurements are reported for common entrapment syndromes (e.g. 10 mm^2 for median nerves at the carpal tunnel entrance).
On the other hand, an important discussion pertains to where/how exactly the measurements are to be taken [14]. There are even some ratios (proximal/distal or median/ulnar) described in the literature. In this sense, like in other pathologies and owing to its convenience, a more simple and reliable suggestion would be to compare with the asymptomatic side in unilateral cases.
Cross-sectional measurements are usually suggested to be perfomed inside the white borders (epineurium) of the nerve.

Dominant sided carpal tunnel syndrome in a 42-year-old carpenter with wrist pain aggravated during manual work and sleep

12.45

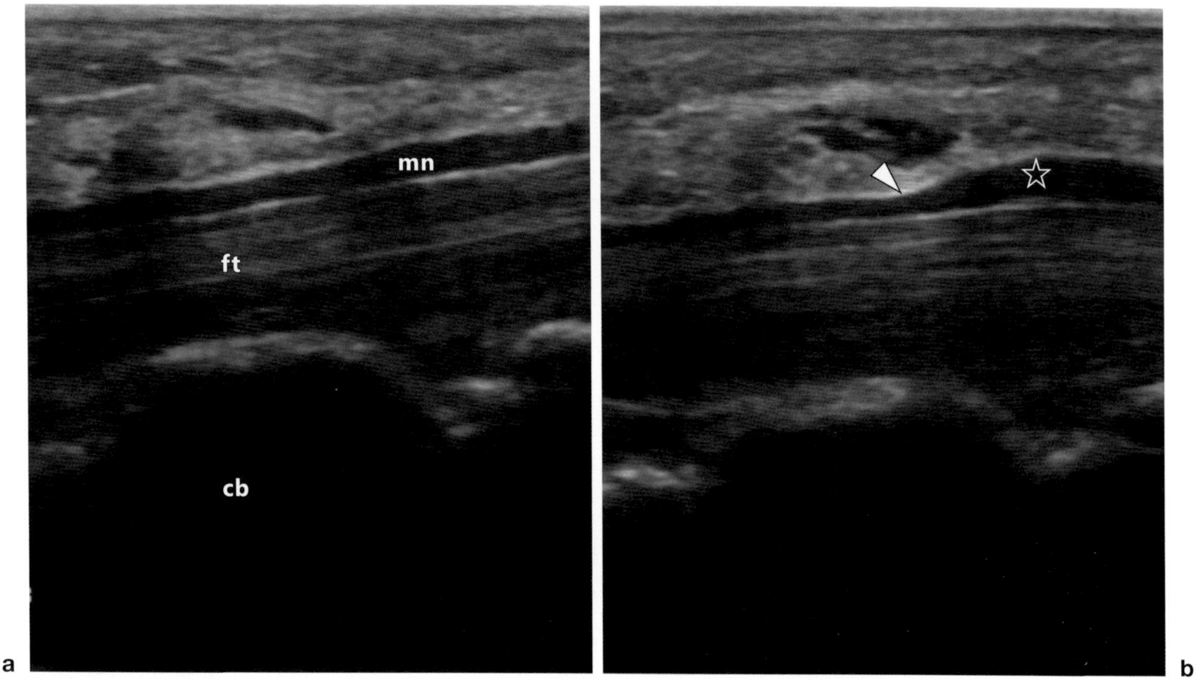

When compared with the normal side (**a**), longitudinal US image through the carpal tunnel (**b**) illustrates swollen (*star*) median nerve (**mn**) just proximal to the compression site (*arrowhead*).

cb carpal bones
ft flexor tendons

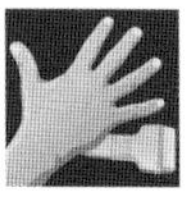

Expert note
This image is sometimes described as a "bottle neck".

12.46 Carpal tunnel syndrome in a 61-year-old woman

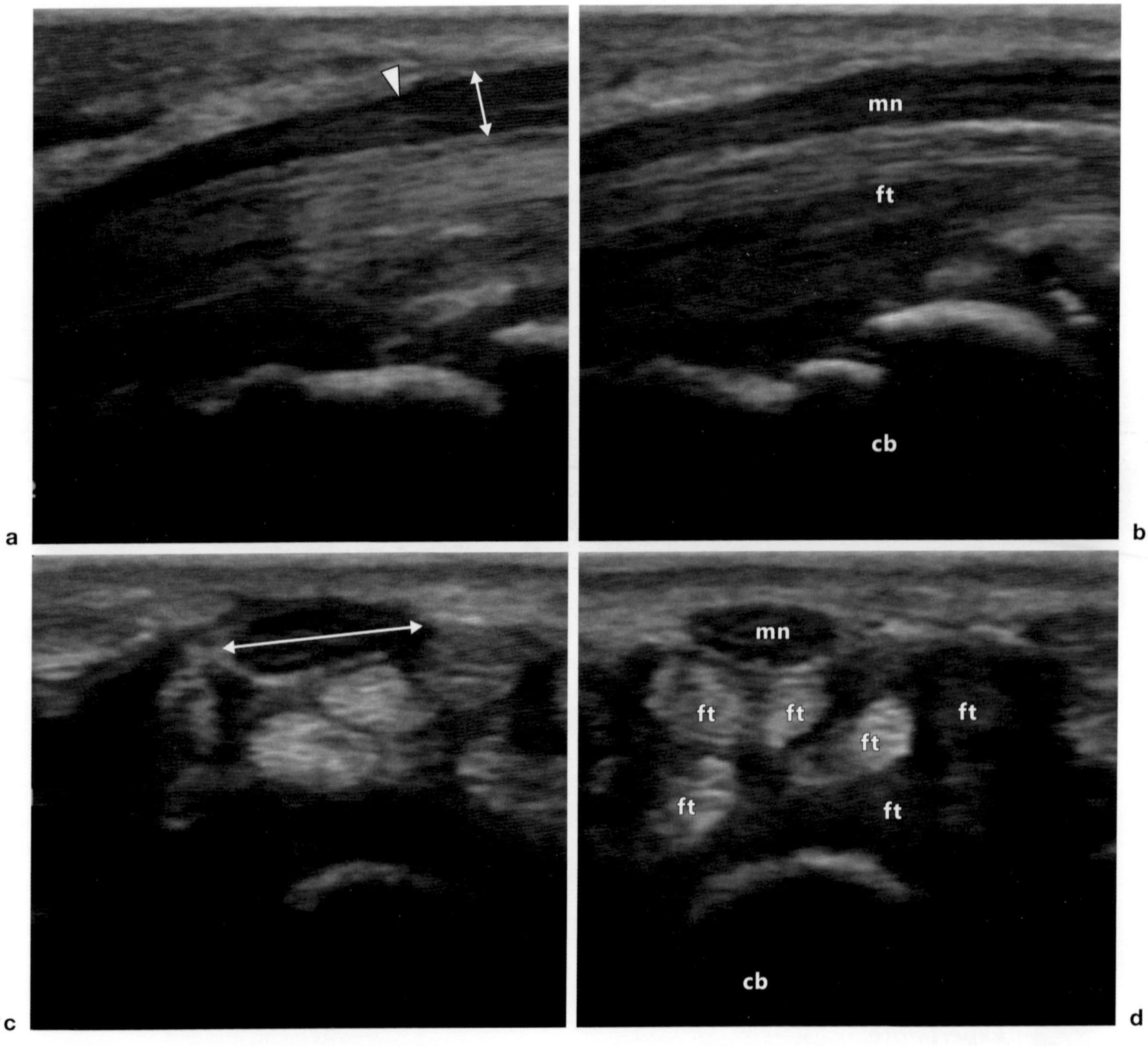

She started to have tingling, numbness and pain in the hand after an episode of strenuous repetitive manual activity.

Longitudinal (**a**) and axial (**c**) US images over the carpal tunnel show mild but diffuse enlargement (*double arrows*) of the median nerve proximal to the entrapment site (*arrowhead*). Normal median nerve (**mn**) and its close relationship with the flexor tendons (**ft**) (**b**, **d**).

cb carpal bones

Flexor tenosynovitis and carpal tunnel syndrome in a 48-year-old patient with rheumatoid arthritis 12.47

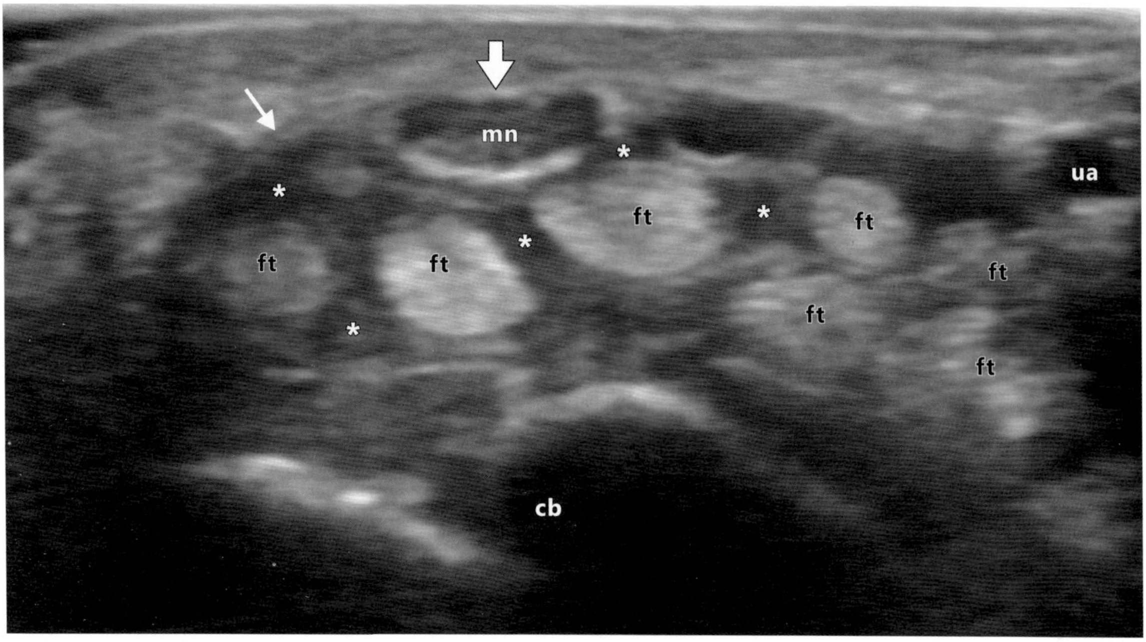

Axial US image shows hypoechoic and edematous (*thick arrow*) median nerve (**mn**) under the flexor retinaculum (*thin arrow*).
Please note that the flexor tendons (**ft**) are seen more hyperechoic than expected possibly due to the synovial effusion (*asterisks*) at the carpal tunnel.

cb carpal bones
ua ulnar artery

Expert note

In cases whereby the carpal tunnel syndrome is found to ensue secondary to other diseases, prompt treatment of the underlying condition is definitely/also necessary. Herewith, again with the help of US imaging/guidance, one can readily "kill two birds with one stone". For instance, precise corticosteroid injection within the tunnel might suffice to treat both problems locally in this patient [15].

12.48 An accessory palmar muscle in a patient with carpal tunnel syndrome

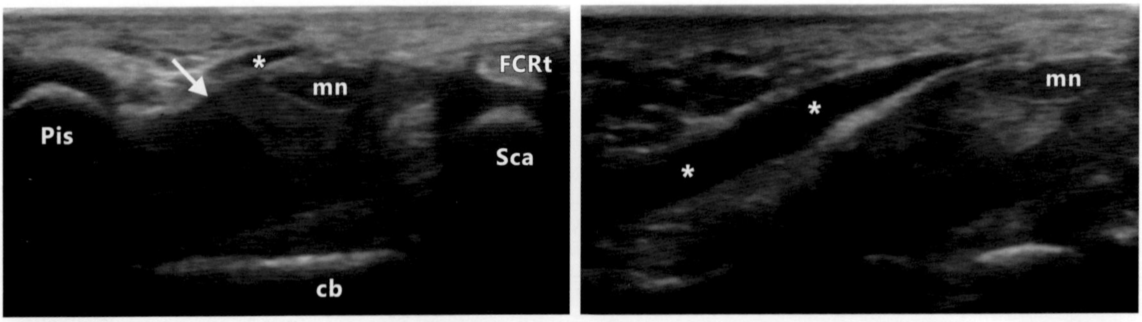

a b

Axial US images at the proximal carpal tunnel (**a**) and at a little more distal (**b**) levels demonstrate an anechoic elongated mass (*asterisks*) reflecting an accessory muscle. Note its attachment over the flexor retinaculum (*arrow*) immediately next to the median nerve (**mn**).

cb carpal bones
FCRt flexor carpi radialis tendon
Pis pisiform bone
Sca scaphoid bone

Expert note

Again, not only the underlying cause of entrapment but also the possible need/approach for surgery can be ascertained with a simple US assessment.

Carpal tunnel syndrome in a patient who had an operation history for the contralateral side one year ago **12.49**

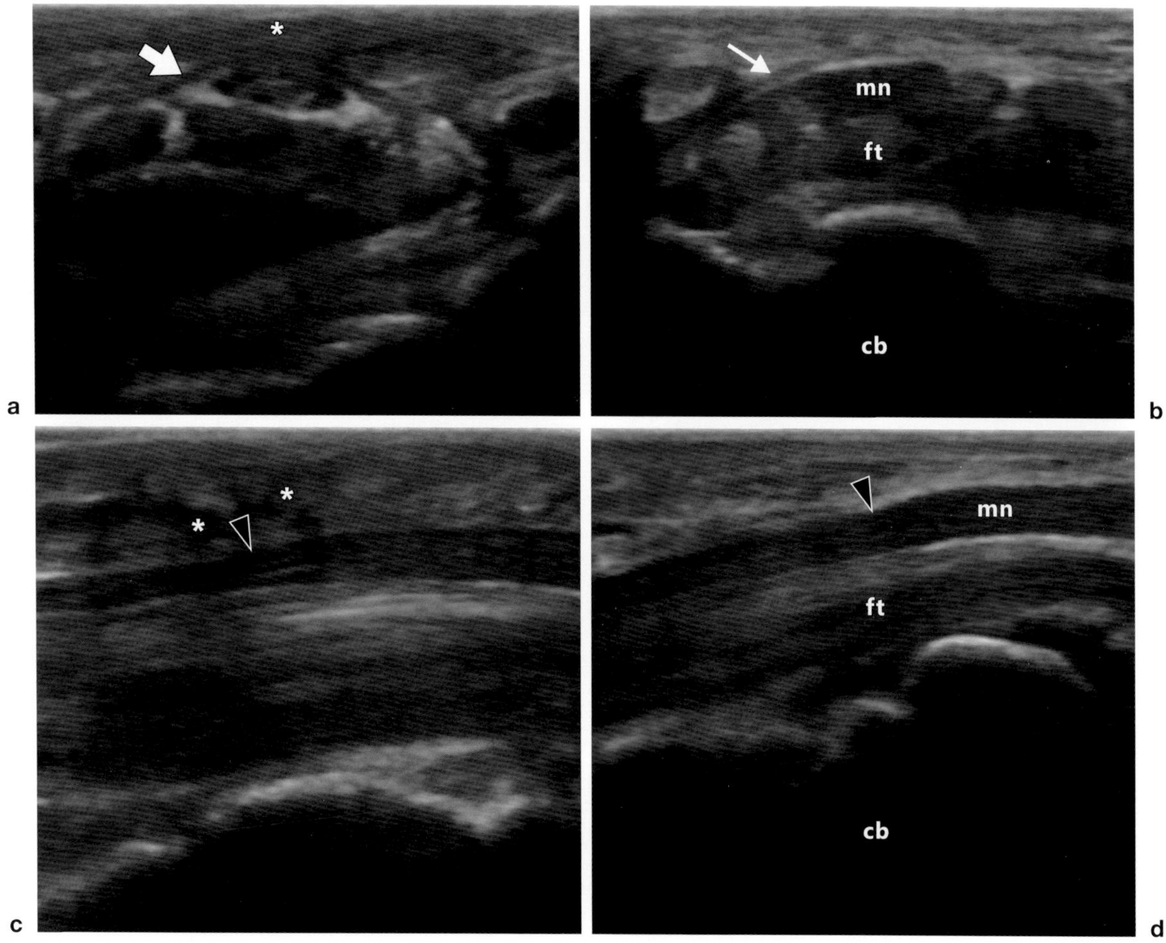

Axial (**a**) and longitudinal (**c**) US scans of the operated wrist demonstrate edematous flexor retinaculum (*thick arrow*) and irregular postsurgical scarring (*asterisks*). While the contralateral symptomatic side (**b**, **d**) shows normal flexor retinaculum (*thin arrow*), there is mild enlargement of the median nerve (**mn**) proximal to the entrapment site (*arrowhead*), reflecting carpal tunnel syndrome. Note that the nerve is also/still edematous (*arrowhead*) on the operated side (**c**).

cb carpal bones
ft flexor tendons

Expert note

When patients are followed postoperatively; like elsewhere, morphological changes might be "exaggerated" and not always correlate with the clinical/electrophysiological findings.

12.50 Carpal tunnel syndrome in 45-year-old housewife 6 months after an operation for the contralateral side

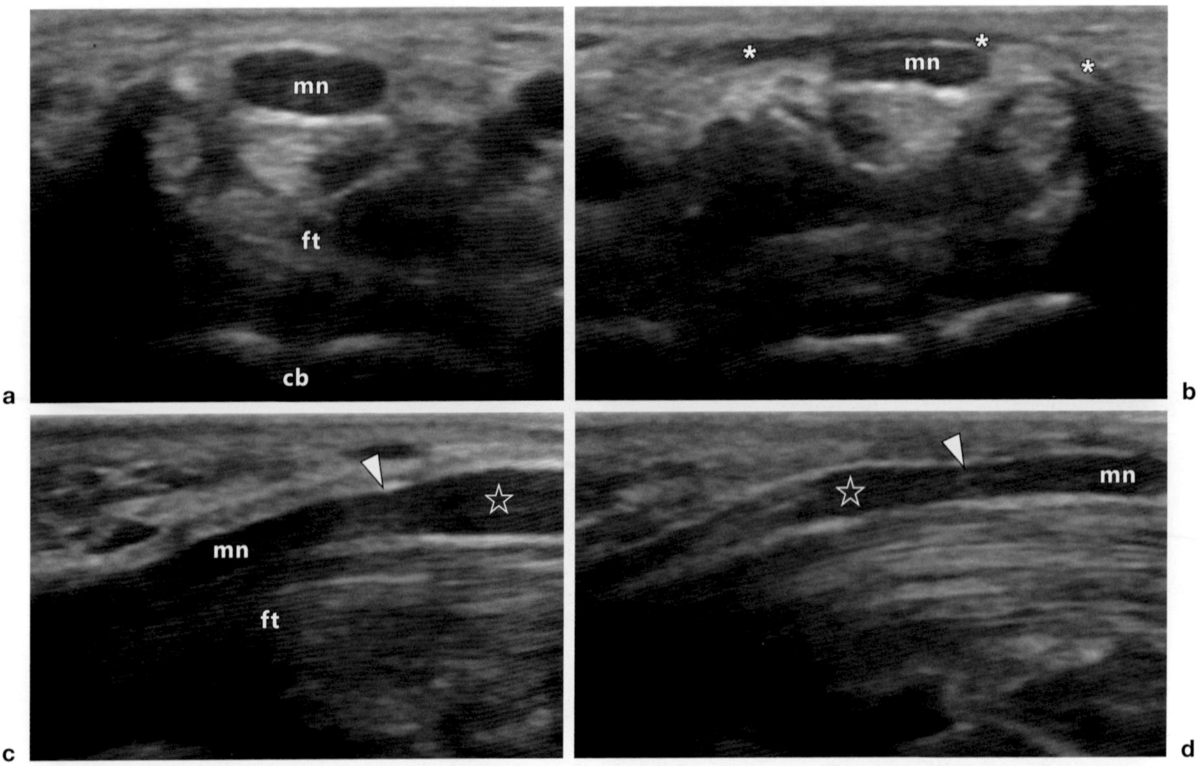

Axial (**a**) and longitudinal (**c**) images obtained over the proximal carpal tunnel show enlarged (*star*) median nerve (**mn**) proximal to the entrapment side (*arrowhead*). On the operated side, thickened and hypoechoic flexor retinaculum (*asterisks*) can be seen together with distal nerve swelling (*star*) (**b**, **d**).

cb carpal bones
ft flexor tendons

Expert note

In contrast/addition to proximal swelling, edema in the distal part of the median nerve can also be observed in the postoperative period [13].

Repaired median nerve and flexor tendons in an 11-year-old girl following a glass injury

12.51

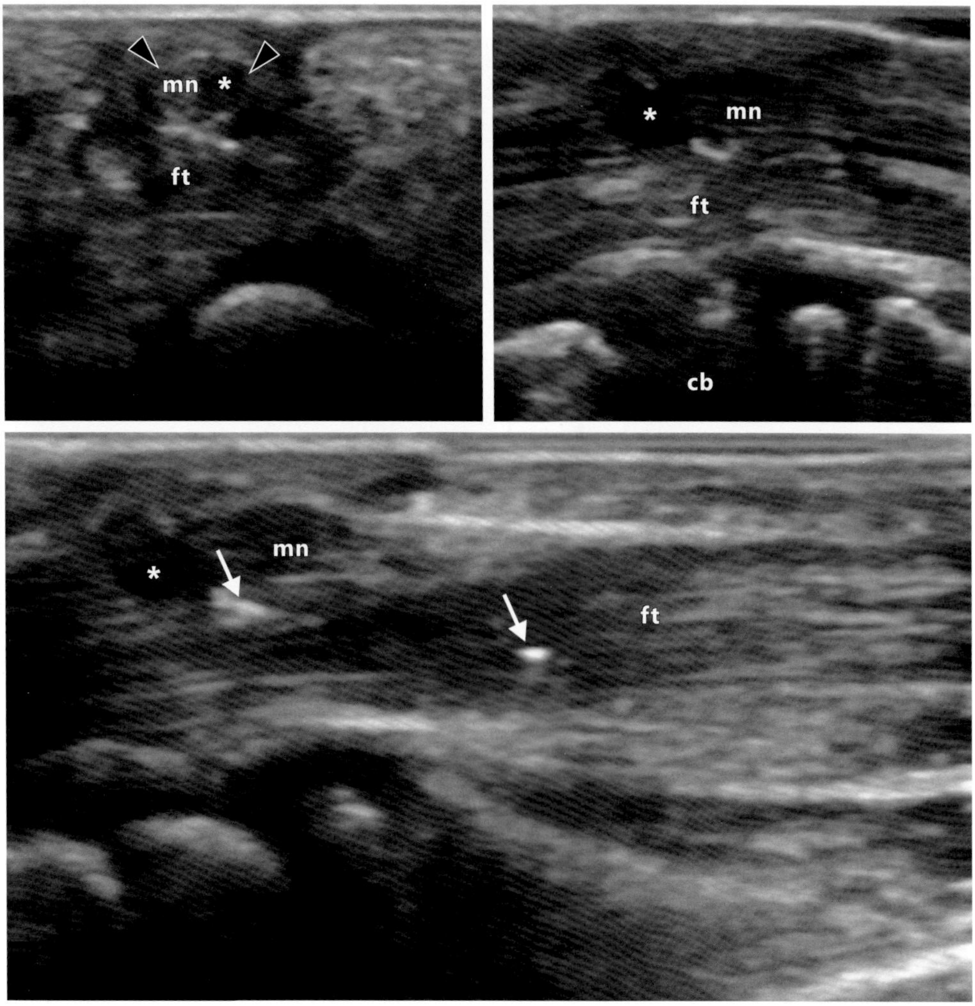

Axial (**a**) and longitudinal (**b**) US images at the wrist level demonstrate the median nerve (**mn**) (*arrowheads*) containing intraneural fluid-filled space (*asterisks*). Suture materials (*arrows*) can be visualized as intratendinous bright specular echoes at the level of the penetrating trauma (**c**).

cb carpal bones
ft flexor tendons

Expert note

Either the intactness of the nerve/tendons or the dynamic relationship in between can substantially be evaluated and followed up.

12.52 Bilateral bifid median nerve in a 42-year-old asymptomatic woman

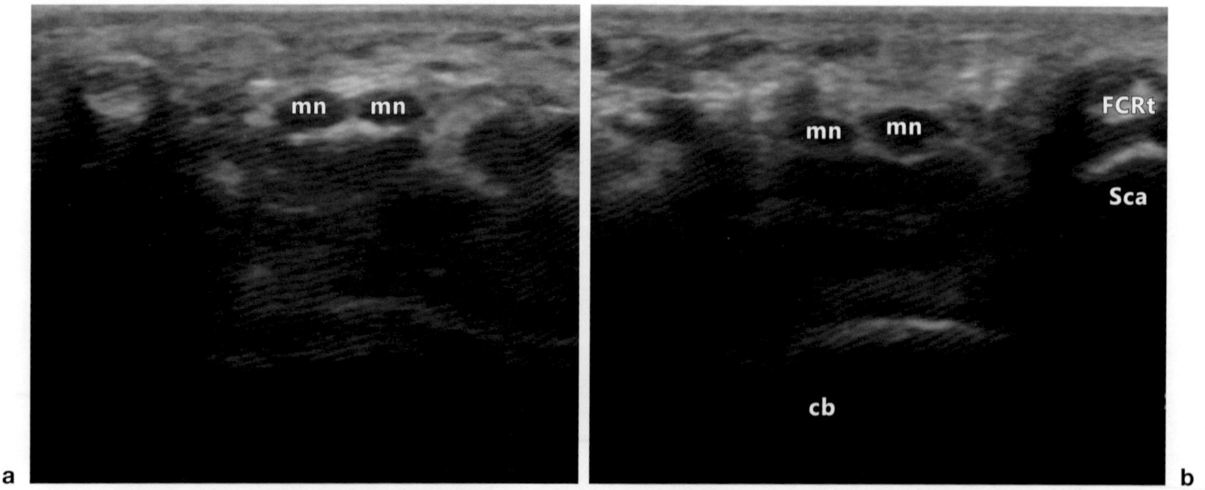

Axial US images obtained at the proximal level of the carpal tunnel reveal bifid median nerve (**mn**) on both sides (**a**, **b**).

cb carpal bones
FCRt flexor carpi radialis tendon
Sca scaphoid bone

Bilateral carpal tunnel syndrome in a 48-year-old man who presented with complaints of numbness and pain in the hands **12.53**

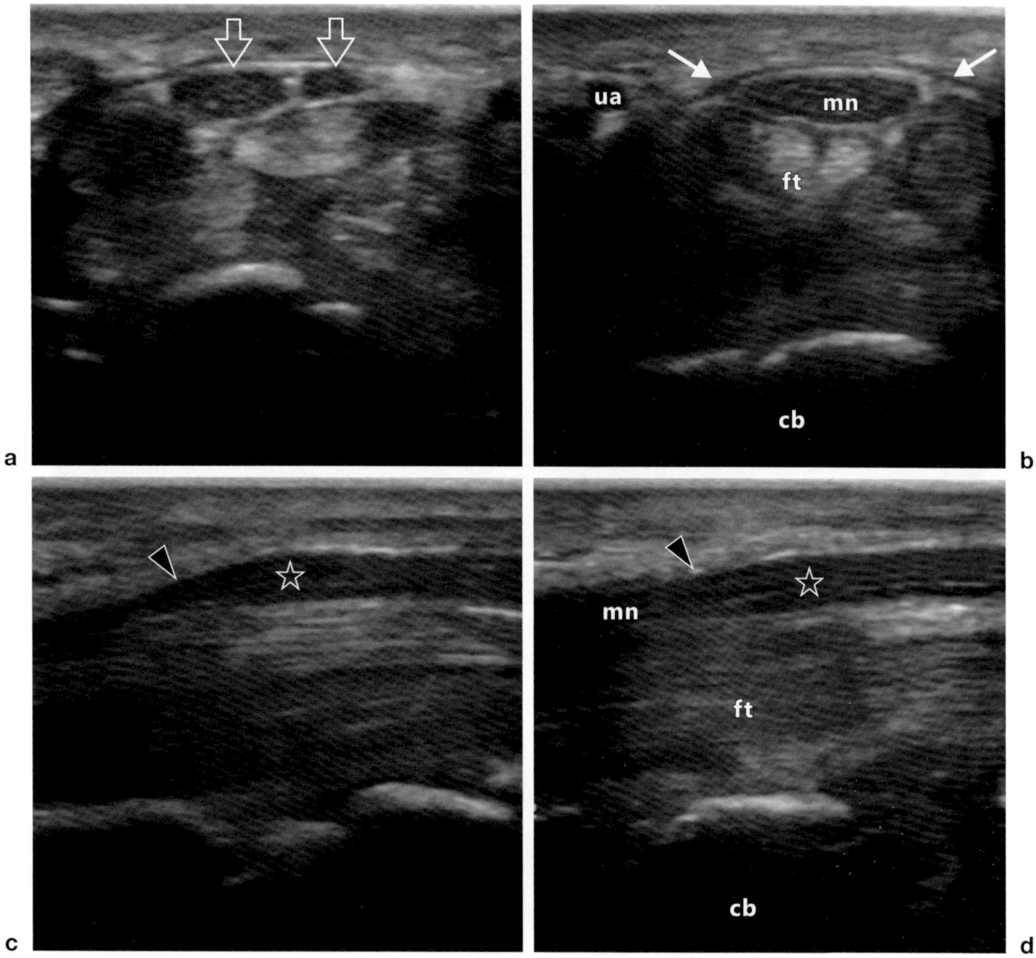

a b c d

Axial US images show bifid median nerve (**mn**) with two paired bundles (*thick arrows*) on one side (**a**) and a single enlarged median nerve beneath the flexor retinaculum (*thin arrows*) on the other side (**b**). Longitudinal US images through the carpal tunnel demonstrate compression sites (*arrowheads*) and proximal swellings (*stars*) (**c**, **d**).

cb carpal bones
ft flexor tendons
ua ulnar artery

Expert note

When measuring the cross-sectional area in case of a bifid nerve, one should measure both bundles and then add the numbers [16, 17].

12.54 Persistent median artery and bifid median nerve in a 30-year-old otherwise asymptomatic man

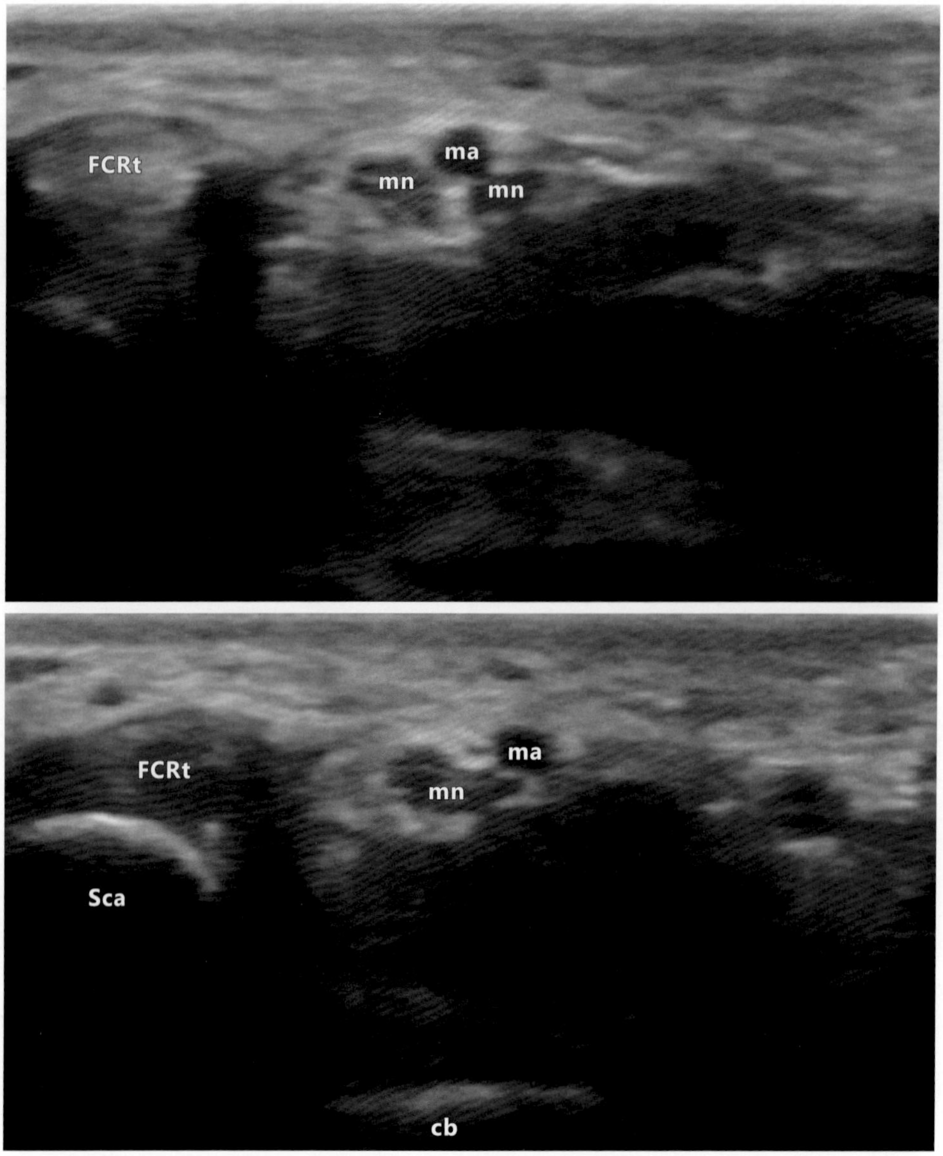

a b

Axial US image obtained over the distal wrist crease reveals an anatomical variant, persistent median artery (**ma**) interposed between the two trunks of a bifid median nerve (**mn**) (**a**). Bifid parts combine and form a single trunk at the proximal carpal tunnel level (**b**).

cb carpal bones
FCRt flexor carpi radialis tendon
Sca scaphoid bone

Persistent median artery in a 43-year-old physician with mild and intermittent pain and paresthesia radiating proximally in the forearm

12.55

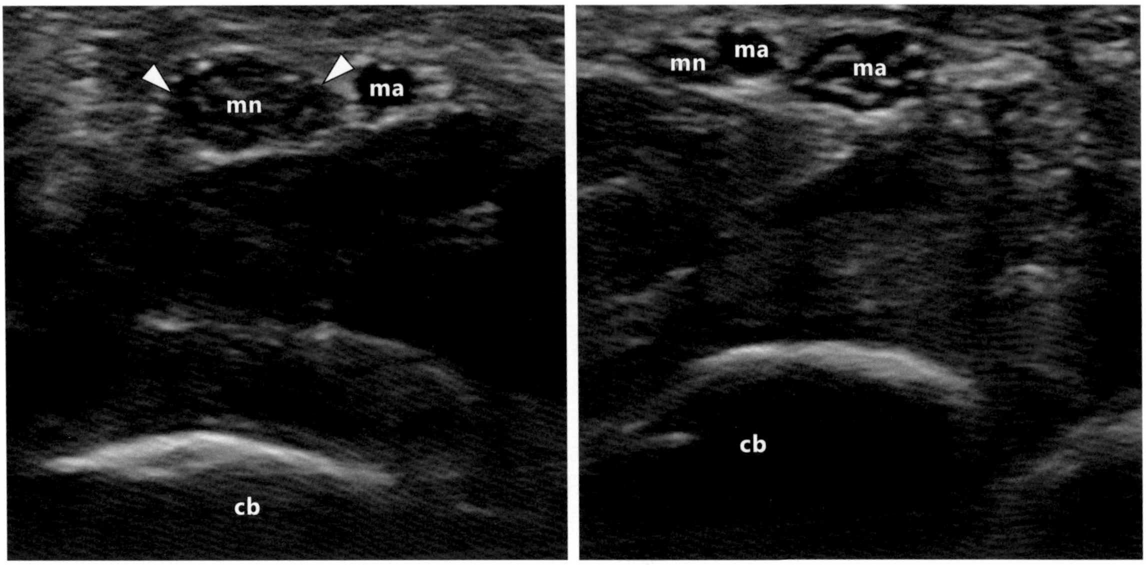

a b

Axial US image demonstrates an edematous (*arrowheads*) median nerve (**mn**) with swollen fascicles and a persistent median artery (**ma**) (**a**). Asymptomatic side also reveals a persistent median artery within the bifid median nerve (**b**).

cb carpal bones

Expert note

It is not uncommon to find various aberrations during US imaging of symptomatic or asymptomatic subjects [18, 19]. Depending on the clinical findings, they can either be (simply) reassured or informed about the underlying/likely anatomical cause as regards the entrapment. The latter is also crucial for the surgeon in case of an onward operation. Herein, if pathological clinical/electrophysiological findings are present, US imaging definitely serves to rename the scenario i.e. no more "idiopathic" carpal tunnel syndrome.

12.56 Bifid median nerve and persistent median artery in a 31-year-old woman who started to drop objects from her hand

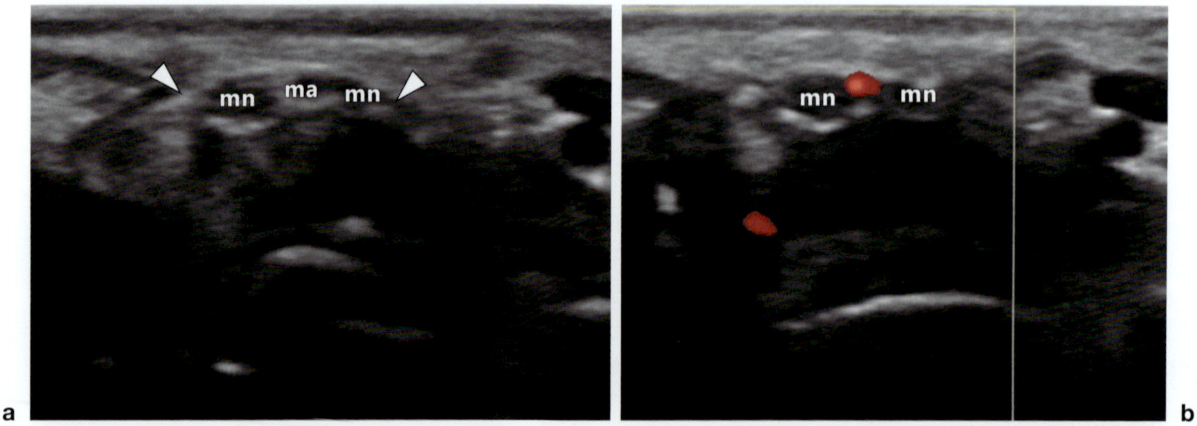

Axial US image reveals persistent median artery (**ma**) located within the bifid median nerve (**mn**) (**a**). Power Doppler imaging is also confirmatory (**b**).
Please note the overlying normal flexor retinaculum (*arrowheads*).

Fibrolipomatous hamartoma of the median nerve in a 38-year-old secretary who had been operated for carpal tunnel syndrome 12.57

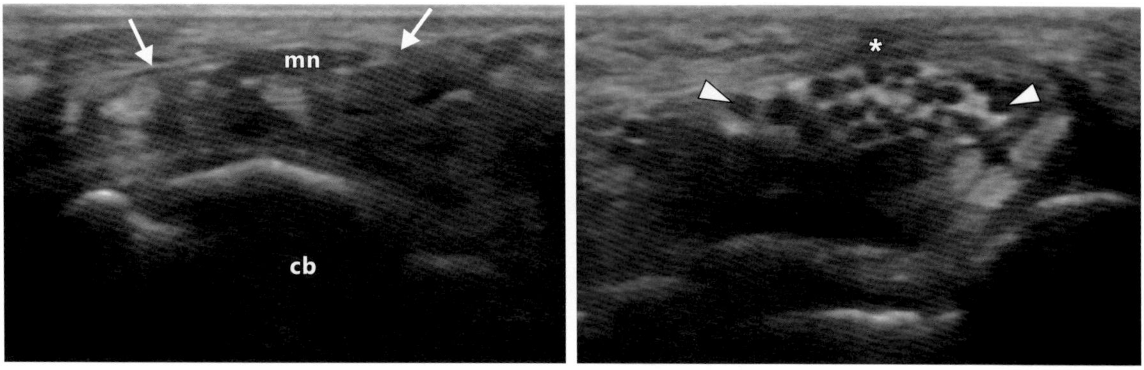

When compared with the normal median nerve (**mn**) beneath the flexor retinaculum (*arrows*) (**a**), axial US image (**b**) shows the significantly enlarged anechoic fascicles (*arrowheads*) embedded within the increased hyperechoic interfascicular fatty tissue. *Asterisk* shows the postsurgical scarring tissue.

cb carpal bones

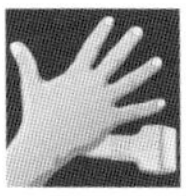

Expert note

US is an indispensable diagnostic tool not only for better guiding the carpal tunnel surgery but also for avoiding irreversible steps at other times. For example, had US imaging been performed before the surgery of this patient, she would have been definitely refrained from an unnecessary operation during which the surgeon thought that the nerve swelling was consistent with a schwannoma. Herein, it would not be incorrect to say that typical appearances of certain pathologies on US imaging can easily help one truly foresee the diagnosis even before another one dissects and inevitably considers the outlook only [20].

12.58 Meralgia paresthetica in an obese woman

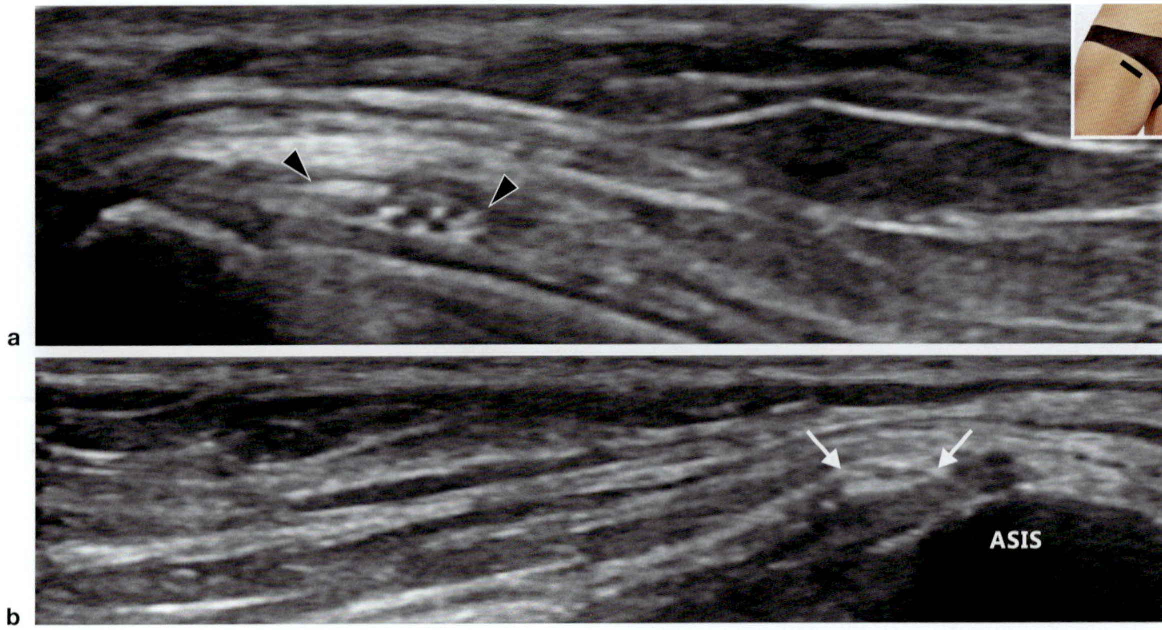

She presented with numbness and paresthesia in the anterolateral region of the thigh where the skin was hypersensitive to touch.

Axial US image demonstrates hypoechoic swelling of the fascicles within the lateral femoral cutaneous nerve (*arrowheads*) as it passes close to the anterior superior iliac spine (**ASIS**) (**a**). Normal nerve (*arrows*) on the contralateral side (**b**).

Expert note

Especially in peripheral nerve entrapment syndromes where electrophysiological studies are hardly conclusive (e.g. meralgia paresthetica), US imaging is invaluable for the diagnosis and the onward interventional procedures [21]. In contrast to what is initially/generally thought, lateral femoral cutaneous nerve can be very nicely imaged with "familiar eyes". Locating the ASIS and the inguinal ligament would be the main landmarks for recognizing the nerve which passes either through, above or beneath the latter structure.

Lateral femoral cutaneous neuropathy in a 55-year-old man with chronic sensory symptoms radiating over the anterolateral region of the thigh

12.59

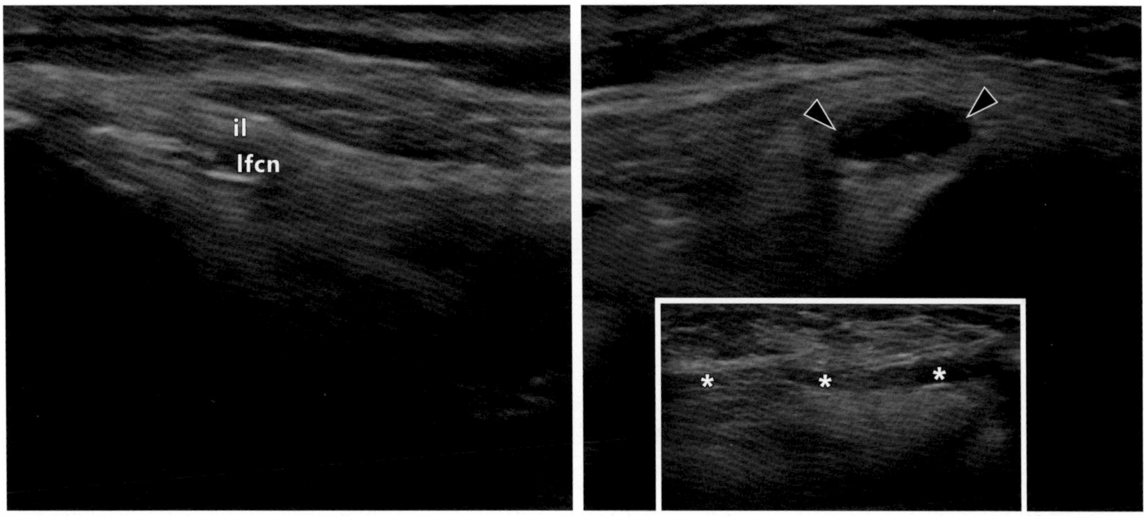

a b

When compared with the normal side (**a**), axial US image (**b**) demonstrate a fusiform, hypoechoic swelling (*arrowheads*) of the lateral femoral cutaneous nerve (**lfcn**). Longitudinal view of the edematous nerve (*asterisks*) (*small figure*).

il inguinal ligament

12.60 Normal longitudinal view of the sciatic nerve

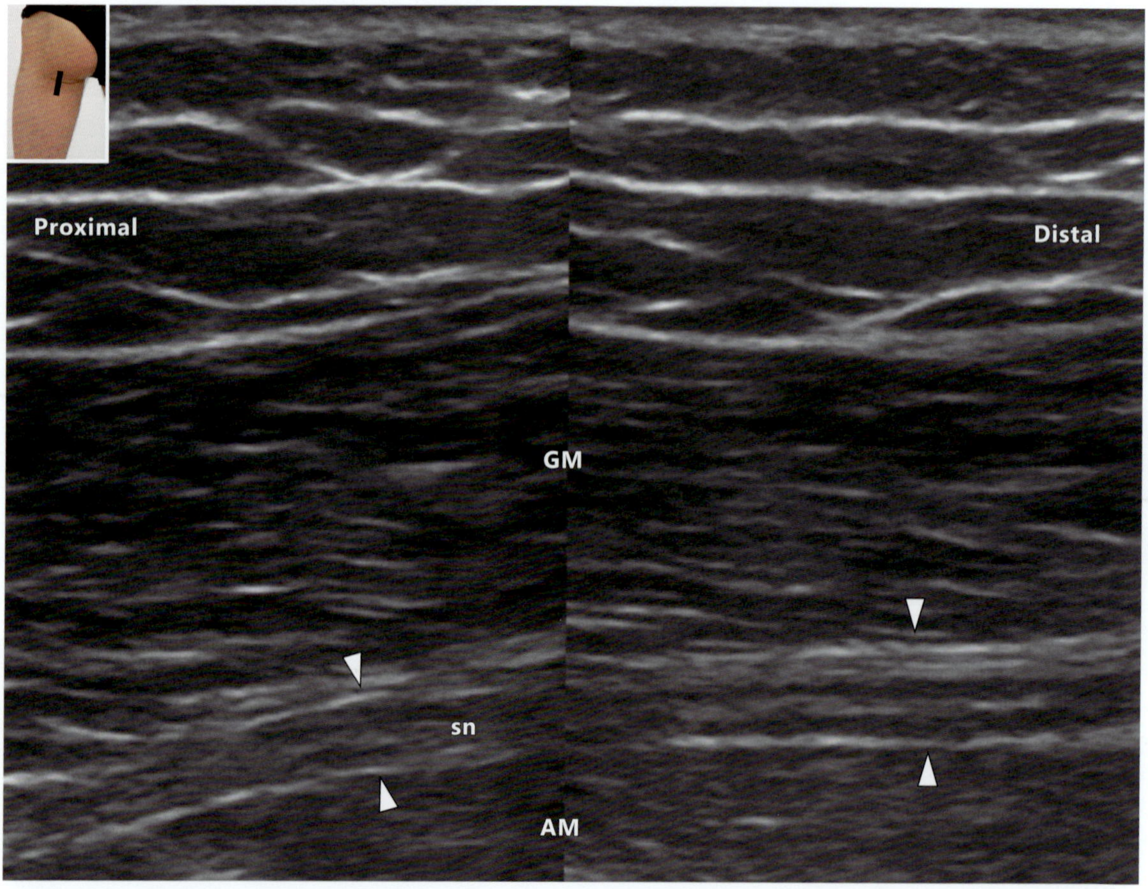

Split-screen longitudinal US image illustrates the normal course (*arrowheads*) and structure of the sciatic nerve (**sn**) between the gluteus maximus (**GM**) and adductor magnus (**AM**) muscles.

Normal axial view of the sciatic nerve between the hamstring and adductor magnus muscles 12.61

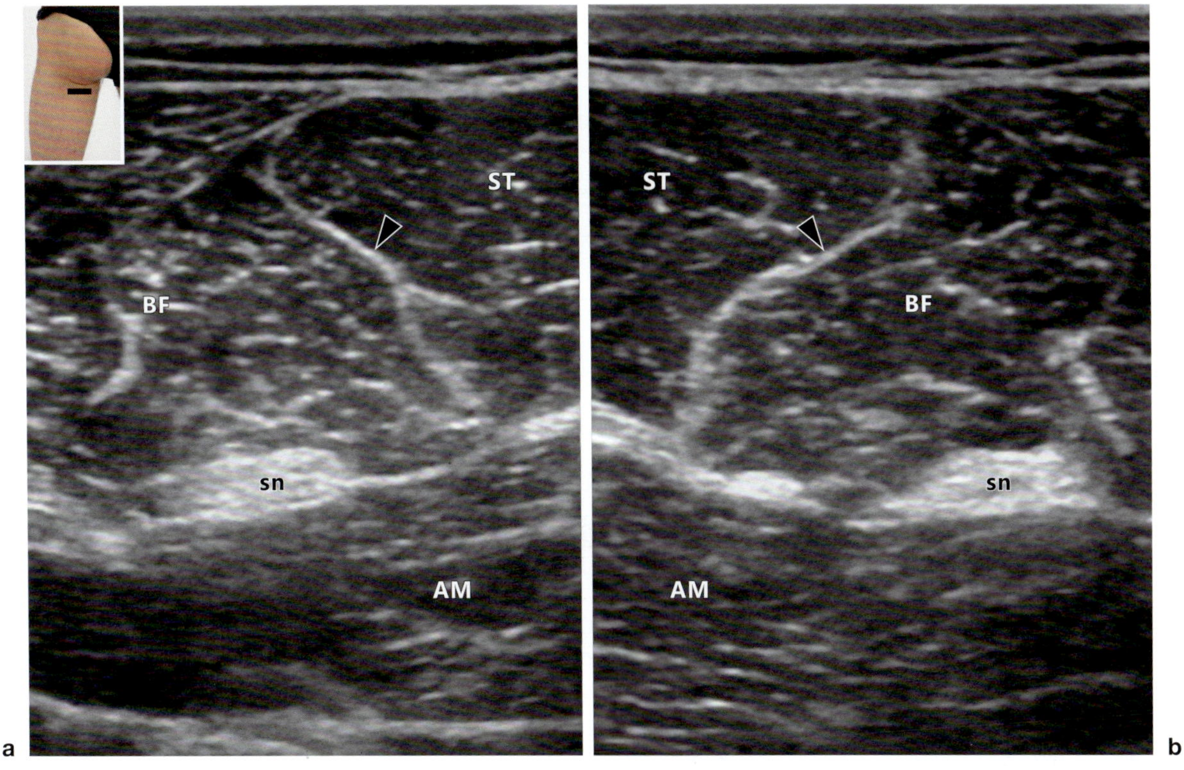

While the sciatic nerve (**sn**) courses between the gluteus maximus and adductor magnus (**AM**) muscles proximally; it is traversing between the long head of the biceps femoris (**BF**) and adductor magnus muscles distally. Bilateral imaging of a normal subject (**a**, **b**).
Please note the hyperechoic appearance of the distal conjoined tendon of the semitendinosus (**ST**)-biceps femoris muscles (*arrowheads*).

12.62 Piriformis syndrome in a 37-year-old man with buttock pain radiating into the posterior thigh (without any trauma)

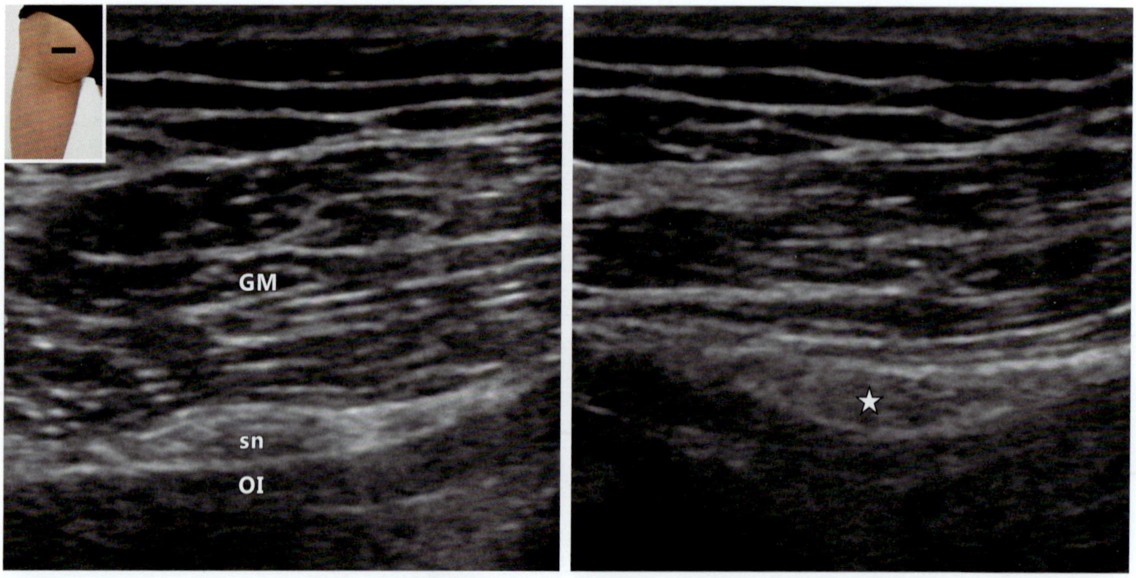

a b

When compared with the normal sciatic nerve (**sn**) (**a**), axial US image (**b**) over the posterior hip just distal to the piriformis muscle demonstrate nerve swelling with hypoechoic appearance (*star*).

GM gluteus maximus
OI obturator internus

Expert note

Aside from detection of focal nerve edema, sono-Tinel (especially eliciting the patient's actual complaints) is definitely helpful for the diagnosis and localization of the possible injection site. Visualization of the nerve in obese patients is often difficult; as such examination while the patient is lying prone with a pillow under the pelvis (with mild hip flexion) can be helpful [22].

Sciatic nerve injury due to heterotopic ossification in a 25-year-old man

12.63

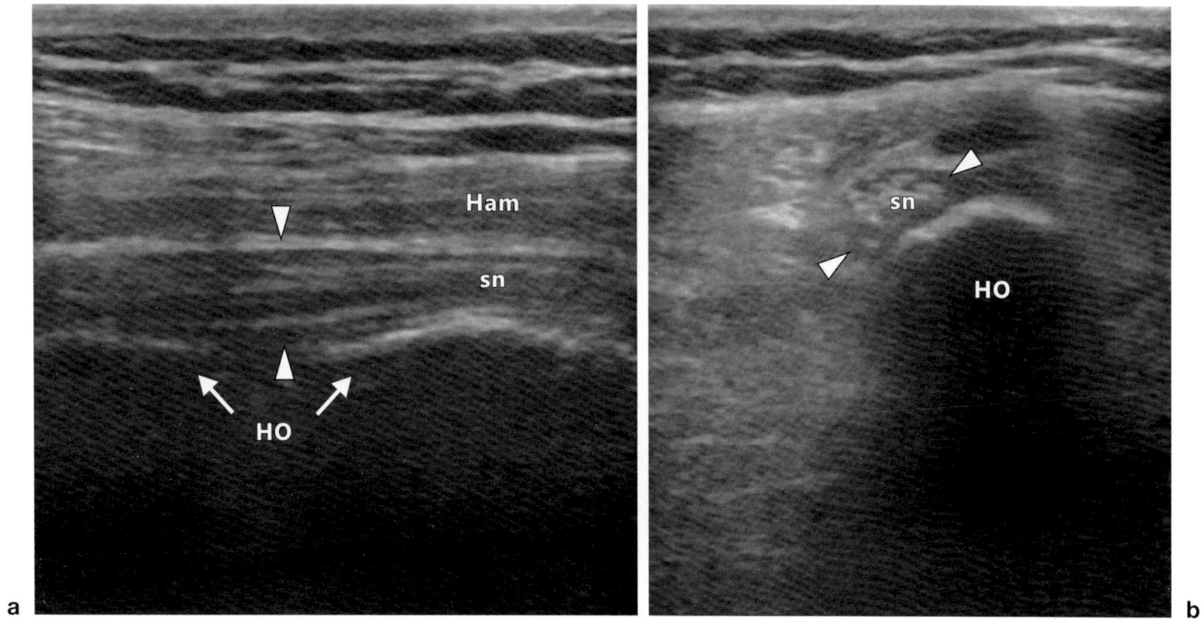

He had a traumatic brain injury who had hypoesthesia in the plantar surface of the foot.

Posterior longitudinal (**a**) and axial (**b**) US images of the proximal thigh show swollen (*arrowheads*) sciatic nerve (**sn**) due to the irritation of the heterotopic ossification (**HO**) (*arrows*).

Ham hamstrings

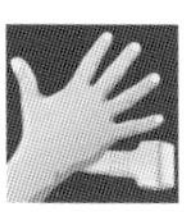

Expert note

Owing to its several advantages, US imaging can display the nerve entrapment and its underlying cause, in this case heterotopic ossification. Herein, it is noteworthy that US seems to be the earliest imaging modality to demonstrate such an association [23].

12.64 Sciatic nerve injury in a 20-year-old man

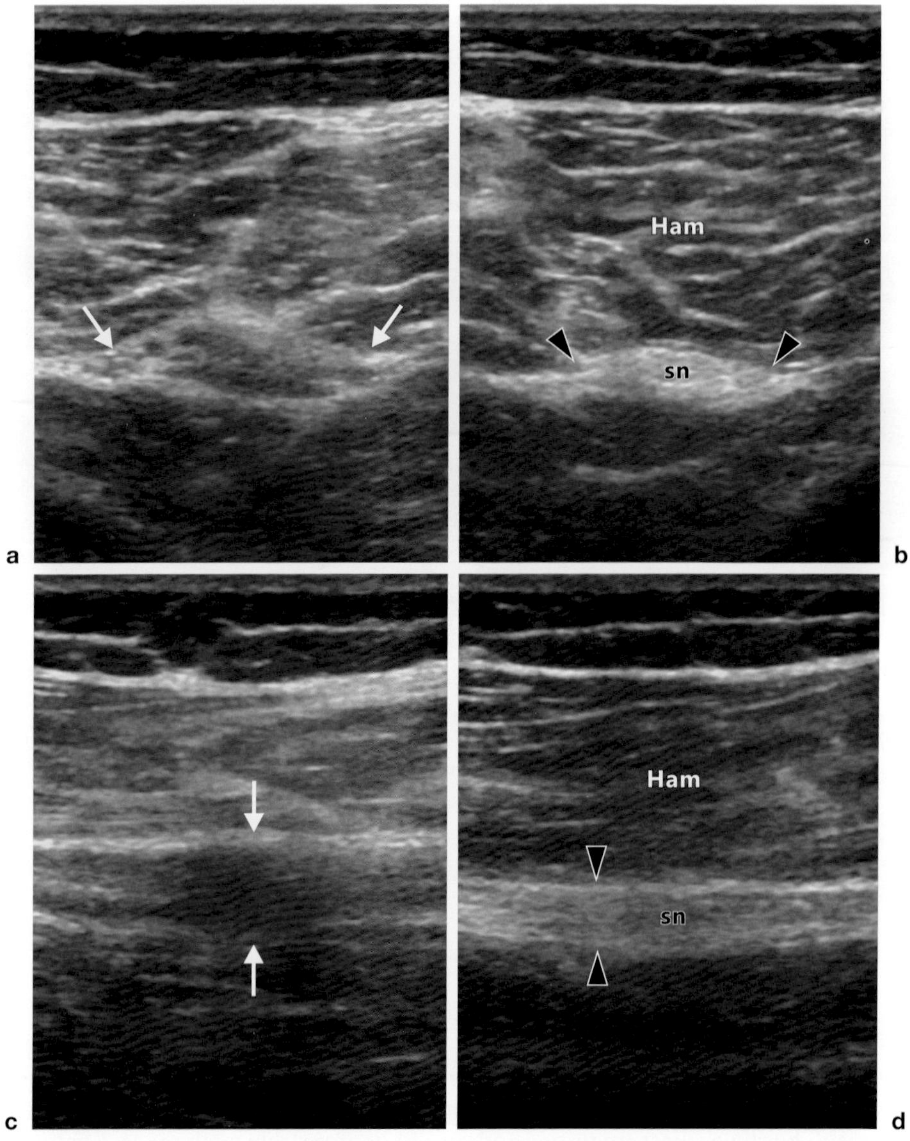

The injury occurred by a sharp object laceration and caused weakness (4/5) in the right foot dorsiflexion.

Axial (**a**) and longitudinal (**c**) US images obtained over the proximal thigh level reveal edematous and hypoechoic sciatic nerve (*arrows*). Normal hyperechoic sciatic nerve (**sn**) with a well-defined fascicular echotexture (*arrowheads*) is seen on the contralateral side (**b**, **d**).

Ham hamstrings

Sciatic nerve injury due to a gluteal injection in a 25-year-old woman **12.65**

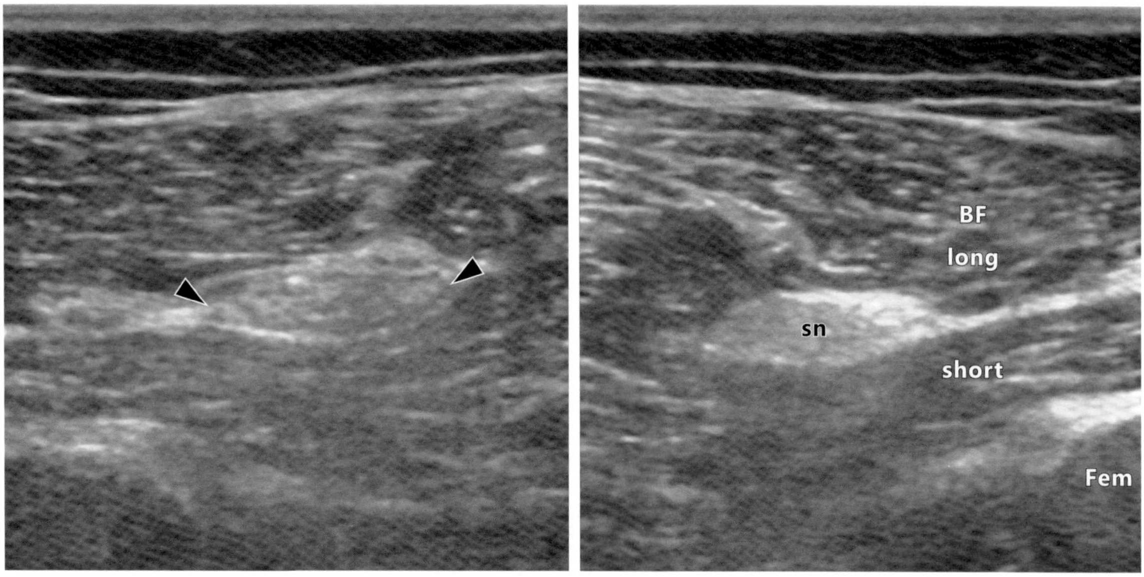

a b

She had complaints of severe neuropathic pain, paresthesia, and weakness in the lower extremity.

Posterior axial US image at the mid-thigh level demonstrates swollen and hypoechoic sciatic nerve (**sn**) (*arrowheads*) (**a**). Normal appearence of the sciatic nerve on the contralateral side (**b**).

BF biceps femoris
Fem femur

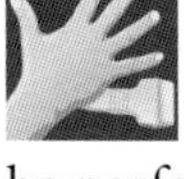

Expert note

Nerve edema can sometimes be observed either distal or proximal to the actual site of the lesion possibly due to impaired axonal transport. Therefore, scanning of the nerve should be performed thoroughly, from proximal to distal or vice versa [24-26].
If direct visualization of the nerve is difficult, one can examine the muscles in its territory, looking for fatty degeneration (in case of denervation).

12.66 Sciatic nerve injury in a 28-year-old woman who had posterior hip pain radiating down to the thigh

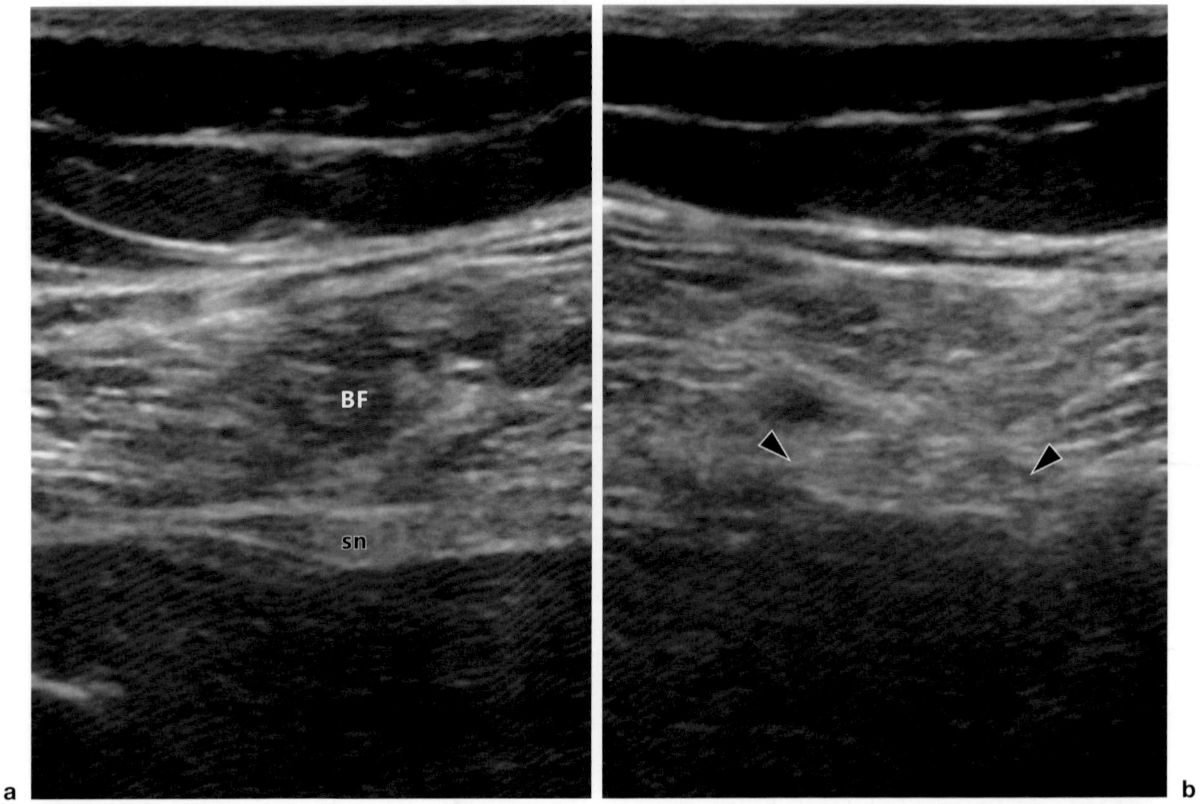

When compared with the normal sciatic nerve (**sn**) and its oval structure (**a**), axial US image reveals grossly edematous nerve (*arrowheads*) on the affected side (**b**).

BF biceps femoris

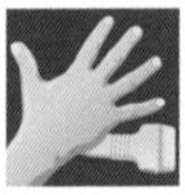

Expert note

One can measure the cross-sectional area of the nerve to quantify swelling and later on for comparison during repeat measurements.

Sciatic nerve injury in a 12-year-old boy who presented with a 5-month history of drop-foot after a gluteal injection

12.67

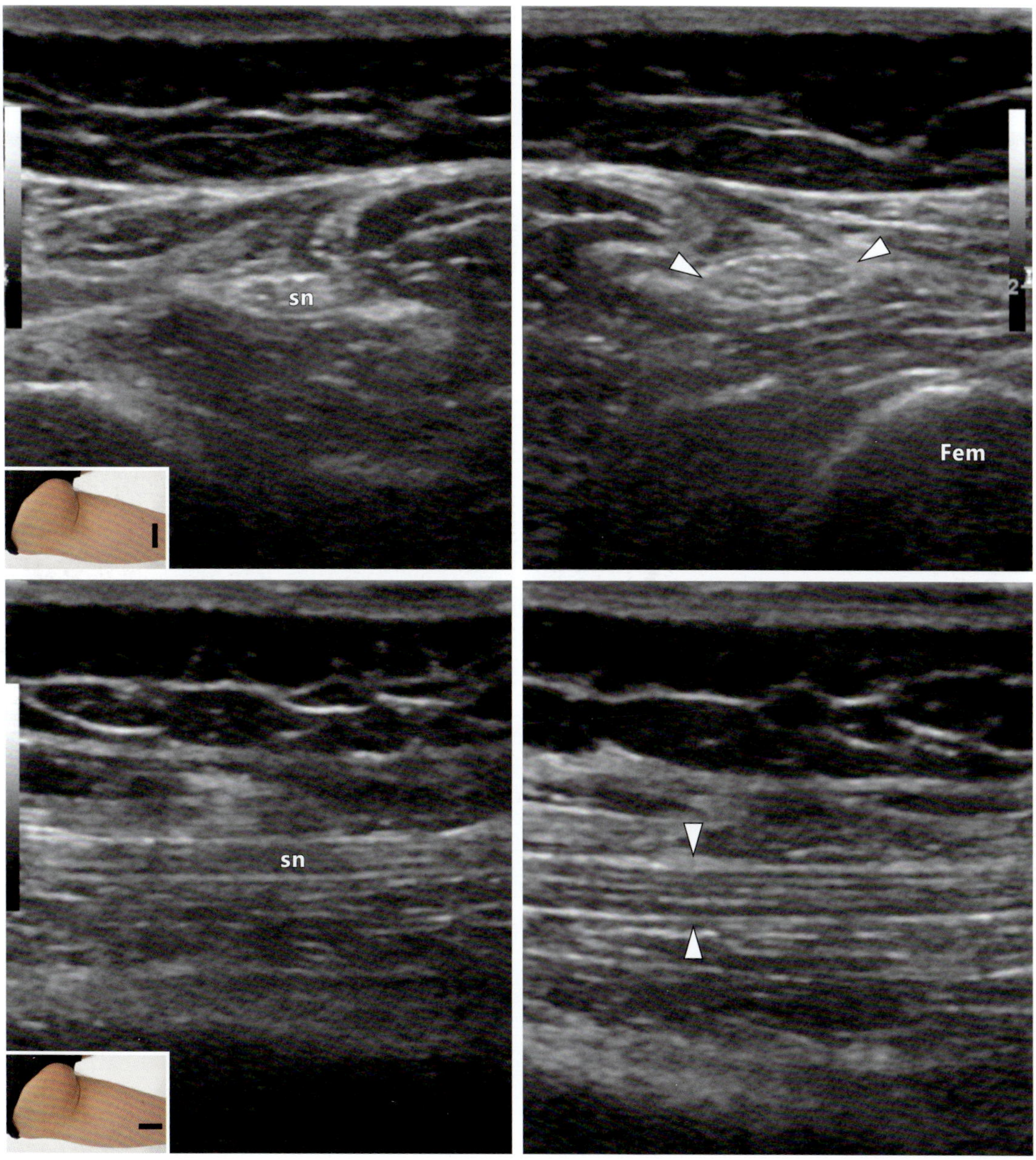

When compared with the normal side (**a**, **c**), axial (**b**) and longitudinal (**d**) US images demonstrate hypoechoic and edematous sciatic nerve (**sn**) (*arrowheads*) proximal to its bifurcation as tibial and common peroneal nerves.

Fem femur

12.68 Healing strain in a middle-aged runner with neuropathic pain at the posterolateral thigh for the last six months

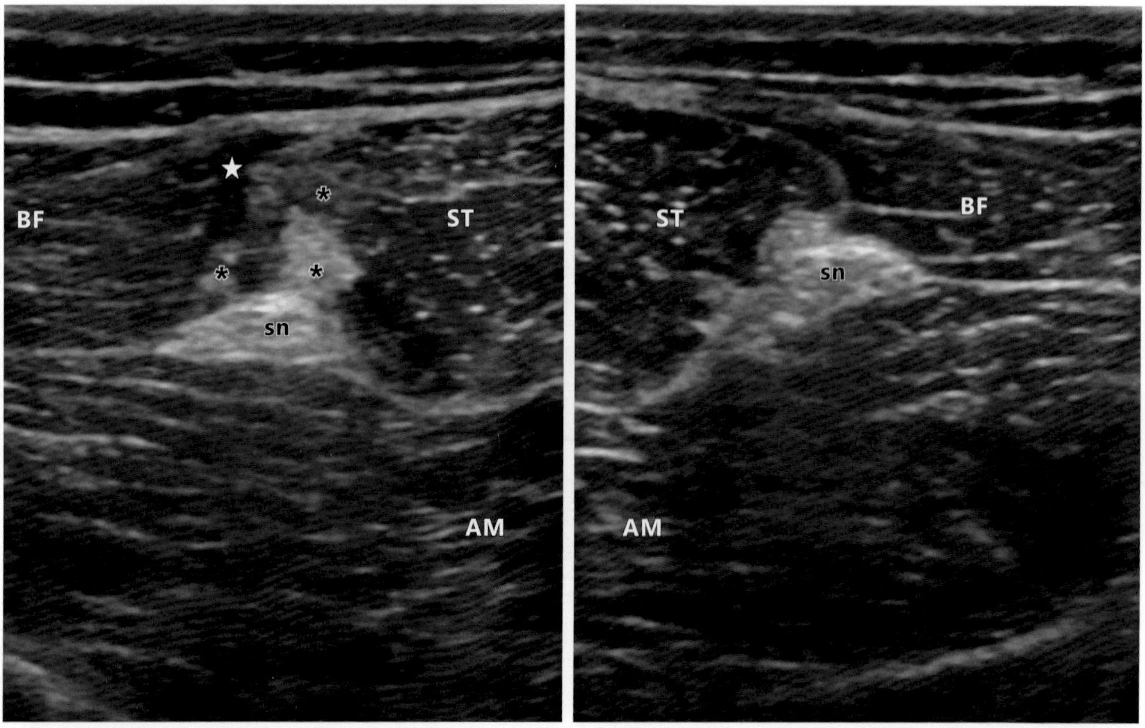

a b

Axial US image (**a**) demonstrates the healing process with an ill-defined hyperechoic area representing perilesional fibrosis (*black asterisks*) and hypoechoic area related to hemorrhagic changes (*star*) immediately neighboring the sciatic nerve (**sn**). Normal contralateral side (**b**).

AM adductor magnus
BF biceps femoris
ST semitendinosus

Expert note

While the nerve does not seem to have been affected much, the close relationship between the strain area and the sciatic nerve is quite explanatory for the patient's clinical findings. Further, the close proximity of the lesion to the nerve would also caution the physician during a possible intervention.

Plexiform neurofibromas in the sciatic nerve of a 45-year-old woman who is otherwise asymptomatic 12.69

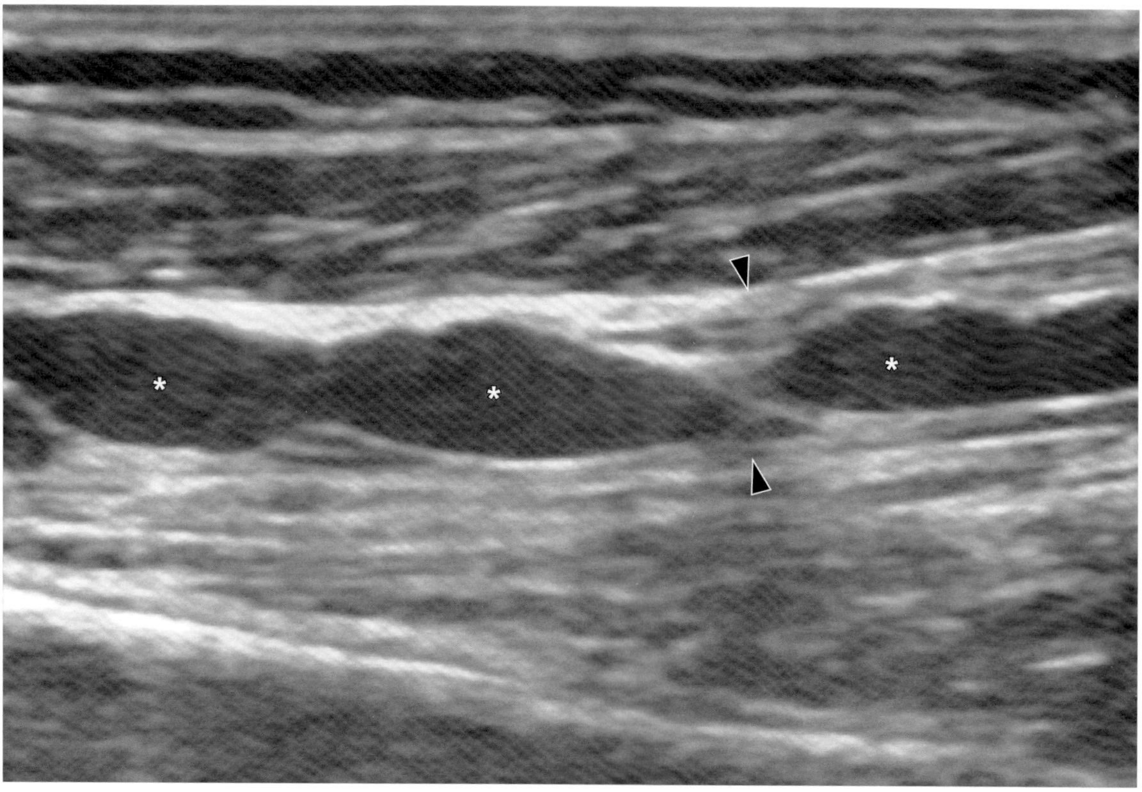

Longitudinal US image shows plexiform neurofibromas (*asterisks*) arising from the fascicles of the of the sciatic nerve (*arrowheads*).

Expert note

In neurofibromatosis, multiple enlargements in the nerve trunk might appear either as irregular (with different sizes) or sometimes -like in this case- as "beads on a string" [5].

Video 19

Nerves

12.70 Normal tibial and common fibular nerve views in a young-aged man

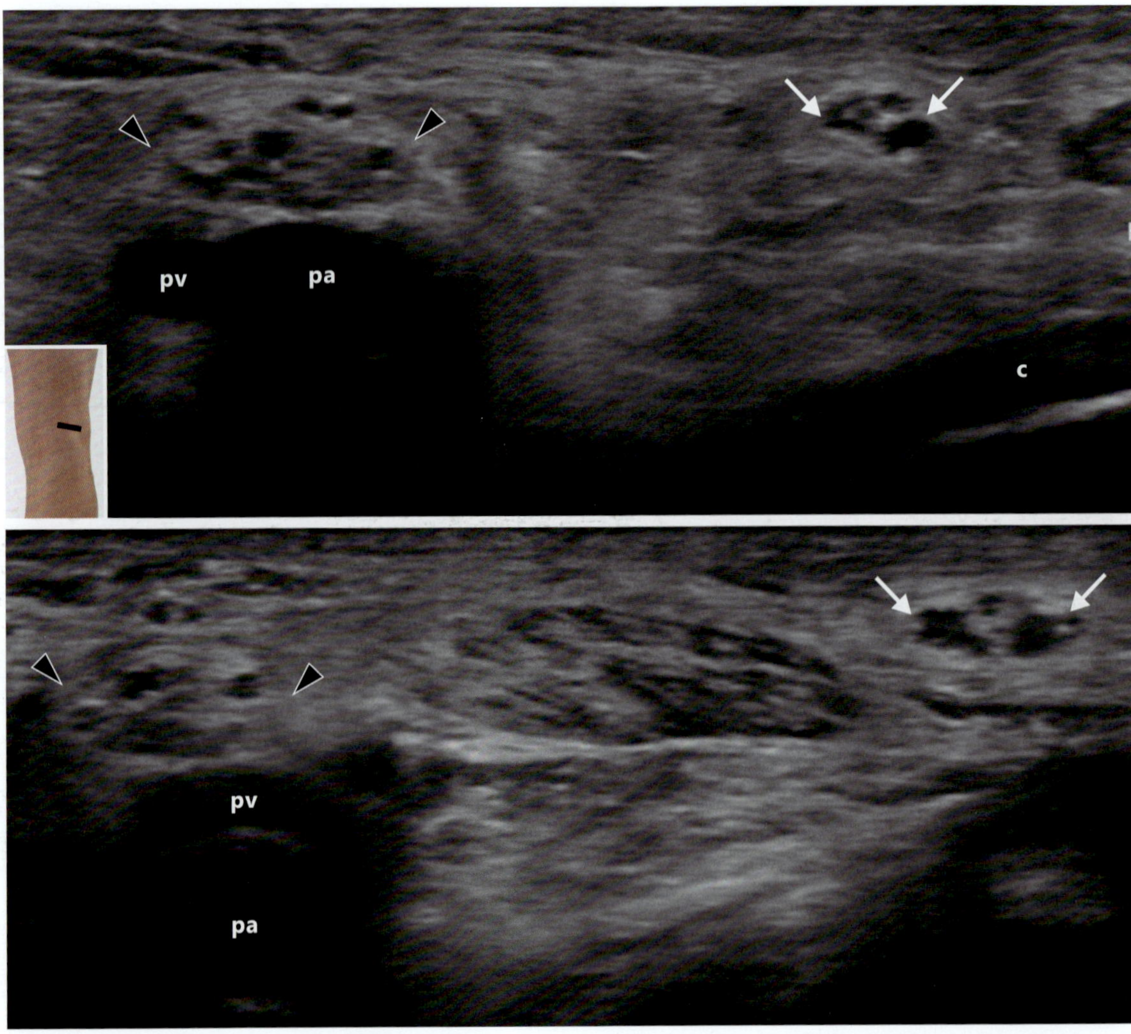

a

b

Axial US images over the popliteal region nicely demonstrate the honeycomb echotexture (small rounded hypoechoic fascicles) of the tibial (*arrowheads*) and fibular (*arrows*) nerves after the bifurcation (**a**) and more distally (**b**).

c cartilage
pa popliteal artery
pv popliteal vein

Charcot-Marie-Tooth disease in a 25-year-old woman

12.71

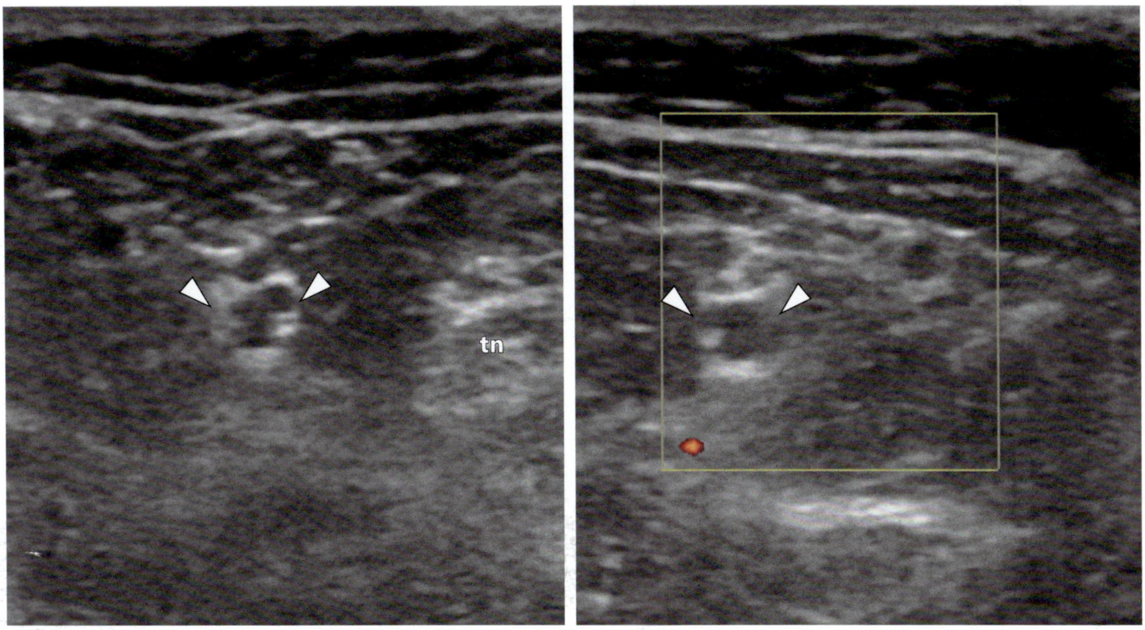

a b

She had difficulty in walking due to progressive distal weakness of the fibular muscles and absence of Achilles tendon reflexes.

Axial US image obtained just proximal to the popliteal region (bifurcation level of the sciatic nerve) demonstrates swollen and hypoechoic fascicles of the fibular nerve (*arrowheads*) (**a**) without any blood flow signal (**b**). At this level, tibial nerve (**tn**) seems to be less affected morphologically.

Expert note

Diffuse enlargement of the fascicles is usually the only but nonspecific finding in Charcot-Marie-Tooth disease [4]. Herewith, the additional value of US imaging is mainly based on its convenient use for scanning any nerve in the body to better understand the extent of involvement.

12.72 Fibular nerve palsy in a young man who had drop-foot for the last six months

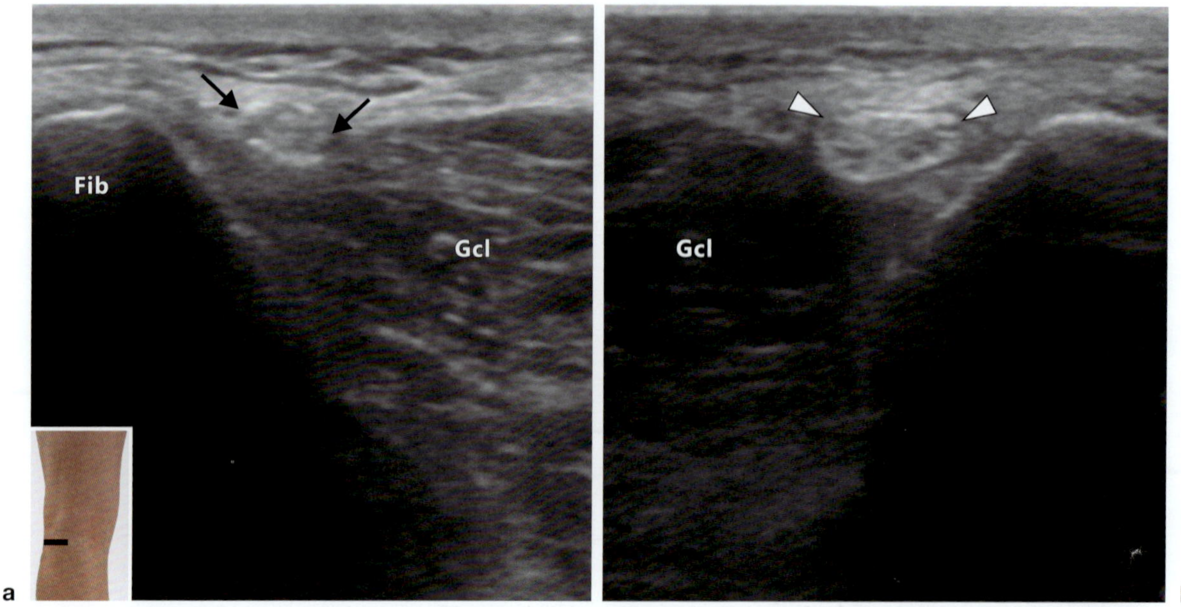

When compared with the normal fibular nerve (*arrows*) on the contralateral side (**a**), axial US image over the fibular head (**Fib**) reveals grossly enlarged nerve (*arrowheads*) (**b**).

Gcl gastrocnemius lateral head

Expert note

Imaging of the fibular nerve around the fibular head is very easy if the sonographer is familiar with its appearance. Otherwise, like in any other nerve, one can start the scanning from a more proximal or distal region. In case of fibular nerve, it would be easier to start with the sciatic nerve proximal to its bifurcation and then follow each (fibular or tibial) nerve separately [22].

US-guided platelet-rich plasma injection in a case of traumatic fibular nerve injury 12.73

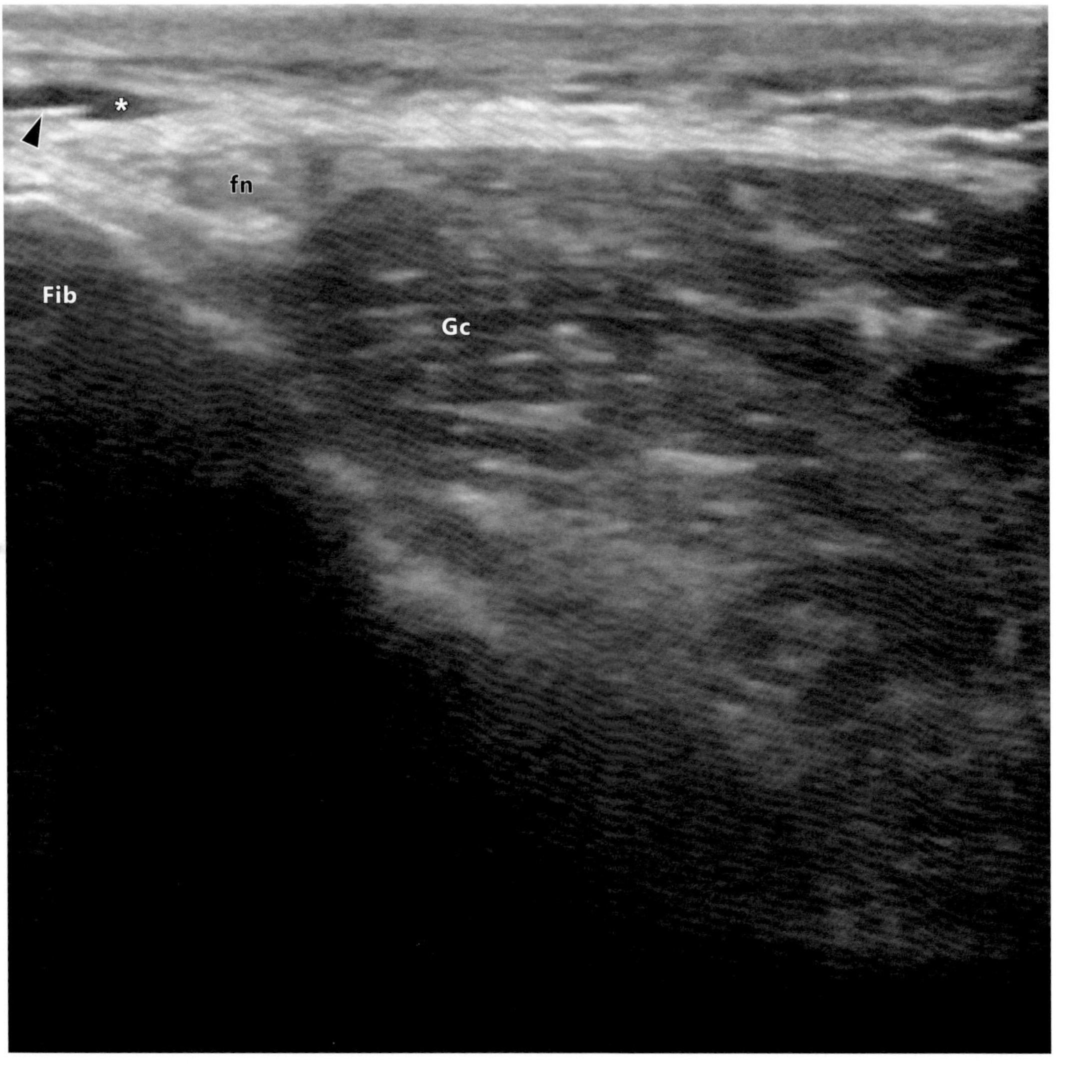

Axial US image shows the swollen fibular nerve (**fn**), the insulin needle (*arrowhead*) and the anechoic injectate (*asterisk*).

Fib fibular head
Gc gastrocnemius

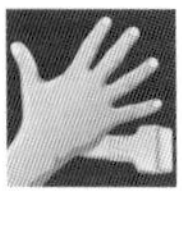

Expert note

Similar to many other conditions, US guidance enables any type of injection as long as the target/pathology can be seen with US imaging.

12.74 Drop-foot in a middle-aged woman after a traumatic tibiofibular fracture

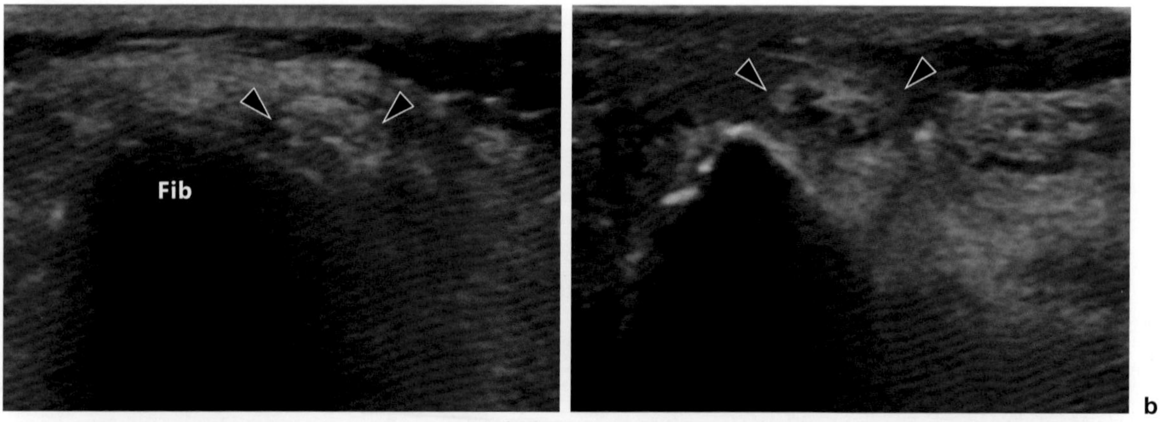

a b

When compared with the normal side (**a**), axial US image over the fibular head region (**Fib**) reveals an abrupt change in the size of the common fibular nerve (*arrowheads*) with a markedly swollen and hypoechoic appearance (**b**).

Superficial fibular neuropathy in a 42-year-old man with leg pain after a fall

12.75

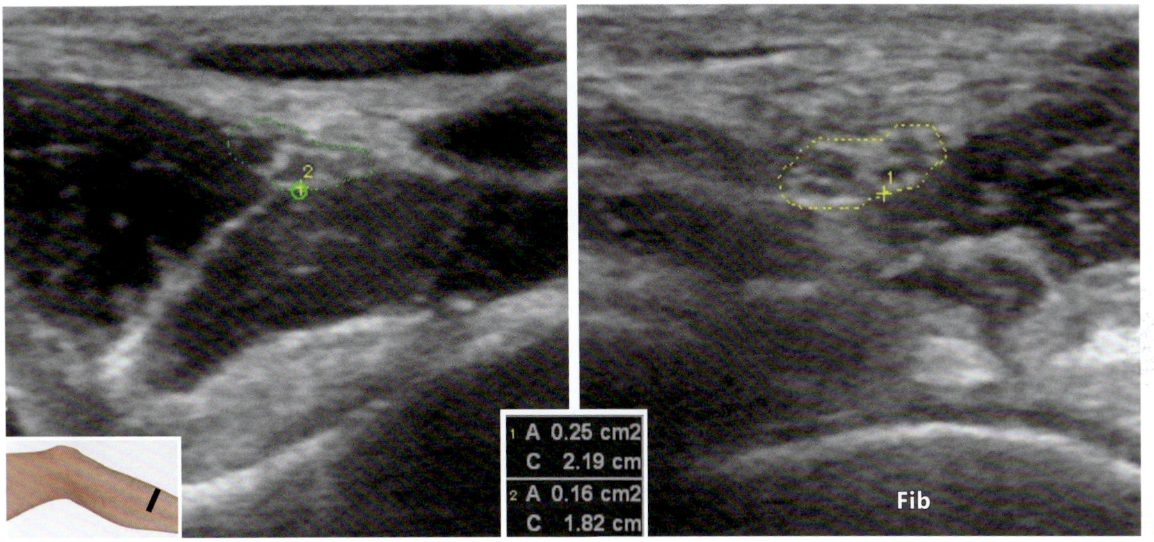

a b

When compared with the normal side (**a**), axial US image over the fibula (**Fib**) illustrates enlargement of the superficial fibular nerve, quantified by cross-sectional area measurements (**b**).

12.76 Ganglion cyst causing tarsal tunnel syndrome in a 41-year-old postal delivery courier man

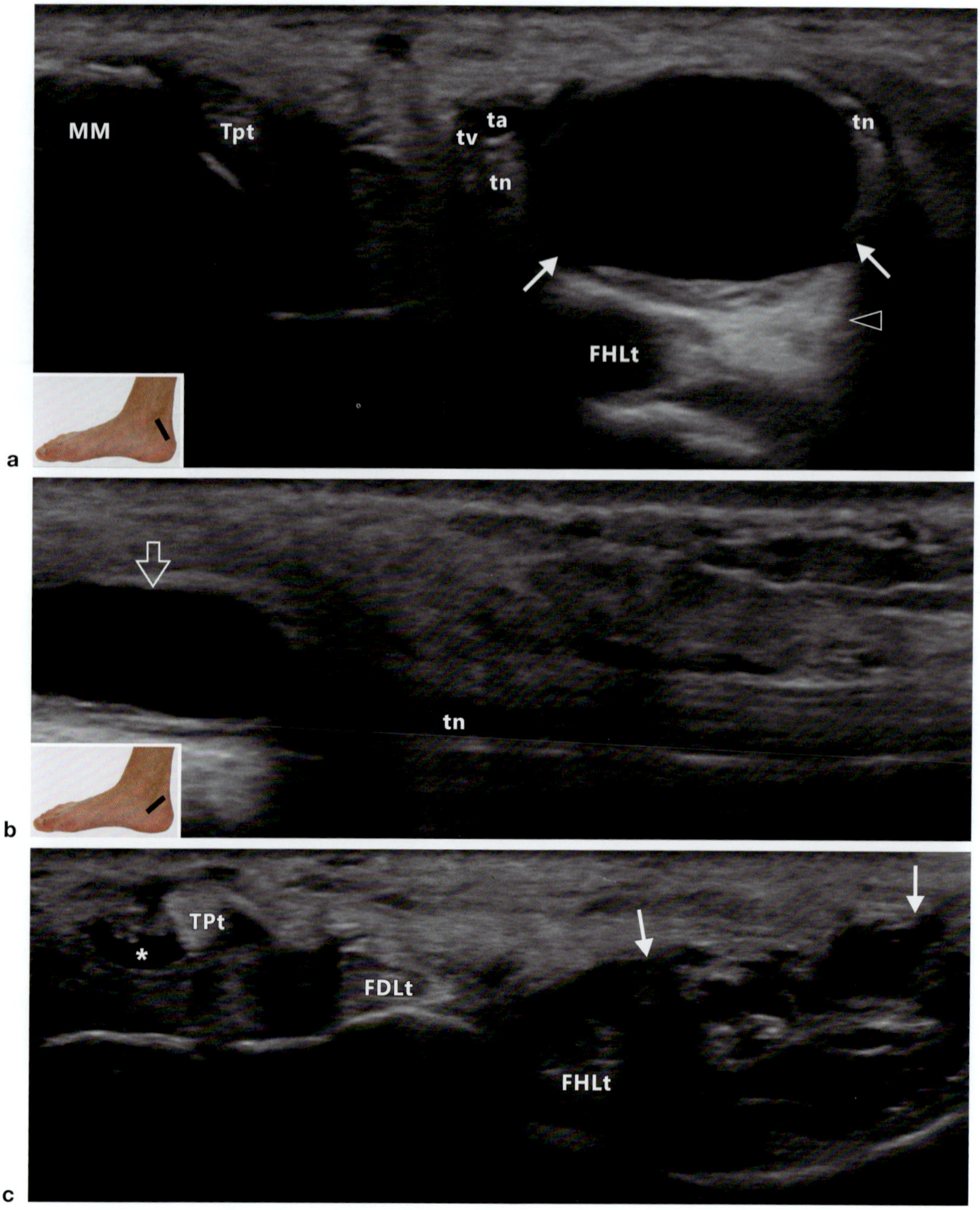

He complained of numbness and tingling in his right foot starting from medial malleolus spreading along his foot sole, worse by physical activity. He had an ankle injury six months ago and a lump occurred near the medial malleolus.

Oblique axial US image at the medial malleolus (**MM**) demonstrates a well-defined, anechoic cystic mass (*arrows*) consistent with a ganglion, in close relationship with the tibial nerve (**tn**). Also, note the posterior acoustic enhancement (*arrowhead*) (**a**). Corresponding longitudinal view confirms the cyst (*arrow*) in close contact with the nerve (**b**).
Axial US image obtained more distally reveals that the ganglion is possibly a chronic one (*arrows*) with septations next to the flexor hallucis longus tendon (**FHLt**). Also, note that there is mild effusion (*asterisk*) around the tibialis posterior tendon (**TPt**) (**c**).

FDLt flexor digitorum longus tendon
ta tibial artery
tv tibial vein

Expert note

Aside from uncovering the details as regards the tarsal tunnel syndrome, US imaging also showed the injury of the TPt possibly due to the preceding ankle injury.

12.77 A 38-year-old woman presenting with dysesthesias in the posterolateral calf region after a diagnostic sural nerve biopsy

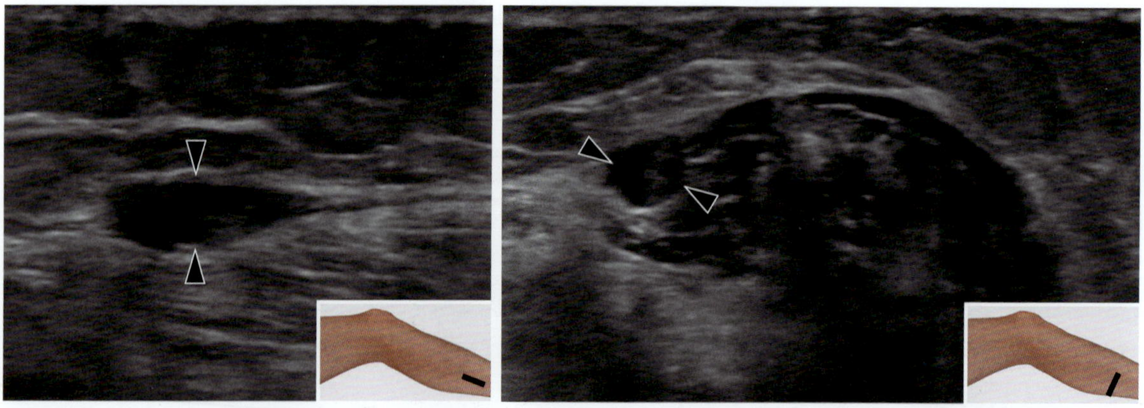

a b

Longitudinal (**a**) and axial (**b**) images obtained over the posterolateral leg show swollen and hypoechoic view of the sural nerve (*arrowheads*).

Morton's neuroma in a patient who defines sharp pain at the base of the web space radiating to the toes **12.78**

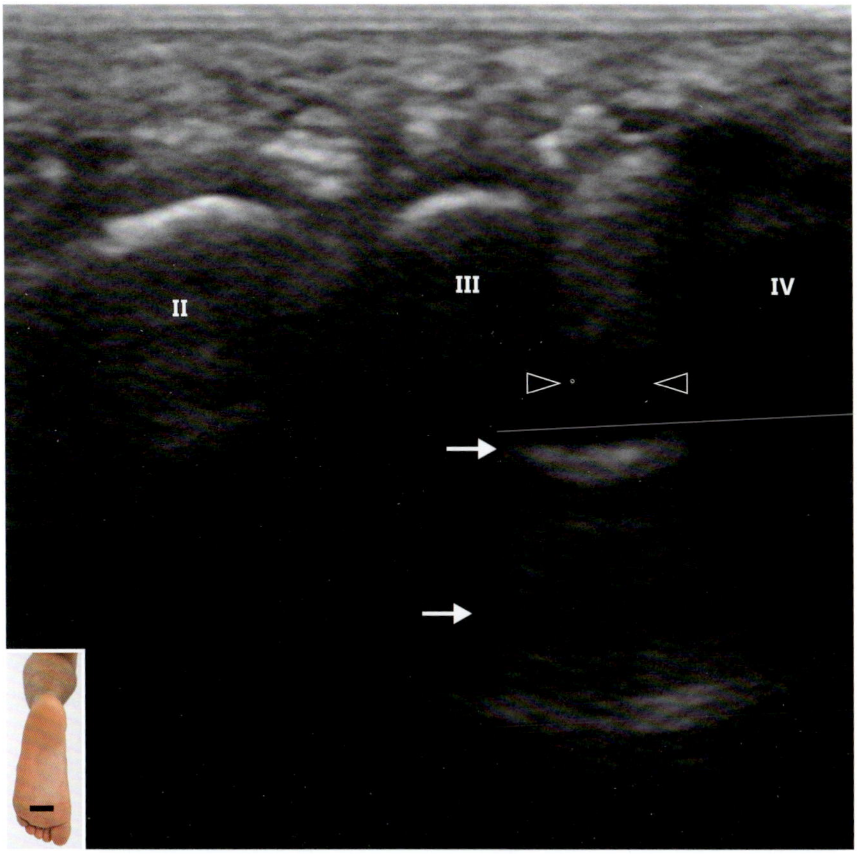

Axial US image obtained from the plantar approach shows an anechoic zone (*arrowheads*) in the third intermetatarsal web space with enhanced through transmission artifact (*arrows*).

Expert note

Commonly, the hypoechoic neuroma itself might not readily be detected at the initial glance. However, the recognition of this relevant artifact which is not seen in the other spaces could be a nice hint leading to a glance in depth. For sure, dynamic imaging with Mulder/squeeze test can also help further demonstrate the neuroma moving from deep to superficial [27]. Looking from the plantar side can be difficult because of callosity of the skin. When looking at the dorsal aspect of the forefoot, the state of the skin is technically no problem. One can push gently from the plantar side to widen the spaces between the metatarsals. Strunsky's sign (bigger space between two toes) can also draw one's attention to the pathological space.
When one neuroma is present, very often more can be found. To differentiate a neuroma from intermetatarsal bursa, compression test is also important -i.e neuromas will not be compressible in contrast to bursae.

Video 20

REFERENCES

1. Chang KV, Lin CP, Hung CY, Özçakar L, Wang TG, Chen WS. Sonographic nerve tracking in the cervical region: a pictorial essay and video demonstration. Am J Phys Med Rehabil. 2016; 95: 862-70.
2. Özçakar L, Yalçin B, Kara M, Yalçin E, Tiftik T, Gülbar S, et al. AnatoMUS-I: ultrasonographic imaging of the peripheral nerves of the upper limb. J Rehabil Med. 2012; 44: 381-2.
3. Kara M, Özçakar L, De Muynck M, Tok F, Vanderstraeten G. Musculoskeletal ultrasound for peripheral nerve lesions. Eur J Phys Rehabil Med. 2012; 48: 665-74.
4. Kara M. Ultrasound imaging for peripheral nerve problems. In: Özçakar L, De Muynck M, editors. Musculoskeletal ultrasound in physical and rehabilitation medicine. Milan: Edi.Ermes; 2014. p. 141-60.
5. Kara M, Akyüz M, Yılmaz A, Hatipoğlu C, Özçakar L. Peripheral nerve involvement in a neurofibromatosis type 2 patient with plexiformneurofibroma of the cauda equina: a sonographic vignette. Arch Phys Med Rehabil. 2011; 92: 1511-4.
6. Wu CH, Chang KV, Özçakar L, Hsiao MY, Hung CY, Shyu SG, et al. Sonographic tracking of the upper limb peripheral nerves: a pictorial essay andvideo demonstration. Am J Phys Med Rehabil. 2015; 94: 740-7.
7. Tok F, Özçakar L, Safaz I, Alaca R. Effects of botulinum toxin-A on the muscle architecture of stroke patients: thefirst ultrasonographic study. J Rehabil Med. 2011; 43: 1016-9.
8. Akyuz M, Yalcin E, Selcuk B, Onder B, Özçakar L. Electromyography and ultrasonography in the diagnosis of a rare double-crushulnar nerve injury. Arch Phys Med Rehabil. 2011; 92: 1914-6.
9. Özçakar L, Cakar E, Kiralp MZ, Dinçer U. Static and dynamic sonography: a salutary adjunct to electroneuromyography for cubital tunnel syndrome. Surg Neurol. 2009; 72: 311-2.
10. Kılıç E, Özçakar L. Ulnar nerve compression possibly due to aberrant veins: sonography is elucidatory for idiopathic cubital tunnel syndrome. Rheumatol Int. 2011; 31: 139-40.
11. Kara M, Yalçın S, Yenigün D, Tiftik T, Malas FÜ, Özçakar L. Heterotopic ossification and cubital tunnel syndrome in traumatic brain injury: Ultrasound 'sees' both. J Back Musculoskelet Rehabil. 2015; 28: 415-7.
12. Özçakar L, Carli AB, Tok F, Tekin L, Akkaya N, Kara M. The utility of musculoskeletal ultrasound in rehabilitation settings. Am J Phys Med Rehabil. 2013; 92: 805-17.
13. Güven SC, Calşkan A, Yasrebi S, Özçakar L. Ultrasound imaging of median and ulnar nerves after carpal tunnel surgery: healing or else? Am J Phys Med Rehabil. 2013; 92: 1035-6.
14. Yu G, Chen Q, Wang D, Wang X, Wang X, Li Z, Zhao J, et al. Diagnosis of carpal tunnel syndrome assessed using high-frequency ultrasonography: cross-section areas of 8-site median nerve. Clin Rheumatol. 2016; 35: 2557-64.
15. Ata AM, Şahin Onat Ş, Kara M, Özçakar L. Ultrasound-guided injection of carpal tunnel: do you mind the retinaculum? Am J Phys Med Rehabil. 2016; 95: e22.
16. Kaymak B, Özçakar L, Cetin A, Candan Cetin M, Akinci A, Hasçelik Z. Acomparison of the benefits of sonography and electrophysiologic measurements aspredictors of symptom severity and functional status in patients with carpaltunnel syndrome. Arch Phys Med Rehabil. 2008; 89: 743-8.
17. Erol O, Özçakar L, Kaymak B. Bifid median nerve revisited: imaging and clinical aspects. Plast Reconstr Surg. 2004; 113: 1289-90.
18. Ekiz T, Onat ŞŞ, Yalçin S, Atik Ç, Özçakar L. Ultrasound ımaging of persistent median artery and veins in an asymptomatic patient with a bifid median nerve. Am J Phys Med Rehabil. 2016; 95: e127-8.
19. Ata AM, Onat ŞŞ, Özçakar L. Ultrasound imaging for diagnosis and follow-up of persistent median artery thrombosis. Muscle Nerve. 2016; 53: 152-4.
20. Kara M, Özçakar L, Ekiz T, Yalçın E, Tiftik T, Akyüz M. Fibrolipomatous hamartoma of the median nerve: comparison of magnetic resonance imaging and ultrasound. PM R. 2013; 5: 805-6.
21. Onat SS, Ata AM, Özçakar L. Ultrasound-guided diagnosis and treatment of meralgia paresthetica. Pain Physician. 2016; 19: E667-9.
22. Hung CY, Hsiao MY, Özçakar L. Sonographic tracking of the lower limb peripheral nerves: a pictorial essay and video demonstration. Am J Phys Med Rehabil. 2016; 95: 698-708.
23. Kara M, Ekiz T, Öztürk GT, Onat ŞŞ, Özçakar L. Heterotopic ossification and peripheral nerve entrapment: ultrasound is a must-use imaging modality. Pain Med. 2015; 16: 1643-4.
24. Kara M, Özçakar L, Tan E, Akıncı A. Ultrasonographic imaging of the sciatic nerve in a patient with knife injury. Muscle Nerve. 2015; 51: 303-4.
25. Kara M, Özçakar L, Tiftik T, Kaymak B, Özel S, Akkuş S, et al. Sonographic evaluation of sciatic nerves in patients with unilateral sciatica. Arch Phys Med Rehabil. 2012; 93: 1598-602.

26. Göktepe AS, Özçakar L, Kömürcü E, Safaz I, Yazicioğlu K. Sonographic evaluation of the sciatic nerve in patients with lower-limb amputations. Muscle Nerve. 2010; 41: 763-6.
27. Ata AM, Onat ŞŞ, Özçakar L. Ultrasound-guided diagnosis and treatment of Morton's neuroma. Pain Physician. 2016; 19: E355-8.

Nerves